Stroke

Stroke: Interventions to Support Occupational Performance

Neurorehabilitation in Occupational Therapy Series, Volume 2

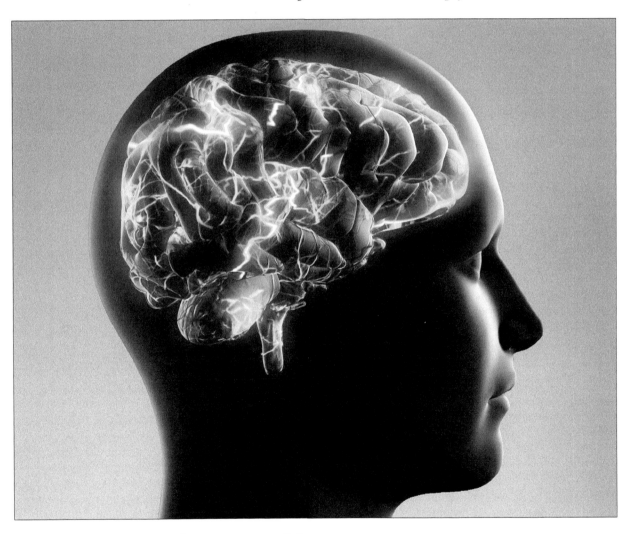

Edited by Timothy J. Wolf, OTD, MSCI, OTR/L
Series Senior Editor: Gordon Muir Giles, PhD, OTR/L, FAOTA

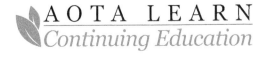

AOTA LEARN
Continuing Education

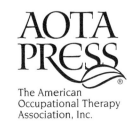

AOTA PRESS

The American
Occupational Therapy
Association, Inc.

AOTA Centennial Vision

We envision that occupational therapy is a powerful, widely recognized, science-driven, and evidence-based profession with a globally connected and diverse workforce meeting society's occupational needs.

Mission Statement

The American Occupational Therapy Association advances the quality, availability, use, and support of occupational therapy through standard-setting, advocacy, education, and research on behalf of its members and the public.

AOTA Staff

Frederick P. Somers, *Executive Director*
Christopher M. Bluhm, *Chief Operating Officer*
Maureen Peterson, *Chief Professional Affairs Officer*

Chris Davis, *Director, AOTA Press*
Caroline Polk, *Digital Publishing Manager*
Ashley Hofmann, *Development/Production Editor*
Barbara Dickson, *Production Editor*
Joe King-Shaw, *AOTA Press Business and Customer Service Administrator*

Kathleen Klein, *Director, Professional Development*
Sarah Hertfelder, *Continuing Education Consultant*

Rebecca Rutberg, *Director, Marketing*
Jennifer Folden, *Marketing Specialist*
Amanda Goldman, *Marketing Specialist*

American Occupational Therapy Association, Inc.
4720 Montgomery Lane
Bethesda, MD 20814
301-652-AOTA (2682)
TDD: 800-377-8555
Fax: 301-652-7711
www.aota.org
To order: 1-877-404-AOTA or store.aota.org

Disclaimers

This publication is designed to provide accurate and authoritative information in regard to the subject matter covered. It is sold or distributed with the understanding that the publisher is not engaged in rendering legal, accounting, or other professional service. If legal advice or other expert assistance is required, the services of a competent professional person should be sought.

—*From the Declaration of Principles jointly adopted by the
American Bar Association and a Committee of Publishers and Associations*

It is the objective of the American Occupational Therapy Association to be a forum for free expression and interchange of ideas. The opinions expressed by the contributors to this work are their own and not necessarily those of the American Occupational Therapy Association/AOTA Press.

ISBN: 978-1-56900-364-0

Library of Congress Control Number: 2014947081

Cover design by Debra Naylor, Naylor Design, Inc., Washington, DC
Composition by Maryland Composition, White Plains, MD
Printed by Automated Graphic Systems, Inc., White Plains, MD
Publication management by Steve Pazdan, College Park, MD

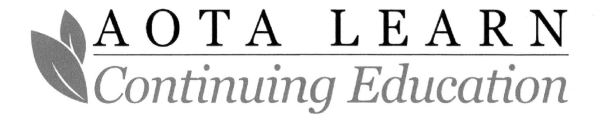

AOTA LEARN
Continuing Education

Make Your Learning Count!

Earn Continuing Education Credit (AOTA CEUs/Contact Hours/NBCOT® PDUs) With This Publication.

SPCC Purchase: If you purchased ***Stroke: Interventions to Support Occupational Performance, Neurorehabilitation in Occupational Therapy Series, Volume 2,*** as an AOTA Self-Paced Clinical Course (SPCC), you are enrolled in the continuing education (CE) activity for this publication. After placing your order, you received information via e-mail to complete the CE activity (exam) for this course at AOTA LEARN (**www.aota.org/learn**), AOTA's online center for professional development.

- The CE exam is available on AOTA LEARN to print and review as you read the SPCC.
- When you finish reading, complete the CE exam on AOTA LEARN.
- Successful completion of the exam requires a minimum passing score of 75%. You are provided with two attempts to pass the exam. If required, additional attempts to pass the exam can be purchased by calling 877-404-AOTA (2682).
- With successful course completion, you will instantly receive a certificate and transcript to download or print to verify your learning for state licensure, certification, employers, or your own professional development.

Publication Purchase: If you purchased the non-CE publication version of ***Stroke: Interventions to Support Occupational Performance, Neurorehabilitation in Occupational Therapy Series, Volume 2,*** you can formally recognize your learning from topic experts and receive CE credit. You may enroll for 20 contact hours (2 AOTA CEUs/25 NBCOT PDUs) addressing the learning objectives listed when you order your CE exam.

Ordering is easy! As a purchaser of this publication, order the SPCC exam only (price will reflect exam only):

- Enter **Order #3033OLE** online at **http://store.aota.org,** or by phone at 877-404-AOTA (2682).
- Once you place an order, you will immediately receive an e-mail with your CE exam access information.

There are even more reasons to learn with an AOTA SPCC:

- Upon successful completion of the SPCC exam, earn **nondegree graduate credits from Colorado State University.** Learn more on the next page.
- This publication may be used to support one of the Knowledge Criteria for appropriate **AOTA Board or Specialty Certifications.** Learn more at **aota.org/certification.**
- Learning with AOTA SPCCs provides a **depth of knowledge from experts** that can assist in achieving clinical excellence. Your colleagues and clients benefit when you apply your enhanced expertise.

Discontinuation: When an AOTA SPCC is discontinued, notification is provided at **aota.org/ce**, in AOTA periodicals, and via e-mail to SPCC learners who have not yet completed the exam. SPCC learners have 1 year from first notification of discontinuation to complete the SPCC exam and receive CE credit.

INTERESTED IN NONDEGREE GRADUATE CREDIT?

Upon successful completion of this Self-Paced Clinical Course (SPCC), you may be eligible for Colorado State University (CSU) nondegree graduate credit. Register with CSU after you successfully complete your online SPCC exam.

Purchasers of this AOTA SPCC who want to obtain nondegree graduate credit from CSU **must register directly with CSU after successful completion of the continuing education (CE) exam.**

To obtain nondegree graduate credit from CSU, do the following:

Contact CSU at the address below to obtain the most current registration form and tuition rate; refer to *OT 590 735 Workshop: Stroke: Interventions to Support Occupational Performance (Neurorehabilitation in Occupational Therapy Series, Volume 2).*

Colorado State University OnlinePlus
Division of Continuing Education
1040 Campus Delivery
Fort Collins, CO 80523-1040
Attn: Contract Courses

Phone (970) 491-5288
E-mail: onlineplus_questions@colostate.edu

You may obtain 2 CSU nondegree graduate credits for completing this course.

- Send CSU your payment and completed registration form with a copy of your AOTA CE transcript indicating a passing grade. The transcript is available online at AOTA LEARN (**www.aota.org/learn**). Retain a copy of the registration form and transcript for your records.
- Upon receipt of your registration form and transcript, CSU will contact AOTA to confirm the grade received for the exam.

The following terms and conditions apply:

- SPCC learners have 7 years from the time of purchase to complete the AOTA SPCC for optional, nondegree graduate credit from CSU.
- You may retake the online exam if you do not complete it successfully on the first attempt. AOTA provides a continuing education certificate of completion and transcript online when the SPCC CE activities have been completed.
- CSU transcripts granting nondegree graduate credits are available from CSU within 1 month from submission of a passing grade.
- Contact CSU directly, at the address above, if assistance is required for the registration process or CSU transcript.
- CSU tuition and fees are subject to change.

Contents

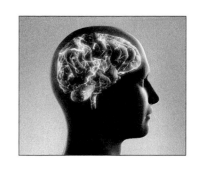

Boxes, Exhibit, Figures, Points to Ponder, Tables, and Appendixes

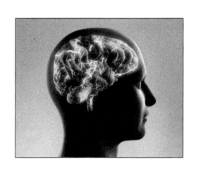

Boxes

Exhibit

Figures

Points to Ponder

Tables

Appendixes

Foreword

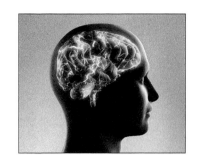

Stroke is the leading cause of adult disability in the United States, and occupational therapists are the leading experts in disability prevention, remediation, and compensation, providing services to the estimated 795,000 Americans who experience a stroke annually. Keeping abreast of advances in neuroscience and their implications for stroke rehabilitation is especially daunting given the accelerating pace of knowledge accumulation. A major objective of the editor in compiling *Stroke: Interventions to Support Occupational Performance* is to facilitate our learning and, more important, our application of that learning to the diversity of clients we treat daily in hospitals, rehabilitation facilities, outpatient clinics, nursing homes, and home health care settings. This Self-Paced Clinical Course and textbook provide an excellent compendium of information and reference tools. It links basic science developments in neuroplasticity to both traditional and nontraditional intervention strategies for stroke-related impairments, limitations in daily living occupations, and restrictions in participation. In so doing, it fosters a science-driven and evidence-based approach to occupational therapy evaluation and intervention for clients with stroke.

Organizationally, the chapters presenting the core concepts explaining stroke-related impairments are preceded by a chapter (Chapter 2) titled "Improving Participation After Stroke: The Transactional Relationship Among the Person, the Environment, and Occupation." This arrangement is judicious because it organizes knowledge of stroke-related impairments around rehabilitation outcomes. Chapter 2 reminds us of the real or long-term goal of stroke rehabilitation from the perspective of clients, their caregivers, and third-party payers. Our attention is directed to reintegration into meaningful societal roles and the community. Although the reduction of impairments is important, activity- or occupation-based interventions that more directly encourage a return to normal living are also needed. By targeting participation as an intervention outcome, the text pushes rehabilitation beyond the rehabilitation setting to the home, workplace, and leisure sites of clients and stakes out a valid claim for occupational therapy's expertise in the delivery of client-centered rehabilitation.

Historically, stroke rehabilitation has focused on motor recovery, and in recent years this focus has been reinforced by the advent of constraint-induced movement therapy (CIMT) and task-specific training. From the perspective of occupational therapy, effective doing requires the physiological and sensorimotor capacity to execute movement, the cognitive capacity to plan and carry out meaningful occupations, and the emotional capacity to want to do the task. Science-driven therapy requires that attention be given to all these capacities. This text provides up-to-date information on recovery from stroke-related impairments in five areas: (1) physiological, (2) sensory, (3) motor, (4) cognitive, and (5) emotional. Equal weight is given to the presentation of knowledge on cognitive and emotional impairments and to that on physiological, sensory, and motor impairments. Just as our understanding of motor recovery was advanced by CIMT, so too our understanding of occupational recovery may well be advanced by novel interventions that combine cognitive and affective strategies with motor strategies. This text positions occupational therapists to think creatively and systematically about combination strategies.

The intervention strategies that are appropriate to use depend on the client's medical and disability status. Using a case-by-case approach, the editor and authors combine client status with components of the continuum of care to discuss application of the occupational therapy process. The second half of this text describes specific evaluation and intervention strategies for clients with differing levels of disability who receive occupational therapy in varied settings, namely acute, inpatient, and outpatient care and the community. Moreover, for outpatient and community settings, the focus moves to the highly relevant instrumental activities of daily living, work, community reintegration, and living with stroke. Thus, this section assists in operationalizing the role of occupational therapy in intervening for participation restrictions.

Stroke: Interventions to Support Occupational Performance takes a science-driven approach to stroke etiology, progression, and recovery by grounding us first in evidence on neuroscientific core concepts, occupational limitations, and participation restrictions. Then, the editor and authors help us to apply these concepts by presenting a variety of clinical cases, assessments, and interventions appropriate for each stage and setting that stroke survivors may experience on the road to recovery. Finally, they solidify our expertise in disability prevention, remediation, and compensation as the chapters focus on community reintegration and living with stroke. This text has utility for the new as well as the seasoned practitioner.

—**Joan C. Rogers, PhD, OTR/L, FAOTA**
Professor of Occupational Therapy and Nursing
Chair of Occupational Therapy
Associate Dean of Graduate Studies
School of Health and Rehabilitation Sciences
University of Pittsburgh

Note From the
Series Senior Editor

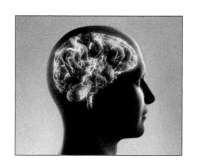

I am grateful to have been asked again by the American Occupational Therapy Association (AOTA) to be senior editor for the Neurorehabilitation Self-Paced Clinical Course (SPCC) and publication series. Titles in this series are intended to serve as textbooks for advanced-level occupational therapy students and to enhance the skills of practicing clinicians. The series also offers excellent continuing education opportunities with the ability to earn AOTA CEUs, contact hours, and NBCOT® PDUs, in addition to nondegree graduate credit through Colorado State University.

Stroke: Interventions to Support Occupational Performance is the second in this series and is fully revised from the 2006 versions of *Core Concepts in Neurorehabilitation* and *Neurorehabilitation for Stroke*. A new edition of *Neurocognitive Disorder (NCD): Interventions to Support Occupational Performance* has been published, and the final text in this series, *Traumatic Brain Injury (TBI): Interventions to Support Occupational Performance,* will follow.

This is an exciting time for the more than 60% of occupational therapists who report working with clients with stroke (National Board for Certification in Occupational Therapy, 2013). The demographics of stroke are changing, and occupational therapists need to be able to respond with new ways to assess and treat clients who are younger and who have expectations of being able to return to work and community engagement (AOTA, 2013; Morrison et al., 2013; Wolf, Baum, & Connor, 2009). The increasing recognition of the role of executive function deficits in compromising the ability of clients with mild stroke to resume vital life roles also presents a challenge and an opportunity for occupational therapists (AOTA, 2013). This work reflects the significant advances in our understanding of stroke and its treatment made over the past decade and provides readers with the information that they need to be current and evidence based in their interventions.

Timothy J. Wolf, OTD, MSCI, OTR/L, of Washington University in St. Louis, agreed to both edit and contribute to this edition, and he has gathered a truly outstanding group of researchers and clinicians from Washington University and beyond to write the chapters. Professor Wolf is an outstanding researcher and author who has made important contributions to the field of stroke rehabilitation. He and his collaborators bring a huge depth of expertise to the development of this publication and here present a valuable resource that has the potential to advance the clinical practice of occupational therapists working with this often demanding population.

—Gordon Muir Giles, PhD, OTR/L, FAOTA

References

American Occupational Therapy Association. (2013). Cognition, cognitive rehabilitation, and occupational performance. *American Journal of Occupational Therapy, 67*(6 Suppl.), S9–S31. http://dx.doi.org/10.5014/ajot.2013.67S9

Morrison, M. T., Giles, G. M., Ryan, J. D., Baum, C. M., Dromerick, A. W., Polatajko, H. J., & Edwards, D. F. (2013). Multiple Errands Test–Revised (MET–R): A performance-based measure of executive function in people with mild cerebrovascular accident. *American Journal of Occupational Therapy, 67,* 460–468. http://dx.doi.org/10.5014/ajot.2013.007880

National Board for Certification in Occupational Therapy. (2013). *2012 practice analysis of the occupational therapist registered: Executive summary.* Gaithersburg, MD: Author.

Wolf, T. J., Baum, C. M., & Connor, L. T. (2009). Changing face of stroke: Implications for occupational therapy practice. *American Journal of Occupational Therapy, 63,* 621–625. http://dx.doi.org/10.5014/ajot.63.5.621

Acknowledgments

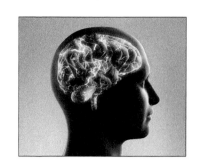

I first thank all of my friends and colleagues who contributed to developing the vision for and the content of this text. For this edition, we started from scratch and collaborated to discuss how we would like to learn about neurorehabilitation for stroke. This meant a lot of extra time, rewrites, and overall effort to make this text what it is. I appreciate the hard work and sacrifice from all of you who made this book possible. Also, I thank the senior editor of this series, Dr. Gordon Muir Giles, the AOTA Press staff, and specifically Sarah Hertfelder, continuing education consultant, for the countless hours they spent keeping this project on target. This was my first endeavor as editor of a text, and Gordon and Sarah were gracious in their mentoring and very patient with their requests and feedback that made my work possible. I thank my students and staff in the Performance, Participation, and Neurorehabilitation Laboratory in the Program in Occupational Therapy at Washington University in St. Louis. They are the ones who kept my work going day to day to allow me to participate in projects such as this and also graciously lent their time to read, review, or provide feedback on content. Finally, I thank my family, especially my wife, Angie, and my son, Will. Their unwavering love and support has been and continues to be the foundation for my life and career.

—**Timothy J. Wolf, OTD, MSCI, OTR/L**

The editor acknowledges and thanks the following professionals who served as invited content reviewers, providing in-depth review of the chapter manuscripts.

Glen Gillen, EdD, OTR, FAOTA
Associate Professor
Rehabilitation and Regenerative Medicine (Occupational Therapy)
   at Columbia University Medical Campus
Columbia University
New York

Naomi Josman, PhD, OT(I)
Professor
Department of Occupational Therapy
Faculty of Social Welfare and Health Sciences
University of Haifa
Haifa, Israel

Dawn M. Nilsen, EdD, OT/L
Assistant Professor
Rehabilitation and Regenerative Medicine (Occupational Therapy)
    at Columbia University Medical Campus
Columbia University
New York

About the Editors and Authors

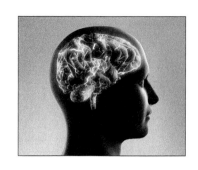

About the Volume Editor

Timothy J. Wolf, OTD, MSCI, OTR/L, is director of the Performance, Participation, and Neurorehabilitation Laboratory in the
Program in Occupational Therapy at Washington University School
of Medicine. Dr. Wolf received his BS in health science–pre-occupa-
tional therapy from Truman State University in Kirksville, Missouri,
and his OTD from the Program in Occupational Therapy at Wash-
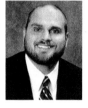
ington University School of Medicine. While pursuing his OTD, he completed the
Predoctoral Interdisciplinary Clinical Research Training Program, a 1-year intensive
clinical investigation training program at Washington University School of Medicine sponsored by a T32 grant from the National Institutes of Health. As a result of
his work in this program, he received his MS in clinical investigation from Washington University School of Medicine.

Dr. Wolf joined the faculty in the Program in Occupational Therapy in 2007
as a clinical instructor and split his time among clinical work, research, and teaching. In 2009, he was awarded an NIH–K12 career development award through the
Comprehensive Opportunities in Rehabilitation Research Training program (http://
www.corrt.pitt.edu), which provides funding for new investigators to acquire the
research skills necessary to become independent investigators in rehabilitation
approaches. After receiving this K12 award, Dr. Wolf switched to an investigator-
track faculty position in the Program in Occupational Therapy. He is currently in
this position as an assistant professor of occupational therapy and neurology at
Washington University School of Medicine. The Performance, Participation, and
Neurorehabilitation Laboratory generates knowledge to guide intervention aimed at
improving participation in work and community activities post–neurological injury.
Currently, Dr. Wolf's research has two primary objectives: (1) to investigate the efficacy of self-management education to improve health and participation outcomes

after stroke, and (2) to identify and manage cognitive deficits after mild stroke and postchemotherapy. Dr. Wolf collaborates with investigators at Washington University in neurology, physical therapy, social work, oncology, radiology, health services, and psychology. He also collaborates with investigators outside of Washington University at the University of Toronto, St. John's Rehabilitation Hospital (Toronto), and the University of Illinois at Chicago.

About the Series Senior Editor

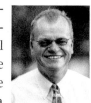

Gordon Muir Giles, PhD, OTR/L, FAOTA, was senior occupational therapist at the first program in the world for behavior disorder after brain injury. He was responsible for developing the clinical program in the first publicly funded neurobehavioral program in the western United States in 1993. Professor Giles is clinically responsible for a 65-bed neurobehavioral program in Fremont, California, and a 165-bed program in Sunnyvale for people whose psychiatric condition complicates the management of their medical condition. In the early 1990s, Professor Giles (in association with Jo Clark-Wilson) developed the Neurofunctional Approach to brain injury rehabilitation, which was demonstrated to be effective in the largest randomized comparison trial of brain injury rehabilitation ever conducted. The Neurofunctional Approach is the only functional approach shown to be effective in people who have had a traumatic brain injury over 10 years previously. His most recent publications and research interests are centered on the role of relationships and on nonaversive intervention in rehabilitation of people with brain injury and behavior disorder. In addition to his clinical responsibilities, Professor Giles teaches at Samuel Merritt University, a health sciences university located in Oakland, California.

About the Authors

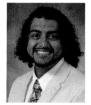

Ganesh Muneshwar Babulal, MOT, OTR/L, is a doctoral student at Washington University School of Medicine. Mr. Babulal's research focuses on the role of emotion and cognition in performance and participation for people with chronic neurological health conditions. His current research focuses on stroke, with the purpose of identifying the relationship between emotion and cognition to better understand their effects on recovery poststroke. He is exploring this relationship through quantitative and qualitative methodologies.

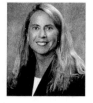

Peggy P. Barco, OTD, OTR/L, SCDCM, is on the faculty of the Program in Occupational Therapy, Washington University School of Medicine in St. Louis, and is certified through the American Occupational Therapy Association as a driving and community mobility specialist. In her faculty position, she is a course master for the cognitive intervention course. Before joining the faculty at Washington University School of Medicine, she was the program coordinator for 15 years for the Head Injury Resource Center (an outpatient day treatment program for people with different types of brain injuries) at St. John's Mercy Medical Center in St. Louis and later was the administrative director of medical services at the Center for Head Injury Services in St. Louis (a not-for-profit comprehensive community reintegration center for people with brain injuries). She has assisted in the development of a model of practice addressing awareness deficits after brain injury that is currently referenced in textbooks and used as part of cognitive intervention programs.

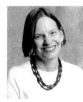

Julie D. Bass, PhD, OTR/L, FAOTA, is professor and past chair of the Department of Occupational Science and Occupational Therapy and founding director of the public health program at St. Catherine University, St. Paul, Minnesota. She is a coeditor of *Occupational Therapy: Performance, Participation, and Well-Being* and a chapter author in *Occupational Therapy for Physical Dysfunction* and *Evaluation: Obtaining and Interpreting Data*. In 2009, she served as a guest editor of the *American Journal of Occupational Therapy* for a special issue on social justice and health disparities. Her teaching and research interests include occupation, health, well-being, task-oriented approaches, community-based practice, research methods, occupational therapy education, and health disparities. She was the chair of two American Occupational Therapy Association (AOTA) task force committees, Health Disparities and Health and Wellness, and served on the AOTA committee that developed the *Blueprint for Entry-Level Education*. Dr. Bass is a fellow of AOTA.

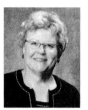

Carolyn M. Baum, PhD, OTR/L, FAOTA, is Elias Michael Director and professor of occupational therapy and neurology, Washington University School of Medicine. Dr. Baum received her BS in occupational therapy at the University of Kansas, Lawrence; her MA in health management at Webster University, St. Louis; and her PhD in social work with a concentration in social policy and aging at the George Warren Brown School of Social Work, Washington University in St. Louis. Dr. Baum directs the Program in Occupational Therapy at Washington University School of Medicine and teaches in the MSOT, OTD, and PhD in Rehabilitation and Participation Science programs. She has twice served as president of the American Occupational Therapy Association, was president of the American Occupational Therapy Certification Board (now the National Board for Certification in Occupational Therapy), and is currently chair of the Research Commission for the American Occupational Therapy Foundation. Dr. Baum's research focuses on enabling older adults to live independently. She and her colleagues have built a measurement model that demonstrates the capacity of a person to engage in activities, tasks, and roles. Since 1996, Dr. Baum has been the principal investigator of a grant supporting the Cognitive Rehabilitation Research Group, an interdisciplinary research group organized to better understand the relationship among brain function, behavior, and performance in people with stroke. The goal of this research is to design interventions that maximize recovery of people after stroke. Since 2009, Dr. Baum has been an investigator on two National Institute on Disability and Rehabilitation Research Rehabilitation Research and Training Center projects (Allen Heinemann and Elliot Roth, principal investigators) and has worked with Joy Hammel on both.

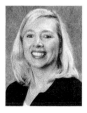

Rebecca L. Birkenmeier, OTD, OTR/L, is a research assistant professor in the Program in Occupational Therapy, Program in Physical Therapy, and Department of Neurology at Washington University in St. Louis. She graduated from Truman State University in 1998 with a bachelor's degree in psychology and earned her master's degree in occupational therapy from Washington University School of Medicine in 2001. She received her occupational therapy doctorate from Washington University School of Medicine in 2010. In her faculty role, she is a course master for the sensorimotor interventions course and is responsible for teaching students evidence-based motor interventions. Dr. Birkenmeier currently works in the Neurorehabilitation Research Lab at Washington University School of Medicine. She provides the occupational therapy perspective for many of the lab projects investigating the loss of upper-extremity function after stroke and the effects of stroke on activity and participation.

Leeanne Carey, PhD, heads the neurorehabilitation and recovery research group at the Florey Institute of Neuroscience and Mental Health and is professor of occupational therapy at La Trobe University in Melbourne, Victoria, Australia. Dr. Carey's research program focuses on stroke rehabilitation and recovery, in particular how the brain adapts and how that potential might be harnessed in rehabili- 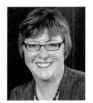 tation. This research has involved development of novel rehabilitation approaches based on neuroscience. Dr. Carey uses tools such as magnetic resonance imaging to investigate changes in the brain and how this knowledge may be used to better understand recovery and target rehabilitation optimally to individual stroke survivors. An important focus is to translate these discoveries into clinical practice and better outcomes for stroke survivors.

Lisa Tabor Connor, PhD, MSOT, is Professor and Chair of the Department of Occupational Therapy at MGH Institute of Health Professions in Boston. Connor is a cognitive neuroscientist who studies stroke recovery. Her research focuses on factors that contribute to successful participation after stroke, including cognitive, emotional, and environmental factors. She received her doctorate in experimental 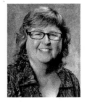 psychology and master's in occupational therapy from Washington University. She completed postdoctoral training in cognitive aging at Georgia Institute of Technology and in adult communicative disorders at Boston University School of Medicine and the Harold Goodglass Aphasia Research Center. She served as assistant professor at Washington University in occupational therapy, neurology, and radiology.

Melissa S. Dappen, MS, OTR/L, is a senior occupational therapist in clinical practice at Rush University Medical Center, Chicago. She works in inpatient physical medicine and rehabilitation and is also the primary clinical therapist in the program's outpatient Day Rehabilitation and Driving Rehabilitation programs. She is active in program planning and development throughout the therapy department. Arti- 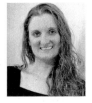 cles on her work have been published in *ADVANCE for Physical Therapy* and *Chicago Health*. Ms. Dappen also serves as a guest lecturer in the master's program in occupational therapy at Rush University. She has completed the Fieldwork Educators Certificate Program, available through the American Occupational Therapy Association, and educates multiple fieldwork students each year. She is currently working toward certification as a driver rehabilitation specialist.

Keri DeGroot, OTD, OTR/L, earned her Doctor of Occupational Therapy degree from Washington University in St. Louis in 2007. She has worked for 5 years as an inpatient occupational therapist mainly in the cerebrovascular accident/brain injury unit of The Rehabilitation Institute of St. Louis. Dr. DeGroot has also been involved in teaching various courses at the Washington University's Program in 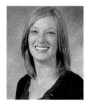 Occupational Therapy since 2007, including "Evaluation: Tools and Process for Measuring Occupational Performance," "Toolbox to Support Professional Practice," and "Community Health and Occupational Therapy." Dr. DeGroot has published two journal articles on wheelchair mobility training. In addition, she has been an interventionist for a research study involving home modifications for older adults.

Fred Feuchter, PhD, received his doctorate in human anatomy from the University of Iowa School of Medicine in 1979. He has held several faculty positions in anatomy, including postdoctoral fellow at the University of Washington School of Medicine (1979–1982), assistant professor of anatomy at the University of New Mexico School of Medicine (1982–1989), director of morphological programs at the 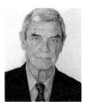 University of New Mexico Allied Health Division (1989–1994), and visiting associate professor of anatomy at the University of California, San Francisco, School of Medicine (1995–2005). He has been at Samuel Merritt University in Oakland, California, since 1994, where he currently serves as professor and chair of the basic sciences department. He has served two terms as president of the faculty organization. Professor Feuchter teaches human anatomy and physiology and functional neurosciences and directs students in research projects. His current research interests include development of interactive media for use in his courses and three-dimensional computer reconstruction of parts of the human brain and spinal cord.

Mary W. Hildebrand, OTD, OTR/L, graduated with an MOT degree from Texas Woman's University in 1993 and worked in a variety of settings for 12 years before attending Washington University in St. Louis and graduating with a postprofessional OTD in 2007. After earning the OTD, she taught in the Washington University in St. Louis Program in Occupational Therapy for 4 years, specializing in interventions with older adults, health promotion for older adults, self-management of chronic conditions, and home health. Dr. Hildebrand has been an assistant professor in the Department of Occupational Therapy at East Carolina University since 2011 and teaches the adult intervention courses in the MSOT program. She has published in the area of participation in physical activities for older adults and people with mild stroke and has presented at several American Occupational Therapy Association Annual Conference & Expos on psychological sequelae of stroke. She has also participated in a randomized controlled trial for and published journal articles on enhancing therapy for older adults in a skilled nursing facility. Dr. Hildebrand is now working on a U.S. Department of Agriculture grant to establish AgrAbility in North Carolina to help farmers with disabilities and chronic conditions continue to participate in farming.

Stroke: Interventions to Support Occupational Performance

Vicki Kaskutas, OTR/L, OTD, FAOTA, received her BS in occupational therapy from the University of Illinois in 1980. After 5 years of providing inpatient rehabilitation and hand therapy, she began working at an underground coal mine, performing on-site rehabilitation and work hardening and administering the light-duty work program. After that, she managed an occupational medicine and rehabilitation center for 8 years, where she performed work hardening, functional capacity evaluations, hand therapy, and ergonomic services. Since 1997, Dr. Kaskutas has been employed at the Program in Occupational Therapy at Washington University School of Medicine. She completed her master's degree in health care services in 2000 and earned a clinical doctorate in occupational therapy in 2008. She helped to develop the Occupational Performance Center at the Rehabilitation Institute of St. Louis and intervention tools and methods used to rehabilitate people with illness and injury that interrupt work participation. In her current role as assistant professor, Dr. Kaskutas performs research regarding work injury prevention, tendon and nerve injuries to the hand, and work assessment. She has been awarded several research grants and authored many peer-reviewed articles and several book chapters or books.

Christina C. Lewis, PhD, received her doctorate in physiology from Colorado State University in 2002. Her doctoral research investigated the mechanisms of airway remodeling in asthma and was conducted at National Jewish Medical and Research Center in Denver. Dr. Lewis conducted her postdoctoral fellowship at the Lung Biology Center at the University of California, San Francisco, where her work focused on using gene expression studies to characterize molecular signatures associated with multiple mouse models of lung disease. Dr. Lewis's current research seeks to understand how airway epithelial biology mediates and regulates the susceptibility and pathogenesis of asthma. Her research has used both human disease studies and murine model systems of asthma and has used genomic approaches to describe the underlying cellular and molecular events of the inflammatory process in allergic airway disease. Previously, she taught courses in anatomy, physiology, genetics and genomics, cellular physiology, and pathology at Earlham College, Richmond, Indiana; the University of California, San Francisco; and the University of California, Berkeley. She is currently on the faculty at Samuel Merritt University in Oakland, California, where she teaches anatomy, physiology, and pathophysiology in the nurse anesthesia, occupational therapy, and physician assistant programs.

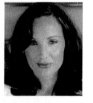

M. Tracy Morrison, OTD, OTR/L, is manager of programs and clinical services for Courage Kenny Rehabilitation Institute Center, Minneapolis, where she works to support the development and delivery of evidence-based programs. Dr. Morrison previously served as a faculty member at Washington University School of Medicine and the University of Kansas Medical Center. In addition to her position at Courage Kenny, Dr. Morrison works as a research scientist and holds an adjunct faculty position in occupational therapy at the University of Kansas Medical Center.

Dr. Morrison's doctoral and postdoctoral training took place at Washington University School of Medicine. She currently leads three research studies focused on the recovery of executive abilities after brain injury. Most recently, she joined a multisite study investigating executive processing after chronic substance abuse.

Becky L. Russell, OTR/L, graduated from Queen's University in Kingston, Ontario, in 1990 and has extensive clinical experience in a variety of settings ranging from inpatient acute care to outpatient therapy and community-based private practice. Ms. Russell currently provides occupational therapy services through the Community Practice Group in-home program at Washington University in St. Louis; works as a lecturer at the Washington University Program in Occupational Therapy; and provides support to research labs. Ms. Russell also provides occupational services at Barnes Jewish Hospital to the acute neurological and neurosurgical population.

Christopher J. Wolf, DO, FAAPMR, is a graduate of the Kirksville College of Osteopathic Medicine. He completed his residency at the University of Missouri in 2008 and is board certified by the American Board of Physical Medicine and Rehabilitation and the American Osteopathic Board of Physical Medicine and Rehabilitation. He currently serves as assistant professor of physical medicine 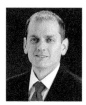 and rehabilitation at the University of Missouri. He is the director of brain injury rehabilitation at the University of Missouri and Rusk Rehabilitation Center in Columbia, Missouri, and serves on the neurorehabilitation team. He also serves as associate residency director and clinic director. Dr. Wolf's practice involves inpatient and outpatient care of people with neurologic injuries, including stroke and brain injury.

Introduction

Timothy J. Wolf, OTD, MSCI, OTR/L

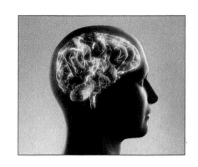

Overall Learning Objectives

After completing this Self-Paced Clinical Course (SPCC) and reading this publication, learners and readers will be able to

- Identify components of the medical management of adults who have sustained a stroke and their importance to successful rehabilitation outcomes;
- Identify components of the Person–Environment–Occupation–Performance (PEOP) model and how each component supports the management of adults with stroke;
- Recognize how neurological deficits after stroke affect performance deficits and how this knowledge can help guide intervention;
- Identify common physiological, sensory, motor, cognitive, and emotional impairments after stroke and the current evidence-based methods for addressing them;
- Recognize how the *Occupational Therapy Practice Framework: Domain and Process* (3rd ed.; American Occupational Therapy Association, 2014) can guide occupational therapy practice across the continuum of care for adults with stroke; and
- Recognize how adults with stroke across the continuum of care and with varying neurological impairments are evaluated and intervention priorities are established.

About This Work

This work is the second edition of the SPCC for **stroke** first published by the American Occupational Therapy Association (AOTA) in 2006. This new edition has benefited from extensive user feedback on the first edition (Beckley, 2006), but it retains many of the innovative features that made the first edition so successful. It has several unique features intended to assist occupational therapists to further develop their clinical competency in working with adults with stroke. Features include "Points to Ponder" (in select chapters), a glossary that corresponds to boldfaced terms in the text, and three case studies in which hypothetical clients (based on common factors identified in real patients) are followed through the various stages of intervention and placement.

Stroke: Interventions to Support Occupational Performance can serve as a textbook for advanced-level occupational therapy students and assist in skill development for practicing clinicians. For this reason, this work is produced for purchase as either a text or an SPCC. For licensed occupational therapists, it can be used to provide either continuing education units or college credit.

This text and SPCC are part of a series of works on neurorehabilitation produced by AOTA with Gordon Muir Giles as senior editor. Texts in the series also include *Neurocognitive Disorder (NCD)* (Corcoran, 2014) and the forthcoming *Traumatic Brain Injury (TBI)* (Golisz & Radomski, 2015).

This text is organized into two sections. The first section provides readers with the core material necessary to work with adults with stroke. Similar to other stroke-related textbooks, each chapter presents a specific content area related to stroke rehabilitation, for example, "Core Concepts in Physiological Impairment and Recovery After Stroke." This information will be valuable to those who are looking to further their knowledge in a particular facet of stroke rehabilitation or to those who are looking for the foundational knowledge necessary to work with adults with stroke.

The second section is organized to mirror the recovery process and the clinical settings in which poststroke rehabilitation for adults takes place. These chapters provide readers with examples of how the foundational knowledge from the first section of the text is applied to patients with stroke whose occupational histories, impairments, skills, and abilities are often complex and multifaceted. Three case studies representing a spectrum of poststroke neurological impairments ranging from mild to severe are used to show how the rehabilitation process may differ at each level of severity. The clinical descriptions of the clients are used to illustrate the principles and intervention techniques involved in the therapeutic process of occupational therapy for people with stroke.

As mentioned, this text is designed for the advanced-level student or the practicing occupational therapist who wants to further explore this important area of competence. Even a large project such as this is selective, and not every topic can be covered. Each chapter is written by practicing clinicians, educators, and researchers, and the topics are intended to reflect the leading edge of current clinical practice and theory in occupational therapy.

Just as with the first edition, we welcome feedback to improve future editions of this work.

References

American Occupational Therapy Association. (2014). Occupational therapy practice framework: Domain and process (3rd ed.). *American Journal of Occupational Therapy, 68*(Suppl. 1), S1–S48. http://dx.doi.org/10.5014/ajot.2014.682006

Beckley, M. N. (Ed.). (2006). *Neurorehabilitation for stroke* (Neurorehabilitation Self-Paced Clinical Course Series). Bethesda, MD: American Occupational Therapy Association.

Corcoran, M. A. (Ed.) (2014). *Neurocognitive disorder (NCD): Interventions to support occupational performance* (Neurorehabilitation in Occupational Therapy Series, Vol. 1). Bethesda, MD: AOTA Press.

Golisz, K., & Radomski, M. (Eds.) (2015). *Traumatic brain injury (TBI): Interventions to support occupational performance* (Neurorehabilitation in Occupational Therapy Series, Vol. 3). Bethesda, MD: AOTA Press.

CHAPTER 1

Stroke Etiology, Symptoms, and Progression

Christopher J. Wolf, DO, FAAPMR

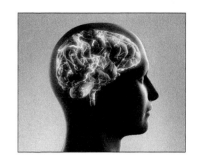

Learning Objectives

After completion of this chapter, readers will be able to

- Identify the differences in hemorrhagic versus ischemic stroke;
- Identify the nonmodifiable and modifiable risk factors associated with stroke;
- Delineate the different symptoms associated with stroke on the basis of the vasculature involved;
- Identify the use of thrombolytic therapy for acute stroke and the exclusion criteria for this treatment;
- Identify common medical concerns that occur in the acute and early post-acute period after a stroke; and
- Identify the National Institutes of Health Stroke Scale and the scoring system it entails.

Introduction

In a moment, a life can change with a stroke of bad luck or bad health. Few afflictions in modern medicine are more familiar and more feared than a stroke. **Stroke,** or **cerebrovascular accident** (CVA), is an injury to the brain caused by **occlusion** or the disruption of the cerebral blood vessels resulting in diminished **perfusion** to the brain tissue. Stroke results in variable and potentially devastating neurologic deficits depending on the severity of the injury and the location in the brain.

Epidemiology

Stroke is the fourth leading cause of death and the main cause of disability in the United States (Go et al., 2013; National Heart, Lung, and Blood Institute [NHLBI], 2006). Population-based studies have estimated the yearly incidence of stroke in the United States to be 795,000, with 610,000 of these being new strokes (Lloyd-Jones et

Key Words

- antiplatelet therapy
- cerebrovascular accident
- constraint-induced movement therapy
- deep vein thrombosis
- hemorrhagic stroke
- hyperlipidemia
- hypertension
- intracerebral hemorrhage
- ischemic stroke
- National Institutes of Health Stroke Scale
- neuromuscular electrical stimulation
- pain
- pulmonary embolism
- spasticity
- subarachnoid hemorrhage
- thrombolytic therapy

al., 2009). African Americans' risk of first stroke is almost twice that of White Americans (NHLBI, 2006). Additionally, stroke mortality rates have been declining since the 1950s, yet age-adjusted death rates in African Americans remain high (Go et al., 2013; Roger et al., 2012). The reasons behind this disparity have not been completely elucidated, but evidence has pointed to not only the increased rate of risk factors but also the increased impact of risk factors on African Americans (Howard, 2013).

In 2009, when separated from the remainder of the cardiovascular causes, stroke accounted for approximately 1 in 19 deaths in the United States and is the fourth leading cause of death after diseases of the heart, cancers, and chronic lower respiratory disease (Centers for Disease Control and Prevention, 2014; Go et al., 2013). The functional deficits and disability resulting from stroke are a target of treatment for many rehabilitation professionals.

Strokes can be classified as *hemorrhagic* or *ischemic*. Ischemic strokes (Figure 1.1) make up approximately 87% of all strokes (Go et al., 2013). They result from vessel occlusion from a **thrombosis** in large and small arteries, most commonly in conjunction with atherosclerosis. Other causes of ischemic stroke include cerebral **embolism,** cerebral vasculitis, and other less common causes. Neurologic injury from ischemic stroke is extremely variable, ranging from transient ischemic attacks (TIAs) with symptoms of very brief duration to severe disability. Cerebral emboli typically have a cardiac source such as valvular disease or atrial fibrillation.

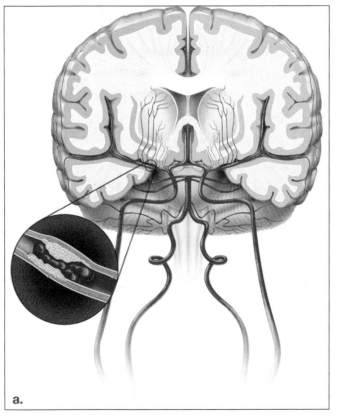
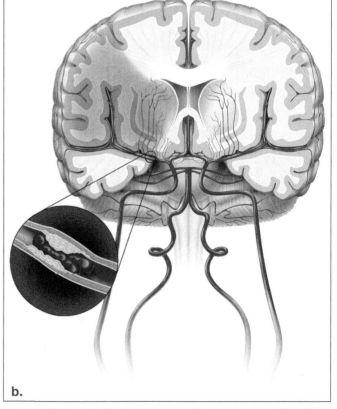

a.   b.

Figure 1.1. Arterial blockage in the brain (a), and ischemic stroke results from lack of oxygen and nutrients resulting from the blockage (b).

Source. Matthew Holt, illustrator. From "Ischemic Stroke," n.d., retrieved from the Internet Stroke Center, http://www.strokecenter.org/patients/about-stroke/ischemic-stroke. Illustrations Copyright © 2002 by Matthew Holt. Used with permission.

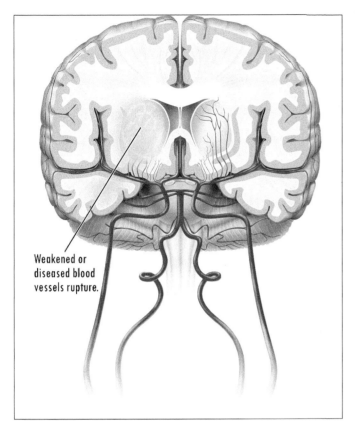 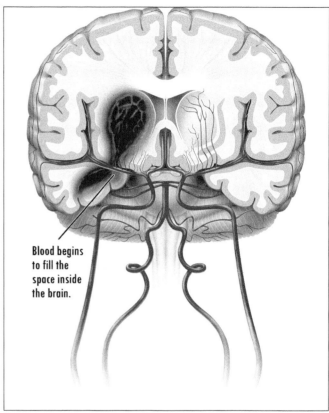

Figure 1.2. Weakened or damaged vessels leading to hemorrhagic stroke.

Source. Matthew Holt, illustrator. From "Intracerebral Hemorrhage," n.d., retrieved from the Internet Stroke Center, http://www.strokecenter.org/patients/about-stroke/intracerebral-hemorrhage/. Illustrations Copyright © 2002 by Matthew Holt. Used with permission.

Hemorrhagic stroke (Figure 1.2) accounts for the other 13% of strokes, with intracerebral hemorrhage (ICH) accounting for the majority of these strokes (10%), and **subarachnoid hemorrhage** (SAH) accounting for the remainder (3%; Go et al., 2013). ICH is caused by **hypertension,** arteriovenous malformation, or tumor. Half of ICHs occur in the **putamen** and the cerebral **white matter.** SAHs (Figure 1.3) are typically due to aneurysmal rupture of a cerebral artery.

Mortality resulting from stroke has decreased (Fang, Alderman, Keenan, & Croft, 2007; Go et al., 2013). However, the rate of hospitalization per 100,000 for stroke increased by 18.6% from 1988 to 1997 (Fang & Alderman, 2001; possibly as a result of decreased mortality and increased quality of care) before falling to 89% of the 1988 rate by 2004 (Fang et al., 2007). Despite the decreasing rate of stroke in the U.S. population, the total number of hospitalizations for stroke in 2010 had reached over a million, with average stay duration of 6.1 days (Go et al., 2013). Many more patients are seen for rehabilitation as outpatients.

Risk Factors

Nonmodifiable risk factors for stroke include history of a previous stroke, age, race, and gender. Women's risk of stroke is higher between ages 55 and 75 at 20% to 21%, whereas the risk for men is between 14% and 17% (Seshadri et al., 2006). The demographics of stroke are shifting, with strokes occurring at an earlier point in life

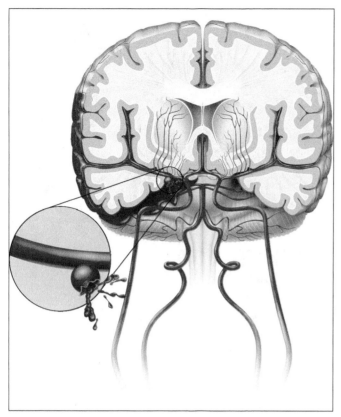

Figure 1.3. Subarachnoid hemorrhage resulting from a ruptured aneurysm.

Source. Matthew Holt, illustrator. From "Subarachnoid Hemorrhage," n.d., retrieved from the Internet Stroke Center, http://www.strokecenter.org/patients/about-stroke/subarachnoid-hemorrhage/. Illustration Copyright © 2002 by Matthew Holt. Used with permission.

(Wolf, Baum, & Connor, 2009). Wolf et al. (2009) followed 7,740 patients and found 45% of patients with stroke were younger than age 65, and nearly 27% were younger than age 55.

Modifiable risk factors include hypertension, smoking, hyperlipidemia, diabetes mellitus, and other smaller contributors. Hypertension is a major player in the risk of stroke. Individuals with blood pressure (BP) less than 120/80 mm Hg have nearly half the lifetime risk of those with hypertension. Lowering these patients' BP has been shown to result in a reduction in risk of stroke (Action to Control Cardiovascular Risk in Diabetes [ACCORD] Study Group, 2010). Smoking is known to be connected to risk of stroke, with recent evidence showing a dose-dependent increase in risk on the basis of how much a person smokes (Shah & Cole, 2010). Indirect evidence has shown that hyperlipidemia may be a risk factor. The use of HMG-CoA reductase inhibitors, which are used to treat elevated lipids, has been shown to decrease the risk of stroke (Byington et al., 2001). Exercise has been connected to a reduction in risk of ischemic stroke (Willey et al., 2009). However, an additional study reported that this decrease in incidence only occurred with moderate- to vigorous-intensity exercise. Low-intensity exercise, such as walking, showed no benefit (Willey et al., 2009).

It has been recognized since the 1980s that diabetes increases the risk of stroke independently of its connection to heart disease and hypertension (Abbott, Donahue, MacMahon, Reed, & Yano, 1987; Hägg et al., 2014). These modifiable risk factors continue to be targets of treatment in the prevention of initial and recurrent stroke.

Symptoms

The symptoms of a stroke are varied depending on the location of the stroke as well as the severity of the event. Although signs and symptoms after a stroke show some variability, constellations of symptoms are associated with the location of the occlusion or bleed. Table 1.1 shows some of the possible symptoms that can be seen in a stroke involving the vasculature listed.

> **Although signs and symptoms after a stroke show some variability, constellations of symptoms are associated with the location of the occlusion or bleed.**

Acute Management

The initial management of stroke involves ensuring the patient's medical stability as well as determining the appropriateness of thrombolytic therapy. Immediately on presentation, the patient needs to be evaluated for medical stability, ensuring adequate airway, breathing, circulation, and hemodynamic stability. When the patient is stable, further evaluation can ensue. Early evaluation for ICH or SAH can be lifesaving (Broderick et al., 2007). **Hemorrhage** is suggested by headache and

Table 1.1. Possible Symptoms After Stroke

Anterior Cerebral Artery	Middle Cerebral Artery	Posterior Cerebral Artery	Vertebrobasilar System
Contralateral weakness or sensory loss (lower extremity > upper extremity)	Contralateral weakness or sensory loss (face, upper extremity > lower extremity)	Visual field cuts	Cranial neuropathies
		Prosopagnosia	Cerebellar signs
Gait impairment	**Homonymous hemianopsia**	**Alexia**	Weakness or sensory impairment
	Dominant hemisphere: Aphasia Apraxia		Classic syndromes: Wallenberg's, Benedikt's, Weber, Millard-Gubler, medial medullary
	Nondominant hemisphere: Hemineglect Visuospatial impairment		

vomiting; however, it is only fully evaluated by means of computerized tomography (CT) or magnetic resonance imaging (MRI) scan.

History and physical examination then focus on evaluating for and reversing any conditions that can be contributing to the situation and screening for any contraindications to thrombolytic therapy. The differential diagnosis of stroke includes the following, which may mimic brain **ischemia:**

- ICH
- Traumatic brain injury
- Severe migraine headaches
- Brain malignancy
- Seizures
- Infectious process
- Hypoglycemia
- Renal failure
- Drug overdose
- Psychiatric disturbance.

The initial workup should include additional laboratory testing, including complete blood count, finger-stick glucose, electrolytes, blood urea nitrogen, creatinine, and coagulation panel.

Thrombolytic therapy with alteplase (t-PA) is recommended for those who meet criteria. Thrombolytic therapy involves administering a medication that can aid in breaking up a clot that may be causing the stroke. This therapy can be considered in the clinical diagnosis of ischemic stroke, causing a known and measurable deficit in symptoms when treatment begins less than 4.5 hours after their onset (Del Zoppo, Saver, Jauch, & Adams, 2009). It is extremely important to remain within this window of time to avoid dangerous bleeding. Specific exclusion criteria include the following (Adams et al., 2007):

- Previous stroke or head injury within the past 3 months
- Major surgery in the past 14 days
- Symptoms suggestive of SAH
- BP elevation with systolic more than 185 mm Hg or diastolic more than 110 mm Hg

- Platelets less than 100,000/mm3
- Serum glucose less than 50 mg/dL
- **International normalized ratio** (INR) more than 1.7
- Evidence of hemorrhage on CT scan.

The ideal timeline is less than 60 minutes from the time of presentation to the emergency department to the time of start of the infusion of t-PA.

BP is known to elevate after a stroke to maintain cerebral perfusion. The consensus is that BP should not be treated acutely unless t-PA is to be used, the systolic BP is higher than 220 mm Hg or the diastolic BP is higher than 120 mm Hg, or if the patient has other comorbidities that require that elevated BP be treated (Adams et al., 2007). If it is to be treated, a slow correction is advised to maintain cerebral perfusion.

Neuroimaging beyond the initial CT scan to exclude intracranial bleeding is used to evaluate the extent of the injury and to determine etiology of stroke. MRI provides more detail and accuracy on the extent of the stroke than CT scan. MRI can also determine the acuity of the stroke. Echocardiogram is an imaging modality of the heart that can show the effectiveness of the heart as a pump and can also reveal cardiogenic and aortic sources of embolism that could cause a stroke. Carotid Doppler ultrasound is used to determine the patency of the carotid arteries because carotid embolic sources can account for strokes as well. Carotid endarterectomy surgery may be considered if the patient has 60% to 99% stenosis of a carotid artery (Chaturvedi et al., 2005).

> **The prevention and treatment of further medical complications are other important goals of early stroke management.**

The prevention and treatment of further medical complications are other important goals of early stroke management. Of all patients admitted to inpatient rehabilitation for stroke, 75% experienced at least one medical comorbidity (Roth et al., 2001). Common comorbidities include hypoalbuminemia, severe neurologic impairment, and a history of hypertension. Other complications in this period can include **deep vein thrombosis** (DVT); **hydrocephalus; aspiration pneumonia;** cardiac problems, including myocardial infarction and heart failure; urinary tract infections; malnutrition; pressure sores; falls; spasticity; pain; **dysphagia;** and debility and deconditioning from hospitalization.

Medical Management of Stroke in the Rehabilitation Period

Medical management after a stroke is a combination of management of the patient's preexisting medical problems that require ongoing care or that may be aggravated by the stroke and management of secondary medical complications after stroke. The medical management that occurs during inpatient rehabilitation can interfere with the patient's actual time with the therapy teams and potentially hinder the patient's progress. Accurate assessment and medical treatment in the early rehabilitation phase can help promote a successful rehabilitation process for the patient.

DVT is a frequent medical concern in the rehabilitation period. Currently, the standard of practice involves prophylactic treatment with early mobilization and low-molecular-weight heparin to prevent DVTs. It has been reported that without this prophylaxis, as many as one-third of patients admitted to rehabilitation can have a nondiagnosed clot, with incidence potentially as high as 75% (Brandstater, 1992; Field & Hill, 2012; Harvey, 2003). DVT can cause edema, immobility, and pain and can lead to a potentially fatal pulmonary embolism (PE). The treatment of DVT involves surgical placement of a filter in the inferior vena cava to prevent PE, long-term anticoagulant therapy if there are no contraindications to such, or both.

There are many causes of pain after stroke. Shoulder pain is a frequent medical complication. Shoulder pain has multiple potential causes, including **subluxation,** rotator cuff injury, neuropathic pain, myofascial pain, spasticity, and many others. Estimates of the prevalence of shoulder pain in the poststroke period vary; however, one study that followed patients for 11 months after stroke found that 72% of patients had shoulder pain at some point (Van Ouwenaller, Laplace, & Chantraine, 1986). Medical workup of shoulder pain is required to determine the etiology of the pain and thus guide treatment. Pain can also occur elsewhere in the body after stroke. The potential of acute musculoskeletal injuries cannot be excluded as a cause, especially as the patient becomes more active in the rehabilitation phase. Central pain can be considered in the event no other cause is found. This pain, previously thought to be mediated by the **thalamus,** can be debilitating and functionally limiting. Treatment for central pain includes pharmacotherapy and possibly a referral to a pain management program.

Spasticity is tightness in the muscles; **functional impairment** can occur as a result of a velocity-dependent resistance to stretching because of an increase in the tonic stretch reflexes. Spasticity is a natural part of the healing process after a stroke. However, it can not only impair function but also be painful. The initial management involves physical and occupational therapy interventions, including daily stretching, splinting, and patient education. When spasticity is severe, medical interventions such as focal treatment with botulinum toxin or phenol may be necessary to prevent **contractures** or improve functional outcomes. For severe generalized spasticity or severe lower-extremity spasticity, medical consideration can be given to surgically implanting an intrathecal baclofen pump, which allows medication to be delivered directly at the spinal cord level to help ameliorate the spasticity.

> Spasticity is a natural part of the healing process after a stroke. However, it can not only impair function but also be painful.

Nutritional status is linked to stroke both before and after the event. Patients who were undernourished prestroke tend to have more medical complications and worse long-term outcome poststroke (Feed Or Ordinary Diet [FOOD] Trial Collaboration, 2003). Poststroke nutrition needs to be monitored carefully. Dysphagia can lead to malnourishment, dehydration, and aspiration pneumonia. *Neglect syndromes,* in which the patient has an inability to perceive various stimuli from one side of the body or environment, and depression can lead to undereating. The patient's nutrition status needs to be followed closely, and medical interventions such as tube feeding, appetite stimulation, and psychotherapy may be necessary. Decreased nutrition can also accompany debility or deconditioning because the patient finds eating effortful and reduces intake as a result. This decreased nutrition can then add to the fatigue, poor tolerance of rehabilitation, diminished motivation, and depression and can potentially worsen outcome.

The sudden life-changing nature of a stroke and the potential disability associated with it can lead to various reactions from the patient psychologically and in a social sense. The range of psychological effects can include **anger,** frustration, depression, **anxiety,** sadness, and a sense of loss. Patients' premorbid psychological health as well as their social support structures play major roles in how they respond to the new stroke. Addressing these issues is vital if the rehabilitation process is to be successful for the patient. Depression, a frequent diagnosis after stroke, can cause

> The sudden life-changing nature of a stroke and the potential disability associated with it can lead to various reactions from the patient psychologically and in a social sense.

fatigue, impaired sleep, frustration, and loss of hope. Thus, it can severely hamper the rehabilitation process. Selective serotonin reuptake inhibitor class medication is the current first-line therapy for depression after stroke despite a lack of solid evidence as to the best course of treatment (Paolucci, 2008). Psychological interventions can be effective as part of the treatment for these disturbances.

Social concerns such as family reactions and interactions after stroke, reintegration into previous life roles, sexual difficulties, vocational concerns, and the transition to home from rehabilitation are among the challenges after a stroke. Community services, case management, psychologists, therapy, and physicians can all play a role in helping the patient cope with and address these concerns.

Many other potential medical concerns exist during the early poststroke period that can typically continue during the rehabilitation period. Physician oversight during this phase is crucial to minimizing the medical impact on the patient's rehabilitation.

Secondary Prevention

The best long-term intervention for a patient after a stroke is to optimize the patient's medical status to minimize the risk of recurrent stroke. Treatment of modifiable risk factors such as diabetes and hypertension is important in this phase, as is providing good education on other lifestyle modifications. Modifications such as stopping smoking to stop ongoing damage to the vasculature and reduce hypercoagulable state and making dietary changes to reduce hyperlipidemia can be extremely beneficial in reducing risk of a recurrent stroke during the poststroke period.

Medical treatment beyond the modification of risk factors includes institution of antiplatelet therapy. Large studies have found a 25% reduction in nonfatal stroke among both men and women when taking antiplatelet therapy after a stroke (Antithrombotic Trialists' Collaboration, 2002). The typical treatment is daily aspirin therapy or clopidogrel, a nonaspirin antiplatelet medication.

Atrial fibrillation is a relatively common **arrhythmia** of the heart; it can promote clot formation in the heart, which can potentially embolize, causing a stroke. Warfarin has been shown to reduce the risk of stroke by approximately 65%, whereas aspirin reduces the risk by only about 20% (Hart et al., 2003).

As mentioned previously, proper selection for surgery for symptomatic or critical stenosis of the carotid arteries can have a significant reduction in the risk of stroke.

Rehabilitation

Rehabilitation considerations should start at the time of admission and progress throughout the acute stay. Current recommendations from the American Heart Association and the American Stroke Association are for poststroke care to occur in a multidisciplinary rehabilitation center or a dedicated stroke unit. Rehabilitation therapies, proactive measures for prevention of venous thrombi, assessment with the **National Institutes of Health Stroke Scale** (NIHSS), and dysphagia screening should be initiated early. A program for active secondary stroke prevention should also be implemented (Bates et al., 2005).

The NIHSS is used by providers and researchers as a tool to objectively quantify impairment related to stroke. The scale uses 11 categories scored between 0 and 4; the total score ranges from 0, meaning *no impairment,* to 42, meaning *severe stroke symptoms and impairment.* The categories of testing include level of **consciousness,** horizontal eye movement, **visual fields,** facial function, motor function of arms and legs, **ataxia,** sensory function, language and **dysarthria,** and inattention or neglect (Brott et al., 1989).

The rehabilitation options for stroke patients depend on the level of impairment as well as the given patient's ability to participate in rehabilitation. Inpatient rehabilitation is intensive and requires that the patient be able to tolerate 3 hours of therapy per day. Additionally, the patient must have ongoing medical issues that require 24-hour nursing care and daily physician interactions. Day treatment programs have similar intensity of therapy with patients who are medically able to be outside the hospital and do not require 24-hour nursing care. Additional options for care include home health care and outpatient therapy services. The decision making as to how to frame the rehabilitation for a stroke patient is a very individualized process, and a general outline is presented in Figure 1.4. The intervention chapters of this text will discuss occupational therapy's role at each of these levels in the continuum of rehabilitation care.

Functional recovery mechanisms after stroke are being studied extensively, with more coming to light on the injured brain's vast potential to reorganize and recover functions that were lost with a stroke. The mechanisms that are understood at this point include

- Diaschisis,
- Reorganization of the peri-infarct region (vicarious reorganization),
- Ipsilateral motor activity, and
- Contralateral hemisphere activity.

Diaschisis refers to the deactivation of undamaged areas that are distant from the actual injured area. Recovery from diaschisis is thought to contribute to recovery after stroke. *Vicarious reorganization* refers to the idea that noninjured areas of the brain can take over the functions of the injured tissue. Ipsilateral increased activation of the motor pathways is thought to contribute to overall motor recovery as well. Early after stroke, **contralateral** sensorimotor activity is increased and aids in the recovery process.

Recovery from stroke has been most studied in the motor system. The classic description from Twitchell (1951) involves **hemiplegia** and loss of tendon reflexes at the time of the stroke, which then progress to increased tendon reflexes on the involved side followed by the onset of spasticity. Most patients are noted to have more upper-extremity flexor and adductor involvement, whereas the lower extremity tends to have more extensor and adductor involvement. Gradually, an increase in voluntary movement occurs as spasticity improves. In his landmark 1970 study, Brunnstrom described the typical stages of motor recovery expected (Table 1.2). Although this pattern is often seen, not all stroke patients recover fully to Stage 7.

Stroke rehabilitation has shifted to a model emphasizing strategies to enhance neurologic recovery rather than just to compensate for lost function. However, despite this shift, the evidence base continues to be insufficient to provide guidance as to the best possible therapy after stroke. Traditional sensorimotor techniques encompass multiple different approaches, but all emphasize strengthening, **range of motion,** balance, and postural control. Brunnstrom (1956) proposed

> The rehabilitation options for stroke patients depend on the level of impairment as well as the given patient's ability to participate in rehabilitation.

> Stroke rehabilitation has shifted to a model emphasizing strategies to enhance neurologic recovery rather than just to compensate for lost function. However, despite this shift, the evidence base continues to be insufficient to provide guidance as to the best possible therapy after stroke.

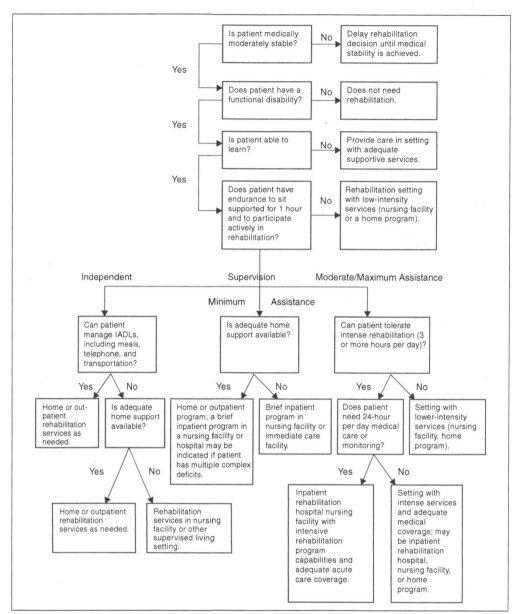

Figure 1.4. Framework for rehabilitation decisions after a stroke.

Source. From "Rehabilitation," by G. E. Gresham et al., 1997. American Heart Association Prevention Conference. IV. Prevention and Rehabilitation of Stroke. *Stroke, 28,* 1522–1526, Figure 1. Used with permission.

Note. IADLs = instrumental activities of daily living.

Table 1.2. Stages of Motor Recovery

Stage	Description
1	Flaccidity—no movement on affected side
2	Appearance of spasticity; movement only in synergy patterns
3	Increasing spasticity; control of movement within synergy patterns increases
4	Decreasing spasticity; voluntary movement outside synergy patterns begins
5	Continued decline of spasticity; more complex movements
6	Spasticity disappears; movement nearly at normal levels
7	Normal movement

Source. From *Movement Therapy in Hemiplegia: A Neurophysiological Approach,* by S. Brunnstrom, 1970, New York: Harper & Row.

techniques encouraging and enhancing the synergy patterns of motor recovery as a way to enhance recovery. This method is contrasted with the methods developed by Bobath (1990), known as *neurodevelopmental technique,* that seek to inhibit the abnormal patterns and movement, focusing on a more normalized muscle control and patterns. Although both Brunnstrom's and Bobath's approaches are still frequently used in rehabilitation, more evidence-based contemporary motor intervention approaches are emerging and becoming more prevalent in rehabilitation. These contemporary motor intervention approaches emphasize meaningful, task-specific, and task-oriented training to promote motor recovery and improve functional independence. A specific example of this approach is **constraint-induced movement therapy** (CIMT).

CIMT is an extension of Edward Taub's theory that a patient has **learned nonuse** of part of the body (Taub, Uswatte, & Pidikiti, 1999). The therapy involves forced use of the affected limb while restraining the unaffected side. This intervention relies on **neuroplasticity** as its basis in treatment. Evidence has shown that this treatment or its modified version, which is less intensive and used over a longer time period, can lead to a moderate reduction in disability by the end of the standard 2-week treatment protocol. However, the evidence that these effects are sustained long term is insufficient (Sirtori, Corbetta, Moja, & Gatti, 2009). CIMT is an option for those with at least some functional control of the affected side.

Neuromuscular electrical stimulation (NMES), however, is an option for those who do not have enough muscle control in an affected limb to perform CIMT. *NMES* involves stimulation of the lower motor **neurons** and thus activation of the associated muscles. This therapy can be used in such a way as to aid motor recovery, but it can also be used functionally to aid movement.

Many other methods are being used to aid in recovery from the neurologic sequelae of stroke. Some focus on one particular aspect of recovery, such as body weight–supported treadmill training, which works to help improve gait function after stroke. Other methods such as noninvasive brain stimulation attempt to maximize outcome and potentially improve the benefits of rehabilitation. The rehabilitation process for a stroke patient should also include a skilled approach to **cognition** and communication.

Aphasia, or the loss of or impairment in communication, can be functionally devastating to a stroke patient. Aphasia has been found to be at its worst early after stroke and tends to improve to a point. However, of those who had aphasia at 7 days poststroke, 40% continued to have aphasia at 6 months, and 60% of those who had been aphasic at 3 weeks continued to be aphasic at 6 months (Wade, Hewer, David, & Enderby, 1986). Dickey et al. (2010) found that 35% of adult patients during the 2004–2005 Ontario stroke audit had aphasia at hospital discharge and that the risk of aphasia was associated with greater age, more severe strokes, and greater disability and that patients with aphasia were more frequently discharged to long-term care or rehabilitation facilities. The speech–language pathology approach to aphasia involves several techniques, with examples including reading, verbalization exercises, oral–motor exercises, melodic intonation, and alternative or augmentative communication. Rehabilitation for **memory** and cognitive impairments involves working to aid in memory recovery and to teach strategies to compensate for the lost memory and cognition. At this time, the evidence base for cognitive

Table 1.3. Adaptive and Assistive Equipment After Stroke

Type	Equipment
Mobility and gait aids	Power or manual wheelchair Walker—standard, rolling, hemi Cane—single-point, quad Transfer board Rocker-bottom shoes Orthoses (e.g., ankle–foot–orthoses)
ADL equipment	Adaptive feeding utensils Adaptive shaving equipment Built-up hairbrushes, toothbrushes, etc. Buttonhooks Long-handled reachers Elastic shoelaces
Tub or shower	Grab bars Shower chair or bench Lift system

Note. ADL = activities of daily living.

Occupational therapy's emphasis on improving the patient's everyday tasks leads to increased independence and can decrease caregiver burden and improve the patient's disposition.

rehabilitation is mixed as to its long-term effectiveness and is addressed in subsequent chapters.

Occupational therapists are critical to the rehabilitation process after a stroke in terms of restoration or improvement in performing everyday life activities. Occupational therapy's emphasis on improving the patient's everyday tasks leads to increased independence and can decrease caregiver burden and improve the patient's disposition. In the later phases of recovery, occupational therapy is vital in other life roles such as return to work and driving. Further discussion of the role of occupational therapy in the rehabilitation of a stroke patient is discussed in Chapter 2.

In addition to augmenting recovery, rehabilitation needs to focus on allowing patients to increase function with their current disabilities. Adaptive and assistive equipment may be necessary and can include but is not limited to those items listed in Table 1.3.

The end goal for rehabilitation of stroke is for patients to transition back to their home and community. Thus, the final phases of the rehabilitation process involve preparing for this. Education of the patient and family with regard to expectations for recovery, risk factors for recurrent stroke, family functioning, **activities of daily living,** and ongoing care is part of this final step in care. It is important to include discussions of more advanced skills such as **instrumental activities of daily living, leisure,** and work activities. These skills are usually very important to the patient but may not yet have been discussed or addressed. Special forms of testing and various programs are available for returning to driving or work after a stroke.

Conclusion

Stroke can be devastating to a person's functional status. Despite the limitations placed on patients, some are able to be discharged home. Looking at the studies regarding discharge to home, it appears that roughly 76% of those who do go home after inpatient rehabilitation remain at home 12 months later (Pettersen, Dahl, & Wyller, 2002). The patients with more medical comorbidities and lower levels of function at the time of discharge have a higher risk of being institutionalized. Medical optimization typically occurs during patients' acute hospitalization. However, optimization continues into inpatient rehabilitation and on throughout patients' transition to home and the rest of their life. This medical rehabilitation is a complement to the therapy team's rehabilitation interventions. The overall goal of recovery includes all the interventions possible to maximize the patient's independence and overall function. The goals for the patient need to be specific to that particular patient's needs and desires and his or her situation.

References

Abbott, R. D., Donahue, R. P., MacMahon, S. W., Reed, D. M., & Yano, K. (1987). Diabetes and the risk of stroke: The Honolulu Heart Program. *JAMA, 257,* 949–952. http://dx.doi.org/10.1001/jama.1987.03390070069025

Action to Control Cardiovascular Risk in Diabetes Study Group. (2010). Effects of intensive blood-pressure control in type 2 diabetes mellitus. *New England Journal of Medicine, 362,* 1575–1585. http://dx.doi.org/10.1056/NEJMoa1001286

Adams, H. P., Jr., del Zoppo, G., Alberts, M. J., Bhatt, D. L., Brass, L., Furlan, A., . . . Wijdicks, E. F.; American Heart Association, American Stroke Association Stroke Council, Clinical Cardiology Council, Cardiovascular Radiology and Intervention Council, Atherosclerotic Peripheral Vascular Disease and Quality of Care Outcomes in Research Interdisciplinary Working Groups. (2007). Guidelines for the early management of adults with ischemic stroke: A guideline from the American Heart Association/American Stroke Association Stroke Council, Clinical Cardiology Council, Cardiovascular Radiology and Intervention Council, and the Atherosclerotic Peripheral Vascular Disease and Quality of Care Outcomes in Research Interdisciplinary Working Groups. *Stroke, 38,* 1655–1711. http://dx.doi.org/10.1161/STROKEAHA.107.181486

Antithrombotic Trialists' Collaboration. (2002). Collaborative meta-analysis of randomised trials of antiplatelet therapy for prevention of death, myocardial infarction, and stroke in high risk patients. *BMJ, 324,* 71–86. http://dx.doi.org/10.1136/bmj.324.7329.71

Bates, B., Choi, J. Y., Duncan, P. W., Glasberg, J. J., Graham, G. D., Katz, R. C., . . . Zorowitz, R.; U.S. Department of Defense; Department of Veterans Affairs. (2005). Veterans Affairs/Department of Defense clinical practice guidelines for the management of adult stroke rehabilitation care: Executive summary. *Stroke, 36,* 2049–2056. http://dx.doi.org/10.1161/01.STR.0000180432.73724.AD

Bobath, B. (1990). *Adult hemiplegia: Evaluation and treatment* (3rd ed.). Waltham, MA: Butterworth-Heinemann.

Brandstater, M. E. (1992). Venous thromboembolism in stroke. *Western Journal of Medicine, 157,* 666–667.

Broderick, J., Connolly, S., Feldmann, E., Hanley, D., Kase, C., Krieger, D., . . . Zuccarello, M.; American Heart Association, American Stroke Association Stroke Council, High Blood Pressure Research Council, Quality of Care and Outcomes in Research Interdisciplinary Working Group. (2007). Guidelines for the management of spontaneous intracerebral hemorrhage in adults: 2007 update: A guideline from the American Heart Association/American Stroke Association Stroke Council, High Blood Pressure Research Council, and the Quality of Care and Outcomes in Research Interdisciplinary Working Group. *Stroke, 38,* 2001–2023. http://dx.doi.org/10.1161/STROKEAHA.107.183689

Brott, T., Adams, H. P., Jr., Olinger, C. P., Marler, J. R., Barsan, W. G., Biller, J., . . . Hertzberg, V. (1989). Measurements of acute cerebral infarction: A clinical examination scale. *Stroke, 20,* 864–870. http://dx.doi.org10.1161/01.STR.20.7.864

Brunnstrom, S. (1956). Associated reactions of the upper extremity in adult patients with hemiplegia: An approach to training. *Physical Therapy Review, 36,* 225–236.

Brunnstrom, S. (1970). *Movement therapy in hemiplegia: A neurophysiological approach.* New York: Harper & Row.

Byington, R. P., Davis, B. R., Plehn, J. F., White, H. D., Baker, J., Cobbe, S. M., & Shepherd, J. (2001). Reduction of stroke events with pravastatin: The Prospective Pravastatin Pooling (PPP) Project. *Circulation, 103,* 387–392. http://dx.doi.org/10.1161/01.CIR.103.3.387

Centers for Disease Control and Prevention, National Center for Health Statistics. (2014, July). Compressed Mortality File 1999–2011 on CDC WONDER Online Database. Data are compiled from Compressed Mortality File 1999–2011 Series 20 No. 2Q, 2014. Accessed at http://wonder.cdc.gov/cmf-icd10.html

Chaturvedi, S., Bruno, A., Feasby, T., Holloway, R., Benavente, O., Cohen, S. N., . . . Wilterdink, J.; Therapeutics and Technology Assessment Subcommittee of the American Academy of Neurology. (2005). Carotid endarterectomy—An evidence-based review: Report of the Therapeutics and Technology Assessment Subcommittee of the American Academy of Neurology. *Neurology, 65,* 794–801. http://dx.doi.org/10.1212/01.wnl.0000176036.07558.82

Del Zoppo, G. J., Saver, J. L., Jauch, E. C., & Adams, H. P., Jr.; American Heart Association Stroke Council. (2009). Expansion of the time window for treatment of acute ischemic stroke with intravenous tissue plasminogen activator: A science advisory from the American Heart Association/American Stroke Association. *Stroke, 40,* 2945–2948. http://dx.doi.org/10.1161/STROKEAHA.109.192535

Dickey, L., Kagan, A., Lindsay, M. P., Fang, J., Rowland, A., & Black, S. (2010). Incidence and profile of inpatient stroke-induced aphasia in Ontario, Canada. *Archives of Physical Medicine and Rehabilitation, 91,* 196–202. http://dx.doi.org/10.1016/j.apmr.2009.09.020

Fang, J., & Alderman, M. H. (2001). Trend of stroke hospitalization, United States, 1988–1997. *Stroke, 32,* 2221–2226. http://dx.doi.org/10.1161/hs1001.096193

Fang, J., Alderman, M. H., Keenan, N. L., & Croft, J. B. (2007). Declining U.S. stroke hospitalization since 1997: National Hospital Discharge Survey, 1988–2004. *Neuroepidemiology, 29,* 243–249. http://dx.doi.org/10.1159/000112857

Feed Or Ordinary Diet Trial Collaboration. (2003). Poor nutritional status on admission predicts poor outcomes after stroke: Observational data from the FOOD trial. *Stroke, 34,* 1450–1456. http://dx.doi.org/10.1161/01.STR.0000074037.49197.8C

Field, T. S., & Hill, M. D. (2012). Prevention of deep vein thrombosis and pulmonary embolism in patients with stroke. *Clinical and Applied Thrombosis/Hemostasis, 18,* 5–19. http://dx.doi.org/10.1177/1076029611412362

Go, A. S., Mozaffarian, D., Roger, V. L., Benjamin, E. J., Berry, J. D., Borden, W. B., . . . American Heart Association Statistics Committee and Stroke Statistics Subcommittee. (2013). Heart disease and stroke statistics—2013 update: A report from the American Heart Association. *Circulation, 127,* e6–e245. http://dx.doi.org/10.1161/CIR.0b013e31828124ad

Gresham, G. E., Alexander, D., Bishop, D. S., Giuliani, C., Goldberg, G., Holland, A., . . . Trombly, C. A. (1997). American Heart Association Prevention Conference. IV. Prevention and rehabilitation of stroke. Rehabilitation. *Stroke, 28,* 1522–1526. http://dx.doi.org/10.1161/01.STR.28.7.1522

Hägg, S., Thorn, L. M., Forsblom, C. M., Gordin, D., Saraheimo, M., Tolonen, N., . . . FinnDiane Study Group. (2014). Different risk factor profiles for ischemic and hemorrhagic stroke in type 1 diabetes mellitus. *Stroke, 45,* 2558–2562. http://dx.doi.org/10.1161/STROKEAHA.114.005724

Hart, R. G., Halperin, J. L., Pearce, L. A., Anderson, D. C., Kronmal, R. A., McBride, R., . . . Marler, J. R.; Stroke Prevention in Atrial Fibrillation Investigators. (2003). Lessons from the Stroke Prevention in Atrial Fibrillation Trials. *Annals of Internal Medicine, 138,* 831–839. http://dx.doi.org/10.7326/0003-4819-138-10-200305200-00011

Harvey, R. L. (2003). Prevention of venous thromboembolism after stroke. *Topics in Stroke Rehabilitation, 10,* 61–69.

Howard, V. J. (2013). Reasons underlying racial differences in stroke incidence and mortality. *Stroke, 44*(Suppl. 1), S126–S128. http://dx.doi.org/10.1161/STROKEAHA.111.000691

Lloyd-Jones, D., Adams, R., Carnethon, M., De Simone, G., Ferguson, T. B., Flegal, K., . . . Hong, Y. (2009). Heart disease and stroke statistics—2009 update: A report from the American Heart Association Statistics Committee and Stroke Statistics Subcommittee. *Circulation, 119,* 480–486. http://dx.doi.org/10.1161/CIRCULATIONAHA.108.191259

National Heart, Lung, and Blood Institute. (2006). *Incidence and prevalence: 2006 chart book on cardiovascular and lung diseases.* Retrieved from http://www.nhlbi.nih.gov/resources/docs/06a_ip_chtbk.pdf

Paolucci, S. (2008). Epidemiology and treatment of post-stroke depression. *Neuropsychiatric Disease and Treatment, 4,* 145–154. http://dx.doi.org/10.2147/NDT.S2017

Pettersen, R., Dahl, T., & Wyller, T. B. (2002). Prediction of long-term functional outcome after stroke rehabilitation. *Clinical Rehabilitation, 16,* 149–159. http://dx.doi.org/10.1191/0269215502cr482oa

Roger, V. L., Go, A. S., Lloyd-Jones, D. M., Benjamin, E. J., Berry, J. D., Borden, W. B., . . . Turner, M. B.; American Heart Association Statistics Committee and Stroke Statistics Subcommittee. (2012). Executive summary: Heart disease and stroke statistics—2012 update: A report from the American Heart Association. *Circulation, 125,* 188–197. http://dx.doi.org/10.1161/CIR.0b013e3182456d46

Roth, E. J., Lovell, L., Harvey, R. L., Heinemann, A. W., Semik, P., & Diaz, S. (2001). Incidence of and risk factors for medical complications during stroke rehabilitation. *Stroke, 32,* 523–529. http://dx.doi.org/10.1161/01.STR.32.2.523

Seshadri, S., Beiser, A., Kelly-Hayes, M., Kase, C. S., Au, R., Kannel, W. B., & Wolf, P. A. (2006). The lifetime risk of stroke: Estimates from the Framingham Study. *Stroke, 37,* 345–350. http://dx.doi.org/10.1161/01.STR.0000199613.38911.b2

Shah, R. S., & Cole, J. W. (2010). Smoking and stroke: The more you smoke the more you stroke. *Expert Review of Cardiovascular Therapy, 8,* 917–932. http://dx.doi.org/10.1586/erc.10.56

Sirtori, V., Corbetta, D., Moja, L., & Gatti, R. (2009). Constraint-induced movement therapy for upper extremities in stroke patients. *Cochrane Database of Systematic Reviews, 2009,* CD004433. http://dx.doi.org/10.1002/14651858.CD004433.pub2

Taub, E., Uswatte, G., & Pidikiti, R. (1999). Constraint-induced movement therapy: A new family of techniques with broad application to physical rehabilitation—A clinical review. *Journal of Rehabilitation Research and Development, 36,* 237–251. http://dx.doi.org/10.1080/16501960310010124

Twitchell, T. E. (1951). The restoration of motor function following hemiplegia in man. *Brain, 74,* 443–480. http://dx.doi.org/10.1093/brain/74.4.443

Van Ouwenaller, C., Laplace, P. M., & Chantraine, A. (1986). Painful shoulder in hemiplegia. *Archives of Physical Medicine and Rehabilitation, 67,* 23–26.

Wade, D. T., Hewer, R. L., David, R. M., & Enderby, P. M. (1986). Aphasia after stroke: Natural history and associated deficits. *Journal of Neurology, Neurosurgery, and Psychiatry, 49,* 11–16. http://dx.doi.org/10.1136/jnnp.49.1.11

Willey, J. Z., Moon, Y. P., Paik, M. C., Boden-Albala, B., Sacco, R. L., & Elkind, M. S. V. (2009). Physical activity and risk of ischemic stroke in the Northern Manhattan Study. *Neurology, 73,* 1774–1779. http://dx.doi.org/10.1212/WNL.0b013e3181c34b58

Wolf, T. J., Baum, C. M., & Connor, L. T. (2009). Changing face of stroke: Implications for occupational therapy practice. *American Journal of Occupational Therapy, 63,* 621–625. http://dx.doi.org/10.5014/ajot.63.5.621

Improving Participation After Stroke: The Transactional Relationship Among the Person, the Environment, and Occupation

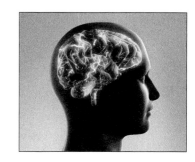

Timothy J. Wolf, OTD, MSCI, OTR/L, and
Carolyn M. Baum, PhD, OTR/L, FAOTA

Learning Objectives

After completion of this chapter, readers will be able to

- Delineate how practice models are applied in occupational therapy practice;
- Identify the components of the Person–Environment–Occupation–Performance (PEOP) model;
- Identify the relationship between occupational performance and the domains of the PEOP model; and
- Apply the PEOP model to the stroke population and be able to recognize how each domain affects overall health and occupational performance.

Key Words

- extrinsic factors
- intrinsic factors
- model
- occupation
- participation
- performance
- quality of life

Introduction

Why do we use models in practice? Models provide the basis to help us develop an understanding of concepts and allow us to track the concepts as evidence brings greater understanding to support our approach to care, and they provide a basis for decision making and support the therapist in being systematic and comprehensive in the collection of information (Turpin & Iwama, 2011). The Person–Environment–Occupation–Performance (PEOP) model is particularly valuable in the management of **stroke** because it serves to bridge the medical and sociocultural models by identifying three relevant domains of knowledge for occupational therapy practice: (1) the person or intrinsic factors, which if used alone would identify impairments; (2) the cultural, social, physical, policy, and technology environment, which introduces the sociocultural model extrinsic to the person; and (3) the occupations of importance to the client's well-being (activities, tasks, roles). It is transactive in that it views everyday occupations as being affected by, and affecting, the client and the environment that supports the client's home, work or school, and community life.

The Person–Environment–Occupation–Performance (PEOP) model is particularly valuable in the management of **stroke** because it serves to bridge the medical and sociocultural models by identifying three relevant domains of knowledge for occupational therapy practice.

PEOP is a model for occupational therapy practice. The knowledge necessary to use the PEOP model in stroke is generated from occupational science, **neuroscience,** environmental science, and other biological and social sciences. The PEOP model was designed to facilitate the development of a collaborative approach with the client and with other professionals in which the occupational therapist offers the knowledge to direct practice that bridges the world of the client who is served in the medical, educational, or community health system. A core assumption of occupational therapists is that to be healthy, one must be able to engage in daily occupations that are meaningful and provide satisfaction. The PEOP model provides the infrastructure to organize knowledge that will support the practitioner in engaging the client in planning the intervention process. Occupational performance is central to the PEOP model and is defined as the complex interactions between people and the environments in which they carry out activities, tasks, and roles that are meaningful to or required of them (Baum & Christiansen, 2005).

Description of the Model

Figure 2.1 provides a graphic representation of the PEOP model. This representation is intended to convey that occupational performance is determined not only by the nature of the activity, task, or role to be performed but also by the characteristics of the person and the environment. Optimal occupational performance occurs when

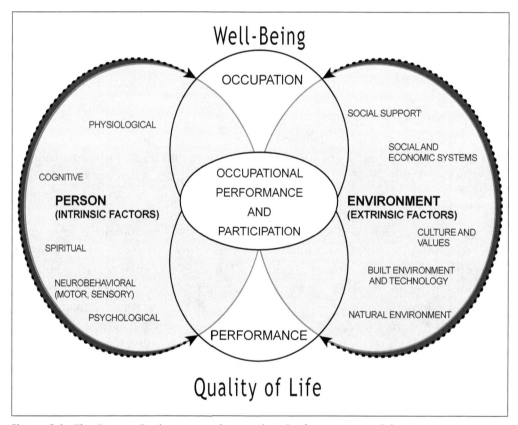

Figure 2.1. The Person–Environment–Occupation–Performance model.

Source. From "Person–Environment–Occupation–Performance: An Occupation-Based Framework for Practice," by C. M. Baum and C. H. Christiansen, in *Occupational Therapy: Performance, Participation, and Well-Being* (3rd ed., p. 246), by C. H. Christiansen, C. M. Baum, and J. D. Bass-Haugen (Eds.), 2005, Thorofare, NJ: Slack. Copyright © 2005 by Slack, Inc. Reprinted with permission.

the person–environment fit supports the client in doing what he or she wants and needs to do. We should note that for a given situation, the applicability or importance of the person and environment factors will vary. The PEOP model presupposes that an assessment to plan intervention will include a consideration of each of the factors because some will offer challenge and others will provide the resources that will make occupational performance possible.

The intrinsic factors in the PEOP model that are central to occupational performance include physiological (strength, endurance, flexibility, inactivity, **stress,** sleep, nutrition, and health); cognitive (organization, reasoning, **attention,** awareness, **executive function,** and **memory**); neurobehavioral (somatosensory, olfactory, gustatory, visual, auditory, proprioceptive, tactile, and motor control; motor planning [praxis]; and postural control); psychological and emotional (emotional state [affect], self-concept, **self-esteem** and sense of identity, **self-efficacy** and theory of mind [social awareness]); and spiritual or that which brings meaning. The extrinsic factors in the PEOP model that are central to occupational performance include social support (practical or instrumental support and informational support); societal factors (interpersonal relationships [groups], social receptivity, laws, and policies); the cultural environment (values, beliefs, customs, and use of time); the built environment (physical properties, tools, assistive technology, and design); and the natural environment (geography, terrain, climate, and air quality). In this chapter, we review these key components of the PEOP model in reference to how they apply to people with stroke.

Using the PEOP Model in the Management of People With Stroke

Occupational therapy is a profession founded on a belief in the fundamental importance of occupation (Christiansen, Clark, Kielhofner, & Rogers, 1995). Engagement in occupation is assumed to be an essential part of living and to have the potential to influence health and well-being (Polatajko, 1992; Yerxa, 1993). Many people who have had a stroke have persistent physical, psychological, and **functional impairments** that have an impact on their daily activities and quality of life, altering both the nature and the extent of their involvement in occupations related to all aspects of life (Desrosiers et al., 2006; Edwards, Hahn, Baum, & Dromerick, 2006; White, MacKenzie, Magin, & Pollack, 2008). The sudden inability to perform valued occupations can undermine a person's identity and self-worth (Clarke & Black, 2005). Many people characterize their roles as changing from "doers" to "receivers," from active to passive—meaning derived from occupational engagement is transformed from themes of autonomy and accomplishment to feelings of insufficiency and frustration. Decreases in occupational engagement and performance result in diminished self-efficacy, which in turn is linked to further withdrawal from valued occupations (Eriksson, Kottorp, Borg, & Tham, 2009).

Although research has continued to confirm decreased participation after stroke, it has also found that many people with stroke are able to return to a life of engagement in meaningful and fulfilling occupations (Cardol et al., 2002; White et al., 2008). A 2001 qualitative study exploring disability's influence on occupations found that it involved a process of reevaluation and reconstruction of values (Magnus, 2001), for example, reducing participation in activities such as applying makeup so as to have the energy and functional reserve to devote to more valued occupations such as parenting. This active choosing, shaping, and orchestrating of one's relationship to occupations aids in asserting a sense of self-control, thereby restoring one's self-efficacy (Bandura, 1997; Pound, Gompertz, & Ebrahim, 1999). The autonomy associated with "typical" adulthood can be characterized as authoring one's own life (Ahlström & Bernspång, 2003). By orchestrating daily occupations, authorship is restored to the adult's life.

Person or Intrinsic Factors

Stroke has traditionally been seen as a medical event. In fact, it is a life-changing event that can affect many aspects of an individual's and his or her family's lives. Occupational therapists must understand the complexity of stroke to identify the impairments that can be addressed in recovery and the capacities that can facilitate a return to daily life. Each of the PEOP concepts is discussed further in this chapter because all are active topics in research. It will be important for readers to further explore these topics in their ongoing learning. Several free resources exist to help practitioners stay current on the existing literature related to stroke **rehabilitation.** Some examples include http://strokengine.ca/, http://www.otseeker.com/, http://scholar.google.com/, and http://www.aota.org. In this section, we introduce the person or intrinsic factors that are known to affect the performance of people with stroke. Figure 2.2 introduces the intrinsic or person factors of the PEOP model.

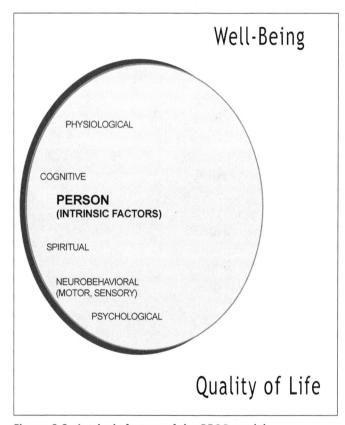

Figure 2.2. Intrinsic factors of the PEOP model.

Source. From "Person–Environment–Occupation–Performance: An Occupation-Based Framework for Practice," by C. M. Baum and C. H. Christiansen, in *Occupational Therapy: Performance, Participation, and Well-Being* (3rd ed., p. 246), by C. H. Christiansen, C. M. Baum, and J. D. Bass-Haugen (Eds.), 2005, Thorofare, NJ: Slack. Copyright © 2005 by Slack, Inc. Reprinted with permission.

Cognitive Factors

Cognitive impairments are common in patients with stroke and often interfere with functional recovery and participation in daily life activities (Alladi, Meena, & Kaul, 2002). According to Katz and Maeir (2011), **cognition** is conceptualized as consisting of basic cognitive skills (i.e., memory, attention, perception) as well as higher-level cognitive functions, including awareness and executive processing. Sachdev et al. (2004) compared a sample of 170 stroke and transient ischemic attack survivors at 3 to 6 months poststroke and 96 age-matched controls. In the study, the factors that contributed most to differentiating impaired from unimpaired participants were abstraction, information-processing speed, **working memory,** and mental flexibility. In addition, others have reported that cognitive dysfunction in stroke patients can be a source of safety concern in nearly all areas of occupational performance, with key areas including mobility, meal preparation, and management of medication (Hyndman & Ashburn, 2003). Although we discuss only a few impairments here, other cognitive impairments are common poststroke. Please see Chapter 7 for more detailed information about cognition.

Unilateral spatial neglect is frequently present in people with stroke (Freeman, 2001). *Unilateral spatial neglect* is a cognitive deficit in which the person is impaired in his or her ability to attend, respond, or orient to stimuli presented unilaterally. Neglect has important implications for occupational therapy practice because of the functional implications of this phenomenon. Decreased attention to one side of extrapersonal space can severely compromise safety and independence with self-care (Nijboer, van de Port, Schepers, Post, & Visser-Meily, 2013). Omitting words on one side of the page when reading can lead to poor comprehension of written materials, and the distorted perception of the world resulting from neglect can contribute to general confusion in daily life (Freeman, 2001). Neglect is a very difficult concept for families to understand because their affected family members can see; it is their brain that cannot allow them to attend to part of their visual field.

Neglect has important implications for occupational therapy practice because of the functional implications of this phenomenon.

Executive dysfunction has important implications for everyday life because affected people appear disorganized while performing complex tasks, may not initiate new activities, and may have difficulties with problem solving, impulse control, and appropriate task shifting (Burgess, 2000; Hanna-Pladdy, 2007). People with executive dysfunction poststroke commonly experience significant self-awareness deficits, which have been shown to be a serious obstacle to successful rehabilitation (Hartman-Maeir, Soroker, Oman, & Katz, 2003; Hartman-Maeir, Soroker, Ring, & Katz, 2002). Patients with stroke who lack awareness of their impairments and disabilities may not be motivated to learn and find it difficult to use compensatory techniques because they do not think they need them (Toglia & Kirk, 2000).

Psychological Factors

Major depression is a common occurrence after a stroke (Paul, Dewey, Sturm, Macdonell, & Thrift, 2006). According to Whyte and Mulsant (2002), the prevalence of depression varies on the basis of time since the injury, with peak prevalence generally reported at 3 to 6 months poststroke. However, a 2006 study by Paul et al. revealed that 45% of stroke survivors were still depressed 5 years poststroke. Such a finding suggests that depression is a chronic issue faced by people with stroke that endures well beyond discharge from rehabilitation and must be assessed and treated as a part of stroke rehabilitation services.

A related psychological issue faced by people with stroke is apathy and altered self-concept. A person with **apathy** may appear listless, passive, unmotivated, and lacking in spontaneity and initiative (Marin, Fogel, Hawkins, Duffy, & Krupp, 1995). After stroke, many people experience a change in self-concept (Ellis-Hill & Horn, 2000). Ellis-Hill and Horn examined the past and present self-concept of 26 people with a first-time stroke who had returned home from the hospital as many as 2 years previously. In their study, people with stroke largely described themselves in more negative terms than they had before their stroke. In particular, they described themselves as being less interested, capable, and independent than before their stroke and as less in control, satisfied, and active; however, respondents still saw themselves as friendly, calm, caring, hopeful, and talkative (Ellis-Hill & Horn, 2000). These changes in self-concept suggest that clinicians need to be aware of the meaning of the stroke in the past, present, and future life of each individual they treat.

Emotional lability is another distressing complication in stroke. ***Emotional lability*** is a condition in which exaggerated and rapid swings of **emotion** occur that can result in outbursts of tears, laughter, and even **anger** (Stroke Association,

2011). Approximately 1 in every 4 people experiences this condition in the first 6 months after a stroke (Stroke Association, 2011). Anger and frustration often emerge as patients realize that they cannot perform activities that they used to be able to perform before the stroke (Santos, Caeiro, Ferro, Albuquerque, & Luísa Figueira, 2006). In a 2006 study, Santos et al. evaluated anger in 202 patients after acute stroke and found anger present in 71 (35%), of whom 26 were classified as severely angry. In a similar study, Kim, Choi, Kwon, and Seo (2002) demonstrated that anger and aggression were still present in 32% of patients at 3 to 12 months poststroke and that anger was strongly related to motor dysfunction, **dysarthria,** and lesions affecting the frontal lenticulocapsular-pontine base areas.

Physiological Factors

Given the high rate of stroke, it is important for health professionals to direct interventions toward reducing patients' risk of future stroke. Many of the cardiovascular risk factors associated with stroke require changes in health behaviors, such as choosing a healthier diet, losing weight, beginning an exercise program, stopping smoking, or adhering to a medication regimen (Michael & Shaughnessy, 2006). Behavior change is closely associated with changing beliefs, which is essential to the adoption and maintenance of self-care and exercise after stroke (Michael & Shaughnessy, 2006; Robinson-Smith & Pizzi, 2003). After stroke, regular exercise can facilitate motor recovery and can also help control the common comorbidities that influence recurrent stroke risk by reducing **hypertension,** enhancing glucose regulation, improving blood lipid profiles, and reducing body fat (Michael & Shaughnessy, 2006).

The role of exercise is especially significant because reduced cardiorespiratory fitness is a well-documented physical impairment in patients with chronic stroke (Kelly, Kilbreath, Davis, Zeman, & Raymond, 2003; Macko et al., 2005). During maximal-effort exercise, patients within 30 days poststroke exhibited peak oxygen uptake that was less than 50% of that obtained by a healthy, age-matched population (Kelly et al., 2003). Submaximal exercise also required increased energy expenditure in those with stroke (Kelly et al., 2003).

Assessment of physiological factors is critical for effective self-management of stroke risk factors. Blood pressure should be evaluated by clinicians on a routine basis to determine clients' cardiovascular status and candidacy for physical exertion. Regarding visceral adiposity, the **body mass index** is a simple calculation for evaluating a person's level of body fat (Kitahara et al., 2014). Finally, clients' cardiorespiratory fitness can be evaluated regularly using heart rate assessments during rest and physical activity (Kelly et al., 2003).

Motor Factors

Recovery of motor function is an important component of the rehabilitation process for survivors of stroke. Patients with stroke experience several primary neurological impairments that affect their movement. These primary impairments include hemiparesis and **hemiplegia,** tonal abnormalities, and deficits in coordination of movement (Ada, O'Dwyer, & O'Neill, 2006). Jørgensen, Nakayama, Raaschou, and Olsen (1995) found that a patient with mild leg paresis on admission was 4 times as likely to show motor recovery as a patient with initial leg paralysis. Approximately

65% of all hospitalized individuals with stroke who have motor deficits at the time of stroke will show some degree of motor recovery (Hendricks, van Limbeek, Geurts, & Zwarts, 2002).

In addition to hemiparesis, people with stroke often experience tonal abnormalities after their injury. **Hypotonicity,** defined as a reduction in passive muscle resistance, occurs early on in stroke and is how the body reacts immediately after loss of corticospinal input. **Hypertonicity,** or increased muscle **tone,** often develops after the initial hypotonicity resolves, frequently in the form of **spasticity** (Watkins et al., 2002).

Patients with stroke also frequently have difficulty with coordination or organization of movement (Ma & Trombly, 2002). Such deficits can take the form of **ataxia,** which is a disorder of coordination. Patients may also have significant problems with tasks as basic as putting on a jacket or shirt. Ataxia is a condition that is difficult for families to grasp, and they therefore need to learn strategies to help their loved one manage its consequences.

Stroke survivors also experience many secondary problems as a consequence of the primary neurological impairments. Because primary impairments take time to resolve, secondary impairments arise as adaptations to the primary deficits (Ada et al., 2006). More specifically, these secondary problems are believed to relate to the immobility that often follows patients' primary impairments (Ada et al., 2006). Secondary problems include disuse atrophy, decreased **active range of motion, contracture, subluxation,** and cardiac deconditioning (Ada et al., 2006).

Sensory Factors

Somatosensory deficits are another frequent outcome of stroke. According to an epidemiologic survey by Sterzi et al. (1993), **somatic sensation** is impaired in 37% of patients with a lesion to the right hemisphere and in 25% of patients with a lesion to the left hemisphere. In addition, a 1996 study by Kim and Choi-Kwon found that 22 of 25 patients initially diagnosed as having pure motor stroke actually had dysfunctional discriminative sensation when evaluated with a comprehensive sensory battery.

Visual dysfunction is another common sensory impairment poststroke. Vision is arguably the most complex sensory function, and this complexity is reflected by the sophisticated neural systems controlling visual processing (Edmans & Hume, 2010). Visual dysfunction has been found in 30% to 85% of the stroke population (Lotery et al., 2000). The most common sensory-related visual impairment poststroke is deficits in the **visual field** (portion of space seen while fixating centrally), estimated to occur in 20% to 57% of the stroke population (Pollock et al., 2011). Visual field deficits (VFDs) are commonly categorized as *hemianopsia* (loss of half of the visual field) and *quadrantanopsia* (loss of the upper or lower quadrant of the visual field; Khan, Leung, & Jay, 2008). People with VFDs have particular difficulties with reading and scanning scenes fast enough to process things as a whole (Pollock et al., 2011). VFDs can have far-reaching repercussions on people's occupational performance.

Although not as prevalent as vision deficits, stroke can affect **olfaction** and gustation. Chronic smell and taste dysfunction resulting from stroke are rare but have been reported after lesions affecting the anterior, posterior, or **middle cerebral arteries** (Heckmann, Heckmann, Lang, & Hummel, 2003; Moo & Wityk,

> Vision is arguably the most complex sensory function, and this complexity is reflected by the sophisticated neural systems controlling visual processing.

1999). Dysfunctions of smell and taste have been categorized as *hyposmia* (diminished sense of smell), *anosmia* (complete loss of smell), and *dysgeusia* (distorted taste; Etoh, Kawahira, Ogata, Shimodozono, & Tanaka, 2008).

Pain is another frequent sensory complication of stroke, with three varieties reported in the literature: (1) central poststroke pain, (2) nociceptive pain mainly in the shoulder and arm, and (3) tension-type headache (Jespersen, Jorgensen, Nakayama, & Olsen, 1995). These three pain conditions have been found to occur in people as many as 2 years poststroke, suggesting that pain is often experienced on a long-term basis (Widar, Samuelsson, Karlsson-Tivenius, & Ahlström, 2002). Studies have reported that chronic pain interferes with many aspects of living, with pain-related problems including disturbed sleep, fatigue, **mood** changes, stress in relationships, and preoccupation with the meaning of pain (Widar, Ek, & Ahlström, 2004; Widar et al., 2002). Deficits in the sensory control of balance are also seen after stroke. According to Bonan et al. (2004), balance control requires the integration of many types of sensory information. Yet, the literature has suggested that motor control theories in rehabilitating balance are overemphasized at the expense of properly acknowledging sensory contributions (Bonan et al., 2004).

Spiritual Factors

A major life event such as a stroke typically leads to a profound change in people's relationship to themselves and to the world around them. This event can and will likely trigger existential questioning (relating to spirituality) as people attempt to modify and re-create their poststroke world (Chow & Nelson-Becker, 2010). As a result of this existential search for meaning, people's spirituality will most likely be affected in one of two ways. The first possibility is that the foundation on which the spirit was built was so greatly affected that one's former spirituality is replaced by doubt and disconnection (Morgenstern et al., 2011). The other possibility is that one's spirituality is fortified. Some literature has supported the notion that strengthened spirituality is more common than a decreased spiritual connection poststroke (Kaye & Raghavan, 2002).

Often, spirituality becomes a valuable **coping** strategy for people poststroke (Kaufman, 1988). Spirituality has been found to help people restore meaning and purpose poststroke, as well as establish new life goals (Johnston et al., 2007). Kalra (2007) found that religious beliefs do not reduce stress and misfortune; however, those who are religious deal with life stressors and misfortunes more effectively (Kalra, 2007). In fact, coping via spirituality has been shown to add a unique effect to the prediction of positive adjustment for people with disabilities after controlling for the effects of other coping strategies (Johnston, Morrison, Macwalter, & Partridge, 1999).

Empirical exploration of spirituality's relationship with health has been limited (Powell, Shahabi, & Thoresen, 2003), although the majority of research has indicated that increased religiosity or spirituality is associated with better health (Crisp, 2009). Specifically, spirituality has been linked to better mental health, better physical health, lower use of health services, and lower mortality (Larson & Larson, 2003). In the stroke population, regular attendance at religious services is associated with better overall physical functioning (Morgenstern et al., 2011).

In addition to being connected to health, spirituality has been linked to other favorable outcomes. An overarching theme appears to be spirituality's association with positive thoughts and behaviors. In addition to positive thought as a coping mechanism, positive thought stemming from spirituality is reported to empower people poststroke to minimize stroke-induced dependency on others, thus transcending the helpless role (Kaye & Raghavan, 2002). Some studies have found spirituality to be a protective factor against **poststroke depression** and general emotional distress (Greenstreet, 2006). Because depression and distress are negatively correlated with stroke outcomes, Haley, Koenig, and Bruchett (2001) surmised that spirituality indirectly promotes recovery of **activities of daily living** (ADL) and **instrumental activities of daily living** (IADL) abilities. Understanding the role of spirituality in stroke recovery is important for promoting well-being and optimizing patient care (Arnaert, Filteau, & Sourial, 2006).

Environment or Extrinsic Factors

The intrinsic factors of stroke can have a pronounced effect on occupational performance and participation levels. Although such component skills contribute to functional outcomes and stroke recovery, it is important that these factors not be overemphasized to the point that ways in which environmental contexts mediate performance are overlooked. The environment is a multifaceted construct and can consist of physical, social, and cultural settings in which people live and conduct their lives (World Health Organization [WHO], 2001). Environmental factors exist outside of the individual and interact with aspects of the person to influence everyday functioning (WHO, 2001). Figure 2.3 introduces the extrinsic or environment factors of the PEOP model.

The occupational therapy literature has acknowledged the importance of the environment for occupational performance and for therapy (Baum & Christiansen, 2005; Law et al., 1996; Nelson, 1988). Occupational therapists understand that environments supporting clients' ability to use their skills can optimize their capabilities. At times, it is easier to modify an environment than to change intrinsic factors. Kielhofner and Forsyth (2002) also recognized the significance of the environment, arguing that occupational therapy consists primarily of using and creating conditions in the environment to support the client's occupational engagement.

In a study of people with stroke living in the community, Hammel, Jones, Gossett, and Morgan (2006) documented environmental and systems-level barriers to community participation. In their study, barriers were extensive and ranged from physical access issues to societal attitudes and beliefs about disability. Similar findings are evident in studies examining people with stroke as they transition to and age in their homes

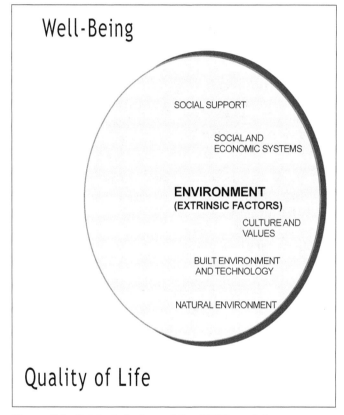

Figure 2.3. Extrinsic factors of the PEOP model.

Source. From "Person–Environment–Occupation–Performance: An Occupation-Based Framework for Practice," by C. M. Baum and C. H. Christiansen, in *Occupational Therapy: Performance, Participation, and Well-Being* (3rd ed., p. 246), by C. H. Christiansen, C. M. Baum, and J. D. Bass-Haugen (Eds.), 2005, Thorofare, NJ: Slack. Copyright © 2005 by Slack, Inc. Reprinted with permission.

**Occupational therapists
routinely provide
social support that
addresses the functional
or informational
dimensions; however,
. . . it is critical that the
occupational therapist
also help the client and
the family identify other
sources of social support.**

(Amarshi, Artero, & Reid, 2006). Amarshi et al.'s study portrayed participation as a dynamic process rather than a static event and pointed to the impact of environmental and societal barriers on participation choice and control. In the discussion that follows, we introduce major environmental factors. Each is central to a person's occupational performance, and it is essential that the occupational therapist address them as he or she enables the person with stroke and the person's family to plan for and support his or her reintegration into family, work, and community life.

Social Support

Social support has been shown to have a positive impact on people's health and well-being, as well as their ability to adjust to trauma or injury (Helgeson, 2003; McKenna & Lau, 2001). According to Friedland and McColl (1992), social support is "the experience or information that one is loved and cared for, valued and esteemed, and able to count on others should the need arise" (p. 574). In their definition, Friedland and McColl delineated three dimensions of social support: (1) a functional or informational dimension outlining different types of support; (2) a structural dimension, including all social network characteristics such as size and sources of support; and (3) an appraisal dimension, including the person's satisfaction and subjective appraisal of received support. Occupational therapists routinely provide social support that addresses the functional or informational dimensions; however, because the strength of a person's social network is known to be related to his or her need for poststroke institutionalization, it is critical that the occupational therapist also help the client and the family identify other sources of social support. In particular, the more securely the patient is embedded in a social network before the stroke, the less likely he or she is to have to live in an institution poststroke (Colantonio, Kasl, Ostfeld, & Berkman, 1993). Such results suggest that social support networks may have a buffering effect on a person's health and need for outside support and underlie the importance of issues such as social capital (Mendes de Leon, Glass, & Berkman, 2003).

Social Capital

Social capital is a term that occupational therapists are just beginning to use. It is important to grasp the concept and to help patients identify their social capital because it is a factor that has been linked to health and may be of particular significance for people as they age and for people with disabilities (Cannuscio, Block, & Kawachi, 2003). According to Putnam (1995), *social capital* refers to the "features of social organization such as networks, norms, and social trust that facilitate coordination and cooperation for mutual benefit" (p. 67).

There are a range of explanations for the positive influence that social capital can have on health. For example, recent studies of the general population have shown that social capital can boost self-esteem, provide social support, help people to access better resources, and buffer against stressful life events and chronic illness (Ahern & Hendryx, 2005; Woolcock & Narayan, 2000). Additionally, other studies have shown that high social capital is associated with lower mortality and fewer accidents and suicides (Dominkus, Grisold, & Jelinek, 1990; Kaplan, Pamuk, Lynch, Cohen, & Balfour, 1996; Kawachi, Kennedy, Lochner, & Prothrow-Stith, 1997).

Clearly, such literature has depicted the importance of social capital and its widespread effects on the overall health of the population and its particular importance for people with stroke who want to reengage in their communities, particularly if they want to return to work.

Culture

Culture is an important issue in contemporary health care and is very important for occupational therapists to understand and incorporate in their interactions with clients and their families. *Culture* is broadly defined as a shared system of values, beliefs, and learned patterns of behaviors (Low, 1984). Occupational therapists and all health care providers face the challenge of caring for people from many cultures who have different languages, levels of acculturation to the dominant U.S. culture, and socioeconomic status and unique ways of understanding illness and health care (Odawara, 2005). Satisfaction and compliance with medical and rehabilitation recommendations are closely related to the effectiveness of communication and the patient–provider relationship (Novack, 1995). Because sociocultural differences between provider and patient can lead to communication and relationship barriers, understanding the concepts inherent to overcoming these challenges is extremely important.

As with many health conditions, the occurrence and management of stroke are clearly influenced by cultural factors. Much literature has documented the ethnic disparities in the epidemiology of stroke in the United States (Cruz-Flores et al., 2011; Stansbury, Jia, Williams, Vogel, & Duncan, 2005). African Americans are disproportionately affected by stroke, with literature demonstrating that African Americans have more residual impairment and greater mortality than White Americans (Cruz-Flores et al., 2011; Stansbury et al., 2005). It is also clear that African Americans tend to have strokes at an earlier age than White Americans (Stansbury et al., 2005).

In addition to disparities in stroke incidence and prevalence, there are also disparities in care. A study by Bhandari, Kushel, Price, and Schillinger (2005) examined outcomes of inpatient stroke rehabilitation across different racial groups. The study found that African Americans achieved less functional improvement at discharge than White Americans and, despite worse **FIM™** scores, were more likely to be discharged to the home environment. Interestingly, Asian American patients did not differ from White patients in terms of functional improvement at discharge but were found to have less improvement at 3-month follow-up (Bhandari et al., 2005).

Cultural issues are undeniably present in stroke care and affect the patient's approach to treatment. A patient enters a therapy setting with certain beliefs, concerns, and expectations about his or her illness and the medical encounter. This conceptualization of the illness experience can be described as the patient's explanatory model (Eisenberg, 1977). The *explanatory model* refers to the patient's understanding of the cause, severity, and prognosis of an illness, as well as his or her expectations for treatment (Eisenberg, 1977). In essence, the explanatory model represents the meaning of the illness to the patient, and it is to a large extent culturally determined (Eisenberg, 1977). Occupational therapists must consider the client's explanatory model to achieve a client-centered approach to goal setting and intervention.

Points to Ponder: Therapy Adaptations

What are some examples of ways you might adapt your therapy session to be more culturally appropriate?

Physical Environment

Several studies have examined the physical environment and its impact on the everyday lives of people with stroke (Hammel et al., 2006). Hammel et al. examined barriers to community participation poststroke. The most frequent barriers to community participation identified were physical and cognitive access to community sites. Physical access issues included inaccessible entryways, bathrooms, and transportation systems, with key barriers including door thresholds and lack of handrails (Hammel et al., 2006). Regarding cognitive access, participants described a lack of environmental aids and supports for **orientation,** navigation, memory, and problem solving (Hammel et al., 2006). Many environments did not offer adequate signage to enable effective use of the setting, and many others failed to provide directions on how to seek assistance if needed. In environments that did provide signage, the signage and directions were often too cognitively and perceptually complex to decipher (Hammel et al., 2006). The occupational therapist must work with the person, the family, and the community to address these barriers. On an individual level, removing barriers may seem impossible, but progress in the removal of barriers on a community level will help all people with disabilities. It is important, however, to know how to help the person with stroke anticipate and overcome barriers that will limit the activities and roles that are important to him or her.

Hammel et al. (2006) reported that some environments have built-in features that promote safety and access for people with stroke (i.e., environmental supports). For example, some environments (corridors and entryways) have grab bars on both sides, entryways with doors that accommodate walkers and canes as well as wheelchairs, built-in visual maps that are easy to use, picture signage, and information resources and instructions (Hammel et al., 2006). In addition to physical supports in the environment, Hammel et al. also described systems-level supports for community participation. For example, transportation policies on national and local levels that provide accessible transport options can support the participation of people with stroke. However, many people are not aware of these options or how to strategize their use depending on the purpose for using them. The occupational therapist can help the person with stroke develop and strategize how to use such supports.

Technology

Assistive technology is conceptually different from other environmental elements because it is intimate to the person (Sanford, 2012). People commonly think of the environment as structures (physical, social, institutional) that exist within a context (e.g., ramps at a building entrance, social support, policies that shape access to service). Assistive technology comes with the person to a situation, affecting how the person performs occupations within the environment.

Assistive technology initially serves as an intervention, as something that enables occupational performance through augmentation or replacement of physical, sensory, or cognitive abilities. On a physical level, assistive technology can enhance or replace the client's strength, endurance, balance, coordination, or **range of motion** (e.g., a mobility or positioning or transfer device, a device to control objects remotely within the environment). At the sensory level, assistive technology can enhance information from the environment and convert it into a form the client is able to use (increased light, spices to enhance taste, thermometer

> On an individual level, removing barriers may seem impossible, but progress in the removal of barriers on a community level will help all people with disabilities.

to be safe with temperature, glasses to enhance vision). Cognitive technologies support numerous cognitive functions such as memory, task sequencing, organization, and attention (complex systems that allow a client to perform occupations or that monitor and cue the client to perform them (Bardram, Mihalidis, & Wan, 2007). Assistive technology becomes one with the person to expand his or her personal environment to be able to do what the person wants and needs to do.

Summary

The PEOP model states that occupational performance is not just the result of person factors but rather is a consequence of an interaction among person, environment, and occupation (Baum & Christiansen, 2005). The PEOP makes explicit the unique contributions of occupational therapists to the management of people with stroke. Occupational therapists' unique contribution to health care is occupational performance. Occupational performance complements the physical therapist's focus on movement and the speech–language pathologist's focus on communication to contribute to a collaborative approach to the rehabilitation of people who have experienced a stroke. Figure 2.1 depicts how all of these factors together support the occupational therapist's unique approach to care. We hope you will find this model helpful in organizing your knowledge to help those with stroke live their lives to the fullest.

> **Occupational performance is not just the result of person factors but rather is a consequence of an interaction among person, environment, and occupation.**

Acknowledgments

Each year our students develop a practice model in partial fulfillment of their OTD. The following students' work contributed to the development of this chapter, and we would like to acknowledge their contributions: Erin Henshaw, OTD 2010; Colleen Fowler, OTD 2012; and Rachel Kravitt, OTD 2012.

References

Ada, L., O'Dwyer, N., & O'Neill, E. (2006). Relation between spasticity, weakness and contracture of the elbow flexors and upper limb activity after stroke: An observational study. *Disability and Rehabilitation, 28,* 891–897. http://dx.doi.org/10.1080/09638280500535165

Ahern, M. M., & Hendryx, M. S. (2005). Social capital and risk for chronic illnesses. *Chronic Illness, 1,* 183–190. http://dx.doi.org/10.1177/17423953050010030201

Ahlström, S., & Bernspång, B. (2003). Occupational performance of persons who have suffered a stroke: A follow-up study. *Scandinavian Journal of Occupational Therapy, 10,* 88–94. http://dx.doi.org/10.1080/11038120310009443

Alladi, S., Meena, A. K., & Kaul, S. (2002). Cognitive rehabilitation in stroke: Therapy and techniques. *Neurology India, 50*(Suppl.), S102–S108.

Amarshi, F., Artero, L., & Reid, D. (2006). Exploring social and leisure participation among stroke survivors: Part two. *International Journal of Therapy and Rehabilitation, 13,* 199–208. http://dx.doi.org/10.12968/ijtr.2006.13.5.21376

Arnaert, A., Filteau, N., & Sourial, R. (2006). Stroke patients in the acute care phase: Role of hope in self-healing. *Holistic Nursing Practice, 20,* 137–146. http://dx.doi.org/10.1097/00004650-200605000-00008

Bandura, A. (1997). *Self-efficacy: The exercise of control.* New York: Freeman.

Bardram, J., Mihalidis, A., & Wan, D. (2007). *Pervasive computing in healthcare.* London: CRC Press.

Baum, C. M., & Christiansen, C. H. (2005). Person–Environment–Occupation–Performance: An occupation-based framework for practice. In C. H. Christiansen, C. M. Baum, & J. Bass-Haugen (Eds.), *Occupational therapy: Performance, participation, and well-being* (3rd ed., pp. 242–267). Thorofare, NJ: Slack.

Bhandari, V. K., Kushel, M., Price, L., & Schillinger, D. (2005). Racial disparities in outcomes of inpatient stroke rehabilitation. *Archives of Physical Medicine and Rehabilitation, 86,* 2081–2086. http://dx.doi.org/10.1016/j.apmr.2005.05.008

Bonan, I. V., Yelnik, A. P., Colle, F. M., Michaud, C., Normand, E., Panigot, B., . . . Vicaut, E. (2004). Reliance on visual information after stroke. Part II: Effectiveness of a balance rehabilitation program with visual cue deprivation after stroke: A randomized controlled trial. *Archives of Physical Medicine and Rehabilitation, 85,* 274–278. http://dx.doi.org/10.1016/j.apmr.2003.06.016

Burgess, P. W. (2000). Strategy application disorder: The role of the frontal lobes in human multitasking. *Psychological Research, 63,* 279–288. http://dx.doi.org/10.1007/s004269900006

Cannuscio, C., Block, J., & Kawachi, I. (2003). Social capital and successful aging: The role of senior housing. *Annals of Internal Medicine, 139,* 395–399. http://dx.doi.org/10.7326/0003-4819-139-5_Part_2-200309021-00003

Cardol, M., de Jong, B. A., van den Bos, G. A., Beelem, A., de Groot, I. J., & de Haan, R. J. (2002). Beyond disability: Perceived participation in people with a chronic disabling condition. *Clinical Rehabilitation, 16,* 27–35. http://dx.doi.org/10.1191/0269215502cr464oa

Chow, E. O. W., & Nelson-Becker, H. (2010). Spiritual distress to spiritual transformation: Stroke survivor narratives from Hong Kong. *Journal of Aging Studies, 24,* 313–324. http://dx.doi.org/10.1016/j.jaging.2010.06.001

Christiansen, C., Clark, F., Kielhofner, G., & Rogers, J. (1995). Position Paper: Occupation. American Occupational Therapy Association. *American Journal of Occupational Therapy, 49,* 935. http://dx.doi.org/10.5014/ajot.49.9.935b

Clarke, P., & Black, S. E. (2005). Quality of life following stroke: Negotiating disability, identity, and resources. *Journal of Applied Gerontology, 24,* 319–336. http://dx.doi.org/10.1177/0733464805277976

Colantonio, A., Kasl, S. V., Ostfeld, A. M., & Berkman, L. F. (1993). Psychosocial predictors of stroke outcomes in an elderly population. *Journal of Gerontology, 48,* S261–S268. http://dx.doi.org/10.1093/geronj/48.5.S261

Crisp, B. (2009). Finding God in illness. *Way, 48,* 41–52.

Cruz-Flores, S., Rabinstein, A., Biller, J., Elkind, M., Griffith, P., Gorelick, P., . . . Valderrama, A. (2011). Racial–ethnic disparities in stroke care: The American experience. *Stroke, 42,* 2091–2116.

Desrosiers, J., Rochette, A., Noreau, L., Bourbonnais, D., Bravo, G., & Bourget, A. (2006). Long-term changes in participation after stroke. *Topics in Stroke Rehabilitation, 13,* 86–96. http://dx.doi.org/10.1310/tsr1304-86

Dominkus, M., Grisold, W., & Jelinek, V. (1990). Transcranial electrical motor evoked potentials as a prognostic indicator for motor recovery in stroke patients. *Journal of Neurology, Neurosurgery, and Psychiatry, 53,* 745–748. http://dx.doi.org/10.1136/jnnp.53.9.745

Edmans, J., & Hume, C. (2010). *Occupational therapy and stroke.* New York: Wiley.

Edwards, D. F., Hahn, M., Baum, C., & Dromerick, A. W. (2006). The impact of mild stroke on meaningful activity and life satisfaction. *Journal of Stroke and Cerebrovascular Diseases, 15,* 151–157. http://dx.doi.org/10.1016/j.jstrokecerebrovasdis.2006.04.001

Eisenberg, L. (1977). Disease and illness: Distinctions between professional and popular ideas of sickness. *Culture, Medicine and Psychiatry, 1,* 9–23. http://dx.doi.org/10.1007/BF00114808

Ellis-Hill, C. S., & Horn, S. (2000). Change in identity and self-concept: A new theoretical approach to recovery following a stroke. *Clinical Rehabilitation, 14,* 279–287. http://dx.doi.org/10.1191/026921500671231410

Eriksson, G., Kottorp, A., Borg, J., & Tham, K. (2009). Relationship between occupational gaps in everyday life, depressive mood and life satisfaction after acquired brain injury. *Journal of Rehabilitation Medicine, 41,* 187–194. http://dx.doi.org/10.2340/16501977-0307

Etoh, S., Kawahira, K., Ogata, A., Shimodozono, M., & Tanaka, N. (2008). Relationship between dysgeusia and dysesthesia in stroke patients. *International Journal of Neuroscience, 118,* 137–147. http://dx.doi.org/10.1080/00207450601044686

Freeman, E. (2001). Unilateral spatial neglect: New treatment approaches with potential application to occupational therapy. *American Journal of Occupational Therapy, 55,* 401–408. http://dx.doi.org/10.5014/ajot.55.4.401

Friedland, J. F., & McColl, M. (1992). Social support intervention after stroke: Results of a randomized trial. *Archives of Physical Medicine and Rehabilitation, 73,* 573–581.

Greenstreet, W. (2006). From spirituality to coping strategy: Making sense of chronic illness. *British Journal of Nursing, 15,* 938–942. http://dx.doi.org/10.12968/bjon.2006.15.17.21909

Haley, K. C., Koenig, H. G., & Bruchett, B. M. (2001). Relationship between private religious activity and physical functioning in older adults. *Journal of Religion and Health, 40,* 305–312. http://dx.doi.org/10.1023/A:1012561909054

Hammel, J., Jones, R., Gossett, A., & Morgan, E. (2006). Examining barriers and supports to community living and participation after a stroke from a participatory action research approach. *Topics in Stroke Rehabilitation, 13,* 43–58. http://dx.doi.org/10.1310/5X2G-V1Y1-TBK7-Q27E

Hanna-Pladdy, B. (2007). Dysexecutive syndromes in neurologic disease. *Journal of Neurologic Physical Therapy, 31,* 119–127.

Hartman-Maeir, A., Soroker, N., Oman, S. D., & Katz, N. (2003). Awareness of disabilities in stroke rehabilitation—A clinical trial. *Disability and Rehabilitation, 25,* 35–44. http://dx.doi.org/10.1080/0963828021000007897

Hartman-Maeir, A., Soroker, N., Ring, H., & Katz, N. (2002). Awareness of deficits in stroke rehabilitation. *Journal of Rehabilitation Medicine, 34,* 158–164. http://dx.doi.org/10.1080/16501970213236

Heckmann, J. G., Heckmann, S. M., Lang, C. J., & Hummel, T. (2003). Neurological aspects of taste disorders. *Archives of Neurology, 60,* 667–671. http://dx.do.org/10.1001/archneur.60.5.667

Helgeson, V. S. (2003). Social support and quality of life. *Quality of Life Research, 12*(Suppl. 1), 25–31. http://dx.doi.org/10.1023/A:1023509117524

Hendricks, H. T., van Limbeek, J., Geurts, A. C., & Zwarts, M. J. (2002). Motor recovery after stroke: A systematic review of the literature. *Archives of Physical Medicine and Rehabilitation, 83,* 1629–1637. http://dx.doi.org/10.1053/apmr.2002.35473

Hyndman, D., & Ashburn, A. (2003). People with stroke living in the community: Attention deficits, balance, ADL ability and falls. *Disability and Rehabilitation, 25,* 817–822. http://dx.doi.org/10.1080/0963828031000122221

Jespersen, H. F., Jorgensen, H. S., Nakayama, H., & Olsen, T. S. (1995). Shoulder pain after a stroke. *International Journal of Rehabilitation Research, 18,* 273–276. http://dx.doi.org/10.1097/00004356-199509000-00010

Johnston, M., Bonetti, D., Joice, S., Pollard, B., Morrison, V., Francis, J. J., & Macwalter, R. (2007). Recovery from disability after stroke as a target for a behavioural intervention: Results of a randomized controlled trial. *Disability and Rehabilitation, 29,* 1117–1127. http://dx.doi.org/10.1080/03323310600950411

Johnston, M., Morrison, V., Macwalter, R., & Partridge, C. (1999). Perceived control, coping and recovery from disability following stroke. *Psychology and Health, 14,* 181–192. http://dx.doi.org/10.1080/08870449908407322

Jørgensen, H. S., Nakayama, H., Raaschou, H. O., & Olsen, T. S. (1995). Recovery of walking function in stroke patients: The Copenhagen Stroke Study. *Archives of Physical Medicine and Rehabilitation, 76,* 27–32. http://dx.doi.org/10.1016/S0003-9993(95)80038-7

Kalra, L. (2007). Faith under the microscope. *Stroke, 38,* 848–849. http://dx.doi.org/10.1161/01.STR.0000257979.08702.b6

Kaplan, G. A., Pamuk, E. R., Lynch, J. W., Cohen, R. D., & Balfour, J. L. (1996). Inequality in income and mortality in the United States: Analysis of mortality and potential pathways. *British Medical Journal, 312,* 999–1003. http://dx.doi.org/10.1136/bmj.312.7037.999

Katz, N., & Maeir, A. (2011). Higher-level cognitive functions enabling participation: Awareness and executive functions. In N. Katz (Ed.), *Cognition, occupation, and participation across the life span: Neuroscience, neurorehabilitation, and models of intervention in occupational therapy* (3rd ed., pp. 13–40). Bethesda, MD: AOTA Press.

Kaufman, S. R. (1988). Toward a phenomenology of boundaries in medicine: Chronic illness experience in the case of stroke. *Medical Anthropology Quarterly, 2,* 338–354. http://dx.doi.org/10.1525/maq.1988.2.4.02a00040

Kawachi, I., Kennedy, B. P., Lochner, K., & Prothrow-Stith, D. (1997). Social capital, income inequality, and mortality. *American Journal of Public Health, 87,* 1491–1498. http://dx.doi.org/10.2105/AJPH.87.9.1491

Kaye, J., & Raghavan, S. K. (2002). Spirituality in disability and illness. *Journal of Religion and Health, 41,* 231–242. http://dx.doi.org/10.1023/A:1020284819593

Kelly, J. O., Kilbreath, S. L., Davis, G. M., Zeman, B., & Raymond, J. (2003). Cardiorespiratory fitness and walking ability in subacute stroke patients. *Archives of Physical Medicine and Rehabilitation, 84,* 1780–1785. http://dx.doi.org/10.1016/S0003-9993(03)00376-9

Khan, S., Leung, E., & Jay, W. M. (2008). Stroke and visual rehabilitation. *Topics in Stroke Rehabilitation, 15,* 27–36. http://dx.doi.org/10.1310/tsr1501-27

Kielhofner, G., & Forsyth, K. (2002). The process of change in therapy. In G. Kielhofner (Ed.), *A Model of Human Occupation: Theory and application.* Baltimore: Williams & Wilkins.

Kim, J. S., Choi, S., Kwon, S. U., & Seo, Y. S. (2002). Inability to control anger or aggression after stroke. *Neurology, 58,* 1106–1108. http://dx.doi.org/10.1212/WNL.58.7.1106

Kim, J. S., & Choi-Kwon, S. (1996). Discriminative sensory dysfunction after unilateral stroke. *Stroke, 27,* 677–682. http://dx.doi.org/10.1161/01.STR.27.4.677

Kitahara, C. M., Flint, A. J., Berrington de Gonzalez, A., Bernstein, L., Brotzman, M., MacInnis, R. J., . . . Hartge, P. (2014). Association between class III obesity (BMI of 40–59 kg/m^2) and mortality: A pooled analysis of 20 prospective studies. *PLOS Medicine, 11,* e1001673. http://dx.doi.org/10.1371/journal.pmed.1001673

Larson, D. B., & Larson, S. S. (2003). Spirituality's potential relevance to physical and emotional health: A brief review of quantitative research. *Journal of Psychology and Theology, 31,* 37–51.

Law, M., Cooper, B., Strong, S., Stewart, D., Rigby, P., & Letts, L. (1996). The Person–Environment–Occupation model: A transactive approach to occupational performance. *Canadian Journal of Occupational Therapy, 63,* 9–23. http://dx.doi.org/10.1177/000841749606300103

Lotery, A. J., Wiggam, M. I., Jackson, A. J., Refson, K., Fullerton, K. J., Gilmore, D. H., & Beringer, T. R. (2000). Correctable visual impairment in stroke rehabilitation patients. *Age and Ageing, 29,* 221–222. http://dx.doi.org/10.1093/ageing/29.3.221

Low, S. M. (1984). The cultural basis of health, illness and disease. *Social Work in Health Care, 9,* 13–23. http://dx.doi.org/10.1300/J010v09n03_02

Ma, H.-I., & Trombly, C. A. (2002). A synthesis of the effects of occupational therapy for persons with stroke, Part II: Remediation of impairments. *American Journal of Occupational Therapy, 56,* 260–274. http://dx.doi.org/10.5014/ajot.56.3.260

Macko, R. F., Ivey, F. M., Forrester, L. W., Hanley, D., Sorkin, J. D., Katzel, L. I., . . . Goldberg, A. P. (2005). Treadmill exercise rehabilitation improves ambulatory function and cardiovascular fitness in patients with chronic stroke. *Stroke, 36,* 2206–2211.

Magnus, E. (2001). Everyday occupations and the process of redefinition: A study of how meaning in occupation influences redefinition of identity in women with a disability. *Scandinavian Journal of Occupational Therapy, 8,* 115–124. http://dx.doi.org/10.1080/110381201750464467

Marin, R. S., Fogel, B. S., Hawkins, J., Duffy, J., & Krupp, B. (1995). Apathy: A treatable syndrome. *Neurosciences, 7,* 23–30.

McKenna, K., & Lau, A. (2001). Conceptualizing quality of life for elderly people with stroke. *Disability and Rehabilitation, 23,* 227–238. http://dx.doi.org/10.1080/096382801750110838

Mendes de Leon, C. F., Glass, T. A., & Berkman, L. F. (2003). Social engagement and disability in a community population of older adults: The New Haven EPESE. *American Journal of Epidemiology, 157,* 633–642. http://dx.doi.org/10.1093/aje/kwg028

Michael, K. M., & Shaughnessy, M. (2006). Stroke prevention and management in older adults. *Journal of Cardiovascular Nursing, 21*(Suppl. 1), S21–S26. http://dx.doi.org/10.1097/00005082-200609001-00006

Moo, L., & Wityk, R. J. (1999). Olfactory and taste dysfunction after bilateral middle cerebral artery stroke. *Journal of Stroke and Cerebrovascular Diseases, 8,* 353–354. http://dx.doi.org/10.1016/S1052-3057(99)80011-1

Morgenstern, L. B., Sánchez, B. N., Skolarus, L. E., Garcia, N., Risser, J. M., Wing, J. J., . . . Lisabeth, L. D. (2011). Fatalism, optimism, spirituality, depressive symptoms, and stroke outcome: A population-based analysis. *Stroke, 42,* 3518–3523. http://dx.doi.org/10.1161/STROKEAHA.111.625491

Nelson, D. L. (1988). Occupation: Form and performance. *American Journal of Occupational Therapy, 42,* 633–641. http://dx.doi.org/10.5014/ajot.42.10.633

Nijboer, T., van de Port, I., Schepers, V., Post, M., & Visser-Meily, A. (2013). Predicting functional outcome after stroke: The influence of neglect on basic activities in daily living. *Frontiers in Human Neuroscience, 7,* 182. http://dx.doi.org/10.3389/fnhum.2013.00182

Novack, D. H. (1995). *Therapeutic aspects of the clinical encounter: The medical interview* (pp. 32–49). New York: Springer.

Odawara, E. (2005). Cultural competency in occupational therapy: Beyond a cross-cultural view of practice. *American Journal of Occupational Therapy, 59,* 325–334.

Paul, S. L., Dewey, H. M., Sturm, J. W., Macdonell, R. A., & Thrift, A. G. (2006). Prevalence of depression and use of antidepressant medication at 5-years poststroke in the North East Melbourne Stroke Incidence Study. *Stroke, 37,* 2854–2855. http://dx.doi.org/10.1161/01. STR.0000244806.05099.52

Polatajko, H. J. (1992). Naming and framing occupational therapy: A lecture dedicated to the life of Nancy B. *Canadian Journal of Occupational Therapy, 59,* 189–200. http://dx.doi. org/10.1177/000841749205900403

Pollock, A., Hazelton, C., Henderson, C. A., Angilley, J., Dhillon, B., Langhorne, P., . . . Shahani, U. (2011). Interventions for visual field defects in patients with stroke. *Cochrane Database of Systematic Reviews, 2011,* CD008388. http://dx.doi.org/10.1002/14651858.CD008388.pub2

Pound, P., Gompertz, P., & Ebrahim, S. (1999). Social and practical strategies described by people living at home with stroke. *Health and Social Care in the Community, 7,* 120–128. http://dx.doi.org/10.1046/j.1365-2524.1999.00168.x

Powell, L. H., Shahabi, L., & Thoresen, C. E. (2003). Religion and spirituality: Linkages to physical health. *American Psychologist, 58,* 36–52. http://dx.doi.org/10.1037/ 0003-066X.58.1.36

Putnam, R. D. (1995). Bowling alone: America's declining social capital. *Journal of Democracy, 6,* 65–78. http://dx.doi.org/10.1353/jod.1995.0002

Robinson-Smith, G., & Pizzi, E. R. (2003). Maximizing stroke recovery using patient self-care self-efficacy. *Rehabilitation Nursing, 28,* 48–51. http://dx.doi. org/10.1002/j.2048-7940.2003.tb02028.x

Sachdev, P. S., Brodaty, H., Valenzuela, M. J., Lorentz, L., Looi, J. C. L., Wen, W., & Zagami, A. S. (2004). The neuropsychological profile of vascular cognitive impairment in stroke and TIA patients. *Neurology, 62,* 912–919. http://dx.doi.org/10.1212/01. WNL.0000115108.65264.4B

Sanford, J. A. (2012). *Universal design as a rehabilitation strategy.* New York: Springer.

Santos, C. O., Caeiro, L., Ferro, J. M., Albuquerque, R., & Luísa Figueira, M. (2006). Anger, hostility and aggression in the first days of acute stroke. *European Journal of Neurology, 13,* 351–358. http://dx.doi.org/10.1111/j.1468-1331.2006.01242.x

Stansbury, J. P., Jia, H., Williams, L. S., Vogel, W. B., & Duncan, P. W. (2005). Ethnic disparities in stroke: Epidemiology, acute care, and postacute outcomes. *Stroke, 36,* 374–386. http:// dx.doi.org/10.1161/01.STR.0000153065.39325.fd

Sterzi, R., Bottini, G., Celani, M. G., Righetti, E., Lamassa, M., Ricci, S., & Vallar, G. (1993). Hemianopia, hemianaesthesia, and hemiplegia after right and left hemisphere damage: A hemispheric difference. *Journal of Neurology, Neurosurgery, and Psychiatry, 56,* 308–310. http://dx.doi.org/10.1136/jnnp.56.3.308

Stroke Association. (2011). *Psychological effects of stroke.* Retrieved from http://www.stroke. org.uk

Toglia, J., & Kirk, U. (2000). Understanding awareness deficits following brain injury. *NeuroRehabilitation, 15,* 57–70.

Turpin, M., & Iwama, M. K. (2011). *Using occupational therapy models in practice: A fieldguide.* Edinburgh: Churchill Livingstone.

Watkins, C. L., Leathley, M. J., Gregson, J. M., Moore, A. P., Smith, T. L., & Sharma, A. K. (2002). Prevalence of spasticity post stroke. *Clinical Rehabilitation, 16,* 515–522. http:// dx.doi.org/10.1191/0269215502cr512oa

White, J. H., MacKenzie, L., Magin, P., & Pollack, M. R. P. (2008). The occupational experience of stroke survivors in a community setting. *OTJR: Occupation, Participation and Health, 28,* 160–167. http://dx.doi.org/10.3928/15394492-20080901-05

Whyte, E. M., & Mulsant, B. H. (2002). Post stroke depression: Epidemiology, pathophysiology, and biological treatment. *Biological Psychiatry, 52,* 253–264. http://dx.doi. org/10.1016/S0006-3223(02)01424-5

Widar, M., Ek, A.-C., & Ahlström, G. (2004). Coping with long-term pain after a stroke. *Journal of Pain and Symptom Management, 27,* 215–225. http://dx.doi.org/10.1016/j. jpainsymman.2003.07.006

Widar, M., Samuelsson, L., Karlsson-Tivenius, S., & Ahlström, G. (2002). Long-term pain conditions after a stroke. *Journal of Rehabilitation Medicine, 34,* 165–170. http://dx.doi. org/10.1080/16501970213237

Woolcock, M., & Narayan, D. (2000). Social capital: Implications for development theory, research, and policy. *World Bank Research Observer, 15,* 225–249. http://dx.doi.org/10.1093/wbro/15.2.225

World Health Organization. (2001). *International classification of functioning, disability and health.* Geneva: Author.

Yerxa, E. J. (1993). Occupational science: A new source of power for participants in occupational therapy. *Journal of Occupational Science, 1,* 3–9. http://dx.doi.org/10.1080/1442759 1.1993.9686373

CHAPTER 3

Neuroanatomy of Stroke

Fred Feuchter, PhD; Christina C. Lewis, PhD; and
Gordon Muir Giles, PhD, OTR/L, FAOTA

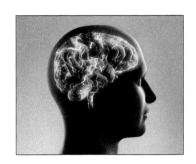

Learning Objectives

After completion of this chapter, readers will be able to

- Identify the components of the central nervous system;
- Recognize the basic components and organization of neurons and glia;
- Identify the basic structure of the cerebrum;
- Identify the basic subcomponents and organization of a neuron;
- Identify the way in which experiences and behavior patterns can affect the expression of genes;
- Identify the layered structure of typical isocortex;
- Identify the primary sensory and motor cortex and the unimodal and heteromodal association cortex;
- Recognize the organization and role of neural networks in brain functioning;
- Identify the brain areas and brain processes fundamental to language functions;
- Identify the brain areas and brain processes fundamental to attention;
- Identify the components and brain structures involved in vision;
- Identify the brain areas and brain processes fundamental to memory;
- Identify the frontal subcortical networks that are important for executive functions and behavioral control; and
- Delineate the organization and key features of the cerebral blood supply.

Key Words

- association cortex
- axon
- basal nuclei
- central nervous system
- cerebral cortex
- cerebrum
- dendrites
- glia
- gray matter
- isocortex
- neural networks
- nucleus
- white matter

Introduction

This chapter provides a review of the organization of the human **central nervous system** (CNS) and focuses specifically on the systems that, when damaged by **stroke**, result in behavior changes that are the focus of occupational therapy intervention.

Although the chapter describes brain regions, it focuses on the interrelated systems underlying the processes that may be affected in stroke. This and the other chapters in this publication and Self-Paced Clinical Course together form a basis for understanding the ways in which performance can break down in stroke and for interventions that may help clients redevelop or compensate for neurological deficits.

Overview of the Central Nervous System

The CNS consists of the brain and the spinal cord. The brain has several anatomical subdivisions including the **cerebrum, diencephalon** (which lies deep within the center of the brain, above the brainstem, but is not represented in the figure below), **brainstem,** and **cerebellum** (Figure 3.1). Each division exhibits a unique morphology and is associated with specific neural activities that are not replicated elsewhere in the CNS. For instance, the primary region that receives input from the retina about what a person sees is located in the far posterior of the cerebrum, and the area that directs automatic aversive movements when the eyes detect an object moving rapidly toward the head is located in the upper regions of the midbrain. Similarly, the area

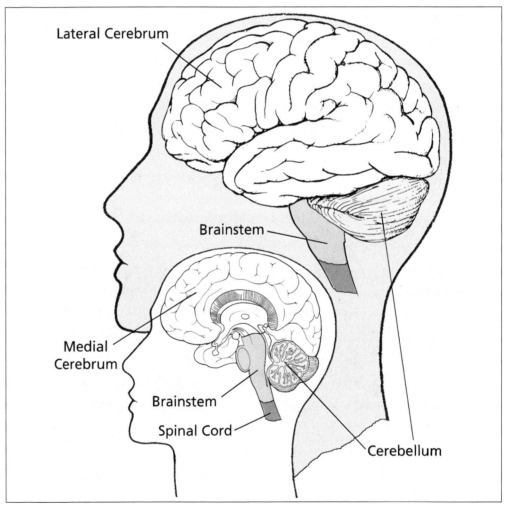

Figure 3.1. Anatomical subdivisions of the brain, including the lateral and medial cerebrum, brainstem, and cerebellum.

Source. F. Feuchter.

that receives pain information from the right big toe is on the inner surface of the left cerebral hemisphere, but the area responsible for creating new memories (say, from stubbing that toe) is buried deep within the hemisphere in the medial temporal lobe.

It is perfectly reasonable to expect that damage to a specific region of the CNS will result in loss of the neurological functions associated with the damaged region. Complex neurological tasks, however, such as the execution of purposeful movements, analysis of competing sensory inputs, and performance of cognitive processes, involve both simultaneous and sequential processing in multiple areas of the CNS. Although specific functions can be localized to specific regions of the CNS, most neurological processing takes place across **neural networks** of interconnected sites in the CNS, each of which processes specific information related to the specific neurological task. Each region may play a role in multiple functions and participate in many separate and distinct networks. Therefore, specific types of neurological dysfunction may be related either to damage to specific CNS sites or to disruptions of the interconnections among those sites.

Specific types of neurological dysfunction may be related either to damage to specific CNS sites or to disruptions of the interconnections among those sites.

Neurons

Nervous tissue consists of **neurons** and their supporting cells, **glia** (also called *neuroglia*). The primary form of neuron-to-neuron communication is through slender cytoplasmic extensions that form **synapses** for the release of **neurotransmitters** (Figure 3.2). The function of the cellular extensions, known as *axons,* is to transmit neural signals, and the function of the **dendrites,** which are typically on the opposite pole of the neuron, is to receive signals. Each neuron communicates with an average of 10^4 to 10^5 other neurons, and many axons are quite long, especially those communicating between the brain and spinal cord. Therefore, much of the volume of the brain and CNS consists of axons and dendrites interconnecting the neurons. Chemical neurotransmitters released from the **presynaptic** neuron bind to dendrites of the **postsynaptic** neuron in the area of the synapse, changing the resting potential of the membrane in the cell body (–70 mV). If the potential changes enough to reach the threshold value (usually –59 mV), an electrical impulse or action potential is initiated, with calcium ions flowing into the neuron and resulting in the release of the neurotransmitter.

The neuronal cell bodies are grouped into layers or clusters at specific sites within the CNS. For instance, in the cerebrum, the neuronal cell bodies are confined to six layers on the external surface, known as the *cerebral cortex,* and to globular clusters deep within the center of the cerebrum, known as *basal nuclei* (historically referred to as *basal ganglia*). The rest of the cerebrum consists of billions of axons interconnecting neurons that are nearby, in the opposite hemisphere, or elsewhere in the CNS (see the "Cytoarchitecture of the Cerebral Cortex" section later in this chapter). Areas of the CNS that consist predominantly of axons and dendrites are known as *white matter* because the abundance of the fat-rich insulating material *myelin* makes it appear light in color. Areas that contain neuronal cell bodies are known as *gray matter* because those areas contain very little or no myelin. Collections of neuronal cell bodies in the CNS are referred to as *nuclei,* and those in the **peripheral nervous system** are referred to as *ganglia* (Purves & Augustine, 2004).

It is generally accepted that the action of one neuron on another is most often unidirectional, propagating a neural signal from the presynaptic axon terminal of

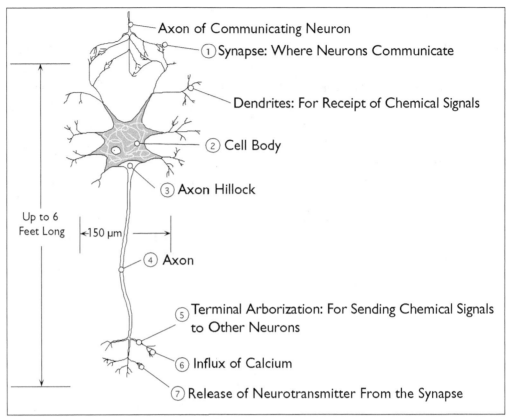

Figure 3.2. The neuron. (1) Chemical neurotransmitters released from neurons bind to dendrites in the area of the synapse. (2) Binding changes the resting potential of the membrane in the cell body (–70 mV). If the potential changes enough to reach the threshold value (usually –59 mV), an action potential is initiated from the axon hillock (3), which travels down the axon (4) to the terminus (5), resulting in calcium ions flowing into the neuron (6). The influx of calcium causes release of the neurotransmitter in the direction of the next neuron's dendrites (7). The activity of neurons can be blocked by blocking the energy supply necessary to maintain membrane potential, blocking the binding of the neurotransmitter to dendrites, or blocking release of the neurotransmitter into the synaptic cleft.

Source. F. Feuchter.

the first (presynaptic) neuron to different sites on the second (postsynaptic) neuron. The postsynaptic neuron can also send information upstream to the presynaptic neuron (retrograde transmission). Examples of substances that can exert their effects via retrograde neurotransmission are endocannabinoids, nitrous oxide, and neurotrophic factors, which can stimulate the **genome** of the presynaptic neuron.

Although the synapse has dominated the conceptual model of neurotransmission, other mechanisms, such as **neuromodulation** and **nonsynaptic diffusion neurotransmission** (NDN), have been considered to support and complement synaptic transmission. In neuromodulation, several classes of neurotransmitters regulate diverse populations of CNS neurons (Stahl, 2008). In contrast to direct synaptic transmission, neuromodulators secreted by a small group of neurons diffuse throughout large areas of the nervous system, thereby exerting their effect on numerous neurons. Examples of neuromodulators include dopamine, serotonin, **acetylcholine,** and histamine. NDN involves the diffusion of neurotransmitters through the **extracellular fluid** and other neuroactive substances released at sites that may be remote from the target cells, with the resulting activation of extrasynaptic receptors (Stahl, 2008).

An example of NDN is dopamine in the prefrontal cortex. Some substances, such as nitrous oxide, diffuse through both the extracellular fluid and cellular membranes to act within the cell. NDN is postulated to play a role in expansive and sustained functions such as **mood** and sleep. Because receptor up-regulation and down-regulation in response to brain damage may be among the methods of compensating for the damage, NDN may have a role in brain plasticity (Bach-y-Rita, 1995).

The timing and pattern of neurotransmission, as well as the type of transmission and the specific neurotransmitter, are all important in brain functioning. Some neurotransmitter signals exhibit a fast onset, starting within milliseconds of the receptors being occupied by the neurotransmitter. Two of the best examples of fast-onset signals are those elicited by the neurotransmitters glutamate and γ-aminobutyric acid (GABA). Glutamate almost uniformly stimulates the neuron it contacts, and GABA almost uniformly inhibits the neuron it contacts. Both glutamate and GABA can cause fast-onset chemical signaling by rapidly altering the excitability of the neurons. Signals from other neurotransmitters (e.g., dopamine, serotonin) can take longer to develop, ranging from many milliseconds to several seconds. Sometimes neurotransmitters with slow onset are also called *neuromodulators* because their actions may last long enough to carry over and modulate a subsequent neurotransmission by another neurotransmitter (Stahl, 2008).

All of this chemical back-and-forth may provoke structural changes at the synapses that increase the ease of neurotransmission and create a mini-network. Neurotransmitters arriving at the cell membrane trigger the actions of second messengers within the cell. The second messengers are signal transducers that pass along the neural signal from the cell membrane to the intracellular environment, eventually reaching the cell nucleus and ultimately resulting in either the initiation or the inhibition of gene expression. Once a change in gene expression has been triggered, a second biochemical cascade is initiated that alters the behavior of the cell. Through this process, patterns of neuronal firing related to a person's experiences or activities can lead to modification of neuronal connections and the development of networks. Thus, the function of chemical neurotransmission is not so much to have a presynaptic neurotransmitter communicate with its postsynaptic receptors as it is to have a presynaptic genome converse with a postsynaptic genome (Stahl, 2008). In this way, chemical neurotransmission may lead to alteration in behavior patterns—that is, people's experiences and what they do can lead to structural brain changes and enduring changes in patterns of thought, **emotion,** and behavior (Stahl, 2008).

Glial Cells

Neurons perform the essential communication functions of the brain, but the glial cells (neuroglia) outnumber them as much as tenfold. Unlike neurons, glial cells are not electrically excitable and do not propagate action potentials. Rather, they maintain the appropriate microenvironment essential for neuronal functions and provide neurons with physical and mechanical support (*glia* means "glue"). Although glial cells do not participate directly in synaptic interactions, their supportive functions help organize synaptic contacts and maintain the signaling abilities of neurons (Sharma & Vijayaraghavan, 2001; Ullian, Sapperstein, Christopherson, & Barres, 2001). The three main varieties of glial cells are (1) **astrocytes,** (2) oligodendrocytes, and (3) microglia.

Chemical neurotransmission may lead to alteration in behavior patterns—that is, people's experiences and what they do can lead to structural brain changes and enduring changes in patterns of thought, **emotion,** and behavior.

Overview of the Cerebrum

The cerebrum is associated with **consciousness** and controls the most complex and highest order functions of the brain, such as language, perception, voluntary movement, understanding of spatial relationships, decision making, memory, and emotions. The cerebrum is more developed in humans than in other animals and is the newest and most highly evolved portion of the brain. It consists of the cerebral cortex, which forms the visible surface of the brain, and the subcortical basal nuclei, which are buried deep within the cerebrum and are not visible except by slicing the brain in horizontal or coronal planes (see the "Basal Nuclei" section later in this chapter).

Cerebral Hemispheres

The cerebrum is divided into left and right hemispheres, which are separated by the deep **longitudinal fissure.** The surface of each hemisphere consists of numerous folds, known as *gyri* (singular ***gyrus***), and intervening grooves, known as *sulci* (singular ***sulcus***). Although certain gyri and sulci are present in almost every human brain, no two brains have exactly the same folding patterns. The outer surface of the cerebrum, the cerebral cortex, is composed of gray matter that is organized into six layers of neurons. The highly folded nature of the cortical surface allows for the presence of many more neurons than could be accommodated if the brain surface were not folded. Loss of gray matter and white matter may occur in the context of poor **perfusion** or several larger strokes. The **lateral ventricles** may show enlargement because of loss of subcortical gray and white matter (i.e., loss of cells in the basal nuclei and loss of axons or myelin in the white matter).

It is noteworthy that the folding of the cerebrum increases in tandem with progression up the phylogenetic tree (i.e., the more complex the animal, the more folded its cerebrum). Brain size generally varies with the size of an animal (i.e., larger animals have larger brains); relative to their size, however, humans have the largest frontal lobe of any animal.

Each **cerebral hemisphere** can be divided into six lobes (Figure 3.3, top). The lateral surface of each hemisphere is split by a deep groove known as the ***lateral sulcus*** (or ***Sylvian fissure***), which gives the hemisphere the shape of a boxing glove. The cortex lying inferior to this groove (i.e., the thumb of the glove) is called the ***temporal lobe*** because it is situated below the temporal bone (and temple region) of the skull. About midway between the anterior and posterior aspects of the cerebrum, another groove, the ***central sulcus (of Rolando),*** runs vertically from the lateral sulcus to the vertex. The cerebrum anterior to the central sulcus is the ***frontal lobe*** and that immediately posterior to the central sulcus is the ***parietal lobe.*** The most posterior region of the cerebrum is the ***occipital lobe,*** which is not very well delineated from the parietal lobe and continues on the lateral and medial surfaces of the posterior aspect of the hemisphere. The remaining two of the six lobes cannot be seen on the surface. However, if the borders of the lateral sulcus are spread apart, more cortex is revealed: the ***insular lobe*** (see Figure 3.3, top). The sixth region, the ***limbic lobe,*** cannot be viewed clearly unless the brain is cut in the midsagittal plane (see Figure 3.3, bottom). The limbic lobe consists of the gyrus immediately surrounding the corpus callosum (the **cingulate gyrus,** described in the "Networks of Attention" section) and the medial surface of the temporal lobe.

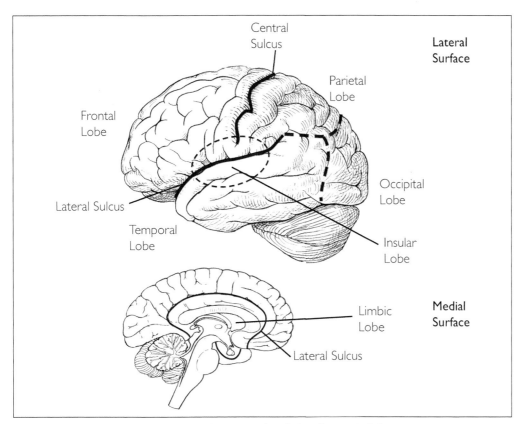

Figure 3.3. Each hemisphere of the brain can be divided into six lobes.
Source. F. Feuchter.

Cytoarchitecture of the Cerebral Cortex

Within the cerebral cortex, two basic types of neurons can be found: (1) neurons with large, pyramidal (i.e., pyramid-shaped) cell bodies and (2) smaller, nonpyramidal neurons with multiple morphologies, often referred to collectively as *granular neurons*. The pyramidal cells represent about 75% of the population of neurons. They have long axons that may leave the cortex and communicate with other brain regions or extend to distant cortical sites. In contrast, many of the granular neurons have shorter axons that do not leave the cerebral cortex and compose the intracortical circuitry.

Most of the cerebral cortex (about 95%) exhibits a well-defined lamellar (i.e., layerlike) organization, with the cells arranged in six layers, numbered I through VI from the surface inward (Figure 3.4). This organization is unique to the evolution of the human brain and therefore is referred to as the *neocortex,* or "new cortex." The multiple layering of neurons is related to the organization of the inputs and outputs. For instance, synapses for receiving nonspecific thalamic input are in Layers I and II, whereas synapses for receiving input from specific thalamic nuclei are in Layer IV. Layer III contains neurons that send information to and receive information from nearby cortical areas and the other cerebral hemisphere. Layer V is the location of large pyramidal cells that send output to distant sites such as the brainstem, spinal cord, and basal nuclei. Cells in Layer VI are the source of **corticothalamic fibers.**

The functional unit of the cerebral cortex at the microscopic level is the **cortical column** (Figure 3.5; Mountcastle, 1998). All the neurons within a column share

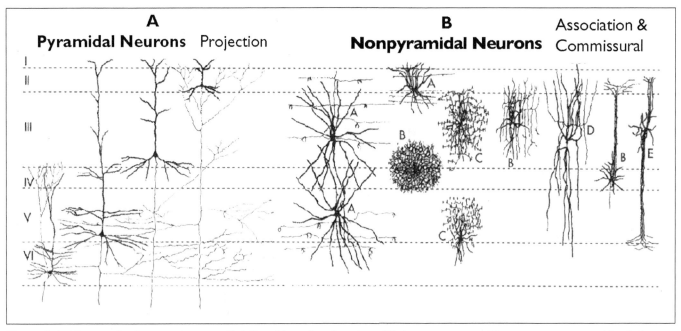

Figure 3.4. The cerebral cortex has a well-defined lamellar (i.e., layerlike) appearance with neurons arranged in six layers, numbered I through VI from the surface inward. (A) Pyramidal neurons in different layers have characteristically different soma sizes and patterns of distribution of axon collaterals. (B) Nonpyramidal neurons come in a variety of sizes and shapes; many have names attributable to their shape. Basket cells (A) are usually large and make basket-shaped endings that partially surround the cell bodies of pyramidal cells. Other kinds of smaller multipolar cells (B) may have elaborate dendritic and axonal arborizations. Chandelier cells (C) have vertically oriented synaptic "candles" that end on the initial segments of pyramidal cell axons. Bipolar cells (D) have dendrites that both ascend and descend, and double bouquet cells (E) have axons that both ascend and descend.

Source. From *The Human Brain* (5th ed., p. 528), by J. Nolte, 2002, St. Louis: Mosby. Copyright © 2002 by Elsevier. Used with permission.

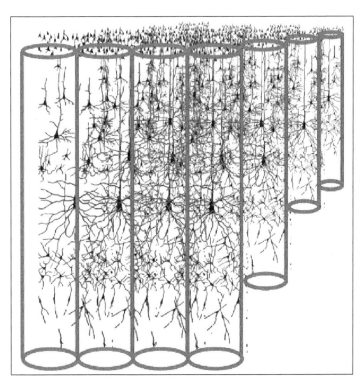

Figure 3.5. Cortical columns. All the neurons within a column are concerned with a single, specific aspect of a neurological task.

Source. F. Feuchter.

in common a specific aspect of a neurological task. For example, a column in the visual cortex may be responsible for detecting an edge at a certain angle at a small spot of the retina. Cortical columns are about 50 to 500 μm in diameter and extend vertically through all six layers of the cortex. Each column contains neurons that receive inputs from extracortical sites (specific and nonspecific) and other areas within the cortex, and each additionally has neurons responsible for sending signals out to other cortical areas. When large numbers of columns in a given region of the cerebral cortex are involved in the specific functions characteristic of that region and span all six well-defined cell layers (i.e., of the neocortex), they are referred to as ***isocortex*** ("same cortex"). Other areas with fewer than six layers are referred to as ***allocortex*** ("other cortex"), whereas those between three and six layers are referred to as ***mesocortex*** ("middle cortex"). Allocortex or mesocortex represent evolutionarily older cortex and are mostly found in the medial portions of the temporal lobe, the insula, and the limbic lobe.

The cell layers are not uniform across the neocortex. Rather, different regions vary in thickness of the layers and relative proportions of pyramidal and granular neurons. Most areas of the isocortex are ***homotypic isocortex;*** that is, they display the prototypical six layers of varying thickness and differing proportions of neurons (Figure 3.6). Certain areas, however, show extreme variations of the homotypic pattern and are referred to as ***heterotypic isocortex.*** Heterotypic cortex of the granular variety contains almost entirely granular neurons and no pyramidal cells, whereas agranular heterotypic cortex consists almost entirely or entirely of pyramidal neurons. Differences in layering can be related to functions within a region. For instance, motor and premotor regions consist almost exclusively of agranular cortex, as one might expect, because the agranular pyramidal cells have long projection axons for carrying motor commands to distant sites where they are needed. The primary motor and sensory cortices are illustrated in Figure 3.7. The primary receptive regions for hearing, vision, and somatosensory functions consist of granular cortex; granular cells typically process information locally and interconnect regional cortical sites.

Most of the remaining cortex is **association cortex,** which shows homotypic structure (see the unshaded portion of Figure 3.7). The association cortex can be further divided into ***unimodal association cortices,*** which process a single kind of sensory modality (e.g., visual, auditory, or somatosensory association areas), and *unimodal motor association cortex,* which deals exclusively with programming movements.

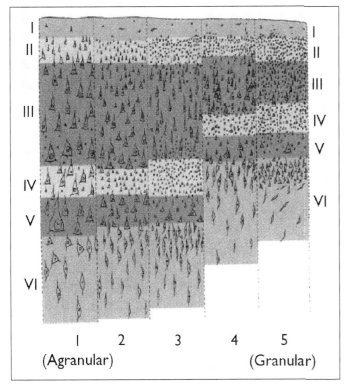

Figure 3.6. Neocortex regions vary in thickness of the layers and relative proportions of agranular (pyramidal) and granular neurons. Most areas of the isocortex are homotypic isocortex; that is, they display the prototypical six layers of varying thickness and differing proportions of neurons.

Source. From *The Human Brain* (5th ed., p. 530), by J. Nolte, 2002, St. Louis: Mosby. Copyright © 2002 by Elsevier. Used with permission.

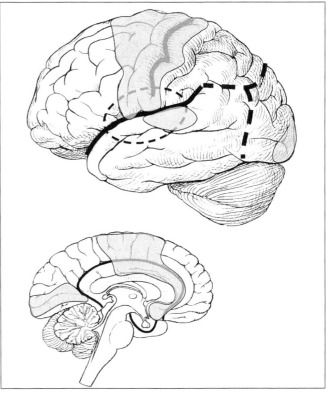

Figure 3.7. The primary motor and sensory cortices. The primary receptive regions for hearing, vision, and somatosensory functions (shaded) consist of granular cortex. The unshaded portion is association cortex, which shows homotypic structure.

Source. F. Feuchter.

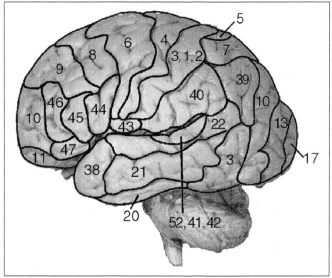

Figure 3.8. Each numbered Brodmann's area denotes a region of the cortex that has a microscopic appearance, cell composition, and thickness of layers that differentiate it from other areas. Many of the Brodmann's areas are used today as a way of describing particular areas of the cortex, but only some of those areas can be associated with a single function.

Source. F. Feuchter.

Although many of the Brodmann's areas are used today as a way of describing particular areas of the cortex, only some of those areas can be associated with a single function, with many apparently serving multiple functions.

Lesions in unimodal association areas lead to complex deficits in sensory perception, but the elemental sensations remain intact. *Heteromodal* association cortex receives input from multiple unimodal areas. Neurons in heteromodal association cortex are responsible for the integration of sensory or sensorimotor material or, in some cases, fire in response to stimuli having some motivational significance. This pattern makes sense when one considers awareness of objects or events in the real world: A person is aware of objects and events not along a single perceptual plane but rather across modes of perception. For example, bacon has a certain odor; tastes salty; and has attributes of shape, color, and texture that are quite specific. **Heteromodal association areas** can be found in prefrontal regions and the posterior parietal and temporal lobes. Lesions in heteromodal areas result in complex deficits involving both cognitive and affective functions.

The concept that the variation in the appearance of the cortex might be related to function has led to use of a map to delineate areas of the cortex that are identical in their microscopic appearance. The map divides the brain into areas on the basis of their cytoarchitecture known as **Brodmann's areas** (Figure 3.8), named after the German scientist Korbinian Brodmann (1868–1918) who developed it. Although many of the Brodmann's areas are used today as a way of describing particular areas of the cortex, only some of those areas can be associated with a single function, with many apparently serving multiple functions. For instance, the primary motor area is Brodmann's area 4; the primary somatosensory areas are Brodmann's areas 1, 2, and 3; and the primary visual area is Brodmann's area 17. The complex tasks of the cerebrum, such as those embodied in higher-level cognitive functions, can be localized to larger regions of cortex that overlap many Brodmann's areas.

Functional Areas of Cerebral Cortex

The current understanding of the cerebral cortex is that local networks of neurons in specific anatomical areas are activated during the performance of mental tasks. Each local network is composed of multiple interconnected cortical columns and performs a particular operation during a mental task. Most mental activity involves sequential processing of information by multiple networks. For example, information from the retina is sent first to the **primary visual cortex,** but this information is coded as edges on certain locations on the retina. The input about edges is passed to other nearby areas of the occipital lobe to generate a representation of the visible object and then to the parietal lobe before an understanding of what is being seen is generated. If the task is to name the visible object, additional networks for the retrieval of the name from memory and for verbalization are involved. Many areas of the cerebral cortex recognized as having a particular functional significance are shown in Figure 3.9, and recognized function–location associations are summarized in Table 3.1.

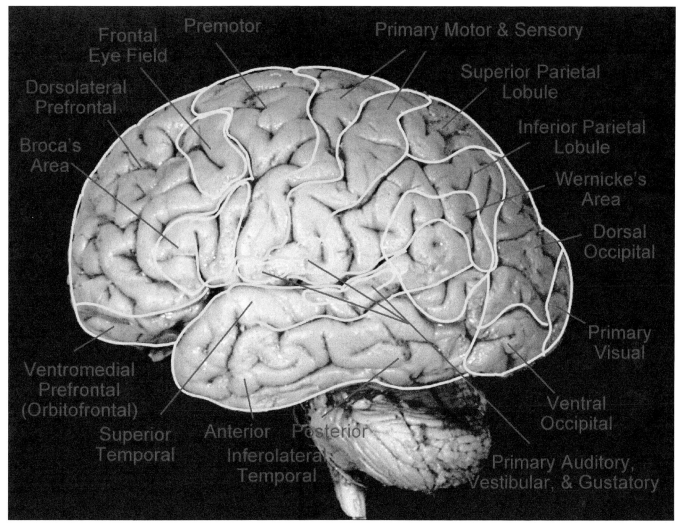

Figure 3.9. Areas of the cerebral cortex recognized as having functional significance.
Source. F. Feuchter.

Lateralization

The issues of lateralization and localization of function in the human brain are complex. Many basic perceptual and motor functions are lateralized—one hemisphere governs the **contralateral** half of the body. Higher order attentional, representational, and processing capacities tend to exhibit *hemispheric specialization,* which is the tendency for one hemisphere to carry out more than 50% of a particular function. Many conditions initially thought to be basic perceptual problems are really disorders of higher order processing and integration. Examples of higher order processing disorders that interfere with basic functions include neglect syndromes and **prosopagnosia.**

> Many conditions initially thought to be basic perceptual problems are really disorders of higher order processing and integration.

Lateralization of Attention

Of particular interest to occupational therapists is the right hemisphere's specialization for **attention.** Damage to the left hemisphere only rarely leads to severe or enduring right neglect, whereas damage to the right hemisphere often leads to profound left neglect. Unilateral visual neglect, **hemianesthesia,** and **hemiplegia**

Table 3.1. Summary of Function of Brain Regions

Region	Function
Frontal Lobe	
Primary motor cortex	Major source of cells (upper motor neurons) for the descending motor pathways that are essential for the voluntary control of movement and that are part of the reflex circuits of brainstem and spinal cord
	Located in the precentral gyrus (Brodmann's area 4)
Premotor cortex	Planning and initiation of voluntary movement, guidance of limb trajectory based on cerebellar input
	Located anterior to the primary motor cortex within the lateral surface of the frontal lobe (part of Brodmann's area 6)
Supplementary motor cortex	Planning of complex movements with motor sequences derived from basal nuclei input, bilateral movements
	Located within the medial surface of the frontal lobe, in the superior frontal gyrus anterior to the primary motor cortex (part of Brodmann's area 6)
Frontal eye field	Direction of eye movement into the contralateral visual hemisphere, volitional saccadic eye movements
	Located in the rostral portion of the premotor cortex and in the posterior portion of the middle frontal gyrus (Brodmann's area 8)
Broca's area	Production of language, both written and spoken
	Located in the inferior frontal gyrus of the dominant hemisphere, usually left (Brodmann's areas 44 and 45)
Area for prosody	Musical aspects of speech, production and recognition of the rhythmic and tonal aspects *(prosody)* of speech that convey much of its emotional meaning, equivalent of Broca's or Wernicke's areas or both
	Located in the inferior frontal gyrus of the nondominant hemisphere, usually right
Prefrontal cortex	Executive functions of the brain; receipt of inputs from sensory, motor association, and limbic areas; decision making, planning, and selection of appropriate responses in social situations; problem solving
	Located anterior to the premotor and supplementary motor cortical areas
Dorsolateral	Critical role in working memory; attention and problem solving; massive connectivity with somatosensory, visual, and auditory association areas of the cortex (Brodmann's areas 8, 9, and 46)
	Left: Verbal intellectual capacities; creative, flexible, verbal thinking; verbal fluency
	Right: Nonverbal intellectual capacities; creative, flexible, nonverbal thinking; design fluency
Ventromedial	Interconnection with limbic structures, emotional aspects of planning and decision making, emotional behaviors and reactions, social conduct, impulse control, judgment, planning, decision making, triggering of bodily states associated with emotions (Brodmann's area 10)
Superomedial	Emotional behavior, emotional aspects of planning and decision making, motivation, basic drive states, maintenance of adaptive state of arousal and alertness, personality characteristics (Brodmann's areas 6, 8, 10, and 12)
Occipital Lobe	
Primary visual cortex	Perception of edges
	Located in the banks of the calcarine sulcus (Brodmann's area 17)
Ventral	*Left:* Perception of shapes and contours (features), color perception and naming, reading, face recognition (features); the "what" recognition system
	Right: Perception of shapes and contours (global), color perception, nonverbal pattern recognition, face recognition (holistic); the "what" recognition system
Dorsal	*Left:* Depth and motion perception, stereopsis, visual attention, recognition of identity from movement; the "where" recognition system
	Right: Depth and motion perception, stereopsis, visual attention, visually guided reaching, recognition of identity from movement, mental rotation; the "where" recognition system
Parietal Lobe	
Primary somatosensory cortex	Primary sensory perception of touch, vibration, temperature, and pain
	Located in the postcentral gyrus (Brodmann's areas 1, 2, and 3)
Superior	Integration of tactile and visual information, sensory and visually guided movements
Inferior	*Left:* Tactile object recognition, verbatim repetition
	Right: Tactile object recognition, self-perception, mapping of physical and emotional states, placement of oneself in space
Wernicke's area	Comprehension of language, both written and spoken
	Located in the posterior part of the superior temporal gyrus of the dominant hemisphere, usually left (Brodmann's area 22)

(Continued)

Table 3.1. Summary of Function of Brain Regions *(cont.)*

Region	Function
	Temporal Lobe
Primary auditory cortex	Primary auditory sensation
	Located in the transverse temporal gyri (Brodmann's areas 41 and 42)
Superior	*Left:* Speech perception and comprehension, processing of temporal aspects of auditory signals
	Right: Processing and comprehension of nonverbal sounds, music, timbre, prosody, perception of spectral aspects of aural signals
Inferolateral	*Posterior:* Visual object recognition, face recognition
	Anterior left: Common and proper noun retrieval, retrieval of verbal information from memory
	Anterior right: Comprehension of emotional meanings of nonverbal stimuli, retrieval of nonverbal information from memory
Medial	*Left:* Anterograde verbal memory, acquisition of new verbal information
	Right: Anterograde nonverbal memory, acquisition of new nonverbal information

are all more pronounced after right-sided stroke than left-sided stroke. Recently, evidence has been mounting that this difference may be accounted for by the attentional disturbance that may follow right-sided stroke. People with right-sided stroke and left neglect may have skin conductance responses and normal somatosensory and visual evoked potentials to stimuli that they fail to report (Sterzi et al., 1993; see the "Lateralized Attention and Related Disorders" section in Chapter 7). This is important because people with neglect have poorer functional outcomes than those without neglect or with left-sided damage (Kinsella & Ford, 1980).

Other Hemispheric Specialization
Table 3.1 provides an overview of lateralization. Lateralized functions include language functions and the hemispheric association of global versus local modes of information processing (Hellige, 1996). There is a tradition of research indicating that the right side of the brain is specialized for the analysis of the gestalt of a figure, outside contour, and global elements, and the left side of the brain is responsible for local detail-by-detail analysis (Hellige, 1996; Kéïta, Bedoin, Burack, & Lepore, 2014). In addition, a lack of awareness is associated with right-sided brain damage, whereas depression is associated with left-sided brain damage (Orfei et al., 2007; Starkstein, Fedoroff, Price, Leiguarda, & Robinson, 1992; Starkstein & Robinson, 1989).

White Matter of the Cerebrum

The bulk of the cerebrum consists of white matter, composed of the axons that interconnect different areas of the cortex with each other and with distant sites. Normal functioning of the cerebral cortex requires intact connections among its component parts and with other parts of the CNS. The fibrous nature of the brain is not apparent on sliced sections but can be seen clearly in specimens that have been pulled apart (Figures 3.10 and 3.11). Three kinds of axons are present in the white matter and are defined by where they travel: (1) projection axons and (2) **long** and (3) **short association fibers.** Projection axons originate either in the cerebrum and synapse in the brainstem or originate in the **thalamus** and synapse in the cerebrum. They carry or project impulses to and from sites outside the cerebrum. The bundle of fibers carrying projection axons is called the *internal capsule;* the internal capsule lies deep within the cerebrum, where it is tightly compacted (see

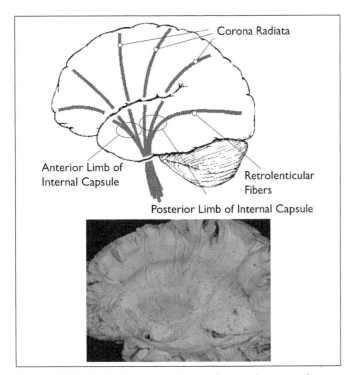

Figure 3.10. Projection axons leave the cerebrum and enter the brainstem or enter the cerebrum from the thalamus. They carry impulses to and from sites outside the cerebrum.

Source. F. Feuchter.

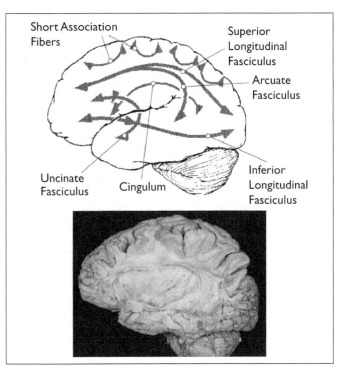

Figure 3.11. Long and short association fibers interconnect various sites within the same cerebral hemisphere. The fibrous nature of the brain is not apparent on sliced sections but can be seen clearly on specimens that have been pulled apart.

Source. F. Feuchter.

Figure 3.10). In locations near the cerebral cortex, the bundle of **projection fibers** is referred to as the ***corona radiata*** because it is expanded and resembles a fan.

Long and short association fibers interconnect various sites within the same cerebral hemisphere. The major long-fiber bundles are known as the *occipitofrontal fasciculus* and the *arcuate fasciculus,* but many other bundles also exist. The fibers connecting one gyrus to another are simply called *short association fibers.* Finally, bundles of fibers interconnect mirror-image sites in the opposite hemisphere; these site-to-site connections across the hemispheres are known as ***commissural fibers,*** the most prominent collection of which is the **corpus callosum** (Figure 3.12).

Cerebral Networks

Our current understanding of information processing in the cerebral cortex is based on the concept of multiple networks. The local networks of cortical columns, which perform a particular operation of a mental task, are interconnected with other sites in the brain that perform other aspects of the task. Thus, multiple brain areas form large networks that are involved in higher cognitive functions. This view expands on the earlier view that the cerebrum operates on the basis of serial, unidirectional processing from primary sensory to association to motor areas in the manner of an elaborate reflex arc. Discoveries about the cortical connections of primates have led to the idea that information processing occurs in simultaneous parallel processes in large-scale networks. This model of cortical functioning takes into account that heteromodal association areas interconnect reciprocally not only with unimodal areas and with each other but also with paralimbic and limbic areas necessary for motivation, learning, and memory. Essentially, simultaneous activation of the various functional areas in a cortical network occurs during task performance. Because many of the functional networks also involve **subcortical** structures, they are discussed later in this chapter (see the "Basal Nuclei" section).

Most of the cerebral surface is classified as association cortex and is responsible for the complex processing that follows the arrival of input from primary sensory cortices and that leads to the generation of behavior via connections to the primary motor cortex. Higher order cerebral functions depend on both local cortical functions and distributed network functions; for example, reading depends on vision and language. Numerous subcortical structures participate in such integrative functions. For example, complex behavioral functions *(executive functions)* are managed via a range of frontal subcortical circuits. Thus, specific neurobehavioral deficits can be caused not only by focal cortical lesions but also by lesions that involve only subcortical structures or by lesions that disrupt cortical–cortical or cortical–subcortical network connections.

Knowledge about the functions of cortical regions comes primarily from observations of patients with damage to one or another of these areas. Noninvasive neuroimaging of neurologically healthy people, functional mapping during neurosurgery, and electrophysiological analysis of comparable brain regions in nonhuman primates have generally confirmed the clinical deductions (Squire & Wixted, 2011). Together, the studies indicate that the parietal association cortex has particular responsibility for attending to stimuli in the external and internal environment, the temporal association cortex is important in identifying the nature of such stimuli, and the frontal association cortex is especially important in planning and controlling appropriate behavioral responses.

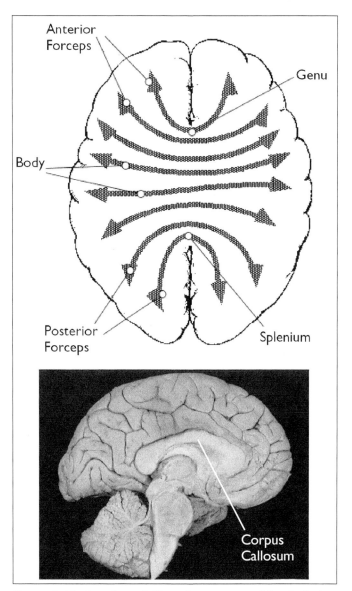

Figure 3.12. Bundles of fibers interconnect identical sites between the two hemispheres. These fibers are known as *commissural fibers,* the most prominent of which is the corpus callosum.

Source. F. Feuchter.

Visual Networks

Among the earliest investigated and best understood of the cerebral networks is the system for processing visual stimuli. The general organizational features of the visual system have been well established in all primates, including human beings, from decades of detailed study of patients with permanently impaired vision and from laboratory experiments with nonhuman primates. Input from the visual system is the trigger for many forms of higher mental activity, such as pattern recognition,

> Knowledge about the functions of cortical regions comes primarily from observations of patients with damage to one or another of these areas.

the construction of mental images in the absence of outside stimuli, and the interpretation of symbols involved in reading.

When examining the specifics of vision, it is useful to divide the **visual fields** into right and left halves because the parts of the retina of each eye that receive light from the left half of the visual field send the information to the right half of the visual cortex through their connections. Similarly, the parts of the retina of each eye that receive light from the right half of the visual field send the information to the left half of the visual cortex (Figure 3.13). Thus, the information from the right visual world is received and analyzed on the left side of the cerebrum, whereas the information from the left visual world is received and analyzed on the right side of the cerebrum. Each cell in the visual cortex receives its input only from a particular part of the retina and, hence, from a particular part of the visual field, which is called the

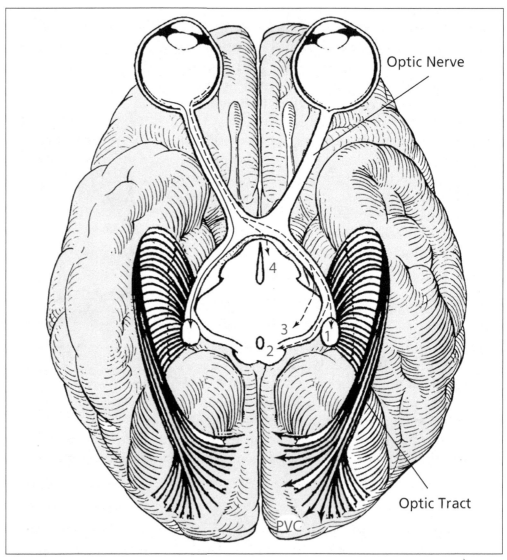

Figure 3.13. Diagram of the optic tract showing how objects on one side of the visual field send information to the contralateral visual cortex. (1) Lateral geniculate nucleus, (2) superior colliculus, (3) pretectal region, (4) hypothalamus.

Source. F. Feuchter.

Note. PVC = primary visual cortex.

receptive field of the cell. Therefore, the cells of the retina and the corresponding cells of the visual cortex to which they report have a precise topographic relationship, called *retinotopic* because it defines a particular place on the retina. In this organizational scheme, adjacent regions of the retina (and thus visual field) are connected to cells in the primary visual cortex that are also located adjacent to each other. Additionally, the cells in the corresponding location on the other retina are also connected to cells in primary visual cortex in areas adjacent to those from the other eye.

The axons in the optic nerve synapse in the **lateral geniculate nucleus** (LGN) of the *thalamus* (the thalamus is the sensory relay center for all sensory inputs except **olfaction**). From the thalamus, the optic tract fibers radiate to the primary visual cortex. Additionally, the optic nerve fibers communicate with three other important areas of the brain: (1) The **superior colliculus** of the brainstem receives input from the optic nerve to coordinate reflexive eye and head movement, (2) the pretectal region of the midbrain receives input from the optic nerve to control the pupillary light reflex, and (3) the **suprachiasmatic nucleus** of the hypothalamus regulates **diurnal rhythms** and hormonal levels.

Information flow from the retina through the optic nerves and tracts appears to follow one of three main data streams on the basis of shape, movement, and color. This organization is preserved in the LGN and passed on to the primary visual area V1 (Brodmann's area 17). However, the color, shape, and movement information from the thalamus is sent to different and specific neurons within V1 for processing and then subsequently sent on to different areas of the occipital lobe known as ***extrastriate visual cortex*** (described later in this section). Within V1, a population of cells known as ***blob cells*** processes information about color, including the perception and discrimination of color and the learning and memory of the color of objects. Also within V1 are the *interblob cells,* which exhibit orientation and location specificity, are not motion sensitive, and are used in object perception, discrimination, learning, and memory or in **spatial orientation.** These interblob cells are the shape- and form-processing cells and the location-processing cells of V1. A second subset of interblob cells respond preferentially to moving stimuli without a preference for the direction of movement. A third subset respond preferentially to movement in a particular direction. The motion-sensitive V1 interblob cells detect object movement, direction, and velocity and guide eye movements. Motion-sensitive interblob cells are the motion-detecting cells of V1.

The medioposterior surfaces of the occipital lobe are devoted to primary vision (Brodmann's area 17; Figure 3.14). Bundles of nerve fibers innervating the primary visual cortex form a clear stripe visible to the naked eye termed the ***striate cortex*** (*striate* means "striped"). The striate cortex is split by a prominent sulcus known as the ***calcarine fissure,*** which marks the division between the inputs received from the upper versus lower halves of the visual field. The input is inverted, with the striate cortex inferior to the calcarine fissure receiving input from the upper half of the visual field and the striate cortex superior to the calcarine fissure receiving input from the lower half of the visual field. Furthermore, the volume of striate cortex receiving input from specific areas of the retina varies depending on the location within the retina. Significantly more striate cortex is devoted to analyzing input from central parts of the retina, especially the *macula lutea*. Peripheral parts of the retina send information about the periphery of the visual field, such as

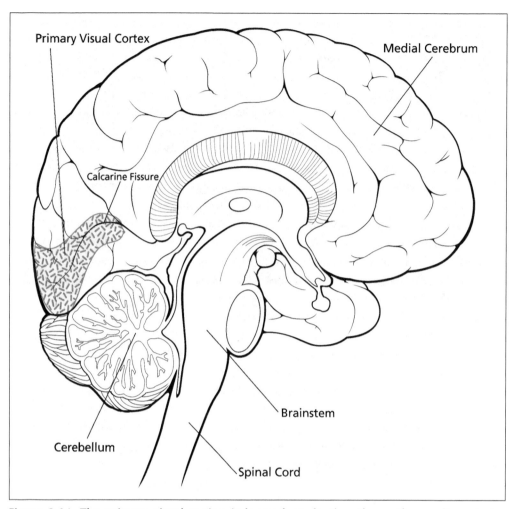

Figure 3.14. The primary visual region is located predominantly on the medioposterior surfaces of the occipital lobe.

Source. F. Feuchter.

moving objects, but visual objects that receive attentional focus are visualized with the macula lutea. The macula lutea occupies about 1% of the entire surface area of the retina, but information from the macula lutea is reported by approximately 50% of the fibers within the optic nerve to cells occupying about 50% of the striate cortex (Figure 3.15).

The most acute vision (i.e., that which occurs at the macula lutea) is analyzed in the visual cortex at the most posterior pole of the occipital lobe, with the *fovea,* the central region of the macula lutea region of the retina, represented on the external surface at the posterior tip of the lobe. Retinal cells located more laterally in the retina report to cortical cells located more anteriorly on the medial surface of the occipital lobe. The most peripheral retinal cells send input to the most anterior portions of the striate cortex.

Recordings from individual cells have shown that the visual system is organized into maps, each of which represents the "picture" viewed by the retina. The maps are organized in a hierarchical manner, each corresponding to a distinct area of the brain responsible for carrying out a particular type of analysis of the visual information sent to the brain. The primary visual cortical cells respond most strongly to

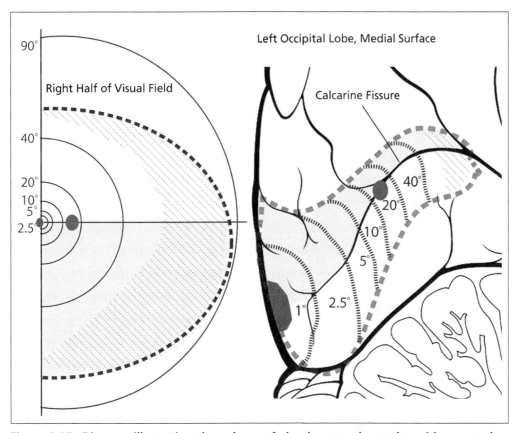

Figure 3.15. Diagram illustrating the volume of visual cortex devoted to either central or peripheral parts of the retina. On the left side of the diagram, the right half of the visual field is shown, with the superior part in light blue and the inferior part in yellow. The red dot indicates the macula lutea, which focuses on objects on which attention is fixed, and the blue dot is the blind spot. The concentric semicircles indicate distance from the macula on the retina in degrees, and the region with hatch lines is the part seen with only one eye. On the right side of the diagram, the corresponding representation of the visual field on the primary visual cortex is shown. The part of the visual field within 40° of the macula is represented on most of the primary visual cortex, with peripheral regions less well represented. The field is inverted, and the area of most acute vision is located on the most posterior part of the lobe.

Source. F. Feuchter.

form, movement, or color. However, complete analysis of the information coming from the visual fields, and therefore pattern recognition, involves sequential processing through several areas that go from the primary visual area in the back of the brain into adjacent areas of the occipital, temporal, and parietal lobes. These areas of visual processing have been referred to as *extrastriate cortex* and *visual association cortex* (Figure 3.16). Researchers have determined that the monkey may have as many as 34 separate extrastriate and visual association regions, each analyzing a different attribute of the visual field.

In humans, the extrastriate cortex includes all of the occipital lobe areas surrounding the primary visual cortex (Brodmann's areas 18 and 19). The extrastriate cortex has been subdivided into as many as three functional visual areas (V2, V3, and V4). Each of these visual areas contains neurons, the receptive fields of which together represent the entire visual field. Visual information enters through the primary visual cortex and travels through the rest of the areas in sequence.

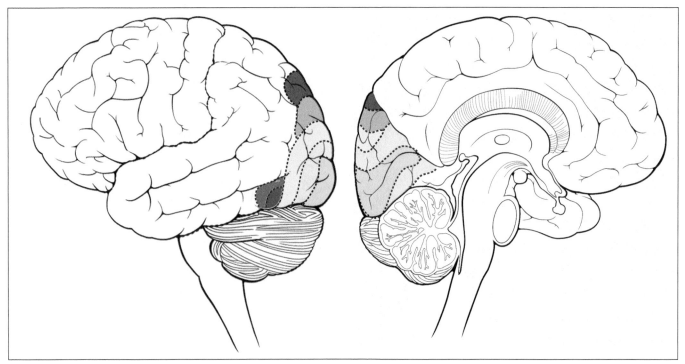

Figure 3.16. Several regions in the visual association and extrastriate cortices, each specialized for carrying out a particular type of analysis of the visual information sent to the brain.

Source. F. Feuchter.

The visual association cortex extends anteriorly from the extrastriate cortex to encompass adjacent areas of the posterior parietal lobe and much of the posterior temporal lobe (Brodmann's areas 7, 20, 37, and 39). These areas receive visual input from the extrastriate cortex, which sends color, shape and form, location, and motion information to different areas of the visual association cortex. Several areas of the visual association cortex have been described in humans, including V5, medial temporal superior, and superior temporal sulcus, all of which analyze various aspects of motion. Other areas analyze faces and specific body parts, and still others analyze various aspects of location and space.

The network of visual analysis in the extrastriate occipital cortex sends out two main streams of information, the *dorsal/where* stream and the *ventral/what* stream. Data regarding attributes of the stimulus, such as the position of an object in space and its movement, are sent anteriorly toward the parietal lobe in the data stream constituting the dorsal/where system (Figure 3.17). Also known as the *dorsal visual pathway,* the dorsal/where stream stretches from the primary visual cortex in the occipital lobe forward into the parietal lobe. The dorsal/where system is believed to be involved in the guidance of actions and the recognition of where objects are in space. The dorsal/where stream commences with purely visual functions in the occipital lobe before gradually transferring to spatial awareness at its termination in the parietal lobe. The posterior parietal cortex is essential for the perception and interpretation of spatial relationships, accurate body image, and learning of tasks involving coordination of the body in space.

The dorsal/where stream is interconnected with the parallel ventral/what stream, which runs anteriorly from V1 into the temporal lobe. The ventral/what

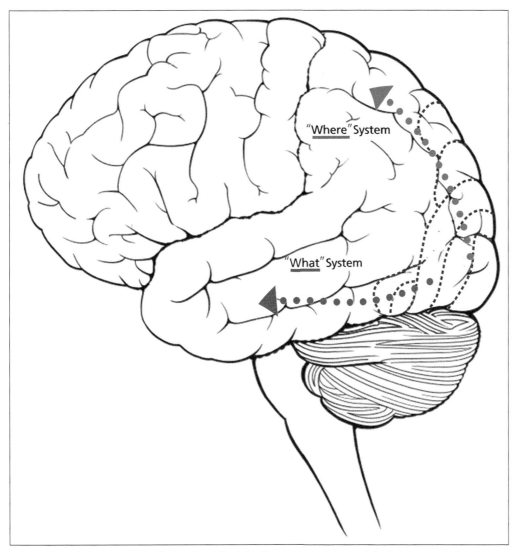

Figure 3.17. The network of visual analysis in the extrastriate occipital cortex sends out two main streams of information, the *dorsal/where* stream and the *ventral/what* stream. Data regarding attributes of the stimulus, such as position of an object in space and its movement, are sent anteriorly toward the parietal lobe in the data stream constituting the where system. The ventral/what stream is associated with object recognition and form representation and has strong connections to the medial temporal lobe (involved in the encoding of explicit memories).

Source. F. Feuchter.

stream is associated with object recognition and form representation and has strong connections to the medial temporal lobe (involved in the encoding of explicit memories), the limbic system (involved in emotions), and the dorsal/where stream (which deals with object location and motion). All the areas in the ventral/what stream are influenced by extraretinal factors in addition to the nature of the stimulus in the receptive field; these factors include attention, working memory, and stimulus salience. Thus, the ventral/what stream does not merely provide a description of the elements in the visual world; it also plays a crucial role in judging the significance of these elements.

Researchers in neurophysiology have emphasized the importance of bidirectional signaling within these systems, with multiple reciprocal connections, and it is postulated that when a visual image of an object is created in the absence of visual stimuli (i.e., in imagination), the extrastriate areas of the brain that are activated are the same as those involved in actively viewing the object when it is physically present. Positron emission tomography studies have provided abundant evidence that multiple visual areas of the human brain contribute to the formation of visual imagery. It is clear that the elements of the ventral/what and dorsal/where pathways within the visual system can be engaged in forming visual imagery.

Additional brain areas outside the visual area can also be activated when forming mental imagery, including the basal nuclei and **anterior cingulate gyrus,** which are elements of the attentional networks of the brain (see the "Networks of Attention" section). Attentional networks are central to the types of top-down processing that occur in many of the brain networks.

Language Networks

Symbolic language, as far as is known, is a uniquely human ability. Much of a person's conscious life consists of concepts represented by words. Therefore, by examining what occurs in the brain as a person understands and expresses words, researchers can examine much of the process of conscious thought.

Figure 3.18 illustrates a model proposed by Norman Geschwind (1926–1984), an important U.S. behavioral neurologist, who described the successive participation of several brain areas as research participants read and spoke a written word (Geschwind, 1979). Although the model is consistent with observed deficits after human brain damage, it does not account for people's flexibility in language-processing strategies during different kinds of language-related tasks. For instance, when research participants were presented with a noun and asked to generate an appropriate verb, different areas of the brain were activated in addition to those activated during the reading task (Figure 3.19). The activated areas included the anterior cingulate region, the left prefrontal and left posterior temporal cortices, and the right half of the cerebellum. The additional demands of verb generation thus appear to be supported by a network of widely separated brain areas not involved in the basic functions of reading. Moreover, the change in brain activity after practice and associated improved performance on the verb-generating task suggest that as the task is learned, the brain regions involved in the task change. The pathway used might depend on the degree to which a task has become automatic because participation of frontal areas typically associated with the management of novel experience diminishes as a task becomes automatized.

> By examining what occurs in the brain as a person understands and expresses words, researchers can examine much of the process of conscious thought.

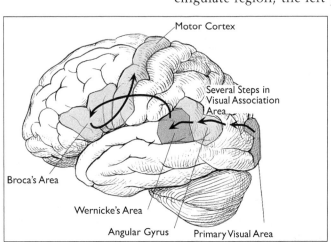

Figure 3.18. The model proposed by Geschwind (1979) is consistent with observed deficits following human brain injury, but it does not account for flexibility in language-processing strategies during different kinds of language-related tasks.

Source. From *Images of Mind* (p. 108), by Michael I. Posner and Marcus E. Raichle. Copyright © 1994, 1997 by Scientific American Library. Reprinted by permission of Henry Holt and Company, LLC.

Networks of Attention

The ability to attend to and identify internal and external stimuli with relevance to the self is a fundamental component of cognitive functioning. Several different but interlinked attentional systems have been examined. The **covert visual orienting network** is

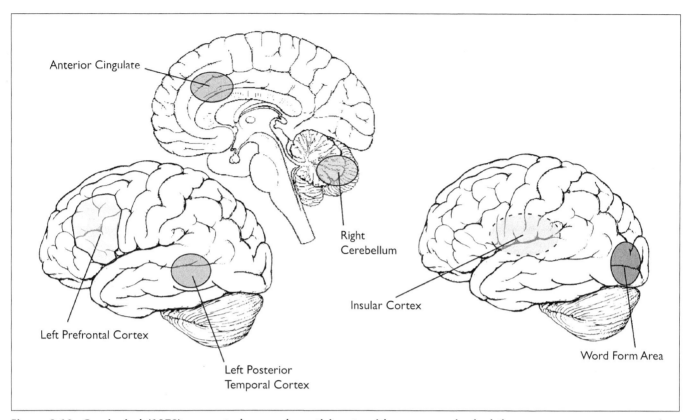

Figure 3.19. Geschwind (1979) presented research participants with a noun and asked them to generate an appropriate verb; different areas of the brain were activated in addition to those activated on the reading task. The activated areas included the anterior cingulate region, the left prefrontal and left posterior temporal cortices, and the right half of the cerebellum. Left diagrams: The generation task requires the combined activation of four brain areas, which may constitute at least part of an executive attention network. Right diagram: When practice has made responses automatic, an entirely different set of areas is activated, including areas in the insular cortex of both hemispheres.

Source. From *Images of Mind* (p. 124), by Michael I. Posner and Marcus E. Raichle. Copyright © 1994, 1997 by Scientific American Library. Reprinted by permission of Henry Holt and Company, LLC.

active in shifting attention from one focus to another in the external environment. When one attends to an object in the environment, one usually looks at that object (i.e., moves the eyes to place the image on the *retinal fovea,* the central region of the macula lutea) (Posner & Petersen, 1990). One can also visually focus attention on objects in the environment without moving the eyes. The circuitry proposed by Posner and Petersen (1990) is shown in Figure 3.20. The right parietal lobe, known for many years to play a significant role in selective attention, initiates movement of the focus of attention to a new location. It seems likely that the superior colliculus in the midbrain plays a role in moving visual covert attention from one location to another, much as it does for eye movements.

The role of the *pulvinar region* of the thalamus (a region known to be involved in visual and attentional processing) is suspected to be that of enhancing input from the new location while filtering out much of the unattended information before passing the information forward to the frontal lobe. Once attention has shifted to a new location and the new content is transmitted forward in the brain, the **executive attention network** is engaged (Figure 3.21). The task of the executive attention network is ***detection***—conscious recognition that an object is present,

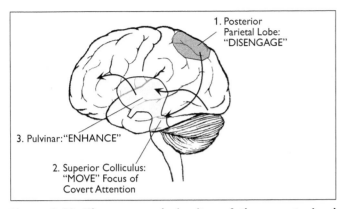

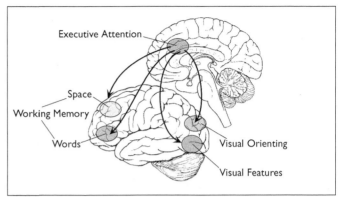

Figure 3.20. The proposed circuitry of the covert visual orienting network, which is active in shifting attention from one focus to another in the external environment. The three areas of the orienting network perform three functions required to orient attention: (1) The focus of attention is first disengaged from a cue, (2) then moved to the expected target location; (3) finally, there is enhanced focus on the new target location.

Source. From *Images of Mind* (p. 168), by Michael I. Posner and Marcus E. Raichle. Copyright © 1994, 1997 by Scientific American Library. Reprinted by permission of Henry Holt and Company, LLC.

Figure 3.21. Once attention has shifted to a new location and the new content is transmitted forward in the brain, the executive attention network is engaged in the task of *detection*—conscious recognition that an object is present, along with recognition of the object's identity and its significance.

Source. From *Images of Mind* (p. 173), by Michael I. Posner and Marcus E. Raichle. Copyright © 1994, 1997 by Scientific American Library. Reprinted by permission of Henry Holt and Company, LLC.

along with recognition of the object's identity and its significance. Detection plays a special role in selecting a target from many alternatives, a process known as *target detection.*

Target detection absorbs attention in a way that resists interference by other signals and thus represents a different kind of attention than merely orienting to a cue. The anterior cingulate gyrus appears to have executive control over information processing and is linked to frontal lobe regions involved in working memory (see the "Networks of Memory" section, which follows) and to posterior regions for visual orienting and feature identification. Damage to medial prefrontal structures (anterior cingulate gyrus) diminishes both the speed and the amount of human activity. The medial sagittal structures are part of a system that includes brainstem structures that are responsible for tonic arousal. Tonic arousal appears to be subserved by pathways originating in the **locus coeruleus** and terminating in frontal areas with the function lateralized to the right (Posner & Petersen, 1990).

Another brain network, the **vigilance network** (Figure 3.22), appears to maintain a sustained state of alertness. Sometimes a person must minimally attend to environmental stimuli to be vigilant about a future event (i.e., maintain a state of expectancy). In this state, physical changes in the brain and body occur that have a quieting effect; heart rate slows, and electrical activity in the brain is reduced. Subjectively, the person feels calm as he or she tries to avoid any stray thoughts. Although total brain activity decreases, activity in the right frontal and right parietal areas increases; these areas may be part of a network responsible for maintaining the alert state. As activation in the right prefrontal and right parietal regions increases, the anterior cingulate region for target detection quiets. In tasks in which a person needs to suspend activity while waiting for infrequent signals, it is important not to carry out any mental activity that might interfere with detecting an external event.

The vigilance network affects activity in both the executive attention network and the covert visual orienting network. During the vigilant state, the orienting system is tuned so that it acts faster. Thus, in highly alert states, response time is reduced.

It is useful to view attention as a set of networks carrying out particular functions. The interactions among the networks, however, suggest that these networks make up a single attentional system that underlies the unity of people's subjective experience of the world.

Networks of Memory

Although memory is often thought of as a single phenomenon, remembering in daily life involves multiple memory systems, each of which is dependent on different sets of neural structures and pathways. **Memory** involves the acquisition, storage, and retrieval of knowledge, and the capabilities of human memory systems for retention are highly varied, ranging from milliseconds to many decades. Additionally, the learning can be intentional or unintentional, and retrieval of information may occur in the presence or absence of awareness that something is being remembered. Thus, memory can be categorized qualitatively, on the basis of whether it is available to introspection, or temporally, depending on the time over which the retention may occur. In this section, memory systems are grouped temporally into immediate, short-term, and working memory types and qualitatively into explicit (declarative) and implicit (nondeclarative) memory types. Table 3.2 summarizes the memory functions and their neuroanatomical correlates.

Immediate, Short-Term, and Working Memory

Immediate memory (also called *sensory memory*) involves the automatic holding of ongoing sensory experiences in mind for very short periods of time (i.e., seconds or even fractions of seconds), maintaining very briefly how a stimulus looked (*iconic* or *visual sensory memory*), sounded (*echoic* or *auditory sensory memory*), or felt (*tactile* or *haptic memory*). The capacity of each sensory memory system is large because each sensory memory system is subserved by its own cortical area (i.e., visual, auditory, sensory, and motor cortices). **Short-term memory** (*active* or *primary memory*) allows the processing and temporary storage of information needed to carry out activities as diverse as understanding, learning, and reasoning for a limited amount of material to be readily accessible for a brief period of time (i.e., several seconds). Simple short-term memory does not require the rehearsal of information but can be extended

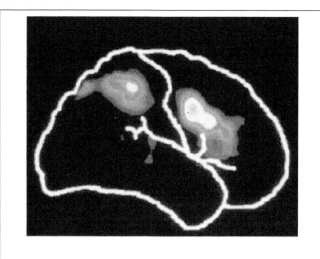

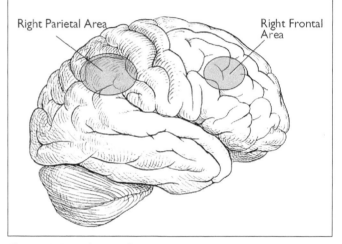

Right Parietal Area

Right Frontal Area

Figure 3.22. The vigilance network appears to maintain a sustained state of alertness. This positron emission tomography (PET) scan (top) shows activity increasing in the right frontal and right parietal lobes, the proposed sites of the vigilance network, when the person was required to maintain a state of alertness. Areas of the right parietal and right frontal lobes (bottom) may constitute a vigilance network that maintains the alert state.

Source. From *Images of Mind* (p. 176), by Michael I. Posner and Marcus E. Raichle. Copyright © 1994, 1997 by Scientific American Library. Reprinted by permission of Henry Holt and Company, LLC.

Remembering in daily life involves multiple memory systems, each of which is dependent on different sets of neural structures and pathways.

Table 3.2. Summary of Memory Systems

Immediate, Short-Term, and Working Memory

Memory Type	Duration Before Decay	Function	Neuroanatomical Components	Description
Immediate (sensory memory)	Iconic (<1 s)	Visual sensory memory	Photoreceptors of retina and visual cortex (occipital lobe)	Is not under conscious control; Awareness is present but cannot be suppressed; Fast-decaying stores of information; Allows retention of information after original stimulus is removed
	Echoic (<4 s)	Auditory sensory memory	Hair cells in inner ear and auditory cortex (superior temporal lobe)	
	Haptic and tactile (<2 s)	Proprioceptive and tactile sensory memory with subcomponents (see final section of the table)	Sensory receptors located throughout body (cutaneous and kinesthetic), primary somatosensory cortex (Harris, Miniussi, Harris, & Diamond, 2002; Zhou & Fuster, 1996), and several distinct areas of parietal lobe (Gallace & Spence, 2009) (see final section of the table)	
Short term	8–10 s, or minutes if rehearsal is used	Simple serial recall (stores 7 ± 2 items; error-free limit 3 items); exhibits temporal decay, but duration may be extended by rehearsal; chunk capacity limits (Camos & Tillmann, 2008)	Prefrontal cortex	Does not correlate with measures of intelligence or aptitude (Cowan, 2008)
Working	8–10 s, or minutes if rehearsal is used (same as short term)	Active maintenance and manipulation of limited amounts of information; function is influenced by passage of time, load, rehearsability, distraction; important to attention, language, reasoning, and problem solving	Prefrontal cortex and posterior regions of association cortex; supported by sustained activity in the brain areas that process the specific perceptual information to be retained (modality-specific cortex; e.g., recall of faces, posterior fusiform gyrus; Ranganath, 2004)	Does correlate with measures of intelligence or aptitude (Cowan, 2008); Not completely distinct from short-term memory; Used to describe both storage and processing components (Smith & Jonides, 1997)
		Phonological loop: Formation and maintenance of memories associated with verbal information (Cowan, 2008)	Frontal cortex, mostly left	
		Visuospatial sketchpad: Formation and maintenance of memories associated with visual and spatial information (Cowan, 2008)	Frontal cortex, mostly right	

Immediate, Short-Term, and Working Memory

(Continued)

Table 3.2. Summary of Memory Systems *(cont.)*

Explicit (Long-Term) Memory

Memory Type	Function	Neuroanatomical Components	Description
Episodic Medium range (0–3 yr)	Memory for events with perceptual and temporal correlates attached	MTL structures, diencephalic (anterior and medial thalamus, mammillary bodies); may be associated with time-dependent dendritic spine formation (Ranganath, 2004; Restivo, Vetere, Bontempi, & Ammassari-Teule, 2009; Squire & Wixted, 2011)	Initially responsible for all supraspan recall of ongoing events (Squire & Wixted, 2011)
Episodic Remote (>3 yr)		MTL structures and cortical areas associated with specific modalities (e.g., visual memory and calcarine cortex). Remote episodic memory may be completely dependent on cortex (the standard model) or contextually rich memories may always involve hippocampus and cortex (multiple trace theory; Nadel & Moscovitch, 1997). Consistent with the standard model, both views suggest prefrontal cortex may be important in integrating multiple cortical regions.	Very remote episodic memories may be more factlike or semantic in quality without spatial or perceptual attributes (Squire & Wixted, 2011)
Semantic	Knowledge of the world (e.g., facts, dates); general knowledge without acquisition context	MTL structures and the same neocortical areas that performed the perceptual processing and analysis at the time of learning; impaired with extensive temporal lobe damage bilaterally	Impairment in initial processing may not be separable from recall; therefore, anterior and retrograde deficits co-occur

Organized by semantic category (e.g., asymmetric ability to recognize animate vs. inanimate objects in category-specific amnesia) |

Explicit (Long-Term) Memory

(Continued)

Table 3.2. Summary of Memory Systems (*cont.*)

	Memory Type	Function	Neuroanatomical Components	Description
Implicit Memory	Perceptual priming	Object identification	Modality-specific cortex	Allows for efficient processing, decreased recognition latency, and improved accuracy when encountering a pre-experienced object or concept
	Conceptual priming	Activation of knowledge structures	Modality-specific cortex	
	Motor skills learning	Motor skills acquisition	Basal nuclei, cerebellum, frontal participation during learning and execution	Acquisition of skills through experience
	Operant conditioning	S–R (stimulus–response)	Putamen; DF cortex (pre- and postcentral); DL striatum (putamen), motor cortex	Allows the automatic initiation of behavioral sequences in the context of a sensory stimulus (Yin & Knowlton, 2006)
		A–O (action–outcome)	VL prefrontal cortex, caudate; DM striatum	Allows for the control of actions according to their anticipated outcomes Knowledge of the causal relationship between action and outcome, goal expectancy (Yin & Knowlton, 2006)
	Associative conditioning (habit learning)	Mapping of relationships established through repetitive pairings	Basal nuclei, dorsal striatum, cerebellum	Actions controlled by goals
	Habituation	Reduction in response to repetitive stimuli	Basal nuclei, cerebellum	Actions controlled by stimuli (Yin & Knowlton, 2006)
	Sensitization	Increased response to repetitive stimuli (Yin & Knowlton, 2006)	Limbic cortex, basal nuclei, cerebellum	
Haptic and Tactile Memory	Haptic and tactile	Roughness, texture, spatial discrimination of stimuli	Cutaneous mechanoreceptors, parietal operculum (Gallace & Spence, 2009)	Long-term structure is poorly understood; it is believed that memory for tactile and haptic information is located in the same areas in which initial processing takes place. Haptic memory has implicit and short-term explicit components (Gallace & Spence, 2009; Zhou & Fuster, 1996).
		Size and shape of stimuli	Cutaneous mechanoreceptors, anterior parietal lobe (Zhou & Fuster, 1996)	
		Location of stimuli	Superior parietal lobe, temporoparietal junction (Gallace & Spence, 2009)	

Note. DF = dorsofrontal; DL = dorsolateral; DM = dorsomedial; MTL = medial temporal lobe (includes the hippocampus and adjacent entorhinal, perirhinal, and parahippocampal cortices); s = second/seconds; VL = ventrolateral; yr = years.

with rehearsal. *Chunking* temporally consolidates information to create spatial or nonspatial contexts that reduce information decay and facilitate encoding. These processes associated with short-term memory occur in the prefrontal cortex.

Working memory (which conceptually overlaps with short-term memory) involves holding knowledge briefly in awareness (seconds to minutes) while it is being used to perform a specific mental operation (e.g., planning, organizing, problem solving, paying attention). Working memory is limited in both duration and capacity, and therefore the relevant information must be maintained via rehearsal. The *phonological loop* is the brain's "inner ear" and "inner voice," which allow the rehearsal of verbal information to prevent its decay, such as when repeating a phone number until the number is dialed. The *visuospatial sketchpad* is the "mind's eye," which allows the brain to visualize something and to place it into context. Working memory engages the frontal cortex, and its ability correlates with intelligence or aptitude, in contrast to short-term memory, which does not.

Explicit and Implicit Memory

Long-term memory entails the retention of information in more permanent forms of storage (i.e., days, weeks, or even a lifetime). Material in working memory can enter into long-term memory in various ways, including by conscious rehearsal or practice. Medium-term (i.e., minutes to hours to years) and long-term (i.e., decades) recall of material is subserved by two fundamental types of memory systems, **explicit memory** and **implicit memory.** These memory systems differ fundamentally in their retrieval processes and accordingly engage distinct neuroanatomical structures and pathways across different time scales (explicit) or under different conditions (implicit; Eustache & Desgranges, 2008).

Explicit memories may be retrieved automatically or through introspective processing because people "know that they know" the information that is being retrieved. In contrast, implicit memories may or may not be associated with introspective processing, and people may or may not be aware that they know the information retrieved. Explicit memory encompasses the retrieval of ***episodic memories*** (i.e., personally experienced events, specific history of what happened where and when in an autobiographical context; Tulving, 2001, 2002) and ***semantic memories*** (i.e., words, concepts, general facts and information about the world, independent of temporal and sensory personal experience and without autobiographical context; Eustache & Desgranges, 2008). *Implicit* (or *procedural*) memory is the memory of actions. It includes **priming,** motor-skill learning, cognitive skills, operant conditioning, associative conditioning, habituation, and sensitization.

The two main regions of the brain that appear to be critical to explicit memory formation are (1) the medial temporal lobe (MTL), including the hippocampus and adjacent entorhinal, perirhinal, and parahippocampal cortical areas, and (2) the medial diencephalic areas, including the thalamic **mediodorsal nucleus, anterior nucleus of the thalamus, mammillary bodies,** and other diencephalic nuclei lining the **third ventricle** (Squire & Wixted, 2011). The medial temporal and medial diencephalic memory areas are interconnected both with each other and with widespread regions of cortex by a variety of pathways, crucial for memory consolidation and retrieval (Eichenbaum, 2001; Frankland & Bontempi, 2005; Polyn, Natu, Cohen, & Norman, 2005).

The MTL seems to have a time-limited role in the storage and retrieval of explicit memories. Over time, memories gradually reorganize and become permanently stored outside the MTL. Engagement of hippocampal–cortical networks leads to gradual strengthening of cortical–cortical connections, which eventually allows memories to become independent of the hippocampus and to be gradually integrated with preexisting cortical memories (i.e., the hippocampus is a fast learner and the cortex a slow one; Frankland & Bontempi, 2005). Thus, hippocampal damage preferentially affects recent but not remote memories (Frankland & Bontempi, 2005). Most authorities view the role of the hippocampus as limited to explicit memory. However, some theorists have suggested that the hippocampus may be involved in all forms of complex, integrative memory functioning and not restricted to memories available to conscious introspection (Henke, 2010). Semantic memories are encoded with the participation of the MTL structure, are believed to be widely distributed throughout the neocortex, and are organized categorically (Polyn et al., 2005).

Implicit memory likely involves the construction of motor patterning that makes an action, behavior, or skill become increasingly automatic.

Implicit memory likely involves the construction of motor patterning that makes an action, behavior, or skill become increasingly automatic. Components of the basal nuclei support learning of the causal relationship between action and outcome and between stimulus and response across trials (i.e., instrumental behaviors or operant conditioning; Klimkowicz-Mrowiec, Slowik, Krzywoszanski, Herzog-Krzywoszanska, & Szczudlik, 2008; Knowlton, Mangels, & Squire, 1996; Simons, Schölvinck, Gilbert, Frith, & Burgess, 2006). Priming depends on several cortical areas. Simple associative learning (i.e., classical conditioning) and nonassociative learning (i.e., habituation and sensitization) appear to involve a variety of structures, including the cerebellum (in classical conditioning), **amygdala** (in conditioned fear), cerebral cortex, brainstem nuclei, and even spinal cord.

Typically, a key distinction between explicit and implicit memory is the number of trials needed for memory formation. For example, the learning of procedures, skills, and habits (implicit memory) typically requires a large number of trials, whereas explicit memory formation requires only one. An additional distinction between explicit and implicit memory is the complexity of the memory itself. For example, episodic memories are complex, involving multiple sensory systems, and therefore elements of the memory can be recalled separately. In contrast, implicit memories, although they may be complex, are typically recalled as a single unit (Henke, 2010).

Frontal Subcortical Networks

Basal Nuclei

The *basal nuclei* are a collection of subcortical masses of neuronal cell bodies located deep within the white matter of the cerebrum that modulate the output of the frontal cortex through multiple parallel circuits (Figure 3.23). They influence the activity of the cerebral cortex through their extensive connections and thus a range of functionally diverse activities, including motor control and movement, **cognition,** emotion, and motivation. The components of the basal nuclei (see Table 3.3) are (1) the *corpus striatum* ("striped body"), consisting of the **caudate nucleus** and **putamen;**

(2) the ***globus pallidus*** (GP; "pale globe") consisting of external and internal segments; (3) the ***substantia nigra*** (SN), consisting of the pars recticulata (SNpr) and pars compacta (SNpc); and (4) the ***subthalamic nucleus*** (STN). Collectively, these components of the basal nuclei are part of a complex network of multiple parallel information loops that extend from the cerebral cortex through the basal nuclei and on to the thalamus and subsequently back to the cortex. This basal nuclei circuitry modulates cortical output (see Box 3.1).

The location of the cortical starting and ending points of each loop determines their function, and the interconnections within the basal nuclei determine whether the activity is released or inhibited. The body of the caudate is separated from the putamen by the *internal capsule,* which is a collection of white matter fibers projecting to and from the cerebral cortex, but remains connected to the putamen via cellular bridges. The GP lies just medial to the putamen and has external (Gpe) and internal (Gpi) segments. The SN lies inferior to the internal capsule and has both ventral components (SNpr) and dorsal components (SNpc). The STN is located ventral and inferior to the thalamus but just above the most rostral aspect of the SN. Overall, afferents reach the basal nuclei from the cortex via the striatum and STN, and efferents leave the basal nuclei via the GP and the SN.

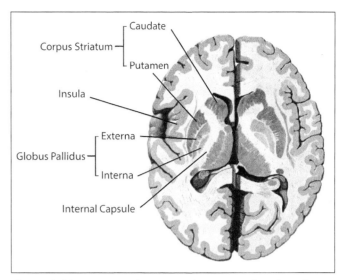

Figure 3.23. Masses of neurons known as *basal nuclei* **are located deep in the cerebrum.** Horizontal (transverse) sections reveal the components of the basal nuclei, surrounded by the white matter and including the internal capsule. The image shown demonstrates the geographical relationship of the basal nuclei to the cerebral cortex and thalamus. The components are the corpus striatum, consisting of the caudate nucleus and putamen; the globus pallidus, consisting of external and internal segments; the substantia nigra, consisting of the pars recticulata and pars compacta (not shown); and the subthalamic nucleus (not shown).

Source. From *Atlas of Human Anatomy* (5th ed., Plate 109), by F. Netter, 2011, Saunders/Elsevier. Netter illustration from http://www.netterimages.com. Copyright © Elsevier Inc. All rights reserved.

The ***prefrontal cortex*** is the anterior portion of the frontal lobe, lying just in front of the motor and premotor cortical areas. The functions of the prefrontal cortex are thought to be accomplished by a division of labor among five distinct and reciprocal subcortical networks that are involved in modulation of motor and cognitive functions in the cerebrum and share the following features: (1) They begin in the anterior frontal gray matter; (2) they have reciprocal connections primarily through the basal nuclei and thalamus; (3) each has its own direct and indirect pathways, which are not exclusive of one another; and (4) they end in the prefrontal cortex, where they began. One circuit is primarily associated with motor control and arises in the supplementary motor area. A second circuit relates primarily to oculomotor control and arises in the frontal eye fields. The remaining three circuits relate to executive control, behavioral inhibition, and skill development (Bonelli & Cummings, 2008; Cummings, 1993; see Tables 3.4 and 3.5).

The dorsolateral prefrontal system is primarily associated with organization, executive planning, and executive attention (Figure 3.24). The orbitofrontal system is primarily associated with response inhibition, reward, and the mediation of empathy and socially appropriate behavior (Figure 3.25). The anterior cingulate system is associated with motivation, error correction, and arousal (Figure 3.26). In general, most cortical areas project afferents to the striatum, which subsequently

Table 3.3. Functions of the Basal Nuclei

Component Nuclei	Summary of Functions
Corpus striatum	The major input zone of the basal nuclei; it receives excitatory (glutamate) inputs from large areas of the cerebral cortex, substantia nigra, and thalamus.
Caudate	The medial part of the striatum, connected with prefrontal and other association areas of cortex. Involved primarily in cognitive functions and less directly in movement.
Putamen	The lateral part of the striatum, involved most prominently in the motor functions of the basal nuclei. Receives input from the primary somatosensory and somatomotor areas of the cortex and from the substantia nigra. The putamen projects output to the globus pallidus, which in turn projects to the premotor and supplementary motor areas via the thalamus.
Globus pallidus	Main output from the basal nuclei; relays information from the striatum to the thalamus.
Externa	Receives inputs from the striatum and sends output to the subthalamic nucleus.
Interna	Receives inputs from the striatum and subthalamic nucleus and sends inhibitory (GABA) projections to the thalamus.
Substantia nigra	Main output from the basal nuclei that sends inhibitory (GABA) projections to the thalamus.
Pars reticulata	Contains loosely arranged neurons that receive input from the striatum and subthalamic nucleus and send output to the thalamus.
Pars compacta	Contains closely packed, pigmented dopaminergic neurons that send their output to the striatum.
Subthalamic nucleus	Located ventral and inferior to the thalamus. Receives input from the striatum as part of the indirect pathway and participates in modulation of motor behavior by sending excitatory (glutamate) inputs to the global pallidus interna or substantia nigra pars reticulata and ultimately the thalamus.

Note. GABA = γ-aminobutyric acid.

funnels them down through the GP and SN and on to the thalamus from which they are then redirected in a loop back to the frontal lobes.

Arterial Supply of the Brain

The vertebral arteries and the internal carotid arteries supply the brain with freshly oxygenated blood (Figure 3.27). The right and left vertebral arteries enter the cranium through the **foramen magnum** and join to form the **basilar artery,** which lies on the anterior surface of the brainstem. This *vertebral–basilar system* constitutes the posterior circulation of the brain and supplies the brainstem and cerebellum, along with the occipital lobe and parts of the parietal and temporal lobes. The internal carotid arteries enter the skull through the **carotid canals** of the temporal bones and emerge into the **middle cranial fossa.** The internal carotid arteries provide blood to anterior brain structures as the anterior circulation of the brain. The right internal carotid supplies the right parietal, temporal, and frontal lobes, and the left internal carotid supplies the parallel structures on the left.

The anterior and posterior circulations meet in an anastomotic ring surrounding the hypothalamus known as the *Circle of Willis* (Figure 3.28). Although the communicating arteries connecting the circle can provide an opportunity for collateral flow among the three arteries, these arteries are fairly small and not capable of carrying much blood; therefore, their effect, if any, may be limited to slowly developing **occlusions.** However, a complete ring is estimated to be present in

Box 3.1. Pathways of the Frontal Subcortical Circuits

Inputs to the basal nuclei arrive via the striatum or the subthalamic nucleus, and outputs leave via the internal segment of the globus pallidus interna (GPi), the closely related substantia nigra pars reticulata (SNpr), or both. Within the basal nuclei are a variety of complex excitatory and inhibitory connections that enable the organism to fine-tune behavior control and mediate learning. Also within the nuclei are several parallel pathways for different functions, including general motor control, eye movements, and cognitive and emotional functions. Inputs from major cortical regions are received by the striatum and subsequently directed to the basal nuclei via one of four distinct pathways: (1) *direct,* (2) *indirect,* (3) *subthalamic,* and (4) *striosomal.* These distinct pathways enable the organism to tailor activity to environmental circumstances and to base behavior on assessment of outcome and reward.

Cortical projections into the striatum are topographically oriented, but multiple cortical neurons terminate on a far more limited number of striatal neurons (i.e., the input compression ratio is high), leading to a considerable reduction in specificity. Certain regions of cerebral cortex may project to more than one region of the striatum, supporting functional integration. Both the regional integration and the reduction from many to few neurons support response pattern formation. Similarities between different patterns of inputs allow for importantly similar events and circumstances to be responded to in the same way. In this way, the same adaptive behavior can occur in the context of different but similar stimulus situations.

Outputs from the basal nuclei arise from the internal segment of the GPi and from the SNpr. Neurons in the GPi have a very high spontaneous firing rate, such that this region is tonically active. The tonic activity in the GPi inhibits activity in the thalamus, preventing the thalamus from activating the downstream cortical neurons to which it connects. Therefore, the basal nuclei can be viewed as inhibiting cortical responsiveness in their normal state. By activating the striatum, cortical activity inhibits the activity in the GPi (which otherwise acts to inhibit thalamic activity), allowing the thalamus to release behavior mediated by the cortex.

Both the direct and the indirect pathways are excitatory in their connections from the cortex to the striatum but ultimately differ in their effects on the GPi or SNpr, the main outputs from the basal nuclei. Thus, these pathways ultimately differ in their ability to activate or inhibit basal nuclei–mediated cortical motor areas. The direct pathway travels from the striatum directly to the GPi or SNpr. The indirect pathway takes a detour from the striatum first to the external segment of the globus pallidus and then to the subthalamic nucleus (STN) before finally reaching the GPi or the SNpr, from which all outputs exit the basal nuclei. The net effect of excitatory input from the cortex via the direct pathway will be excitation of the thalamus, which will in turn facilitate behavior through its cortical connections. In contrast, the net effect of excitation of the indirect pathway will be inhibition of the thalamus, resulting in inhibition of behavior through its connections with the cortex. The two pathways are believed to operate in opposite directions but in balance. Activation of the direct pathway causes the GPi to release inhibition on the thalamus and thus to ultimately enable release behavior of wanted actions. In contrast, activation of the indirect pathway causes the STN to activate the GPi, which suppresses thalamic activity, preventing release behavior, and thus ultimately inhibits closely related but unwanted actions.

The subthalamic pathway connects cortical regions directly to the STN. The striosomal pathway connects certain regions of the cortex to "islands" of neurons or *striosomes* (hence, *striosomal*) to the substantia nigra via the putamen. These pathways operate at a much faster rate because they have fewer synapses. When the subthalamic or "hyperdirect" pathway is active, it suppresses all behavior and thus enables the organism to not respond. When the striosomal pathway is active, it allows information about rewards and behavioral states to be integrated with information about behavioral control. The interaction between cortical and subcortical structures in some ways mirrors the integration of automatic with higher-order control. Because most behaviors involve some level of automatic responsiveness but may from time to time require adaptation or change because of different circumstances, it is possible to see how cortically mediated adaptation and subcortically mediated automatic behaviors can interact to facilitate the accomplishment of adaptive behaviors in a person.

only approximately 25% of the population. Contrast angiograms of cerebral arteries confirm that the brain has three separate arterial circulations and that little mixing of blood occurs among the three. Thus, half of the cerebrum can be rendered unconscious with the use of anesthesia so that the functions of the other half can be examined.

The major arteries that supply the brain arise from the Circle of Willis (Figure 3.28). The arterial supply to the brain differs from that of many other organs in that rather

Table 3.4. Frontal Subcortical Circuits Involved With Behavior Control

Frontal Subcortical Circuit	Dorsolateral Prefrontal System		Orbitofrontal System		Anterior Cingulate System	
Neuronal groups	1. Brodmann's areas 9, 10 (DL) 2. DL caudate 3. DM globus pallidus; substantia nigra 4. VA & DM thalamic nuclei		1. Brodmann's areas 10 (IM), 11 2. VM caudate 3. DM globus pallidus; substantia nigra 4. VA & DM thalamic nuclei		1. Brodmann's area 24 2. Ventral striatum (VM caudate, ventral putamen, nucleus accumbens, olfactory tubercle) 3. RM & V globus pallidus 4. DM thalamic nuclei	
Circuit-specific behaviors	Organization, executive planning, attention		Inhibition, reward; mediates socially appropriate behavior & empathy		Motivated behavior, error correction, wakefulness, arousal	
Cognitive & behavioral abnormalities associated with pathology	Executive dysfunction; poor planning; inability to generate hypotheses; inability to change tasks, filter environmental distractions, or organize or plan		Disinhibition, impulsivity, tactlessness, inability to shift responses		Impaired motivation (abulia), apathy, reduced creative thought, poor response inhibition, impaired emotional display	
Vascular supply (rostral to caudal)	DL caudate	MCA (lenticulostriate aa.)	VM caudate	ACA (Heubner's a.)	Caudate nucleus: accumbens ventral striatum	ACA (Heubner's a. & penetrating aa.)
	Internal capsule (inferior-medial head of caudate)	ACA (Heubner's a.)	Internal capsule (inferior-medial head of caudate)	ACA (Heubner's a.)	Internal capsule (inferior-medial head of caudate)	ACA (Heubner's a.)
	Internal capsule: inferior genu	ACA (Heubner's a.)	Caudate: entire head	ACA & MCA (penetrating aa.)	Caudate: entire head	ACA & MCA (penetrating aa.)
	Caudate: entire head	ACA & MCA (penetrating aa.)	V & VA thalamus	Posterior communicating (tuberothalamic a.)		
	Globus pallidus	MCA (lenticulostriate aa.) ACA (ant. choroidal a.)	DM thalamus	Posterior communicating (paramedian aa.)	Globus pallidus	MCA (lenticulostriate aa.) ACA (ant. choroidal a.)
	V & VA thalamus	Posterior communicating (tuberothalamic a.)			DM thalamus	Posterior communicating (paramedian aa.)
	DM thalamus	Posterior communicating (paramedian aa.)			DM thalamus & mammillothalamic tracts	ICA (paramedian a.)
	DM thalamus & mammillo-thalamic tracts	ICA (paramedian a.)				

Note. a. = arteria (artery); aa. = arteriae (arteries); ACA = anterior cerebral artery; ant. = anterior; DL = dorsolateral; DM = dorsomedial; ICA = internal carotid artery; IM = inferomedial; MCA = middle cerebral artery; MD = medial dorsal; PCA = posterior cerebral artery; RM = rostromedial; V = ventral nucleus; VA = ventral anterior; VM = ventromedial.

Table 3.5. Basal Nuclei Circuitry

	Direct Pathway	Indirect Pathway	Subthalamic	Striosomal
Role	*Cortical input into striatum:* Initiation of action; establishing adaptive patterns; releases behavior or movement	*Cortical input into striatum:* "Braking"; switching from one action to the next; inhibits closely related unwanted behavior or movement	*"Hyperdirect pathway":* Response inhibition; enables nonresponse; suppresses all behavior; stops response faster than indirect pathway owing to fewer synapses	Allows for evaluation of information for reward; influences similar behavior in the future; instrumental learning
Overall circuitry	Cortex → striatum → pallidus → thalamus → cortical motor areas	Cortex → striatum → pallidus → thalamus → cortical motor areas	Cortex → subthalamic nucleus → pallidus or substantia nigra → thalamus → cortical motor areas	Cortex → striatum → pallidus → cortical motor areas
Effects of cortical input to the basal nuclei	Cortex activates striatum	Cortex activates striatum	Cortex activates subthalamic nucleus	Cortex activates putamen
Specific route through the basal nuclei	1. Cortex ↓ 2. striatum ↓ 3. GPi/SNpr ↓ 4. thalamus ↓ 5. cortical motor areas	1. Cortex ↓ 2. striatum ↓ 3. GPe ↓ 4. STN ↓ 5. GPi, SNpr ↓ 6. thalamus ↓ 7. cortical motor areas	1. Cortex ↓ 2. STN ↓ 3. GPi or SNpr ↓ 4. thalamus ↓ 5. cortical motor areas	1. Cortex ↓ 2. putamen ↓ 3. SNpc/SNpr ↓ 4. back through basal nuclei
Effects of basal nuclei (GPi, SNpr) on thalamus	Excitatory	Inhibitory	Inhibitory	No direct involvement with thalamus
Effects of thalamus on cortex	Thalamus activated. Results in release of behavior; releases inhibition of cortex; cortex activated	Thalamus not activated. Results in suppression of behavior; cortex not activated	Thalamus not activated. Results in suppression of behavior; cortex not activated	No direct connection. Evaluation of reward influences future behavior
Summary of activity	Active when required, depending on the circumstances or needs of the organism; allows wanted behavior	Active when required, depending on the circumstances or needs of the organism; inhibits unwanted behavior	Allows person to think before responding; therefore, important in impulse control	Assessment of the value of behavior for the organism; allows instrumental learning

Note. Green type = excitatory, activation via glutamate; red type = inhibitory, inactivation via γ-aminobutyric acid; GPe = globus pallidus externa; GPi = globus pallidus interna; SNpc = substantia nigra pars compacta; SNpr = substantia nigra pars reticulata; STN = subthalamic nuclei.

than penetrating the brain, the arteries remain on the surface. Penetrating arteries branch at right angles from the surface vessels to support deeper brain structures.

The **anterior cerebral artery** (ACA) from each side sweeps across the medial surface of the hemisphere in the longitudinal fissure, supplying the medial surface of the frontal and anterior parietal lobes (Figure 3.29). The **middle cerebral artery** (MCA) turns laterally and enters the lateral sulcus (Sylvian fissure; Figure 3.30). The MCA bifurcates into a *superior division* (shown but not labeled), which provides blood to the lateral surface of the frontal and anterior parietal lobes, and an *inferior division* (shown but not labeled), which supplies the superior

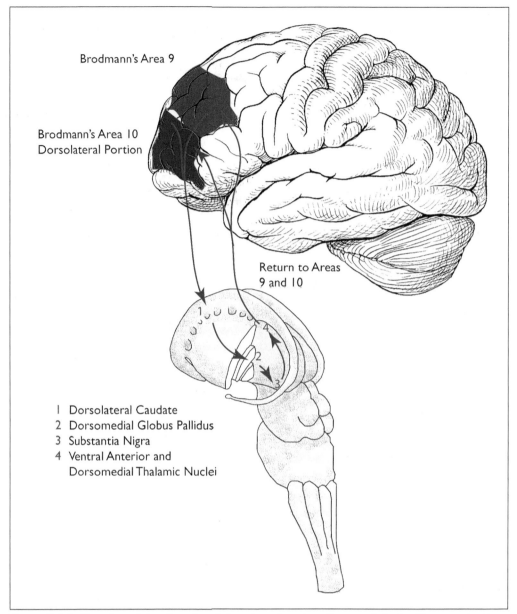

Figure 3.24. The dorsolateral prefrontal system is primarily associated with organization, executive planning, and executive attention.

Source. F. Feuchter.

part of the temporal lobe. Early branches of the MCA, known as *lenticulostriate arteries,* penetrate deeply and supply the basal nuclei and internal capsule (Figure 3.31). These small arteries are the most common site for a stroke. Although the lenticulostriate arteries are small, an occlusion of a lenticulostriate artery can be devastating because of the strategic importance of the internal capsule, which is like a funnel through which all sensory and motor information on one side of the head and body is routed.

The basilar artery ends by dividing into the two (left and right) **posterior cerebral arteries** (PCA). The PCA supplies the inferior portions of the temporal lobe

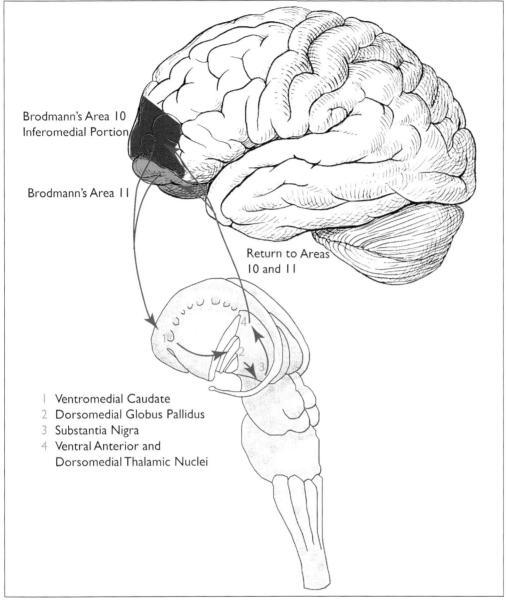

Brodmann's Area 10
Inferomedial Portion

Brodmann's Area 11

Return to Areas
10 and 11

1 Ventromedial Caudate
2 Dorsomedial Globus Pallidus
3 Substantia Nigra
4 Ventral Anterior and
   Dorsomedial Thalamic Nuclei

Figure 3.25. The orbitofrontal system is primarily associated with response inhibition, reward, and the mediation of empathy and socially appropriate behavior.

Source. F. Feuchter.

and all of the occipital lobe. The basilar and vertebral arteries have branches that supply regions of the brainstem and cerebellum (Figure 3.32).

Disruption of the arterial supply to an area of the brain by any of these cerebral arteries for more than a few minutes will result in a stroke, or death of the neural tissue as a result of a lack of oxygen consequential to the reduced blood flow. Strokes can result from several factors that disrupt blood flow to the brain, including (1) atherosclerotic build-up and blockage (thrombotic; 50% of all strokes), (2) blockage from a dislodged mass or embolus traveling in the bloodstream (embolic; 30% of all strokes), or (3) via bleeding out from a ruptured vessel (hemorrhagic; 20% of all strokes). Because the major cerebral arteries have consistent distributions, strokes

Disruption of the arterial supply to an area of the brain by any of these cerebral arteries for more than a few minutes will result in a stroke, or death of the neural tissue as a result of a lack of oxygen consequential to the reduced blood flow.

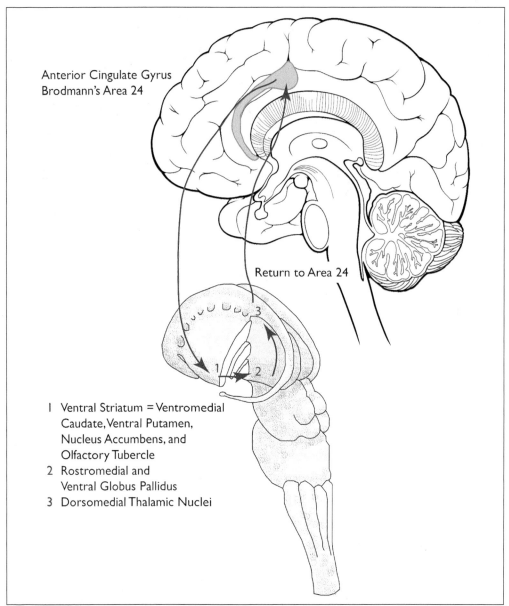

Figure 3.26. The anterior cingulate system is associated with motivation, error correction, and arousal.

Source. F. Feuchter.

involving particular arteries will produce a distinctive spectrum of clinical signs and symptoms (see Table 3.6).

The brain is particularly susceptible to deprivation of its blood supply because the arteries that branch off the Circle of Willis are end arteries and have few, if any, anastomotic connections with each other (watershed areas). Occlusion of any branch deprives a specific region of its blood supply and produces deficits related to the functions of that area. The primary motor and sensory cortices can be mapped relative to the portion of the body controlled by each region (Figure 3.33). The **somatotopic map** indicates that the lateral surface of the cerebrum (primary

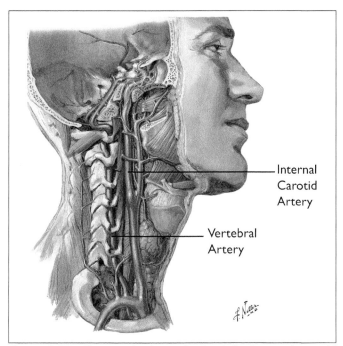

Figure 3.27. The vertebral arteries and the internal carotid arteries supply the brain with blood. The vertebral arteries extend through the foramen magnum and join to form the basilar artery, which lies on the anterior surface of the brainstem.

Source. From *Atlas of Human Anatomy* (5th ed., Plate 135), by F. Netter, 2011, Philadelphia: Saunders/Elsevier. Netter illustration from http://www.netterimages.com. Copyright © Elsevier Inc. All rights reserved.

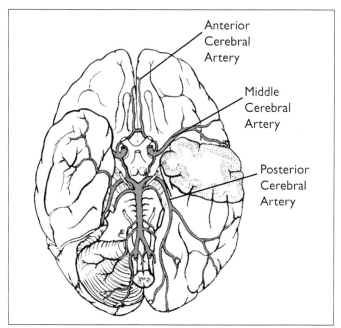

Figure 3.28. The Circle of Willis, in which the anterior and posterior circulations meet in an anastomotic ring surrounding the hypothalamus.

Source. F. Feuchter.

motor and sensory cortices) is related to the contralateral upper half of the body and the medial surface of the hemisphere is related to the contralateral lower half of the body. Therefore, blockage of the MCA could produce sensory and motor loss (*hemianesthesia* and *hemiplegia,* respectively) on the contralateral upper limb, upper body, and face. In addition, occlusion of the MCA proximal to the lenticulostriate arteries, or occlusion of the lenticulostriate arteries themselves, may cause hemiplegia and sensory loss over the entire contralateral half of the body and head. These vessels supply the internal capsule, which conveys motor fibers from the entire hemisphere and sensory fibers from all of half of the body and head. In contrast, blockage of the ACA could produce sensory and motor loss on the contralateral lower body and limb.

The PCA supplies the primary visual cortex in the occipital lobe, and infarcts of the PCA most frequently cause visual deficits. Like the motor and sensory systems, the visual system is linked to the contralateral side, but not in the same way. The right and left visual cortices each receive information about the content of the contralateral visual

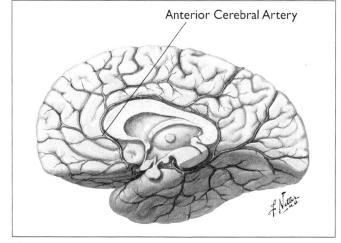

Figure 3.29. The anterior cerebral artery from each side crosses the medial surface of the hemisphere in the longitudinal fissure and supplies the medial surface of the frontal and anterior parietal lobes.

Source. From *Atlas of Human Anatomy* (5th ed., Plate 140), by F. Netter, 2011, Philadelphia: Saunders/Elsevier. Netter illustration from www.netterimages.com. Copyright © Elsevier Inc. All rights reserved.

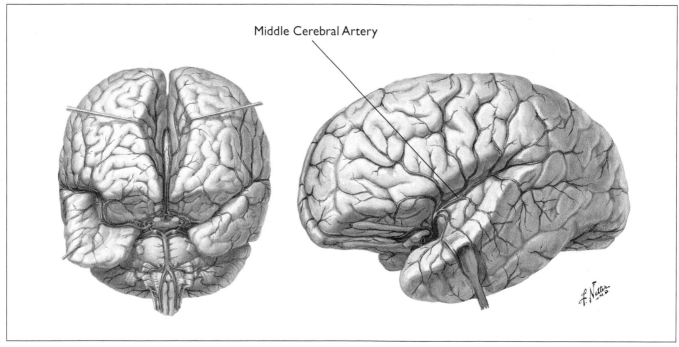

Middle Cerebral Artery

Figure 3.30. The middle cerebral artery turns laterally and enters the lateral fissure.

Source. From *Atlas of Human Anatomy* (5th ed., Plates 139, 140), by F. Netter, 2011, Philadelphia: Saunders/Elsevier. Netter illustration from http://www. netterimages.com. Copyright © Elsevier Inc. All rights reserved.

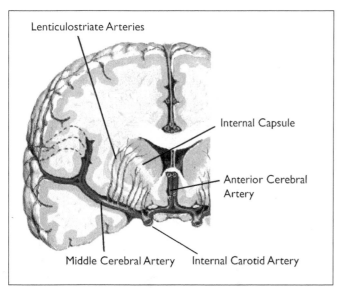

Lenticulostriate Arteries

Internal Capsule

Anterior Cerebral Artery

Middle Cerebral Artery   Internal Carotid Artery

Figure 3.31. Vascular supply to the deep structures of the brain. The coronal (frontal) section of the brain shows the lenticulostriate arteries that arise from the middle cerebral artery and penetrate the brain to supply the basal nuclei and the internal capsule. Because of the importance of these deep cerebral structures, damage to the small lenticulostriate arteries can result in neurological deficits that appear out of proportion to the arteries' size.

Source. From *Atlas of Human Anatomy* (5th ed., Plate 139), by F. Netter, 2011, Philadelphia: Saunders/Elsevier. Netter illustration from http://www. netterimages.com. Copyright © Elsevier Inc. All rights reserved.

field from each eye. In other words, the right primary visual cortex receives information from the left half of the visual field of both the right and the left eyes. Therefore, loss of the PCA will result not in blindness in one eye but in an identical loss of half of the visual field in each eye (i.e., *homonymous hemianopsia*).

The second most common site for stroke in the brain is the **posterior inferior cerebellar artery** (PICA) in the vertebral–basilar system. The PICA supplies the lateral medulla and much of the inferior portion of the cerebellum, and people experiencing PICA stroke therefore exhibit both cerebellar signs (i.e., **ataxia, dysmetria**) and lateral medullary signs (i.e., nausea, dizziness, facial numbness, **dysarthria,** and **dysphagia**).

Microinfarcts are defined as microscopic regions of cellular death or tissue necrosis that may develop a fluid-filled cavity and range in size from 0.2 to 2.9 mm (typically, however, they range in size from 0.2 to 1.0 mm, which is below the resolution of conventional MRI). Microinfarcts have increasingly been recognized as being associated with loss of cognitive ability (Smith, Schneider, Wardlaw, & Greenberg,

2012). The actual mechanisms by which microinfarcts cause cognitive impairment are not well understood but may be the result of diffuse hypoperfusion, hypoxia, oxidative stress, and inflammation, particularly in the watershed areas of the tertiary association cortex (Damasceno, 2012).

Arteriosclerosis involves thickening and narrowing of the arteries leading to hypoperfusion and loss of brain tissue. *Binswanger's disease,* also called *subcortical arteriosclerotic encephalopathy,* is the name given to a clinicopathological condition associated with **hypertension** and lacunar infarctions. The symptoms associated with Binswanger's disease are related to damage in subcortical white matter and the disruption of frontal subcortical circuits and result in executive dysfunction, psychomotor slowness, forgetfulness, gait disturbance with frequent falls, other difficulties with motor control, changes in personality or mood (most likely in the form of **apathy,** irritability, and depression), and urinary incontinence (Ogata, 1999). Onset is between ages 44 and 75 years (Ogata, 1999).

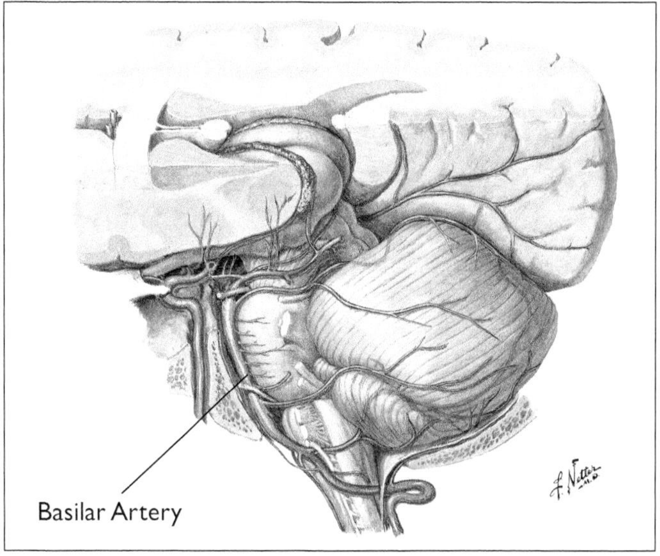

Basilar Artery

Figure 3.32. The basilar artery ends by dividing into two posterior cerebral arteries, which supply the inferior portions of the temporal lobe and all of the occipital lobe. The basilar and vertebral arteries have branches that supply regions of the brainstem and cerebellum.

Source. From *Atlas of Human Anatomy* (5th ed., Plate 141), by F. Netter, 2011, Philadelphia: Saunders/Elsevier. Netter illustration from http://www.netterimages.com. Copyright © Elsevier Inc. All rights reserved.

In cerebral amyloid angiopathy, beta-amyloid deposits develop in the blood vessel walls, weakening them and making them prone to rupture, causing hemorrhagic stroke. Cerebral amyloid angiopathy may occur in the presence or absence of **Alzheimer's disease** and may partially account for the frequent overlap of vascular major neurocognitive disorder (previously termed *vascular dementia*) and major neurocognitive disorder due to Alzheimer's disease. Risk factors for **vascular neurocognitive disorder** are similar to those for stroke and include increasing age, high blood pressure, diabetes, smoking, obesity, excessive alcohol consumption, and high cholesterol.

Conclusion

Neurons are dependent on their arterial supply, and diminution of blood flow can result in loss of function in the area with decreased perfusion. The brain is particularly vulnerable to an interruption in blood supply because it is supplied by end arteries with few, if any, anastomotic connections. Pathologies that obstruct blood flow can occur in major vessels, such as a clot in the MCA, and produce motor, sensory, and neurocognitive deficits. Microscopic damage may be present in slowly progressing occlusion, such as arteriosclerosis, particularly in watershed areas, in which multiple foci of microinfarcts may be present. Other diseases, such as cerebral amyloid angiopathy, may cause weakening of vessels and make them susceptible to rupture. Whatever the process, insufficient blood supply to brain regions leads to loss of neuronal function, and the function that is lost depends on the specific brain region or pathway affected.

Table 3.6. Arterial Supply, Major Clinical Consequences, and Frequency of Stroke

	Anterior Cerebral Artery	Middle Cerebral Artery	Posterior Cerebral Artery
Anatomical distribution	The most anterior terminal branch of the internal carotid artery; supplies most of the superior and medial aspects of the cerebral hemisphere (frontal and parietal lobes).	The posterior terminal branch of the internal carotid artery that supplies most of the lateral aspects of the cerebral hemisphere (frontal, parietal, and temporal lobes); also supplies the insula, basal nuclei, and most of the internal capsule.	Arises from the bifurcation of the basilar artery at the level of the midbrain; forms the posterior aspect of the Circle of Willis and supplies all of the occipital lobe, as well as most of the inferior aspect of the cerebral hemisphere (inferior and medial temporal lobe). Supplies most of the deep structures of the brain, including midbrain, thalamus, and the posterior portion of the internal capsule.
Frequency of stroke affecting cerebrum	<2%–3%; frequency reduced possibly because of collateral circulation provided by anterior communicating artery	≥70%; most common at least in part because of its expansive territory	5%–10%
Possible spectrum of clinical presentations	• Weakness characteristic of upper motor neuron damage and sensory-loss patterns that reflect cortical anatomical distributions • Variable frontal lobe dysfunction, depending on size of infarct • **Contralateral hemianesthesia and contralateral hemiplegia (leg > face and arm)** • Urinary incontinence • Grasp reflex, impaired judgment, flat affect, apraxia, abulia • Damage to supplementary motor area and other regions of the frontal lobe sometimes leads to "alien hand syndrome," characterized by involuntary and semiautomatic movements of contralateral arm.	• Weakness characteristic of upper motor neuron damage and sensory-loss patterns that reflect cortical anatomical distributions • **Contralateral hemianesthesia and contralateral hemiplegia (face and arm > leg)** • Wernicke's aphasia (if occurring in dominant hemisphere) • Hemineglect and apraxia (if occurring in nondominant hemisphere) • Visual field deficits; contralateral homonymous hemianopsia • Large infarcts often associated with marked visual neglect	• **Often associated with occipital cortex** • **Visual field deficits; contralateral homonymous hemianopsia** • Small infarcts may cause smaller homonymous visual field defects. • Contralateral hemianesthesia and contralateral hemiparesis • Involvement of smaller penetrating vessels leading to infarcts in the thalamus or posterior limb of the internal capsule, causing aphasia

Note. **Bold** text indicates the symptoms most frequently encountered and the most specific signs and symptoms associated with the anatomical distribution.

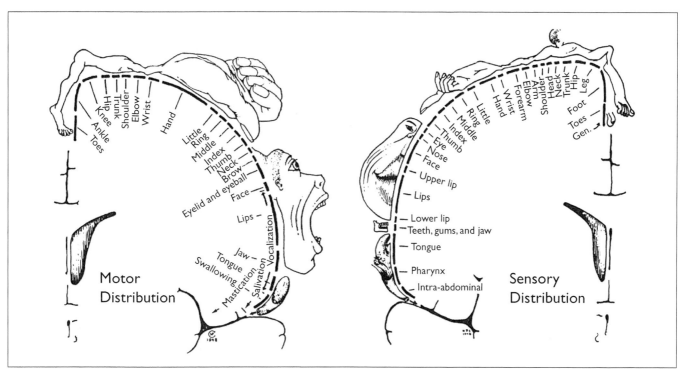

Figure 3.33. The somatotopic map illustrating the proportion of cerebral surface area devoted to motor (left) and sensory (right) functions on the lateral and medial cerebral surfaces.

Source. From *The Human Brain* (3rd ed., p. 308), by J. Nolte, 1993, St. Louis: Mosby. Copyright © 1993 by Elsevier. Used with permission.

References

Bach-y-Rita, P. (1995). *Nonsynaptic diffusion neurotransmission and late brain reorganization.* New York: Demos Medical.

Bonelli, R. M., & Cummings, J. L. (2008). Frontal–subcortical dementias. *Neurologist, 14,* 100–107. http://dx.doi.org/10.1097/NRL.0b013e31815b0de2

Camos, V., & Tillmann, B. (2008). Discontinuity in the enumeration of sequentially presented auditory and visual stimuli. *Cognition, 107,* 1135–1143. http://dx.doi.org/10.1016/j.cognition.2007.11.002

Cowan, N. (2008). What are the differences between long-term, short-term, and working memory? *Progress in Brain Research, 169,* 323–338. http://dx.doi.org/10.1016/S0079-6123(07)00020-9

Cummings, J. L. (1993). Frontal–subcortical circuits and human behavior. *Archives of Neurology, 50,* 873–880. http://dx.doi.org/10.1001/archneur.1993.00540080076020

Damasceno, B. P. (2012). Relationship between cortical microinfarcts and cognitive impairment in Alzheimer's disease. *Dementia and Neuropsychologia, 6,* 131–136.

Eichenbaum, H. (2001). The hippocampus and declarative memory: Cognitive mechanisms and neural codes. *Behavioural Brain Research, 127,* 199–207. http://dx.doi.org/10.1016/S0166-4328(01)00365-5

Eustache, F., & Desgranges, B. (2008). MNESIS: Towards the integration of current multisystem models of memory. *Neuropsychology Review, 18,* 53–69. http://dx.doi.org/10.1007/s11065-008-9052-3

Frankland, P. W., & Bontempi, B. (2005). The organization of recent and remote memories. *Nature Reviews Neuroscience, 6,* 119–130. http://dx.doi.org/10.1038/nrn1607

Gallace, A., & Spence, C. (2009). The cognitive and neural correlates of tactile memory. *Psychological Bulletin, 135,* 380–406. http://dx.doi.org/10.1037/a0015325

Geschwind, N. (1979). Specializations of the human brain. *Scientific American, 241,* 180–199. http://dx. doi.org/10.1038/scientificamerican0979-180

Harris, J. A., Miniussi, C., Harris, I. M., & Diamond, M. E. (2002). Transient storage of a tactile memory trace in primary somatosensory cortex. *Journal of Neuroscience, 22,* 8720–8725.

Hellige, J. B. (1996). Hemispheric asymmetry for visual information processing. *Acta Neurobiologiae Experimentalis, 56*, 485–497.

Henke, K. (2010). A model for memory systems based on processing modes rather than consciousness. *Nature Reviews Neuroscience, 11*, 523–532. http://dx.doi.org/10.1038/nrn2850

Kéïta, L., Bedoin, N., Burack, J. A., & Lepore, F. (2014). Switching between global and local levels: The level repetition effect and its hemispheric asymmetry. *Frontiers in Psychology, 5*, 1–9. http://dx.doi.org/10.3389/fpsyg.2014.00252

Kinsella, G., & Ford, B. (1980). Acute recovery from patterns in stroke patients: Neuropsychological factors. *Medical Journal of Australia, 2*, 663–666.

Klimkowicz-Mrowiec, A., Slowik, A., Krzywoszanski, L., Herzog-Krzywoszanska, R., & Szczudlik, A. (2008). Severity of explicit memory impairment due to Alzheimer's disease improves effectiveness of implicit learning. *Journal of Neurology, 255*, 502–509. http://dx.doi.org/10.1007/s00415-008-0717-x

Knowlton, B. J., Mangels, J. A., & Squire, L. R. (1996). A neostriatal habit learning system in humans. *Science, 273*, 1399–1402. http://dx. doi.org/10.1126/science.273.5280.1399

Mountcastle, V. B. (1998). *Perceptual neuroscience: The cerebral cortex*. Cambridge, MA: Harvard University Press.

Nadel, L., & Moscovitch, M. (1997). Memory consolidation, retrograde amnesia, and the hippocampal complex. *Current Opinion in Neurobiology, 7*, 217–227. http://dx.doi.org/10.1016/S0959-4388(97)80010-4

Nolte, J. (1993). *The human brain* (3rd ed.). St. Louis: Mosby.

Nolte, J. (2002). *The human brain* (5th ed.). St. Louis: Mosby.

Ogata, J. (1999). Vascular dementia: The role of changes in the vessels. *Alzheimer Disease and Associated Disorders, 13*(Suppl. 3), S55–S58.

Orfei, M. D., Robinson, R. G., Prigatano, G. P., Starkstein, S., Rusch, N., Bria, P., . . . Spalletta, G. (2007). Anosognosia for hemiplegia after stroke is a multifaceted phenomenon: A systematic review of the literature. *Brain, 130*, 3075–3090. http://dx.doi.org/10.1093/brain/awm106

Polyn, S. M., Natu, V. S., Cohen, J. D., & Norman, K. A. (2005). Category-specific cortical activity precedes retrieval during memory search. *Science, 310*, 1963–1966. http://dx.doi.org/10.1126/science.1117645

Posner, M. I., & Petersen, S. E. (1990). The attention system of the human brain. *Annual Review of Neuroscience, 13*, 25–42. http://dx.doi.org/10.1146/annurev.ne.13.030190.000325

Posner, M. I., & Raichle, M. E. (1997). *Images of mind*. New York: Henry Holt.

Purves, D., & Augustine, G. J. (2004). *Neuroscience* (3rd ed.). Sunderland, CT: Sinauer Associates.

Ranganath, C. (2004). The 3-D prefrontal cortex: Hemispheric asymmetries in prefrontal activity and their relation to memory retrieval processes. *Journal of Cognitive Neuroscience, 16*, 903–907. http://dx.doi.org/10.1162/0898929041502625

Restivo, L., Vetere, G., Bontempi, B., & Ammassari-Teule, M. (2009). The formation of recent and remote memory is associated with time-dependent formation of dendritic spines in the hippocampus and anterior cingulate cortex. *Journal of Neuroscience, 29*, 8206–8214. http://dx.doi.org/10.1523/JNEUROSCI.0966-09.2009

Sharma, G., & Vijayaraghavan, S. (2001). Nicotinic cholinergic signaling in hippocampal astrocytes involves calcium-induced calcium release from intracellular stores. *Proceedings of the National Academy of Sciences of the United States of America, 98*, 4148–4153. http://dx.doi.org/10.1073/pnas.071540198

Simons, J. S., Schölvinck, M. L., Gilbert, S. J., Frith, C. D., & Burgess, P. W. (2006). Differential components of prospective memory? Evidence from fMRI. *Neuropsychologia, 44*, 1388–1397. http://dx.doi.org/10.1016/j.neuropsychologia.2006.01.005

Smith, E. E., & Jonides, J. (1997). Working memory: A view from neuroimaging. *Cognitive Psychology, 33*, 5–42. http://dx.doi.org/10.1006/cogp.1997.0658

Smith, E. E., Schneider, J. A., Wardlaw, J. M., & Greenberg, S. M. (2012). Cerebral microinfarcts: The invisible lesions. *Lancet Neurology, 11*, 272–282. http://dx.doi.org/10.1016/S1474-4422(11)70307-6

Squire, L. R., & Wixted, J. T. (2011). The cognitive neuroscience of human memory since H. M. *Annual Review of Neuroscience, 34*, 259–288. http://dx.doi.org/10.1146/annurev-neuro-061010-113720

Stahl, S. M. (2008). *Stahl's essential psychopharmachology* (3rd ed.). Cambridge, England: Cambridge University Press.

Starkstein, S. E., Fedoroff, J. P., Price, T. R., Leiguarda, R., & Robinson, R. G. (1992). Anosagnosia in patients with cerebrovascular lesions: A study of causative factors. *Stroke, 23,* 1446–1453. http://dx.doi.org/10.1161/01.STR.23.10.1446

Starkstein, S. E., & Robinson, R. G. (1989). Affective disorders and cerebral vascular disease. *British Journal of Psychiatry, 154,* 170–182. http://dx.doi.org/10.1192/bjp.154.2.170

Sterzi, R., Bottini, G., Celani, M. G., Righetti, E., Lamassa, M., Ricci, S., & Vallar, G. (1993). Hemianopia, hemianaesthesia, and hemiplegia after right and left hemisphere damage: A hemispheric difference. *Journal of Neurology, Neurosurgery, and Psychiatry, 56,* 308–310. http://dx.doi.org/10.1136/jnnp.56.3.308

Tulving, E. (2001). Episodic memory and common sense: How far apart? *Philosophical Transactions of the Royal Society of London, Series B: Biological Sciences, 356,* 1505–1515. http://dx.doi.org/10.1098/rstb.2001.0937

Tulving, E. (2002). Episodic memory: From mind to brain. *Annual Review of Psychology, 53,* 1–25. http://dx.doi.org/10.1146/annurev.psych.53.100901.135114

Ullian, E. M., Sapperstein, S. K., Christopherson, K. S., & Barres, B. A. (2001). Control of synapse number by glia. *Science, 291,* 657–661. http://dx.doi.org/10.1126/science.291.5504.657

Yin, H. H., & Knowlton, B. J. (2006). The role of the basal ganglia in habit formation. *Nature Reviews Neuroscience, 7,* 464–476. http://dx.doi.org/10.1038/nrn1919

Zhou, Y. D., & Fuster, J. M. (1996). Mnemonic neuronal activity in somatosensory cortex. *Proceedings of the National Academy of Sciences of the United States of America, 93,* 10533–10537. http://dx.doi.org/10.1073/pnas.93.19.10533

CHAPTER 4

Core Concepts in Physiological Impairment and Recovery After Stroke

Vicki Kaskutas, OTR/L, OTD, FAOTA

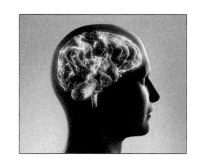

Learning Objectives

After completion of this chapter, readers will be able to

- Identify physiological issues that may occur after stroke;
- Identify physiological functions that the occupational therapist should consider after stroke, methods to assess these functions, and guidelines for vital signs;
- Identify common client comorbidities and the importance of integrating these into poststroke rehabilitation;
- Identify the activity level that provides the appropriate amount of stress to the physiological systems while allowing the poststroke client to resume meaningful daily occupations; and
- Identify methods to improve physical fitness after stroke.

Introduction

The complicated relationship between **stroke** and physiological functioning has been explored for decades, with new findings constantly emerging. The series of events leading to stroke involve physiological functions, as do the cascade of physiological issues that occur during the stroke and continue long after it. The damage to brain tissue caused by stroke results in loss of motor and sensory innervation, cognitive and perceptual functions, emotional control, and language skills. However, stroke also affects cardiac and respiratory functions. Peak oxygen consumption has been found to be reduced to half in many people poststroke in comparison to age-matched controls, making performance of even light self-care tasks exhausting (Ivey, Hafer-Macko, & Macko, 2006).

Stroke is a leading cause of disability that results in severe physical deconditioning that "propagates disability and worsens cardiovascular risk" (Ivey et al., 2006,

Key Words

- **body mass index**
- **cardiorespiratory endurance**
- **hypertension**
- **hypoglycemia**
- **isometric**
- **isotonic**
- **metabolic equivalent**
- **peak oxygen consumption**
- **rating of perceived exertion**
- **Specific Adaptation to Imposed Demand principle**

p. 439). After stroke, many young people and active Baby Boomers aspiring to return to an active lifestyle are unable to perform meaningful instrumental, **leisure,** or work activities that require more than 3 to 4 **metabolic equivalents.** As a result, return to work after stroke is often limited, with fatigue a contributing factor (Andersen, Christensen, Kirkevold, & Johnsen, 2012).

Occupational therapists must be prepared to assess, monitor, and design intervention programs to address the wide range of physiological issues encountered in clients with stroke, whether the impairments were present before the stroke or developed because of the stroke. Earlier chapters explained physiological changes in the nervous system during and after stroke. In this chapter, I explore physiological issues that are important for the occupational therapy practitioner to consider in assessment and intervention, including comorbidities, vital signs, and fitness. I present physiological guidelines that occupational therapy practitioners can use to help patients resume meaningful occupations in a safe manner while providing the "just-right" amount of stress required of the body systems (Mueller & Maluf, 2002). Occupational therapy practitioners must be equipped to address the cascade of physiological changes that occur before, during, and after stroke.

Case Study

Emma is a 58-year-old proud mother of 4 and grandmother of 12. She runs a day care center on the second floor of her home. Emma is 5 feet 9 inches tall and weighs 285 pounds. Her diabetes and hypertension have been poorly managed with oral medications for the past several years. Last fall, Emma gave up her 20-year habit of smoking one pack of cigarettes per day. Emma has a happy demeanor, but she is stressed as a result of financial problems and family turmoil. She loves to cook, and most foods she prepares are high in saturated fats. Emma struggles to carry children and supplies to the second floor because of shortness of breath and low-back pain.

Emma had a stroke 4 weeks ago and has left hemiparesis with moderate weakness in the left upper and lower extremities. She is able to walk short distances with a wide-based quad cane and can transfer from bed to chair with minimal assistance. She needs assistance to dress and bathe her lower body and wash her hair but can manage upper body and chest with standby assist. Emma fatigues easily, especially with upper-extremity activity higher than chest height and position changes. Resting heart rate is 92 beats per minute, and it increases quickly to past predicted maximum with moderate activity. She sweats and becomes short of breath quickly.

Physiological Systems Affected by Stroke

The effects of stroke on the voluntary nervous system, including decreased muscle strength, abnormal muscle **tone,** and impaired sensation, are well known to occupational therapists. Fine and gross motor coordination, balance, joint mobility, and cardiovascular endurance can be directly or indirectly affected by stroke. Occupational therapy practitioners spend much time addressing these impairments with clients after stroke; however, decreases in cardiovascular function may be neglected. Stroke also results in changes in the autonomic system, including changes in blood flow, heart rate, blood pressure, respiratory function, body temperature and sweat production, bowel and bladder control, and sexual functioning (impotence). Bladder and bowel dysfunction affect approximately 25% to 50% of stroke survivors

---

Occupational therapists must be prepared to assess, monitor, and design intervention programs to address the wide range of physiological issues encountered in clients with stroke, whether the impairments were present before the stroke or developed because of the stroke.

Points to Ponder: What Are the Physiological Concerns for Emma?

What are the physiological concerns for occupational therapy at this time? How might these physiological concerns affect Emma's occupational performance?

(Teasell, Foley, Salter, & Bhogal, 2008). **Dysphagia** occurs in 30% to 64% of the general stroke population (Martino et al., 2005).

The pathophysiology of these conditions in people with stroke is beyond the scope of this chapter; however, occupational therapy practitioners need to be alert to these changes in autonomic nervous function. In addition to the obvious task of monitoring heart rate and blood pressure after stroke and during recovery, the occupational therapy practitioner should consider the effects of these autonomic system changes on the person's ability to perform daily tasks, participate in meaningful occupations, and tolerate environmental conditions. For example, in addition to considering the strength and balance issues associated with sexual activity, the occupational therapy practitioner must consider heart rate and blood pressure (both their effect on sexual performance and the effect of sexual performance on them), ability to tolerate increased temperature and to sweat, and ability of the sexual organs to respond and function.

Premorbid Conditions

Stroke does not usually occur in isolation; the prevalence of associated medical problems is high. These conditions may predate the stroke, occur as complications after the stroke, or present as manifestations of preexisting medical conditions after stroke (Roth, 1993). The occupational therapy practitioner must know the client's medical history and understand the potential impact of all of the client's health conditions on participation in therapy and keep these in mind during treatment planning. The practitioner should also understand the numerous risk factors and integrate management of them into treatment. For example, a greater number of motor units may need to be recruited for Emma to lift her upper extremity because it is so heavy, low-back pain may limit Emma's ability to walk, and cooking may involve learning about new ways to prepare foods to limit sugars, fats, and salt. The occupational therapy practitioner will need to use a variety of treatment approaches to address these issues, including methods to restore, compensate, modify, and prevent.

Musculoskeletal Conditions

Musculoskeletal conditions are common throughout the life course, but the incidence increases with age. Twenty million people (9.3% of the adult U.S. population) are projected to report arthritis-attributable activity limitations by 2030 (Hootman & Helmick, 2006). Common musculoskeletal conditions include sprains, strains, osteoarthritis, degenerative joint disease, bulging discs, fractures, tendinitis, rheumatic conditions, plantar fasciitis, or nerve impingement. The 12-month prevalence of upper-extremity musculoskeletal disorders has been reported to be as high as 41% in some populations (Huisstede, Bierma-Zeinstra, Koes, & Verhaar, 2006). Pain is a common symptom of musculoskeletal conditions. In the general population ages 25 to 64 years, 39% of men and 45% of women report chronic musculoskeletal pain (Wijnhoven, de Vet, & Picavet, 2006).

People with stroke who have one or more of these musculoskeletal conditions may have known how to manage their symptoms before stroke through positioning, exercise, rest, splints, or activity patterns. However, after stroke these conditions may become aggravated as a result of muscular weakness, biomechanical issues, changes in movement patterns, sensory loss, or overuse. The occupational therapy practitioner needs to understand the client's musculoskeletal condition and methods used to manage it before the stroke and help the client learn how to prevent problems that will limit participation in **rehabilitation** and daily living.

Hypertension

Hypertension, increased blood pressure in the arterial system, is a common risk factor for stroke. Blood pressure must be below 120/80 to be classified as normal. According to the American Heart Association (2014), hypertension is present if systolic blood pressure is persistently at or above 140 mm Hg or diastolic pressure is at or above 90 mm Hg. Blood pressures between 120/80 and 140/90 are characterized as prehypertension; they should be regularly monitored and treatment should be instituted if readings remain in this range.

In hypertension, the heart must work harder than normal to circulate blood through the constricted artery system. Left untreated, it can lead to cardiomegaly, hypertensive heart disease, stroke, heart failure, myocardial infarction, peripheral artery disease, chronic kidney disease, and impaired vision. In Emma's case, she was medicated for hypertension, but medication was not keeping her blood pressure in the normal range. It is not unusual for more than one medication to be prescribed to control hypertension. Emma's blood pressure may have been under control at one time, but weight gain, inactivity, diet changes, or **stress** may have led to a gradual elevation of her blood pressure. Because people with hypertension rarely experience symptoms unless blood pressure is severely elevated, it is important for blood pressure to be monitored regularly. Occupational therapy practitioners should monitor blood pressure during activity performance and ensure that the Valsalva maneuver is avoided.

Cardiac Conditions

Cardiac conditions can be a risk factor for stroke and limit the ability of people with stroke to participate fully in meaningful activities and occupational roles. *Coronary heart disease* is present in more than one-third of the adult population. In coronary heart disease, atherosclerotic plaques build up in the arteries and can limit blood flow, which can lead to tissue damage in the target organ, be it the brain, heart, kidneys, eyes, or extremities. More than 795,000 people experience a *myocardial infarction* annually (American Heart Association, 2014), and the incidence of stroke increases markedly within the 1st month after myocardial infarction, especially in people who are older, female, diabetic, or hypertensive (Witt et al., 2005).

Other cardiac conditions may also be present in people with stroke, including **atrial fibrillation,** congestive heart failure, valvular heart disease, and cardiomyopathies. As with the brain, many areas of the heart are fed by only one artery, so treatment is essential to avoid life-threatening emergencies.

When working with people with stroke who have concomitant cardiac conditions, the occupational therapy practitioner should closely monitor vital signs and symptoms. If the client is on telemetry, the professionals at the monitoring station should be informed of activities that the client is performing in occupational therapy to observe for abnormal heart rhythms that can arise with certain positions, tasks, and conditions.

As with the brain, many areas of the heart are fed by only one artery, so treatment is essential to avoid life-threatening emergencies.

Diabetes Mellitus

Diabetes mellitus affects 8.5% of the U.S. adult population (Centers for Disease Control and Prevention [CDC], 2013); the incidence of both Type 1 and Type 2 diabetes is increasing. Diabetes affects the body's ability to produce insulin or respond to the insulin that is produced. Long-term diabetes can affect the circulatory system, leading to cardiovascular disease, myocardial infarction, peripheral vascular disease, and stroke. Diabetes can also affect the visual, urinary, and nervous systems. People with diabetes have an increased risk of stroke; among people who have had diabetes for 10 years or longer, the risk can be as much as 3 times as high (Banerjee et al., 2012).

Symptoms of diabetes mellitus that the occupational therapy professional should be aware of during treatment include thirst, hunger, and frequent urination. Communication and awareness problems after stroke may limit people's ability to share their symptoms; therefore, the therapist should watch for signs of low or high blood sugar. Blood glucose can change quickly as a result of changes in eating, exercise, or activity. Hypoglycemia needs to be addressed quickly by giving the person carbohydrates; loss of **consciousness** and diabetic shock can occur if left untreated. It is important that the occupational therapy professional address the person's ability to perform daily monitoring, injections and medication management, and decision making to maintain a safe level of insulin.

Metabolic Syndrome and Obesity

Currently, approximately 34% of U.S. adults meet the criteria for ***metabolic syndrome*** (CDC, 2013), a cluster of major cardiovascular risk factors related to obesity, insulin resistance, and dyslipidemia. This is an increase from 23.7% for adult men and 21.8% for adult women in 2002 (Ford, Giles, & Dietz, 2002). Metabolic syndrome affects 44% of the U.S. population older than age 50. Approximately one-third of people with obesity have metabolic syndrome.

Obesity, cardiovascular disease, and diabetes are closely associated. Excess body fat underlies 64% of cases of diabetes in men and 77% of cases in women. Currently, nearly 35% of U.S. adults and 16.9% of children are obese, defined as having a **body mass index** (BMI) of 30 or higher (American Heart Association, 2014). Obesity can affect resting and exercise heart rate, respiration rate, flexibility, **range of motion,** and aerobic endurance. As a result, fatigue may occur when performing metabolically demanding tasks such as washing hair, climbing stairs or hills, housecleaning, and participating in sports.

Residual weaknesses after stroke may make it difficult for people who are obese to perform bed mobility, self-care tasks, transfers, and ambulation because the heavy mass of the body and extremities requires high force generation. When working with clients who are obese, the occupational therapy practitioner must maintain his or her safety at all times, using additional assistance, lifting devices, and equipment designed to protect the clinician and ensure the client's safety.

Drug Abuse

Drug abuse accounts for an increasing number of strokes each year. Cocaine and amphetamines are strongly linked to stroke (Esse, Fossati-Bellani, Traylor, & Martin-Schild, 2011). Ecstasy, heroin and opiates, phencyclidine (PCP), lysergic acid diethylamide (LSD), cannabis and marijuana, performance-enhancing steroids, tobacco, and ethanol have also been found to have a relationship with stroke. Each drug has unique interactions with the brain and vasculature that predispose healthy people to ischemic or hemorrhagic stroke. Drug use may be the most common predisposing condition for stroke in people younger than age 35. In addition to dealing with the stroke, the person will most likely need to go through detoxification from the drug, which can be a painful process lasting several days. Admittance to a drug rehabilitation program may be warranted. The occupational therapy practitioner will need to call on psychosocial training to address the social and environmental issues associated with drug abuse in addition to the effects of the stroke. Treatment must be client centered, which can be difficult when the client wants to pursue habits such as drug, alcohol, and tobacco use that are detrimental to his or her health.

Measurement of Physiological Functions After Stroke

Stroke has been shown to decrease vital signs in some people. Some people who experience stroke may have abnormal vital signs as a result of comorbid conditions, lifestyle, or fitness level. The resting heart rate of an obese person with poor physical fitness will most likely be elevated, and it will increase quickly with activity. Vital signs may also be affected by medications and environmental conditions; it is therefore important to monitor vital signs frequently while the client performs activities after stroke, including before, during, immediately after, and several minutes after activity performance. Disease status and health conditions, including fever and infection, also affect vital signs, as can many other factors, such as age, drug use, altitude, distended bladder, time since eating, food, caffeine, smoking, fear, pain, sleep disturbances, and **emotions.** Table 4.1 lists normal and abnormal blood pressure categories with the corresponding pressures in millimeters of mercury; Table 4.2 lists normal and abnormal heart and respiration rates.

Drug use may be the most common predisposing condition for stroke in people younger than age 35.

Table 4.1. Blood Pressure Categories

Category	Systolic (mm Hg)		Diastolic (mm Hg)
Hypotension	<90	or	<60
Normal	<120	and	<80
Prehypertension	120–139	or	80–89
Hypertension Stage 1	140–159	or	90–99
Hypertension Stage 2	≥160	or	≥100

Source. Adapted from "Global Burden of Hypertension: Analysis of Worldwide Data," by P. M. Kearney, M. Whelton, K. Reynolds, P. Muntner, P. K. Whelton, and J. He, 2005, *Lancet, 365,* pp. 217–223.

Table 4.2. Heart and Respiration Rate Categories

Category	Heart Rate	Respiration Rate
Below normal	<60 beats/min *(bradycardia[a])*	<10 breaths/min
Normal	60–100 beats/min	10–20 breaths/min
Above normal	>100 beats/min *(tachycardia)*	>20 breaths/min

Source. From *Physical Examination and Health Assessment* (6th ed.), by C. Jarvis, 2011, Philadelphia: Saunders/Elsevier.

[a]Unless the individual is exceptionally fit or is on rate-limiting medication or heart rate is not being regulated by the sinoatrial node.

Points to Ponder: What Should the Therapist Do With Emma?

If Emma's resting blood pressure while sitting is consistently in the range of 150/100, what should the occupational therapy practitioner do?

- Perform planned housekeeping activity of cleaning the kitchen.
- Ensure that Emma has been taking her hypertension medication consistently.
- Ask Emma what she had been doing and thinking about just before the practitioner's visit.
- Leave Emma without performing any intervention.
- Retake Emma's blood pressure.
- If Emma had been resting comfortably without any emotional strain, have her call her physician to tell him or her of the blood pressure readings.

Rating of perceived exertion (RPE) is a way of measuring physical activity intensity level on the basis of a total feeling of exertion and fatigue. Although RPE is a subjective measure, a person's exertion rating may provide a fairly good estimate of the actual heart rate during physical activity (Borg, 1998). Clients rate exertion on a scale ranging from 6 to 20 with behavioral anchors describing exertion levels (6 = *no exertion at all*, 20 = *maximal exertion*). A high correlation exists between RPE and actual heart rate (RPE multiplied by 10, so RPE can be an estimate of the actual heart rate during activity; Borg, 1998). RPE is the preferred method to assess intensity in people taking medications that control heart rate.

According to Borg (1998), for a healthy person, 9 corresponds to very light exercise, which is like walking slowly at his or her own pace for some minutes; 13 corresponds to somewhat hard exercise, but the person still feels okay to continue; and 17 corresponds to very hard, or very strenuous, exercise. A healthy person can still go on but really has to push himself or herself. A rating of 19 corresponds to extremely strenuous exercise; for most people, this is the most strenuous exercise they have ever experienced.

Many standardized assessments are available to measure fatigue in people who have experienced stroke. The Multidimensional Fatigue Inventory (Smets, Garssen, Bonke, & De Haes, 1995) is a 20-question self-report survey that measures fatigue in 5 domains: (1) general fatigue, (2) physical fatigue, (3) reduced activity, (4) reduced motivation, and (5) mental fatigue. However, this scale does not result in an overall fatigue score.

The Multidimensional Assessment of Fatigue is a 16-item self-report questionnaire that measures fatigue severity, distress, and degree of interference with daily activities on a 10-point scale; it also measures frequency of and change in fatigue (Belza, Henke, Yelin, Epstein, & Gilliss, 1993). A 50-point Global Fatigue Index that ranges from *no fatigue* to *severe fatigue* is computed and can be compared with results from other studies of people with cancer, neurological and orthopedic conditions, and rheumatic and other systemic disorders.

The Fatigue Severity Scale is a 9-item self-report survey that measures interference with daily activities and fatigue severity on a 7-point scale, with higher scores suggesting greater fatigue severity (Krupp, LaRocca, Muir-Nash, & Steinberg, 1989). The Fatigue Scale for Motor and Cognitive Functions has been found to differentiate between lesion localization and subdomains of fatigue after stroke, suggesting that separate assessment of motor and cognitive fatigue should be performed after stroke

(Hubacher et al., 2012). Use of a standardized assessment of fatigue can identify people who are experiencing activity-related fatigue and measure changes in fatigue over time.

Using Physiology to Drive Activity Choice in Occupational Therapy

Activity initiated must be safe for the patient at his or her current status. Because the energy demands of tasks vary widely, the occupational therapy practitioner uses metabolic equivalents (METs) to select therapeutic activities for assessment and treatment. A *MET* represents the activity metabolic rate divided by the resting metabolic rate; it indicates the intensity of physical activities. One MET is equivalent to the consumption of 3.5 milliliters of oxygen per kilogram of body mass per minute or expending approximately 1 kilocalorie per kilogram of body weight per hour. This correlates with lying or sitting quietly; MET values range from 1 to 18 (running at 17.5 kilometers per hour or at a pace of 1 mile in 5 minutes, 31 seconds). A 3-MET activity requires 3 times the energy expenditure as being at rest. Intensity categories are broadly interpreted as *light* (<3 METs), *moderate* (3 to 6 METs), and *vigorous* (>6 METs; Pate, 1995).

Actual energy expenditure during an activity depends on the person's body mass and resting metabolic rate; therefore, the energy cost of the same activity will be different for people of different weights (Byrne, Hills, Hunter, Weinsier, & Schutz, 2005). Grooming and dressing are classified as 2.1 METs, meal preparation and cleanup as 2.32 METs, and interior cleaning as 3.01 METs (Tudor-Locke, Washington, Ainsworth, & Troiano, 2009).

People's definitions of tasks vary widely, as do their methods of performing the task, tools used, and environmental conditions. The occupational therapy professional discusses the task with the patient and analyzes it on the basis of contextual and personal factors. After stroke, the energy demands of these tasks may increase substantially depending on the patient's impairment level. The occupational therapy professional helps the client gradually return to activities with higher energy requirements as time progresses, monitoring responses along the way. Patients who were performing higher energy–demanding tasks before the stroke and who are deemed safe to resume these activities may be able to progress back to more demanding tasks more quickly than those who were sedentary and deconditioned before the stroke. Extremely deconditioned patients will begin at a much lower level. The occupational therapy professional should keep in mind that maximal workload is lower after stroke, but oxygen uptake at a given submaximal workload is greater. Of course, this depends on the impairments associated with the stroke. The MET charts were revised in 2009 (Tudor-Locke et al., 2009), with a resultant website that lists the MET level for all activities, including job classifications (http://riskfactor.cancer.gov/tools/atus-met).

For the client to participate in **activities of daily living** (ADLs), **instrumental activities of daily living** (IADLs), leisure, work, and exercise, vital signs should be within a safe zone, and patients should be monitored closely while performing occupational therapy activities to ensure that changes in vital signs remain in that zone. The occupational therapy practitioner should ask the referring physician for specific parameters for the patient. Because guidelines after stroke have not been established, the American Heart Association has suggested using submaximal

> Patients who were performing higher energy–demanding tasks before the stroke and who are deemed safe to resume these activities may be able to progress back to more demanding tasks more quickly than those who were sedentary and deconditioned before the stroke.

protocols and following guidelines similar to those recommended after myocardial infarction. Peak heart rate should not exceed 120 beats per minute or 70% of the age-predicted maximum heart rate, a peak MET level of 5 (Gordon et al., 2004a, 2004b).

It is important to remember that people who have had a stroke will have significantly lower heart rate and blood pressure responses to exercise and activity. A safe rate of activity or exercise will allow the heart rate to return to resting level 2 minutes after stopping the activity. Heart rate will increase more rapidly in deconditioned patients because the heart is not trained to deliver large volumes of blood and hence oxygen. Keep in mind that the maximum heart rate a person should achieve during activity or exercise decreases with age (220 – age = maximum heart rate); therefore, normal exercise heart rates vary by age, with older people able to exercise at a lower heart rate than younger people.

The American College of Sports Medicine's guidelines to participate in exercise (Thompson, Gordon, & Pescatello, 2010) are useful; however, they are not specifically intended for people with stroke. The guidelines state that resting systolic blood pressure should be between 80 and 180 mm Hg, diastolic blood pressure should be between 60 and 100 mm Hg, respiration rate should be less than 35 breaths per minute, oxygen saturation readings should be more than 85% (supplemental oxygen required if less than 90%), and pulse should be 51 to 109 beats per minute. Resting systolic blood pressure readings of more than 180 mm Hg are a caution for exercise, and clients should not exercise if systolic blood pressure is more than 200 mm Hg or less than 80 mm Hg. Diastolic blood pressure of more than 100 mm Hg is classified as a caution for exercise, and no exercise should occur if diastolic readings are more than 110 mm Hg or less than 60 mm Hg (Thompson et al., 2010).

Fitness Before and After Stroke

It is important to know the client's level of fitness before the stroke. Fitness varies greatly in the general population but may be reduced in many people who have had a stroke. Many of the conditions mentioned earlier can be associated with poor fitness, including obesity, substance abuse, and cardiovascular disease. Cardiorespiratory fitness requires the heart, lungs, blood vessels, and skeletal muscles to work together to deliver oxygen and remove metabolic by-products during activity, and it has been found to be reduced by as much as 50% after stroke (Mackay-Lyons & Makrides, 2002).

Whether this reduction is primarily the result of premorbid conditions, direct effects of the stroke itself, or physical inactivity after the stroke is unclear (Billinger, Coughenour, Mackay-Lyons, & Ivey, 2012). Cardiac complications poststroke may result in lower heart rates and higher oxygen consumption at peak effort. Respiratory changes after stroke can also lead to decreased exercise endurance, shortness of breath, sedentary behavior, and increased risk of recurrent stroke (van der Palen et al., 2004). After stroke, peak oxygen consumption decreases significantly, making it difficult to perform moderate or vigorous activities. Fatigue is common when performing low-level self-care skills; therefore, interventions to improve respiratory muscle strength and pulmonary function should be encouraged.

Research has suggested that people with stroke retain the capacity to adapt physiologically to an exercise training stimulus (Billinger et al., 2012). Aerobic fitness has been shown to promote vascularization after stroke and is associated with neuronal viability in the frontal cortex of older adults (Erickson et al., 2012). Improved aerobic fitness can also reduce the risk for recurrent stroke and cardio-vascular events. The American Heart Association has recommended fitness training after stroke to (1) prevent complications of prolonged inactivity, (2) decrease recurrent stroke and cardiovascular events, and (3) increase aerobic fitness (Gordon et al., 2004a, 2004b). Unfortunately, interventions to improve fitness are underused in the general stroke population. Fitness training after stroke has many physiological benefits, including enhanced glucose regulation and decreased body weight, fat stores, blood pressure, C-reactive protein, total blood cholesterol, serum triglycerides, and low-density lipoprotein cholesterol (Franklin & Sanders, 2000). Exercise has been shown to increase high-density lipoprotein cholesterol and improve blood rheology, hemostatic variables, and coronary artery endo-thelial function (Hambrecht et al., 2000). People who sustain stroke experience marked reduction in physical activity and fitness; therefore, regular physical fit-ness training early after stroke is indicated to optimize long-term recovery (Mead & Bernhardt, 2011).

Growing evidence has indicated that fitness can improve after stroke. Before stroke patients begin a fitness program, however, a complete medical history, physi-cal examination, and graded exercise testing with electrocardiograph monitoring are suggested to identify complications from stroke, other medical conditions, and contraindications to exercise (Gordon et al., 2004a, 2004b). This is important because exercise can precipitate ventricular **arrhythmias,** cardiac arrest, and sud-den cardiac death. After discussing the client's perceived impairments and current activity level and exercise tolerance, standardized assessments of the five compo-nents of fitness are performed: (1) body composition, (2) flexibility, (3) muscle strength, (4) muscle endurance, and (5) cardiorespiratory endurance (Thompson et al., 2010). Because impairments may exist as a result of the stroke or comorbid conditions, accommodations may be needed during the assessment to ensure safety.

BMI, a measure of body fat based on height and weight, is a common method for estimating the body composition of adult men and women. BMI is computed as the weight in pounds times 703 divided by the height in inches squared (or weight in kilograms divided by height in meters squared). A BMI of less than 18.5 is classi-fied as underweight; 18.5 to 24.9, as normal weight; 25 to 29.9, as overweight; and more than 30, as obese. However, BMI does not account for muscle mass.

Flexibility is assessed by evaluating the range of motion of several joints in unison, commonly by having the client reach into postures such as touching toes and back of head and rotating trunk and neck to each side. The sit-and-reach test (Thompson et al., 2010) is one common standardized test of flexibility of the lower extremities and trunk.

Strength is commonly assessed in a fitness assessment using isotonic methods, such as sit-ups and bench press. Most fitness programs target isotonic strength, so assessment should be performed isotonically per the principle of Specific Adaptation to Imposed Demand (SAID). Isotonic muscle strength is easily measured by asking the client to lift a light weight for one to three repetitions through the available range of motion and increasing the load gradually until failure to lift through exist-ing range of motion is observed. Strength can be assessed isometrically with manual muscle testing.

Points to Ponder: What Assessments Are Necessary for Emma?

An isotonic strength assessment is performed by having the client lift a light load through range of motion and gradually increasing the load until the client is unable to lift through the full range of motion. What are the benefits of performing this type of strength assessment instead of a standard isometric test as is required in manual muscle testing?

Given Emma's current impairments, would it be safe to administer the YMCA 3-minute step test, which requires stepping up and down on a 12-inch step at the pace of 96 beats per minute on the metronome? Defend your answer.

Muscle endurance is assessed by asking the client to repetitively lift 33% to 50% of the maximum load lifted during isotonic strength testing, commonly 10 repetitions. Depending on level of impairment, level of conditioning, and concomitant conditions, cardiorespiratory endurance assessment may need to be modified to ensure the client's safety poststroke. Common measures of cardiorespiratory endurance are the YMCA 3-minute step test (Golding, 2000), staged treadmill testing, and the Rockport Walking Test (Rockport Walking Institute, 1986). All principles discussed previously about vital signs and safety apply.

Results of the fitness assessment are used to plan the fitness intervention. Depending on the client's level of fitness, 20 to 60 minutes of aerobic conditioning is recommended 3 to 7 days per week, and strengthening, flexibility, and neuromuscular activities (balance and coordination) are recommended 2 to 3 days per week (Gordon et al., 2004a, 2004b). Aerobic conditioning should include 20 to 60 minutes of large-muscle activities (several bouts of 10 minutes or more), such as walking, treadmilling, or using a stationary bicycle, with 40% to 70% maximal heart rate (Thompson et al., 2010) and ratings of perceived exertion of 11 to 14 on Borg's 6 to 20 scale (Gordon et al., 2004a, 2004b).

Strengthening of the major muscle groups (8 to 10 exercises) through graded activity, circuit training, or use of weight machines or free weights is recommended. Recent literature has suggested that strength training can increase upper-limb strength and function without increasing tone or pain in people with stroke (Harris & Eng, 2010). Refer to Chapter 6 for details regarding specific strengthening protocols appropriate for people who have sustained a stroke. Clients with stroke should use lower levels of resistance and more repetitions (1–2 sets of 10–15 repetitions). Stretching before or after aerobic or strength training is recommended, with stretches held for 10 to 30 seconds.

The American Heart Association (2014) has recommended coordination and balance activities after stroke; however, it has not provided parameters for these activities. A recent randomized controlled trial found that balance training in traditional rehabilitation did not provide any additional benefits (Eser, Yavuzer, Karakus, & Karaoglan, 2008); alternative methods, such as yoga and tai chi, should possibly be explored in the stroke population. Most people with stroke have deficits in postural control, balance, hemiparesis, and neuromuscular incoordination of the extremities (Miller et al., 2010). These deficits can predispose the person to falls as a result of the inability to use the hemiparetic upper extremity to prevent a fall, trunk instability, and decreased lower-extremity function (Ashburn, Hyndman, Pickering, Yardley, & Harris, 2008). Fall rates as high as 50% have been documented in community-dwelling people with stroke (Kerse et al., 2008). Therefore, it is important to include coordination and balance activities in a poststroke fitness program.

Application of Physiology to the Case Study

Emma has several health conditions that may complicate her recovery from stroke, including diabetes, hypertension, low-back pain, obesity, and history of smoking. Her level of fitness was most likely significantly decreased before the stroke. Emma's BMI is 42.08, which is in the obese range. Because Emma is 58 years old, her maximum predicted heart rate is 162 beats per minute, and her maximum exercise heart rate should be 113 (70%) at this point in time. Her resting pulse is 92 beats per minute, and it quickly increases to beyond her maximum exercise heart rate. Muscle weakness in the left extremities taxes her right extremities, limits independence with ADLs and IADLs, and makes fitness challenging. Low-back pain will need to be monitored because Emma's movement patterns have changed, and postural changes may lead to increased low-back pain. Activities will initially be limited to 2.0 to 2.5 METS owing to deconditioning, with vital signs monitored regularly. Fatigue management will be an important issue to address with Emma; this can be done via self-management training, use of fatigue rating scales during activity performance, and use of pacing and work simplification.

It will be important for occupational therapy practitioners to use many treatment approaches to help Emma perform daily life activities, resume meaningful daily roles, improve strength and motor control, adapt her home environment, assume emotional control, improve fitness, modify her diet, learn to manage her diabetes, and increase quality of life. Preventive approaches will also be needed to ensure that Emma proactively **self-manages chronic conditions** and does not put herself at risk for further impairments or injuries.

Summary

Stroke affects the physiological functioning of many body systems. Many of the premorbid risk factors for stroke can perpetuate reduced fitness and disability. Occupational therapy practitioners must provide interventions to remediate, compensate, maintain, and prevent these physiological issues from causing occupational performance deficits that can impair quality of life. We must expand our view of rehabilitation after stroke.

References

American Heart Association. (2014). *What is high blood pressure?* Retrieved May 29, 2013, from http://www.heart.org/HEARTORG/Conditions/HighBloodPressure/AboutHighBloodPressure/What-is-High-Blood-Pressure_UCM_301759_Article.jsp

Andersen, G., Christensen, D., Kirkevold, M., & Johnsen, S. P. (2012). Post-stroke fatigue and return to work: A 2-year follow-up. *Acta Neurologica Scandinavica, 125,* 248–253. http://dx.doi.org/10.1111/j.1600-0404.2011.01557.x

Ashburn, A., Hyndman, D., Pickering, R., Yardley, L., & Harris, S. (2008). Predicting people with stroke at risk of falls. *Age and Ageing, 37,* 270–276. http://dx.doi.org/10.1093/ageing/afn066

Banerjee, C., Moon, Y. P., Paik, M. C., Rundek, T., Mora-McLaughlin, C., Vieira, J. R., . . . Elkind, M. S. (2012). Duration of diabetes and risk of ischemic stroke: The Northern Manhattan Study. *Stroke, 43,* 1212–1217. http://dx.doi.org/10.1161/STROKEAHA.111.641381

Belza, B. L., Henke, C. J., Yelin, E. H., Epstein, W. V., & Gilliss, C. L. (1993). Correlates of fatigue in older adults with rheumatoid arthritis. *Nursing Research, 42,* 93–99. http://dx.doi.org/10.1097/00006199-199303000-00006

Billinger, S. A., Coughenour, E., Mackay-Lyons, M. J., & Ivey, F. M. (2012). Reduced cardiorespiratory fitness after stroke: Biological consequences and exercise-induced adaptations. *Stroke Research and Treatment, 2012*, 959120. http://dx.doi.org/10.1155/2012/959120

Borg, G. (1998). *Borg's Perceived Exertion and Pain Scales*. Champaign, IL: Human Kinetics.

Byrne, N. M., Hills, A. P., Hunter, G. R., Weinsier, R. L., & Schutz, Y. (2005). Metabolic equivalent: One size does not fit all. *Journal of Applied Physiology, 99*, 1112–1119. http://dx.doi.org/10.1152/japplphysiol.00023.2004

Centers for Disease Control and Prevention. (2013). *Crude and age-adjusted percentage of civilian, noninstitutionalized adults with diagnosed diabetes, United States, 1980–2011*. Retrieved from http://www.cdc.gov/diabetes/statistics/prev/national/figageadult.htm

Erickson, K. I., Weinstein, A. M., Sutton, B. P., Prakash, R. S., Voss, M. W., Chaddock, L., . . . Kramer, A. F. (2012). Beyond vascularization: Aerobic fitness is associated with N-acetylaspartate and working memory. *Brain and Behavior, 2*, 32–41. http://dx.doi.org/10.1002/brb3.30

Eser, F., Yavuzer, G., Karakus, D., & Karaoglan, B. (2008). The effect of balance training on motor recovery and ambulation after stroke: A randomized controlled trial. *European Journal of Physical and Rehabilitation Medicine, 44*, 19–25.

Esse, K., Fossati-Bellani, M., Traylor, A., & Martin-Schild, S. (2011). Epidemic of illicit drug use, mechanisms of action/addiction and stroke as a health hazard. *Brain and Behavior, 1*, 44–54. http://dx.doi.org/10.1002/brb3.7

Ford, E. S., Giles, W. H., & Dietz, W. H. (2002). Prevalence of the metabolic syndrome among US adults: Findings from the third National Health and Nutrition Examination Survey. *JAMA, 287*, 356–359. http://dx.doi.org/10.1001/jama.287.3.356

Franklin, B. A., & Sanders, W. (2000). Reducing the risk of heart disease and stroke. *Physician and Sportsmedicine, 28*, 19–26. http://dx.doi.org/10.3810/psm.2000.10.1240

Golding, L. A. (Ed.). (2000). *YMCA fitness testing and assessment manual* (4th ed.). Champaign, IL: Human Kinetics.

Gordon, N. F., Gulanick, M., Costa, F., Fletcher, G., Franklin, B. A., Roth, E. J., & Shephard, T. (2004a). Physical activity and exercise recommendations for stroke survivors: An American Heart Association scientific statement from the Council on Clinical Cardiology, Subcommittee on Exercise, Cardiac Rehabilitation, and Prevention; the Council on Cardiovascular Nursing; the Council on Nutrition, Physical Activity, and Metabolism; and the Stroke Council. *Circulation, 109*, 2031–2041.

Gordon, N. F., Gulanick, M., Costa, F., Fletcher, G., Franklin, B. A., Roth, E. J., & Shephard, T.; American Heart Association Council on Clinical Cardiology, Subcommittee on Exercise, Cardiac Rehabilitation, and Prevention; Council on Cardiovascular Nursing; Council on Nutrition, Physical Activity, and Metabolism; and Stroke Council. (2004b). Physical activity and exercise recommendations for stroke survivors: An American Heart Association scientific statement from the Council on Clinical Cardiology, Subcommittee on Exercise, Cardiac Rehabilitation, and Prevention; the Council on Cardiovascular Nursing; the Council on Nutrition, Physical Activity, and Metabolism; and the Stroke Council. *Stroke, 35*, 1230–1240. http://dx.doi.org/10.1161/01.STR.0000127303.19261.19

Hambrecht, R., Wolf, A., Gielen, S., Linke, A., Hofer, J., Erbs, S., . . . Schuler, G. (2000). Effect of exercise on coronary endothelial function in patients with coronary artery disease. *New England Journal of Medicine, 342*, 454–460. http://dx.doi.org/10.1056/NEJM200002173420702

Harris, J. E., & Eng, J. J. (2010). Strength training improves upper-limb function in individuals with stroke: A meta-analysis. *Stroke, 41*, 136–140. http://dx.doi.org/10.1161/STROKEAHA.109.567438

Hootman, J. M., & Helmick, C. G. (2006). Projections of U.S. prevalence of arthritis and associated activity limitations. *Arthritis and Rheumatism, 54*, 226–229. http://dx.doi.org/10.1002/art.21562

Hubacher, M., Calabrese, P., Bassetti, C., Carota, A., Stöcklin, M., & Penner, I. K. (2012). Assessment of post-stroke fatigue: The Fatigue Scale for Motor and Cognitive Functions. *European Neurology, 67*, 377–384. http://dx.doi.org/10.1159/000336736

Huisstede, B. M., Bierma-Zeinstra, S. M., Koes, B. W., & Verhaar, J. A. (2006). Incidence and prevalence of upper-extremity musculoskeletal disorders: A systematic appraisal of the literature. *BMC Musculoskeletal Disorders, 7*, 7. http://dx.doi.org/10.1186/1471-2474-7-7

Ivey, F., Hafer-Macko, C., & Macko, R. (2006). Exercise rehabilitation after stroke. *NeuroRx, 3*, 439–450.

Jarvis, C. (2011). *Physical examination and health assessment* (6th ed.). Philadelphia: Saunders/ Elsevier.

Kearney, P. M., Whelton, M., Reynolds, K., Muntner, P., Whelton, P. K., & He, J. (2005). Global burden of hypertension: Analysis of worldwide data. *Lancet, 365,* 217–223.

Kerse, N., Flicker, L., Pfaff, J. J., Draper, B., Lautenschlager, N. T., Sim, M., . . . Almeida, O. P. (2008). Falls, depression and antidepressants in later life: A large primary care appraisal. *PLoS ONE, 3,* e2423. http://dx.doi.org/10.1371/journal.pone.0002423

Krupp, L. B., LaRocca, N. G., Muir-Nash, J., & Steinberg, A. D. (1989). The Fatigue Severity Scale: Application to patients with multiple sclerosis and systemic lupus erythematosus. *Archives of Neurology, 46,* 1121–1123. http://dx.doi.org/10.1001/ archneur.1989.00520460115022

Mackay-Lyons, M. J., & Makrides, L. (2002). Exercise capacity early after stroke. *Archives of Physical Medicine and Rehabilitation, 83,* 1697–1702. http://dx.doi.org/10.1053/ apmr.2002.36395

Martino, R., Foley, N., Bhogal, S., Diamant, N., Speechley, M., & Teasell, R. (2005). Dysphagia after stroke: Incidence, diagnosis, and pulmonary complications. *Stroke, 36,* 2756–2763. http://dx.doi.org/10.1161/01.STR.0000190056.76543.eb

Mead, G., & Bernhardt, J. (2011). Physical fitness training after stroke, time to implement what we know: More research is needed. *International Journal of Stroke, 6,* 506–508. http:// dx.doi.org/10.1111/j.1747-4949.2011.00679.x

Miller, E. L., Murray, L., Richards, L., Zorowitz, R. D., Bakas, T., Clark, P., & Billinger, S. A.; American Heart Association Council on Cardiovascular Nursing and the Stroke Council. (2010). Comprehensive overview of nursing and interdisciplinary rehabilitation care of the stroke patient: A scientific statement from the American Heart Association. *Stroke, 41,* 2402–2448. http://dx.doi.org/10.1161/STR.0b013e3181e7512b

Mueller, M. J., & Maluf, K. S. (2002). Tissue adaptation to physical stress: A proposed "Physical Stress Theory" to guide physical therapist practice, education, and research. *Physical Therapy, 82,* 383–403.

Pate, R. R. (1995). Physical activity and health: Dose–response issues. *Research Quarterly for Exercise and Sport, 66,* 313–317. http://dx.doi.org/10.1080/02701367.1995.10607917

Rockport Walking Institute. (1986). *Rockport Fitness Walking Test.* Marlboro, MA: Author.

Roth, E. J. (1993). Heart disease in patients with stroke: Incidence, impact, and implications for rehabilitation: I. Classification and prevalence. *Archives of Physical Medicine and Rehabilitation, 74,* 752–760. http://dx.doi.org/10.1016/0003-9993(93)90038-C

Smets, E. M. A., Garssen, B., Bonke, B., & De Haes, J. C. (1995). The Multidimensional Fatigue Inventory (MFI) psychometric qualities of an instrument to assess fatigue. *Journal of Psychosomatic Research, 39,* 315–325. http://dx.doi.org/10.1016/0022-3999(94)00125-O

Teasell, R., Foley, N., Salter, K., & Bhogal, S. (2008). Medical complications post stroke. *Evidence-based review of stroke rehabilitation* (12th ed.). Retrieved from http://www.ebrsr. com/reviews_details.php?Medical-Complications-Post-Stroke-17

Thompson, W., Gordon, N., & Pescatello, L. (Eds.). (2010). *American College of Sports Medicine's guidelines for exercise testing and prescription* (8th ed.). Philadelphia: Lippincott Williams & Wilkins.

Tudor-Locke, C., Washington, T. L., Ainsworth, B. E., & Troiano, R. P. (2009). Linking the American Time Use Survey (ATUS) and the Compendium of Physical Activities: Methods and rationale. *Journal of Physical Activity and Health, 6,* 347–353.

van der Palen, J., Rea, T. D., Manolio, T. A., Lumley, T., Newman, A. B., Tracy, R. P., . . . Psaty, B. M. (2004). Respiratory muscle strength and the risk of incident cardiovascular events. *Thorax, 59,* 1063–1067. http://dx.doi.org/10.1136/thx.2004.021915

Wijnhoven, H. A., de Vet, H. C., & Picavet, H. S. (2006). Prevalence of musculoskeletal disorders is systematically higher in women than in men. *Clinical Journal of Pain, 22,* 717–724. http://dx.doi.org/10.1097/01.ajp.0000210912.95664.53

Witt, B. J., Brown, R. D., Jr., Jacobsen, S. J., Weston, S. A., Yawn, B. P., & Roger, V. L. (2005). A community-based study of stroke incidence after myocardial infarction. *Annals of Internal Medicine, 143,* 785–792. http://dx.doi.org/10.7326/0003-4819-143-11-200512060-00006

CHAPTER 5

Core Concepts in Sensory Impairment and Recovery After Stroke

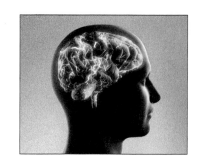

Leeanne Carey, PhD

Learning Objectives

After completion of this chapter, readers will be able to

- Identify factors that affect perception and describe the optimal exploratory procedures used to explore the different somatosensory attributes of objects;
- Recognize key features of central processing of sensory information and how they may affect the nature of sensory impairment and recovery;
- Identify the nature of sensory impairment after stroke and its effect on function;
- Identify appropriate methods to assess sensory loss and its functional implications;
- Differentiate factors that may be structured in a functional activity to assess the presence and functional implications of sensory loss in a patient;
- Match sensory rehabilitation interventions described in the literature with current models of recovery and rehabilitation; and
- Outline methods of treating sensory loss relative to current principles of neuroscience.

Key Words

- perception
- sensation
- sensory processing
- somatosensation
- vision

Introduction

Our senses are part of who we are and how we perceive and interact with our environment. They include vision, touch, hearing, and **olfaction,** and their integration. In this chapter, I focus on body sensations *(somatosensations),* such as touch. In addition, I highlight concepts related to sensory functioning that have relevance to other senses that are commonly impaired after **stroke,** such as vision, and provide some examples and points of comparison. For a fuller description of anatomical and physiological knowledge important to understanding the function of these senses and the impact of impaired sensation on performance and participation, see Carey (2015).

Sensation for Perception and Action in Daily Life

Our senses are important for perception as well as for action. In their own right, they are important for us to be able to perceive ourselves and the world around us. Lyons (2010), a person with somatosensory loss after stroke, said, "I may look alright but I feel all left . . . and half lost" (p. 81) and "To reach out, connect and make contact with another person is to feel alive and part of the human race" (p. 58). The senses are also important in the context of one's actions—they provide people with the information they need to direct their actions as well as provide feedback on their actions. As such, the senses have an important and ongoing influence on one's ability to respond to and participate in daily activities.

> After my stroke, I had quite good movement in my stroke-affected hand but very little sense of touch. My hand felt like it was blind. Everyday tasks were very clumsy and required so much concentration. . . . Things like picking up and using a fork were labored, and tasks where my hand was out of sight, like doing up a bra, putting on jewelry, and tying up my hair, were beyond me. (personal communication, Karen, mother of two young children, who experienced somatosensory loss after cortical stroke)

Definitions

Somatosensory function is the ability to interpret bodily sensation (Puce & Carey, 2010). This function involves the **detection,** discrimination, and recognition of body *(somato)* sensations. It includes submodalities of touch sensation such as light touch (on the surface of the skin), vibration, firm pressure, texture discrimination, ***proprioception*** involving sensing the location and movement of body parts, temperature sensation, and pain *(nociception)*. The experience of sensing often involves a more complex integration of somatosensory inputs (e.g., haptic recognition of objects) or somatosensory and emotional components (e.g., pain) and may be influenced by emotional and social contexts (e.g., perception of tickle; Dunn et al., 2013). It enables humans to identify tactile characteristics of surroundings, create meaning around sensations, and formulate body actions related to the sensations (Dijkerman & de Haan, 2007; Puce & Carey, 2010).

Vision is a complex sensation that provides information about one's surrounding environment. The visual system interprets information from visible light to build a representation of the surrounding world. This process involves reception of light, formation of monocular representations, construction of binocular perception, identification and categorization of visual objects, assessing distances to and between objects, and guiding body movements in relation to visual objects (Carey, 2015; Tovée, 2008). Intact vision supports occupational performance particularly in areas such as reading, mobility (including driving), and visually guided motor behavior and manipulation (Carey, 2015; Massof et al., 2007).

Sensation for Perception

One of the major roles of people's senses is to sense and appreciate themselves in the world around them. Without the senses, people cannot process the world around them. People's perceptions of the world are influenced not only by the stimuli in their environment but also by their current internal state and past experiences.

Sensory information is constantly available from the environment, but people's integrated perception of this information is what forms the interface between themselves and their environment. Thus, sensation is dynamic; it is guided by the goal of the task and has potential to be influenced and modified.

When people perceive an object or stimulus in their environment, that object or stimulus has features that define it relative to the sense through which they are experiencing it. For example, a fork has a visual luminance, color, and intensity. It also has a visual shape (distinctive of a fork) and a texture that can be perceived visually to be smooth and made of metal (based on past experience). Visual perception of the fork will also be influenced by the lighting, contrast with the surface on which it may be resting (e.g., table), other objects around it (e.g., plate or other cutlery in a cluttered drawer), and so forth. The fork also has a shape, texture, weight, and temperature that can be perceived through the sense of touch. Depending on the part of the fork touched, the distinctive shape of the prongs might be perceived or its long flat handle. The texture may be felt as smooth and metal-like, or it may have a part that is made of another material, such as a wooden handle. The weight may be perceived as relatively heavy or light (for a fork), and the metal may be cold (depending on the surrounding environment). Again, these perceptions will be influenced by the person's prior experience with cutlery and this type of fork in particular, the surrounding environment, and the person's need or ability to attend to particular features of the fork. Even the very early stages of information processing of the fork's sensory features will be influenced by prior experience and current expectation (Boly et al., 2007).

Most important, the person's perception of the fork will be influenced by his or her perceptual goal or proposed use of the object. For example, if the person's goal is to recognize what the object is without vision, he or she will most likely focus on the fork's distinctive shape to identify it as a fork. This can be most optimally achieved through the sense of touch by using the exploratory procedure of contour following (Lederman & Klatzky, 1993). *Contour following* involves moving (or "walking") the fingers around the object to perceive its shape. In comparison, if the goal is to identify the texture or material of the fork, the person will typically use *lateral motion* (i.e., side-to-side movement) of the fingertip over the surface of the fork to feel the smooth and metal-like properties of the surface.

Sensation for Action

Alternatively, if the purpose is to use the fork to stabilize food for cutting, the goal might be first to tactually find the handle of the fork and position the fingers at the edges of the handle and rise of the prongs to hold the fork in a stable and comfortable position of the hand for use. To use the fork for this purpose also requires perception of the fork's shape, in particular the distinctive parts of its tactual shape that are needed for a stable grip. It also involves the tactual perception of those features of the object during movement of the hand to grasp, hold, and manipulate the fork, as well as updating of those features in response to the movement or slip of the fork in the hand, to achieve the goal of controlled use of the fork in the daily task of cutting food and eating it.

Multilevel and Integrated Systems to Support Sensory Function

It is important that therapists have a good appreciation of the role of sensation as well as of the multilevel and integrated systems that contribute to the processing of sensory information in daily life. Knowledge of the impact of interruption on different parts of the networks that subserve somatosensory processing is important not only to appreciate the nature of the deficit but also to appreciate remaining strengths in connected networks that have the potential to be accessed in therapy.

Processing of sensory information occurs at multiple levels of the peripheral and central nervous systems and is further integrated with other senses to achieve the sensory function people use in everyday tasks.

Processing of sensory information occurs at multiple levels of the **peripheral** and **central nervous systems** and is further integrated with other senses to achieve the sensory function people use in everyday tasks. Processing of sensory stimuli from the periphery to central nervous system is described in detail in seminal texts such as *Principles of Neural Science* (Kandel, Schwartz, & Jessell, 2000; see Chapter 22, "The Bodily Senses," and Chapter 23, "Touch"). Here, I focus on central processing of sensory information, in particular in relation to somatosensory information.

Models of Sensory Processing Linked With Perception and Action

Models of sensory processing recognize the dual roles of the senses. Pathways involved in processing sensation for perception and sensation for action have been described in relation to both vision (Goodale & Milner, 1992) and somatosensations (Dijkerman & de Haan, 2007). These models help us to better understand the complexities of sensory processing and the interaction between parts of the systems that subserve these capacities. This is important to understanding the nature of impairment after stroke as well as the potential for recovery and identification of pathways and systems that may support recovery. By way of example, I describe information processing for somatosensory function, highlighting the importance of this information in the context of understanding impairment and its impact on performance, recovery, and **rehabilitation** after stroke.

The brain consists of an integrated system of brain regions and functional brain networks involved in information processing. Key regions within the *somatosensory network* include primary **somatosensory cortex** (SI), secondary somatosensory cortex (SII), **thalamus** (in particular, the ventroposterior lateral area of the thalamus), insula, posterior parietal cortex, and **cerebellum** (Carey, 2012c; Dijkerman & de Haan, 2007). These core regions are part of a more distributed network, including **attention** and visual networks, that are involved in conscious processing of somatosensory information (see Chapter 3, "Neuroanatomy of Stroke," for more information). Dijkerman and de Haan (2007) described a model of somatosensory processing that relates to the purpose of the information processing: sensation for perception and sensation for action. The model involves parallel and serial processing across distinct processing streams. Sensation for conscious perception and memory of that perception is reported to be processed by SI and SII to the posterior insula (ventral stream). In comparison, sensation for action (guidance of movement) primarily involves SI, SII, and posterior parietal cortex (dorsal stream). Processing of information increases in complexity from feature detection, primarily involving SI, to higher order recognition involving SII, insula, and posterior parietal cortex (Dijkerman & de Haan, 2007).

Key Features of Central Sensory Information Processing

Knowledge of key features of central processing of somatosensory information is important in understanding the nature of the somatosensory processing deficit experienced after stroke as well as the potential for recovery and identification of residual capacities in information processing that may be targeted in therapy (Carey, 2012c).

First, somatosensory information is processed via *modality-specific serial pathways* as well as *parallel pathways* (Kaas & Pons, 2006). Parallel pathways allow for convergence of somatosensory information within the central nervous system as well as provide a rich framework for neural plastic changes. Second, *multiple* and *multimodal representations of sensory maps,* such as SI and SII, play an important role in sensory processing and integration (Driver & Noesselt, 2008). Matching of sensory maps can influence information processing (Frey et al., 2011), even in early stages, and input from multiple modalities can increase firing rate and improve signal (Becker, 1996). Third, *functional* and *structural interhemispheric connections* and the balance of excitatory and inhibitory activity between hemispheres are critical in processing of somatosensory information (Carey, 2012c; Hlushchuk & Hari, 2006). Finally, sensory signals and thresholds are also affected by top-down influences from attention networks and bottom-up influences from multisensory processing of information (Carey, 2012c; Corbetta, 2012; Talsma, Senkowski, Soto-Faraco, & Woldorff, 2010).

A Network Approach, With Links to Related Networks

The importance of understanding brain function at the level of brain networks and connectivity between networks is increasingly highlighted given that the brain operates as a functional unit with behaviors represented in distributed functional networks (Carey, 2012b; Carey & Seitz, 2007). This is particularly evident in the context of stroke; stroke has an impact beyond the focal lesion and involves viable brain networks in recovery (Carey, 2012b; Carey & Seitz, 2007; Carey et al., 2013; Cramer et al., 2011). Processing of somatosensory information therefore needs to be considered in relation to both the core somatosensory network and related networks. Interactions with related networks such as attention and vision are critical in understanding the central processing of somatosensory information (Corbetta, 2012).

The brain operates as a functional unit with behaviors represented in distributed functional networks.

Sensory signals are buried in noise. Perceptual awareness results from an interaction between specialized sensory regions and a higher order frontoparietal attention network (Boly et al., 2007; Goldberg, Harel, & Malach, 2006). Attention operates across different sensory modalities to facilitate selection of relevant information and multisensory integration. Top-down influences can help to optimize the detection of novel or hard-to-sense stimuli (Nicolelis, 2005). In addition, stimulus-driven, bottom-up mechanisms can influence attention to multisensory processing (Talsma et al., 2010). Strong links are particularly evident between touch and vision (Sathian, 2006). In fact, it has been suggested that visual cortical processing may be necessary for normal tactile perception (Sathian, 2006).

Prevalence and Nature of Sensory Impairment After Stroke

A stroke may lead to impairment in any of the senses. It is therefore important to appreciate the prevalence and nature of impairment of body sensations, vision, and other senses, such as audition, vestibular, olfactory, and gustatory, after stroke, given the impact of these senses on people's ability to interact with their environment and participate in meaningful life occupations (Carey, 2015). Moreover, the impact of impairment across multiple senses needs to be considered. Integration of information across multiple senses is central to adaptive behavior and will have an impact on the ability to adequately process information in complex, multisensory environments. I next describe the prevalence and nature of impairment for two commonly impaired senses, somatosensation and vision.

Prevalence and Nature of Somatosensory Impairment

Studies that have used standardized quantitative measures have reported frequency of somatosensory loss to be 50% to 85% (Carey & Matyas, 2011; Kim & Choi-Kwon, 1996; Tyson, Hanley, Chillala, Selley, & Tallis, 2008; Winward, Halligan, & Dade, 2002), with an average of 50% to 60% reported in reviews and clinical studies that have used either quantitative or nonstandardized, subjective assessments (Carey, 1995; Carey & Matyas, 2011; Connell, Lincoln, & Radford, 2008; Sullivan & Hedman, 2008). Loss of discriminative sensibility in at least one modality has been reported to be as high as 85% in the acute setting (Kim & Choi-Kwon, 1996) and 67% in a subacute rehabilitation sample after unilateral stroke (Carey & Matyas, 2011). Impaired touch sensation has been reported in approximately half of patients tested and impaired proprioception in 27% to 52% (Carey & Matyas, 2011; Tyson et al., 2008; Winward et al., 2002). Approximately 20% of those with impairment in the expected **contralateral** limb also experienced impaired sensation in the hand ipsilateral to the lesion (Carey & Matyas, 2011; Kim & Choi-Kwon, 1996). Ipsilateral impairments are usually less severe.

Loss of body sensations may be observed across different modalities (e.g., touch, proprioception), at different levels of information processing (e.g., detection, discrimination, recognition), and in relation to integration of multiple body sensations. Impairment of the ability to discriminate touch and limb position is the more frequent clinical scenario (Carey, 1995; Kim & Choi-Kwon, 1996; Tyson et al., 2008).

Touch provides information on external objects touching the skin as well as on one's body touching other objects or itself. Impaired touch sensation may be observed as anesthesia, reduced detection of light touch or deep pressure, through to poor texture discrimination. The ability to know where one's limbs are in space, known as *proprioception* or *limb position sense,* may also be impaired. This impairment may include reduced ability to perceive the location or movement of a limb. Temperature and pain sensations may be affected after stroke, with either a loss of these protective sensations or hypersensitivity to them. Impaired recognition and integration of one's body senses is evident in the reduced ability to tactually recognize objects, a capacity often referred to as *haptic object recognition.*

Impaired body sensations are most typically experienced in the half of the body contralateral to the lesion and may involve a total **hemianesthesia** involving face, trunk, and upper and lower limbs or a partial loss in one or more body parts. Although impairment across more than one modality is common (e.g., 67% across touch and limb position sense in the upper limb; Carey & Matyas, 2011), a person may experience quite specific loss within or across a particular modality (or submodality, such as texture discrimination).

The natural history of sensory loss after stroke has not been well characterized. Loss may persist for many years after the stroke, or hypersensitivity may develop over time (Carey, 1995). Improvement in somatosensations has been reported across a range of measures including touch detection, texture and proprioceptive discrimination, and object recognition (see Carey, 1995, for a review). However, the extent of recovery is varied, ranging from lasting deficits to quite remarkable improvement in capacities such as haptic object recognition. Researchers have suggested that recovery is most marked within the first 3 months after stroke, although ongoing recovery has been observed at 6 months and later, but is variable across individuals (Winward, Halligan, & Wade, 2007). Evidence from sensory rehabilitation studies has indicated the potential for marked recovery months and even years poststroke (Carey, Macdonell, & Matyas, 2011).

Prevalence, Nature, and Impact of Visual Impairment

Visual impairment after stroke is common and includes a wide range of different types of impairment such as eye alignment and movement impairment (68%), **visual field** impairment (49%), low vision (26.5%), and perceptual difficulties (20.5%), as identified in a prospective sample (N = 323) with suspected visual difficulty (Rowe et al., 2009). Visual impairment is reported to have the most impact on reading, outdoor mobility, participation in **leisure** activities, and shopping (Lamoureux, Hassell, & Keeffe, 2004), as well as on a person's psychological well-being and quality of life.

In older adults, even mild levels of decreased vision have been associated with lower participation in instrumental, leisure, and social activities (Perlmutter, Bhorade, Gordon, Hollingsworth, & Baum, 2010). Visual field defects have a serious impact on functional ability and quality of life after stroke (Jones & Shinton, 2006). People with hemianopsia report difficulty completing personal hygiene or grooming and feeding and several **instrumental activities of daily living** (IADLs), including driving, shopping, financial management, telephone usage, and meal preparation (Warren, 2009). Patients with visual field deficits also have an increased risk of falling, impaired ability to read, poor **mood,** and higher levels of institutionalization (Rowe et al., 2013a). Rowe et al. (2009, 2013b) have highlighted the need for assessment of visual impairment after stroke.

Impact of Somatosensory Loss After Stroke

Given the central role of sensation in perception and action, one can appreciate how sensory capacities, or their loss, may affect a person's occupational performance, participation, and well-being. Sensory loss may have an ongoing impact on a wide range of daily activities, from being able to communicate through a handshake to knowing the position of one's limb for safety; dressing, especially doing up buttons or tying fasteners out of view; finding coins in a wallet; using objects with confidence, such as drinking from a crushable cup; and returning to previous work and social roles. Yet, loss of body sensations is a somewhat hidden problem and is often not fully appreciated by health professionals, caregivers, and family members. Moreover, the impact of somatosensory loss is hard to understand and is often underrated (Carey, 1995; Robles-De-La-Torre, 2006). It is therefore often not detected. The impact of the loss may be compounded by this lack of awareness and recognition.

> Loss of body sensations is a somewhat hidden problem and is often not fully appreciated by health professionals, caregivers, and family members.

Impact on Perception, Action, and Occupational Performance

Sensation is important in its own right. People need intact body sensations to sense and confidently explore their environment and make quick adjustments. People's senses are part of who they are as human beings—they want to be able to feel. Sensations such as touch and pain are important to being able to experience pleasure or be alerted to danger. They are a part of the way people learn and adapt.

Body sensations are also important in the context of movement and action. In particular, touch and proprioceptive sensibility have an important role in control of pinch grip (Blennerhassett, Matyas, & Carey, 2007), the ability to sustain and adapt appropriate force without vision (Blennerhassett, Carey, & Matyas, 2006), object manipulation (Hermsdörfer, Hagl, Nowak, & Marquardt, 2003), combining component parts of movement such as transport and grasp (Gentilucci, Toni, Daprati, & Gangitano, 1997), and adjustment to sensory conflict conditions (e.g., a rough surface; Carey, 2012c). Thus, people with sensory loss after stroke will have particular difficulty with these tasks. This difficulty is greater than that attributable to motor deficits alone. For example, greater impairment was evident in the timing and adjustment of forces during the fundamental pinch-grip lift-and-hold task in a controlled investigation of the impact of impaired friction discrimination ability on pinch grip poststroke (Blennerhassett et al., 2007).

Somatosensations, in particular proprioception, also have a role in the learning of any new movement or skill. In fact, despite relatively intact movement, the person with somatosensory loss may learn not to use the limb (Dannenbaum & Dykes, 1988), with further deterioration of motor function after nonuse. Finally, tactile input and activity in somatosensory brain regions have been linked to motor recovery poststroke (Schaechter et al., 2012).

Impact on Daily Activities and Rehabilitation Outcome

Somatosensory loss and its associated impact on performance often have an ongoing and negative impact on the person. People with sensory loss may experience difficulty in routine daily tasks such as dressing (e.g., doing up buttons), using a fork, cooking, washing the dishes, making a bed, handling money, sewing, writing, using a computer, walking on uneven ground, driving, and many other daily activities. In a sample of 258 people 3 to 8 months poststroke, the presence of somatosensory loss was associated with return to fewer previous life activities across domestic, social, and leisure domains (Carey, Jacobs, Baum, & Connor, 2010). Return to previous life roles as a worker or mother, for example, may also be negatively affected.

Loss of body sensations after stroke is associated with poorer function and rehabilitation outcomes. For example, presence of somatosensory deficits, in addition to motor deficits, had a significant, negative effect on time taken to regain functional capacity and likelihood of achieving higher levels of function in personal **activities of daily living** (ADLs) and IADLs, as observed in a prospective cohort of 459 patients (Patel, Duncan, Lai, & Studenski, 2000). Loss of body sensations was also a factor contributing to inferior results in independence and mobility (Tyson et al., 2008), reduced independence in relation to discharge destination, and longer rehabilitation in several stroke outcome studies (Carey, 1995; Sullivan & Hedman, 2008). Patient groups with hemiparesis, hemihypesthesia, or hemianopsia compared with those with hemiparesis alone have shown significantly poorer function and time to maximal recovery (Dromerick & Reding, 1995). Loss of sensation also has a negative impact on personal safety, return to sexual and leisure activities, and reacquisition of skilled movements (Carey, 1995; Schaechter et al., 2012; Sullivan & Hedman,

2008). Finally, somatosensory loss has been associated with poorer motor outcome in clinical studies (Tyson et al., 2008), and the sensory system has been identified as important for motor recovery in imaging studies (Schaechter et al., 2012). The high prevalence of somatosensory and visual impairments poststroke, and the impact of these impairments on daily activities and rehabilitation outcome, reinforces the importance of adequately detecting these impairments and addressing their functional consequences in rehabilitation.

Evaluation of Sensory Function After Stroke

Sensory assessment may be undertaken for several reasons: to assess performance capacity; to determine the impact of sensory loss on ability to participate in daily activities and life roles; for diagnosis; for prognosis; to inform treatment planning and education; to monitor progress; and as a criterion for treatment effectiveness. It is recommended that evaluation of somatosensory function after stroke occur at three levels: (1) patient's perception and awareness of sensory loss and its impact on daily activities; (2) quantitative evaluation of somatosensory performance across different modalities, levels of information processing, and body locations; and (3) evaluation in the context of everyday activities, especially those of importance to the patient. Here, I focus on tools that have application for use with people with stroke and, where possible, have the evidence base to support their use.

Patient's Perception and Awareness of Somatosensory Loss

It is useful to start an evaluation of somatosensory loss by determining the extent to which the patient is aware of changes in body sensations after stroke and the potential impact of these changes on motor function and daily activities. Although this part of the evaluation has not been empirically tested, I provide some suggested questions that may help in exploring the patient's awareness. Some of these questions have been developed for use in the SenScreen Sensory Screening tool developed by Carey, Mak, and Tan (2011), which is currently being tested in clinical settings.

- Can you tell me how your arm feels since your stroke?
- Have you noticed any changes in your feeling in any other parts of your body?
- How would you rate your sensory ability now compared with before you had a stroke?
- How does this change in your ability to feel affect your movement?
- How does this change in your ability to feel affect your ability to perform daily activities?

It is also useful to take a history of the patient's sensory function since the stroke. This history may include time since stroke, nature and severity of loss, whether the patient has noticed improvement or deterioration in impairment or performance, and so forth. The patient's strengths and capacities should also be identified and may include the motivation and attention capacities involved in an intensive learning-based training program or problem-solving abilities needed to work through different challenges in different environments.

Quantitative Evaluation of Somatosensory Performance

Several screening tools and clinical and quantitative measures have been used to assess somatosensory function. Identification and review of these measures has been undertaken by several authors (Carey, 1995; Dellon, 2000; Winward, Halligan, & Wade, 1999). It is important that therapists select appropriate measures according to their purpose for testing; taking into account the type and nature of sensory loss is important to assess the functional implications. It is also important that therapists critically evaluate current and future measures by asking the following questions:

- What is the measure designed to assess (e.g., discrimination, severity, impact of loss)?
- Is it suitable for use with stroke patients?
- Are stimuli objectively defined?
- Is it quantitative?
- Does it have a standardized protocol?
- Is it valid?
- Is it reliable?
- Does it have appropriate age-matched norms?
- Is it sensitive to change?

Measures should be quantitative and standardized and have objectively defined stimuli, small intervals in assessment points, and a defined criterion of abnormality (Carey, 1995). They should also have high test–retest reliability and strong theoretical and psychometric foundations (Carey, 1995).

The need for quantitative evidence-based measures of somatosensation has been highlighted (Carey, 1995; Carey, Matyas, & Oke, 2002; Winward et al., 1999). Clinical measures commonly used, such as light touch using the fingertip and limb position sense using up–down movements of the thumb, are largely subjective; lack a standardized protocol; use gross scales such as *normal, impaired,* or *absent;* and have variable reliability and no defined criterion of abnormality (Carey, 1995; Carey, Matyas, & Oke, 2002; Winward et al., 1999). Moreover, these measures are often insensitive or inaccurate. For example, in the acute setting discriminative body sensations remained in only 3 of 25 stroke patients who were reported as having no sensory impairment on the basis of conventional sensory tests (Kim & Choi-Kwon, 1996). Similarly, in a rehabilitation sample, impaired proprioception in the upper limb was missed in 67% of patients when the clinical test was used as compared with the statistically defined abnormal performance found when the quantitative Wrist Position Sense Test was used (Carey, Matyas, & Oke, 2002). In addition, texture discrimination impairment was missed in 25% of patients and inaccurately reported in 40% when using the clinical test rather than the quantitative, norm-referenced Tactile Discrimination Test (TDT; Carey, Matyas, & Oke, 2002).

A few sensory screening tools have been developed for use in the clinical setting after stroke. The Nottingham Sensory Assessment (Lincoln, Jackson, & Adams, 1998) uses methods consistent with clinical practice but has relatively poor empirical foundations. The revised assessment reports acceptable ($\kappa \geq .6$) agreement for only 12 of 86 items (Lincoln et al., 1998), and interrater reliability is 0.38 to 1.00 for the ***stereognosis*** (or object recognition) component. The Rivermead Assessment of Somatosensory Performance (Winward et al., 2002) was developed to address some of the limitations in clinical assessment of somatosensations. It uses standard protocols, uses seven subtests of touch and proprioception, and includes three new instruments—the neurometer, neurotemp, and two-point neurodiscriminator. Intrarater and interrater reliability are high ($r = .92$); however, the scale's sensitivity is limited because many of the items are scored as correct or incorrect, consistent with clinical protocols, and then summed across body parts. Focus is on sharp–dull, pressure, temperature, proprioception, and two-point discrimination rather than on texture discrimination and object recognition.

In clinical settings, therapists need information not only on thresholds of detection but also on the ability to make accurate discriminations and recognize objects with multiple sensory attributes. Detection of light touch and deep pressure may be measured using calibrated monofilaments such as the Semmes–Weinstein monofilaments or Weinstein Enhanced Sensory Test hand monofilaments (Weinstein, 1993). Measures such as these can provide an indication of touch detection and protective sensibility across different body locations. Normative data are available to facilitate interpretation.

The ability to detect hot and cold is also likely to be important from a safety perspective. A hot–cold discrimination kit that consists of two insulated cups with a thermometer and metal test tubes is available and commonly used in clinical settings, although standard protocol, reliability, and normative standards are not typically used. Other tools, such as the Pfizer thermal tester, are available (Dellon, 2000) but are not often used.

Discrimination of tactile stimuli, such as precisely defined texture gratings, may be quantitatively assessed using the TDT (Carey, Oke, & Matyas, 1997). This measure has been developed for use with stroke patients. The patient is required to discriminate the texture that is different from a triplet set of grids using a three-alternative forced-choice design. The TDT has good reliability ($r = .92$; standard error of measurement < 10% of the scale), discriminative validity, and normative standards (Carey et al., 1997). A brief version of the test that takes approximately 5 minutes and involves a reduced number of trials ($n = 12$) has been developed for clinical use (sensitivity = 85%, specificity = 94%). Other quantitative measures of touch discrimination are the grating orientation discrimination test (Van Boven & Johnson, 1994), the AsTex test of touch sensibility (Miller et al., 2009), and the shape–texture identification test (Rosén & Lundborg, 1998).

Assessment of proprioception, also known as *limb position sense,* is important after stroke given its impact on safety and motor function. Clinical measures of proprioception typically involve moving the joint, such as the metacarpophalangeal joint of the thumb, up or down and asking the patient to respond whether the joint is up or down or asking the patient to mirror copy a limb position that the examiner has taken him or her into. A few quantitative measures have been developed for use with people with stroke in clinical settings. The Wrist Position Sense Test (Carey, Oke, & Matyas, 1996) is a quantitative measure of limb position sense at the wrist that has high test–retest reliability ($r = .88$ to $.92$, standard error of measurement = 2.8°), good discriminative validity, and normative standards (Carey et al., 1996). Using a lever and hand splint, the examiner moves the person's wrist to a defined test angle out of view. The patient is required to judge the angle of the wrist within the flexion–extension plane using a response pointer and protractor scale. A brief version of the test (10 trials) has a sensitivity of 93% and a specificity of 95% (Mak, 2010).

In clinical settings, therapists need information not only on thresholds of detection but also on the ability to make accurate discriminations and recognize objects with multiple sensory attributes.

Recognition of objects through the sense of touch *(haptic object recognition)* requires integration of information across somatosensory modalities. Relatively few quantitative standardized tests are available that are suitable for use in clinical settings. Quantitative measures of object recognition that have been developed and may be considered for use with people with stroke are the Manual Form Perception test (Ayres 1980), the Hand Active Sensation Test (Williams, Basso, Case-Smith, & Nichols-Larsen, 2006), and modified Moberg pick-up test (Dellon, 2000). One test that has been used in clinical settings with people with stroke and uses common everyday objects and a standard protocol is the functional Tactile Object Recognition Test (Carey, Nankervis, LeBlanc, & Harvey, 2006). This test uses object sets that vary in the seven diagnostic attributes of sensation defined by Lederman and Klatzky (1993): (1) texture, (2) temperature, (3) shape, (4) size, (5) hardness, (6) weight, and (7) function. The patient is required to recognize the test object through the sense of touch and identify it from a poster of visual representations of the object. Each item is scored on a 4-point scale. The test has good discriminative validity and normative data to guide interpretation. A brief version involving seven items has been adapted for use in clinical settings. In each of these tests, the potential confound of poor movement resulting from paresis needs to be considered (Carey, 2015).

Evaluation in Context of Functional Activities

The impact of sensory loss on hand function, performance of daily activities, and return to previous life activities may be assessed in several ways (e.g., the Hand Function Survey; Blennerhassett, Avery, & Carey, 2010). The Hand Function Survey involves a structured interview that measures self-reported ability to use the affected hand in 13 everyday tasks that are commonly encountered in hospital and rehabilitation settings (e.g., drink water from a cup; button a shirt). The interview includes questions regarding the impact of loss on unilateral and bilateral tasks, level of independence, nature of difficulties (e.g., clumsiness), and use of compensatory techniques. Test–retest reliability is high (ρ = .99; κ = .97), and the test shows moderate agreement with change scores on the Action Research Arm Test (Blennerhassett et al., 2010). Quantitatively defined sensory impairment and pinch-grip deficit after stroke have also been correlated with poor performance on the Jebsen–Taylor Test of Hand Function, particularly the test component that requires timed placement of small objects in a tin can (Blennerhassett, Carey, & Matyas, 2008). Given the association between these tools and sensory loss under controlled conditions, these clinical tools may be useful in assessing hand function, particularly as it relates to poststroke sensory loss.

The Canadian Occupational Performance Measure (COPM; Law et al., 2005) is a structured interview that may be used to help identify activities across self-care, productivity, and leisure domains with which the person with stroke has difficulty and that are perceived by the person to be associated with the sensory loss. Using the tool, patients identify the activities that are important to them and rate their performance and satisfaction with performance of these activities. This tool can be used to identify activities that may be targeted in therapy as well as to evaluate change in performance and satisfaction. Using this information, it is possible to match patients' needs and goals with knowledge of evidence-based interventions that may be appropriate. Clinically significant improvements in performance and satisfaction of patient-selected activities have been found with sensory rehabilitation (Mastos & Carey, 2010).

As yet there is no standardized test of the impact of sensory loss on daily activities. In the absence of standardized measures of sensory disorders on functional activities, the therapist may engage in clinical hypothesis testing. A task of relevance to the person can be used to assess occupational performance outcomes and the impact of sensory loss on task performance. Sensory demands of the task can be manipulated, based on knowledge of the impact of sensory loss on perception and action, in a hypothesis-testing manner. For example, the occupational task of relevance may be eating, which involves use of cutlery and cutting up food. Steps involved would include

1. Identifying occupational performance issues for the patient;
2. Identifying somatosensory demands of the task in relation to touch–texture, proprioception, and tactile object recognition; and
3. Manipulating the sensory demands of the task to assess presence and impact of sensory loss on the task, that is, structuring the task to vary sensory demands and observe relative improvement or deterioration in performance (hypothesis testing).

Tools such as the Activity Card Sort (Baum & Edwards, 2008) may also be useful to define the percentage of activities retained after stroke.

Evaluation of Visual Impairment

Similar levels of evaluation are recommended in relation to visual impairment after stroke. Visual acuity and visual fields are key components of vision that are commonly tested in clinical settings. A recommended and standardized quantitative measure of visual acuity is the Early Treatment of Diabetic Retinopathy Study chart (Vector Vision, n.d.). Visual fields are commonly assessed to detect dysfunction in central and peripheral vision. This assessment may be done clinically using the confrontation visual fields test or using quantitative perimetry testing (Rowe et al., 2013b). The most common type of visual field loss is **homonymous hemianopsia,** which occurs in approximately two-thirds of those with visual field loss (Rowe et al., 2009).

In assessing vision, one must also be aware of the impact of the environment and lighting. The impact of vision loss on function may be assessed using questionnaires such as the National Eye Institute's Visual Functioning Questionnaire–25 or the Impact of Vision Impairment Questionnaire (Lamoureux, Pallant, Pesudovs, Hassell, & Keeffe, 2006). The vision-related quality of life scales may also be used. Vision may also need to be assessed in the context of particular occupations, such as driving (Unsworth et al., 2012). The World Health Organization classifies *visual impairment* as socially significant visual impairment, visual impairment, severe visual impairment, or blindness (Lamoureux et al., 2006). Useful resources for the evaluation of vision are the National Institutes of Health Toolbox site (http://www.nihtoolbox.org/WhatAndWhy/Sensation/Pages/default.aspx; click "Vision") and the visABILITIES® Rehab Services site (http://www.visabilities.com). This site provides continuing education for rehabilitation professionals and is an approved provider program of the American Occupational Therapy Association.

The most common type of visual field loss is **homonymous hemianopsia,** which occurs in approximately two-thirds of those with visual field loss.

Models of Recovery and Rehabilitation for Sensory Impairment After Stroke

Evidence of neural plastic changes associated with somatosensory processing in animals and humans has supported the potential for active, restorative approaches to rehabilitation. Neural plastic changes occur in response to injury but also as part of normal learning and development (Carey, 2012c).

Neural Plasticity as a Model of Somatosensory Recovery and Rehabilitation

The evidence of plasticity within the somatosensory system is growing (Carey, 2012c). For example, animal models have demonstrated large-scale reorganization in the somatosensory cortex and thalamus after sensory loss in macaque monkeys (Kaas & Pons, 2006). Involvement of the thalamus suggests that gating of sensory inputs, rather than cortical representation alone, may be important in recovery. The benefit of experience and task-specific learning in facilitating brain reorganization has been demonstrated in models of recovery in monkeys (Nudo, Wise, SiFuentes, & Milliken, 1996). Similarly, in the somatosensory domain, Recanzone, Jenkins, Hradek, and Merzenich (1992) demonstrated changes in cortical sensory representations associated with improvement in discriminative abilities.

Neural correlates of sensory recovery after stroke have been described in humans, although studies are still relatively few and sample sizes are typically small (Carey, Abbott, et al., 2011; Rossini et al., 2007). Studies of patients with lesions of **subcortical** thalamic sensory regions have shown relative sparing of activation in ipsilesional SI, return of activation in ipsilesional SI and bilateral SII with good recovery, or both (Carey, Abbott, et al., 2002; Rossini et al., 2007). Disruption to interhemispheric activity in SI has also been demonstrated and may be important in recovery. In comparison, patients with cortical lesions involving SI and SII show more distributed and variable patterns (Carey, Abbott, et al., 2011). An interesting finding was that activation in contralesional thalamus was associated with somatosensory recovery in those with lesions of cortical or subcortical sensory regions (Carey, Abbott, et al., 2011). Changes in structural and functional connections in the somatosensory network may also be observed (Carey, 2012c).

My colleagues and I have proposed a **neuroscience**-based model of somatosensory recovery based on this information, although we recognize that the data are still limited and the model requires further development (see Carey & Seitz, 2007, Figure 8). In this model, both hemispheres are involved, consistent with the role of interhemispheric connections in sensory processing and motor recovery. On the basis of this model and studies in somatosensory recovery, we expect recovery to be associated with changes involving transcallosal connections between primary somatosensory regions and thalamocortical connections. More important, new connections with the related visual system are also proposed on the basis of evidence of cross-modal plasticity and activity in visual cortical regions during tactile perception.

Learning-Based Models of Recovery and Rehabilitation

Carey, Polatajko, Connor, and Baum (2012) have advocated learning-based models of stroke rehabilitation. These models are supported by cognitive neuroscience of learning and evidence of neural plastic changes after stroke and require identification of core principles that underlie these changes. One such model is the Rehabilitation Learning Model of stroke rehabilitation (Carey et al., 2012). In this model, Carey et al. defined *rehabilitation* as "an active process focused on facilitation of adaptive learning" (p. 12). The role of the therapist is to facilitate reacquisition of performance capacities and skills that may be relearned or learned in a new way. Learning is synonymous with neural plastic changes in the brain. The question remains: How can therapeutic intervention build on and shape the ability of the brain to adapt and learn after injury such as a stroke?

The question remains: How can therapeutic intervention build on and shape the ability of the brain to adapt and learn after injury such as a stroke?

One approach to sensory rehabilitation that has been systematically developed over the past 20 years and is based on theories of learning and neural plasticity is known as *SENSe* (based on the acronym given to the randomized controlled trial that tested its effectiveness, the Study of the Effectiveness of Neurorehabilitation on Sensation; Carey, Macdonell, & Matyas, 2011). The program includes core principles of active facilitated learning as well as principles specific to somatosensory function. Three key principles of training are operationalized in the SENSe approach: (1) goal-directed attention and deliberate anticipation, (2) calibration across and within modality, and (3) graded progression within and across sensory attributes and tasks (Carey, 2012c; Carey, Macdonell, & Matyas, 2011). The program also uses principles of learning specifically designed to facilitate transfer of training effects (Carey & Matyas, 2005). In addition to clinical outcomes, our research group has demonstrated changes in brain activity associated with sensory recovery (Carey, Abbott, et al., 2002; Carey, Abbott, et al., 2011) and sensory rehabilitation (Carey, 2012c). Improvement in touch discrimination capacity has been associated with return to more typical task-related patterns of activation and intrinsic brain connectivity in primary and secondary somatosensory cortices. Involvement of attention and vision networks has also been observed.

Further development and integration of neuroscience and learning-based models of rehabilitation are needed. A model that incorporates learning and neural plasticity would need to identify core brain networks involved in processing goal-directed somatosensory information, as well as related networks (such as visual and attention networks) that have a role in processing sensory information under certain conditions, particularly with learning. Identifying these networks will help to build a model of interconnected networks that may be targeted in therapy, while taking into account the impact of the infarct (Carey, 2012c).

Compensatory Approaches

In addition to models that focus on restoration of capacities and skills, addressing issues related to ongoing and residual performance limitations is needed from a safety and lifestyle perspective. Here it is important to integrate the person's goals and take into account the environmental context. Compensatory models may include changing the environment, performing the task in an alternative way (e.g., using the other hand), and educating the patient on how to approach the task in a different way (e.g., testing the temperature of the bath water using the unaffected hand).

Current Approaches to Sensory Rehabilitation After Stroke

The number of documented and tested somatosensory retraining programs designed for use with stroke patients is relatively limited (Carey, 1995, 2006, 2012c; Doyle,

Bennett, Fasoli, & McKenna, 2010; Schabrun & Hillier, 2009). These approaches may be grouped according to major principles of training, the underlying models of recovery and rehabilitation, or both (Carey, 2012c). To date, only a few interventions are supported by empirical evidence and a strong scientific foundation.

Passive Stimulation and Bombardment

Early approaches that used sensory bombardment and passive stimulation (e.g., high-intensity touch and vibration stimuli) did not show a positive outcome (Fox, 1964) or showed only limited effect (De Jersey, 1979). More recent approaches have used sensory stimulation, such as electrical stimulation, in the context of improving motor function. Some of these approaches have been included in systematic reviews of sensory retraining as methods of passive sensory training (Doyle et al., 2010; Schabrun & Hillier, 2009). However, as argued by Carey and colleagues (McCluskey, Logan, Carey, Blennerhassett, & Matyas, 2010), these should not be viewed as approaches to sensory rehabilitation on the basis that most did not directly retrain sensation but were focused on movement, most patients did not show sensory impairment, and stimulation was transient with only short-term outcomes that were short-lived. Moreover, caution has been recommended in relation to use of suprasensory threshold stimulation (Conforto et al., 2010). A bombardment–passive stimulation approach does not involve attentive processing of sensory information and has an unknown effect on interhemispheric balance of activity (Carey, 2012c). Patients frequently report that the approach, which may include being asked to retrieve objects from bowls of rice, is frustrating and confusing (Lyons, 2010). On this basis, passive stimulation and bombardment approaches are not recommended.

Graded Sensory and Sensorimotor Exercises With Feedback

A few approaches have used graded somatosensory and sensorimotor exercises, with and without vision, in which the patient is required to attend to the sensation during the task and feedback is provided, often via the other hand (Byl et al., 2003; Yekutiel & Guttman, 1993). Sensory tasks include identification of number of touches or letters drawn on the arm; "find your [plegic] thumb" while blindfolded; discrimination of weight, shape, and texture of objects; and passive drawing with the finger (Yekutiel & Guttman, 1993). Yekutiel and Guttman's approach was based on perceptual learning and provided guidance on the tactics of perception. Training was conducted 3 times a week for 6 weeks. Byl et al.'s (2003) approach focused more on sensorimotor exercises to achieve outcomes of improved accuracy and speed in relation to sensorimotor function. Sensory exercises included playing board games and learning to read braille books, retrieving objects from a box filled with rice, exercises in graphesthesia, localization, stereognosis, and kinesthesia, and use of hook-and-loop fasteners on objects. The hand was used in functional activities, and both mental rehearsal and constraint of the unaffected limb were used. In addition, patients were educated regarding the potential for neural plasticity, and tasks were used to "quiet" the nervous system. Principles of training were linked to theories of neural plasticity (Byl & Merzenich, 2000) and included matching tasks to the patient's ability and use of attention, repetition, feedback on performance, and progression in difficulty. Supervised sensory training was conducted for 1.5 hours per week over 4 weeks. Smania, Montagnana, Faccioli, Fiaschi, and Aglioti (2003) conducted a study of sensorimotor exercises in four case studies. Focus was on sensory and motor functions and incorporated practice of functional tasks. Overall, using this approach patients were reported to show improvement in one or more of the sensory tasks and in related tasks not trained.

Perceptual Learning and Neuroscience-Based Approach: Stimulus-Specific and Transfer-Enhanced Training

Carey and colleagues have systematically developed an approach to sensory rehabilitation that is derived from theories of learning and neural plasticity and operationalized into stimulus-specific (Carey, Matyas, & Oke, 1993) and transfer-enhanced (Carey, Macdonell, & Matyas, 2011; Carey & Matyas, 2005) training approaches. Seven principles of training have been defined and operationalized in the program (Carey, 2012c; Carey, Macdonell, & Matyas, 2011), with three of these being identified as core (Carey, 2012c). These three principles are (1) use of goal-directed attentive exploration and anticipation trials to enhance sensory thresholds and processing; (2) calibration of the patient's impaired touch sensation internally by reference to more normal touch sensation experienced through the unaffected hand and via vision; and (3) graded progression of training across a matrix of somatosensory tasks that vary in degree of difficulty and sensory attribute trained. This training program has demonstrated effectiveness in a randomized controlled trial (Carey, Macdonell, & Matyas, 2011) and a meta-analysis of 30 single-case experiments (Carey, 2006).

Stimulus-specific training (Carey, 2006; Carey et al., 1993) uses learning-based discrimination training of specific sensory stimuli, such as texture grids and limb positions (Carey et al., 1993). Outcomes were clinically and statistically effective in improving sensory tasks trained on the basis of a meta-analysis of 30 controlled single-case experiments ($z = -8.6$, $p < .0001$; Carey, 2006). The training approach was then developed to enhance transfer of training effects to novel stimuli not trained. Transfer-enhanced training (Carey & Matyas, 2005) involves training of a variety of sensory attributes such as roughness across a matrix of sensory tasks, including common textures with varying surface characteristics or training of limb position sense across different movement ranges such as flexion–extension and ulnar–radial deviation at the wrist. A variety of stimuli and learning conditions, tuition in training principles, and feedback on the act of transfer to novel stimuli are used to facilitate transfer (Carey & Matyas, 2005). Transfer-enhanced training significantly improved transfer to novel stimuli not trained ($z = -5.7$, $p < .0001$; Carey, 2006; Carey & Matyas, 2005).

The transfer-enhanced training approach has since been incorporated into SENSe, a clinical package to train texture discrimination, limb position sense, and tactile object recognition. This training program, discussed earlier in the "Learning-Based Models of Recovery and Rehabilitation" section, was tested in a randomized controlled trial performed by our research group with positive outcomes in sensory capacity and upper-limb function (Carey, Macdonell, & Matyas, 2011). A further development has been to apply the principles in the context of training occupational tasks identified as important by the patient (Carey, 2012c; Mastos & Carey, 2010).

Stroke patients with varying characteristics, including side of lesion and age, were able to benefit from SENSe training (Carey, Matyas, Walker, & Macdonell, 2010).

A training manual and video have been developed to demonstrate how the training principles are operationalized (Carey, 2012a). Training modules are described for texture discrimination using a wide range of surface characteristics; limb position sense at elbow, wrist, and finger; and tactile object recognition that involves discrimination of shape, size, texture, hardness, weight, temperature, and functional motion. The steps involved in applying the SENSe training principles to occupational tasks are also described. Finally, examples of how to plan a treatment program and further examples of application to everyday tasks are provided.

One person with stroke who participated in the SENSe learning-based approach to sensory rehabilitation made the following comment after training:

> Since undertaking sensory retraining, all tasks using my stroke-affected hand are easier and require less concentration. It still doesn't feel as though I have as much sense of touch in my stroke-affected hand but obviously my brain is making very good sense of a lot of information as I am now quite competently performing most tasks. Because things require less concentration, I am less frustrated and fatigued, leaving more brain space and energy for enjoying life and assisting others. I am able to celebrate more things I can do rather than feel the setbacks of the things I can't do or struggle with.

Current Approaches to Rehabilitation of Visual Functions

Rehabilitation approaches for visual field loss include restitution, substitution, and compensatory options (Pollock et al., 2011; Romano, 2009; Rowe, 2013a). Treatment of the hemianoptic patient may include (1) teaching the patient basic strategies to overcome the hemianopsia, such as boundary marking (i.e., use of the finger or cues to mark the edge of print) and encouraging the patient to look first in the direction of the field loss before trying to search for an object; (2) using optical devices to shift the visual field over, including the Gottlieb Visual Field Awareness System (http://www.hemianopsia.net/the-gottlieb-visual-field-awar); and (3) using scanning therapy to train the patient to better compensate for the loss of visual field (Carey, 2015; Rowe, 2013a). A comparison of these approaches indicated that the greatest improvement in function occurs after visual search training (Pollock et al., 2011).

Significant improvements in overall quality of life, emotional well-being, and reading and accessing information were found in people with low vision after a multidisciplinary low-vision rehabilitation program.

Significant improvements in overall quality of life, emotional well-being, and reading and accessing information were found in people with low vision after a multidisciplinary low vision rehabilitation program that included occupational therapists and orientation and mobility, orthoptics, and welfare specialists (Lamoureux et al., 2007). Compensatory options, in particular, have shown favorable effects on improved visual scanning into the hemianopic side (Pambakian, Currie, & Kennard, 2005; Roth et al., 2009). Fresnel Prism glasses (15 diopter) have also been investigated as a means of improving visual function in people with homonymous hemianopsia (Rossi, Kheyfets, & Reding, 1990).

Visual restitution training has potential (Henriksson, Raninen, Näsänen, Hyvärinen, & Vanni, 2007) but is not currently being used in rehabilitation settings

(Rowe, 2013a). Visual restorative therapy aims to restore the visual field, and treatment options may include computer-based visual restitution training (Kasten, Wüst, Behrens-Baumann, & Sabel, 1998) or flicker stimulation of the blind field (Henriksson et al., 2007). Improvement has been reported in locating moving flickering objects in the blind field, navigation skills, reading ability, and visual sensitivity (Mueller, Mast, & Sabel, 2007). Involvement of spouses and other family members in rehabilitation may be important given the negative impact of the visual impairment on them in addition to the visually impaired person (Strawbridge, Wallhagen, & Shema, 2007). Further information and guidelines for the application of rehabilitation interventions may be found at the visABILITIES Rehab Services site (http://www.visabilities.com). Web-based therapies are also freely available as compensatory visual search and scanning training (http://www.readright.ucl.ac.uk, http://www.eyesearch.ucl.ac.uk).

Stroke Guidelines

Clinical guidelines for stroke rehabilitation, for example from Australia, support the use of sensory-specific training (Byl et al., 2003; Carey et al., 1993; Hillier & Dunsford, 2006; Yekutiel & Guttman, 1993) and sensory training designed to facilitate transfer (Carey & Matyas, 2005) for people with stroke who have somatosensory loss (National Stroke Foundation, 2010). This approach is further supported by the more recent randomized controlled trial known as SENSe (Carey, Macdonell, & Matyas, 2011). In relation to visual impairment, stroke guidelines (National Stroke Foundation, 2010) have indicated some support for Fresnel Prism glasses (15 diopter) to improve visual function in people with homonymous hemianopsia (Rossi et al., 1990). Computer-based visual restitution training may also be used to improve visual function in people with visual field deficits (Kasten et al., 1998).

Summary

Impairment of sensation, including somatosensations and vision, after stroke is common and has a significant impact on an individual and his or her ability to reengage in previous life activities. Sensations are interpreted in the context of the goal of the perceiver in his or her environment. This is important in relation to how people use their senses, the affordances they provide for action, and how therapists should guide stroke survivors to reinterpret their altered sensations during training. Quantitative measures are available to assess sensory loss. Presence and implications of this loss should be assessed within the context of functional activities important to the individual. Approaches to sensory rehabilitation based on neural plasticity and learning are supported by growing evidence in animal models of recovery as well as in humans. Current approaches to rehabilitation of sensory functions should be reviewed, in relation to both current theory and empirical outcomes. Therapists can now help stroke survivors regain lost body sensations through evidence-based interventions, such as SENSe, that have operationalized neuroscience and learning principles into empirically tested specific therapeutic protocols. It is critical that therapists adopt an evidence-based approach to assessment and treatment in this important area of clinical practice.

References

Ayres, A. J. (1980). *Southern California Sensory Integration Tests*. Los Angeles: Western Psychological Services.

Baum, C. M., & Edwards, D. F. (2008). *Activity Card Sort* (2nd ed.). Bethesda, MD: AOTA Press.

Becker, S. (1996). Mutual information maximization: Models of cortical self-organization. *Network: Computations in Neural Systems, 7*, 7–31. http://dx.doi.org/10.1088/0954-898X/7/1/003

Blennerhassett, J. M., Avery, R. M., & Carey, L. M. (2010). The test–retest reliability and responsiveness to change for the Hand Function Survey during stroke rehabilitation. *Australian Occupational Therapy Journal, 57*, 431–438. http://dx.doi.org/10.1111/j.1440-1630.2010.00884.x

Blennerhassett, J. M., Carey, L. M., & Matyas, T. A. (2006). Grip force regulation during pinch grip lifts under somatosensory guidance: Comparison between people with stroke and healthy controls. *Archives of Physical Medicine and Rehabilitation, 87*, 418–429. http://dx.doi.org/10.1016/j.apmr.2005.11.018

Blennerhassett, J. M., Carey, L. M., & Matyas, T. A. (2008). Clinical measures of handgrip limitation relate to impaired pinch grip force control after stroke. *Journal of Hand Therapy, 21*, 245–252, quiz 253. http://dx.doi.org/10.1197/j.jht.2007.10.021

Blennerhassett, J. M., Matyas, T. A., & Carey, L. M. (2007). Impaired discrimination of surface friction contributes to pinch grip deficit after stroke. *Neurorehabilitation and Neural Repair, 21*, 263–272. http://dx.doi.org/10.1177/1545968306295560

Boly, M., Balteau, E., Schnakers, C., Degueldre, C., Moonen, G., Luxen, A., . . . Laureys, S. (2007). Baseline brain activity fluctuations predict somatosensory perception in humans. *Proceedings of the National Academy of Sciences of the United States of America, 104*, 12187–12192. http://dx.doi.org/10.1073/pnas.0611404104

Byl, N., & Merzenich, M. M. (2000). Principles of neuroplasticity: Implications for neurorehabilitation and learning. In E. S. Gonzalez, S. Myers, J. Edelstein, J. S. Liebermann, & J. A. Downey (Eds.), *Downey and Darling's physiological basis of rehabilitation medicine* (pp. 609–628). Boston: Butterworth-Heinemann.

Byl, N., Roderick, J., Mohamed, O., Hanny, M., Kotler, J., Smith, A., . . . Abrams, G. (2003). Effectiveness of sensory and motor rehabilitation of the upper limb following the principles of neuroplasticity: Patients stable poststroke. *Neurorehabilitation and Neural Repair, 17*, 176–191. http://dx.doi.org/10.1177/0888439003257137

Carey, L. M. (1995). Somatosensory loss after stroke. *Critical Reviews in Physical and Rehabilitation Medicine, 7*, 51–91.

Carey, L. M. (2006). Loss of somatic sensation. In M. Selzer, S. Clarke, L. Cohen, P. Duncan, & F. H. Gage (Eds.), *Textbook of neural repair and rehabilitation: Vol. II. Medical neurorehabilitation* (pp. 231–247). Cambridge, England: Cambridge University Press.

Carey, L. M. (2012a). *SENSe: Helping stroke survivors regain a sense of touch; A manual for therapists*. Melbourne, Victoria: Florey Neuroscience Institutes.

Carey, L. M. (2012b). *Stroke rehabilitation: Insights from neuroscience and imaging*. New York: Oxford University Press.

Carey, L. M. (2012c). Touch and body sensations. In L. M. Carey (Ed.), *Stroke rehabilitation: Insights from neuroscience and imaging* (pp. 157–172). New York: Oxford University Press.

Carey, L. M. (2015). Person factors: Sensory. In C. H. Christiansen, C. M. Baum, & J. Bass-Haugen (Eds.), *Occupational therapy: Performance, participation, and well-being* (4th ed.). Thorofare, NJ: Slack.

Carey, L. M., Abbott, D. F., Harvey, M. R., Puce, A., Seitz, R. J., & Donnan, G. A. (2011). Relationship between touch impairment and brain activation after lesions of subcortical and cortical somatosensory regions. *Neurorehabilitation and Neural Repair, 25*, 443–457. http://dx.doi.org/10.1177/1545968310395777

Carey, L. M., Abbott, D. F., Puce, A., Jackson, G. D., Syngeniotis, A., & Donnan, G. A. (2002). Reemergence of activation with poststroke somatosensory recovery: A serial fMRI case study. *Neurology, 59*, 749–752. http://dx.doi.org/10.1212/WNL.59.5.749

Carey, L. M., Jacobs, S., Baum, C., & Connor, L. (2010). *Loss of somatosensation and its impact on activity participation following stroke*. Paper presented at the 2010 European Stroke Conference, Barcelona, Spain.

Carey, L. M., Macdonell, R., & Matyas, T. A. (2011). SENSe: Study of the Effectiveness of Neurorehabilitation on Sensation: A randomized controlled trial. *Neurorehabilitation and Neural Repair, 25*, 304–313. http://dx.doi.org/10.1177/1545968310397705

Carey, L. M., Mak, Y., & Tan, A. M. (2011). *SenScreen: Sensory Screening Tool administration manual*. Melbourne, Victoria, Australia: Florey Neuroscience Institutes.

Carey, L. M., & Matyas, T. A. (2005). Training of somatosensory discrimination after stroke: Facilitation of stimulus generalization. *American Journal of Physical Medicine and Rehabilitation, 84,* 428–442. http://dx.doi.org/10.1097/01.PHM.0000159971.12096.7F

Carey, L. M., & Matyas, T. A. (2011). Frequency of discriminative sensory loss in the hand after stroke in a rehabilitation setting. *Journal of Rehabilitation Medicine, 43,* 257–263. http://dx.doi.org/10.2340/16501977-0662

Carey, L. M., Matyas, T. A., & Oke, L. E. (1993). Sensory loss in stroke patients: Effective training of tactile and proprioceptive discrimination. *Archives of Physical Medicine and Rehabilitation, 74,* 602–611. http://dx.doi.org/10.1016/0003-9993(93)90158-7

Carey, L. M., Matyas, T. A., & Oke, L. E. (2002). Evaluation of impaired fingertip texture discrimination and wrist position sense in patients affected by stroke: Comparison of clinical and new quantitative measures. *Journal of Hand Therapy, 15,* 71–82. http://dx.doi.org/10.1053/hanthe.2002.v15.01571

Carey, L. M., Matyas, T. A., Walker, J., & Macdonell, R. (2010). SENSe: Study of the Effectiveness of Neurorehabilitation on Sensation: Individual patient characteristics that predict favourable outcomes. *International Journal of Stroke, 5*(Suppl.), 1–45. http://dx.doi.org/10.1111/j.1747-4949.2010.00496.x

Carey, L. M., Nankervis, J., LeBlanc, S., & Harvey, L. (2006). *A new functional Tactual Object Recognition Test (fTORT) for stroke clients: Normative standards and discriminative validity.* Paper presented at the 14th International Congress of the World Federation of Occupational Therapists, Sydney, New South Wales, Australia.

Carey, L. M., Oke, L. E., & Matyas, T. A. (1996). Impaired limb position sense after stroke: A quantitative test for clinical use. *Archives of Physical Medicine and Rehabilitation, 77,* 1271–1278. http://dx.doi.org/10.1016/S0003-9993(96)90192-6

Carey, L. M., Oke, L. E., & Matyas, T. A. (1997). Impaired touch discrimination after stroke: A quantitative test. *Neurorehabilitation and Neural Repair, 11,* 219–232. http://dx.doi.org/10.1177/154596839701100404

Carey, L. M., Polatajko, H. J., Connor, L. T., & Baum, C. M. (2012). Stroke rehabilitation: A learning perspective. In L. M. Carey (Ed.), *Stroke rehabilitation: Insights from neuroscience and imaging* (pp. 11–23). New York: Oxford University Press.

Carey, L. M., & Seitz, R. J. (2007). Functional neuroimaging in stroke recovery and neurorehabilitation: Conceptual issues and perspectives. *International Journal of Stroke, 2,* 245–264. http://dx.doi.org/10.1111/j.1747-4949.2007.00164.x

Carey, L. M., Seitz, R. J., Parsons, M., Levi, C., Farquaharson, S., Tournier, J.-D., . . . Connelly, A. (2013). Beyond the lesion: Neuroimaging foundations for post-stroke recovery. *Future Neurology, 8,* 507–524. http://dx.doi.org/10.2217/fnl.13.39

Conforto, A. B., Ferreiro, K. N., Tomasi, C., dos Santos, R. L., Moreira, V. L., Marie, S. K., . . . Cohen, L. G. (2010). Effects of somatosensory stimulation on motor function after subacute stroke. *Neurorehabilitation and Neural Repair, 24,* 263–272. http://dx.doi.org/10.1177/1545968309349946

Connell, L. A., Lincoln, N. B., & Radford, K. A. (2008). Somatosensory impairment after stroke: Frequency of different deficits and their recovery. *Clinical Rehabilitation, 22,* 758–767. http://dx.doi.org/10.1177/0269215508090674

Corbetta, M. (2012). Functional connectivity and neurological recovery. *Developmental Psychobiology, 54,* 239–253. http://dx.doi.org/10.1002/dev.20507

Cramer, S. C., Sur, M., Dobkin, B. H., O'Brien, C., Sanger, T. D., Trojanowski, J. Q., . . . Vinogradov, S. (2011). Harnessing neuroplasticity for clinical applications. *Brain, 134,* 1591–1609. http://dx.doi.org/10.1093/brain/awr039

Dannenbaum, R. M., & Dykes, R. W. (1988). Sensory loss in the hand after sensory stroke: Therapeutic rationale. *Archives of Physical Medicine and Rehabilitation, 69,* 833–839.

De Jersey, M. C. (1979). Report on a sensory programme for patients with sensory deficits. *Australian Journal of Physiotherapy, 25,* 165–170. http://dx.doi.org/10.1016/S0004-9514(14)61039-4

Dellon, A. L. (2000). *Somatosensory testing and rehabilitation.* Baltimore: Institute for Peripheral Nerve Surgery.

Dijkerman, H. C., & de Haan, E. H. (2007). Somatosensory processes subserving perception and action. *Behavioral and Brain Sciences, 30,* 189–201, discussion 201–239. http://dx.doi.org/10.1017/S0140525X07001392

Doyle, S., Bennett, S., Fasoli, S. E., & McKenna, K. T. (2010). Interventions for sensory impairment in the upper limb after stroke. *Cochrane Database of Systematic Reviews, 2010,* CD006331.

Driver, J., & Noesselt, T. (2008). Multisensory interplay reveals crossmodal influences on "sensory-specific" brain regions, neural responses, and judgments. *Neuron, 57,* 11–23. http://dx.doi.org/10.1016/j.neuron.2007.12.013

Dromerick, A. W., & Reding, M. J. (1995). Functional outcome for patients with hemiparesis, hemi-hypesthesia, and hemianopsia: Does lesion location matter? *Stroke, 26,* 2023–2026. http://dx.doi.org/10.1161/01.STR.26.11.2023

Dunn, W., Griffith, J. W., Morrison, M. T., Tanquary, J., Sabata, D., Victorson, D., . . . Gershon, R. C. (2013). Somatosensation assessment using the NIH Toolbox. *Neurology, 80*(Suppl. 3), S41–S44. http://dx.doi.org/10.1212/WNL.0b013e3182872c54

Fox, J. V. (1964). Cutaneous stimulation: Effects on selected tests of perception. *American Journal of Occupational Therapy, 18,* 53–55.

Frey, S. H., Fogassi, L., Grafton, S. T., Picard, N., Rothwell, J. C., Schweighofer, N., . . . Fitzpatrick, S. M. (2011). Neurological principles and rehabilitation of action disorders: Computation, anatomy, and physiology (CAP) model. *Neurorehabilitation and Neural Repair, 25*(Suppl.), 6S–20S. http://dx.doi.org/10.1177/1545968311410940

Gentilucci, M., Toni, I., Daprati, E., & Gangitano, M. (1997). Tactile input of the hand and the control of reaching to grasp movements. *Experimental Brain Research, 114,* 130–137. http://dx.doi.org/10.1007/PL00005612

Goldberg, I. I., Harel, M., & Malach, R. (2006). When the brain loses its self: Prefrontal inactivation during sensorimotor processing. *Neuron, 50,* 329–339. http://dx.doi.org/10.1016/j.neuron.2006.03.015

Goodale, M. A., & Milner, A. D. (1992). Separate visual pathways for perception and action. *Trends in Neurosciences, 15,* 20–25. http://dx.doi.org/10.1016/0166-2236(92)90344-8

Henriksson, L., Raninen, A., Näsänen, R., Hyvärinen, L., & Vanni, S. (2007). Training-induced cortical representation of a hemianopic hemifield. *Journal of Neurology, Neurosurgery, and Psychiatry, 78,* 74–81. http://dx.doi.org/10.1136/jnnp.2006.099374

Hermsdörfer, J., Hagl, E., Nowak, D. A., & Marquardt, C. (2003). Grip force control during object manipulation in cerebral stroke. *Clinical Neurophysiology, 114,* 915–929. http://dx.doi.org/10.1016/S1388-2457(03)00042-7

Hillier, S., & Dunsford, A. (2006). A pilot study of sensory retraining for the hemiparetic foot post-stroke. *International Journal of Rehabilitation Research, 29,* 237–242. http://dx.doi.org/10.1097/01.mrr.0000210052.32539.22

Hlushchuk, Y., & Hari, R. (2006). Transient suppression of ipsilateral primary somatosensory cortex during tactile finger stimulation. *Journal of Neuroscience, 26,* 5819–5824. http://dx.doi.org/10.1523/JNEUROSCI.5536-05.2006

Jones, S. A., & Shinton, R. A. (2006). Improving outcome in stroke patients with visual problems. *Age and Ageing, 35,* 560–565. http://dx.doi.org/10.1093/ageing/afl074

Kaas, J. H., & Pons, T. P. (2006). Plasticity of mature and developing somatosensory systems. In M. Selzer, S. Clarke, L. G. Cohen, P. W. Duncan, & F. H. Gage (Eds.), *Textbook of neural repair and rehabilitation: Neural repair and plasticity* (pp. 97–108). Cambridge, England: Cambridge University Press.

Kandel, E. R., Schwartz, J. H., & Jessell, T. M. (2000). *Principles of neural science.* New York: McGraw-Hill.

Kasten, E., Wüst, S., Behrens-Baumann, W., & Sabel, B. A. (1998). Computer-based training for the treatment of partial blindness. *Nature Medicine, 4,* 1083–1087. http://dx.doi.org/10.1038/2079

Kim, J. S., & Choi-Kwon, S. (1996). Discriminative sensory dysfunction after unilateral stroke. *Stroke, 27,* 677–682. http://dx.doi.org/10.1161/01.STR.27.4.677

Lamoureux, E. L., Hassell, J. B., & Keeffe, J. E. (2004). The determinants of participation in activities of daily living in people with impaired vision. *American Journal of Ophthalmology, 137,* 265–270. http://dx.doi.org/10.1016/j.ajo.2003.08.003

Lamoureux, E. L., Pallant, J. F., Pesudovs, K., Hassell, J. B., & Keeffe, J. E. (2006). The Impact of Vision Impairment Questionnaire: An evaluation of its measurement properties using Rasch analysis. *Investigative Ophthalmology and Visual Science, 47,* 4732–4741. http://dx.doi.org/10.1167/iovs.06-0220

Lamoureux, E. L., Pallant, J. F., Pesudovs, K., Rees, G., Hassell, J. B., & Keeffe, J. E. (2007). The effectiveness of low-vision rehabilitation on participation in daily living and quality of life. *Investigative Ophthalmology and Visual Science, 48,* 1476–1482. http://dx.doi.org/10.1167/iovs.06-0610

Law, M., Baptiste, S., Carswell, A., McColl, M. A., Polatajko, H., & Pollock, N. (2005). *The Canadian Occupational Performance Measure* (4th ed.). Ottawa, Ontario: CAOT Publications.

Lederman, S. J., & Klatzky, R. L. (1993). Extracting object properties through haptic exploration. *Acta Psychologica, 84,* 29–40. http://dx.doi.org/10.1016/0001-6918(93)90070-8

Lincoln, N. B., Jackson, J. M., & Adams, S. A. (1998). Reliability and revision of the Nottingham Sensory Assessment for stroke patients. *Physiotherapy, 84,* 358–365. http://dx.doi.org/10.1016/S0031-9406(05)61454-X

Lyons, W. (2010). *Left of tomorrow.* Glen Waverley, Victoria, Australia: Sid Harta.

Mak, Y. K. (2010). *Development of a sensory screening tool for use with rehabilitation patients post stroke: Evaluation of quantitative measures for inclusion.* Unpublished honors thesis, Latrobe University, Bundoora, Victoria, Australia.

Massof, R. W., Ahmadian, L., Grover, L. L., Deremeik, J. T., Goldstein, J. E., Rainey, C., . . . Barnett, G. D. (2007). The Activity Inventory: An adaptive visual function questionnaire. *Optometry and Vision Science, 84,* 763–774. http://dx.doi.org/10.1097/OPX.0b013e3181339efd

Mastos, M., & Carey, L. (2010). *Occupation-based outcomes associated with sensory retraining post-stroke.* Paper presented at the 21st Annual Scientific Meeting of the Stroke Society of Australasia, Melbourne, Victoria, Australia.

McCluskey, A., Logan, P., Carey, L., Blennerhassett, J., & Matyas, T. A. (2010). Evidence for the retraining of sensation after stroke remains limited. *Australian Occupational Therapy Journal, 57,* 200–202. http://dx.doi.org/10.1111/j.1440-1630.2010.00867.x

Miller, K. J., Phillips, B. A., Martin, C. L., Wheat, H. E., Goodwin, A. W., & Galea, M. P. (2009). The AsTex: Clinimetric properties of a new tool for evaluating hand sensation following stroke. *Clinical Rehabilitation, 23,* 1104–1115. http://dx.doi.org/10.1177/0269215509342331

Mueller, I., Mast, H., & Sabel, B. A. (2007). Recovery of visual field defects: A large clinical observational study using vision restoration therapy. *Restorative Neurology and Neuroscience, 25,* 563–572.

National Stroke Foundation. (2010). *Clinical guidelines for stroke management 2010.* Melbourne, Victoria: Author.

Nicolelis, M. A. (2005). Computing with thalamocortical ensembles during different behavioural states. *Journal of Physiology, 566,* 37–47. http://dx.doi.org/10.1113/jphysiol.2005.083709

Nudo, R. J., Wise, B. M., SiFuentes, F., & Milliken, G. W. (1996). Neural substrates for the effects of rehabilitative training on motor recovery after ischemic infarct. *Science, 272,* 1791–1794.

Pambakian, A., Currie, J., & Kennard, C. (2005). Rehabilitation strategies for patients with homonymous visual field defects. *Journal of Neuro-Ophthalmology, 25,* 136–142.

Patel, A. T., Duncan, P. W., Lai, S.-M., & Studenski, S. (2000). The relation between impairments and functional outcomes poststroke. *Archives of Physical Medicine and Rehabilitation, 81,* 1357–1363. http://dx.doi.org/10.1053/apmr.2000.9397

Perlmutter, M. S., Bhorade, A., Gordon, M., Hollingsworth, H. H., & Baum, M. C. (2010). Cognitive, visual, auditory, and emotional factors that affect participation in older adults. *American Journal of Occupational Therapy, 64,* 570–579. http://dx.doi.org/10.5014/ajot.2010.09089

Pollock, A., Hazelton, C., Henderson, C. A., Angilley, J., Dhillon, B., Langhorne, P., . . . Shahani, U. (2011). Interventions for visual field defects in patients with stroke. *Cochrane Database of Systematic Reviews, 2011,* CD008388.

Puce, A., & Carey, L. (2010). Somatosensory function. In I. B. Weiner, W. E. Craighead, & C. B. Nemeroff (Eds.), *The Corsini encyclopedia of psychology* (4th ed., pp. 1678–1680). New York: Wiley.

Recanzone, G. H., Jenkins, W. M., Hradek, G. T., & Merzenich, M. M. (1992). Progressive improvement in discriminative abilities in adult owl monkeys performing a tactile frequency discrimination task. *Journal of Neurophysiology, 67,* 1015–1030.

Robles-De-La-Torre, G. (2006). The importance of the sense of touch in virtual and real environments. *IEEE MultiMedia, 13,* 24–30. http://dx.doi.org/10.1109/MMUL.2006.69

Romano, J. G. (2009). Progress in rehabilitation of hemianopic visual field defects. *Cerebrovascular Diseases, 27*(Suppl. 1), 187–190. http://dx.doi.org/10.1159/000200458

Rosén, B., & Lundborg, G. (1998). A new tactile gnosis instrument in sensibility testing. *Journal of Hand Therapy, 11,* 251–257. http://dx.doi.org/10.1016/S0894-1130(98)80020-3

Rossi, P. W., Kheyfets, S., & Reding, M. J. (1990). Fresnel prisms improve visual perception in stroke patients with homonymous hemianopia or unilateral visual neglect. *Neurology, 40,* 1597–1599. http://dx.doi.org/10.1212/WNL.40.10.1597

Rossini, P. M., Altamura, C., Ferreri, F., Melgari, J.-M., Tecchio, F., Tombini, M., . . . Vernieri, F. (2007). Neuroimaging experimental studies on brain plasticity in recovery from stroke. *Europa Medicophysica, 43,* 241–254.

Roth, T., Sokolov, A. N., Messias, A., Roth, P., Weller, M., & Trauzettel-Klosinski, S. (2009). Comparing explorative saccade and flicker training in hemianopia: A randomized controlled study. *Neurology, 72,* 324–331. http://dx.doi.org/10.1212/01.wnl.0000341276.65721.f2

Rowe, F. J.; VIS Group UK. (2013a). A prospective profile of visual field loss following stroke: Prevalence, type, rehabilitation, and outcome. *BioMed Research International, 2013,* 719096. http://dx.doi.org/10.1155/2013/719096

Rowe, F. J.; VIS Group UK. (2013b). Symptoms of stroke-related visual impairment. *Strabismus, 21,* 150–154. http://dx.doi.org/10.3109/09273972.2013.786742

Rowe, F. J., Brand, D., Jackson, C. A., Price, A., Walker, L., Harrison, S., . . . Freeman, C. (2009). Visual impairment following stroke: Do stroke patients require vision assessment? *Age and Ageing, 38,* 188–193. http://dx.doi.org/10.1093/ageing/afn230

Sathian, K. (2006). Cross-modal plasticity in sensory systems. In M. Selzer, S. Clarke, L. G. Cohen, P. W. Duncan, & F. H. Gage (Eds.), *Textbook of neural repair and rehabilitation: Neural repair and plasticity* (pp. 180–193). Cambridge, England: Cambridge University Press.

Schabrun, S. M., & Hillier, S. (2009). Evidence for the retraining of sensation after stroke: A systematic review. *Clinical Rehabilitation, 23,* 27–39. http://dx.doi.org/10.1177/0269215508098897

Schaechter, J. D., van Oers, C. A., Groisser, B. N., Salles, S. S., Vangel, M. G., Moore, C. I., & Dijkhuizen, R. M. (2012). Increase in sensorimotor cortex response to somatosensory stimulation over subacute poststroke period correlates with motor recovery in hemiparetic patients. *Neurorehabilitation and Neural Repair, 26,* 325–334. http://dx.doi.org/10.1177/1545968311421613

Smania, N., Montagnana, B., Faccioli, S., Fiaschi, A., & Aglioti, S. M. (2003). Rehabilitation of somatic sensation and related deficit of motor control in patients with pure sensory stroke. *Archives of Physical Medicine and Rehabilitation, 84,* 1692–1702. http://dx.doi.org/10.1053/S0003-9993(03)00277-6

Strawbridge, W. J., Wallhagen, M. I., & Shema, S. J. (2007). Impact of spouse vision impairment on partner health and well-being: A longitudinal analysis of couples. *Journals of Gerontology, Series B: Psychological Sciences, 62,* S315–S322. http://dx.doi.org/10.1093/geronb/62.5.S315

Sullivan, J. E., & Hedman, L. D. (2008). Sensory dysfunction following stroke: Incidence, significance, examination, and intervention. *Topics in Stroke Rehabilitation, 15,* 200–217. http://dx.doi.org/10.1310/tsr1503-200

Talsma, D., Senkowski, D., Soto-Faraco, S., & Woldorff, M. G. (2010). The multifaceted interplay between attention and multisensory integration. *Trends in Cognitive Sciences, 14,* 400–410. http://dx.doi.org/10.1016/j.tics.2010.06.008

Tovée, M. J. (2008). *An introduction to the visual system.* Cambridge, England: Cambridge University Press.

Tyson, S. F., Hanley, M., Chillala, J., Selley, A. B., & Tallis, R. C. (2008). Sensory loss in hospital-admitted people with stroke: Characteristics, associated factors, and relationship with function. *Neurorehabilitation and Neural Repair, 22,* 166–172. http://dx.doi.org/10.1177/1545968307305523

Unsworth, C. A., Baker, A., Taitz, C., Chan, S. P., Pallant, J. F., Russell, K. J., & Odell, M. (2012). Development of a standardised Occupational Therapy–Driver Off-Road Assessment Battery to assess older and/or functionally impaired drivers. *Australian Occupational Therapy Journal, 59,* 23–36. http://dx.doi.org/10.1111/j.1440-1630.2011.00979.x

Van Boven, R. W., & Johnson, K. O. (1994). The limit of tactile spatial resolution in humans: Grating orientation discrimination at the lip, tongue, and finger. *Neurology, 44,* 2361–2366. http://dx.doi.org/10.1212/WNL.44.12.2361

Vector Vision. (n.d.). *ETDRS acuity testing.* Greenville, OH: Author. Retrieved from http://www.vector-vision.com/html/educationETDRSAcuity

Warren, M. (2009). Pilot study on activities of daily living limitations in adults with hemianopsia. *American Journal of Occupational Therapy, 63,* 626–633. http://dx.doi.org/10.5014/ajot.63.5.626

Weinstein, S. (1993). Fifty years of somatosensory research: From the Semmes–Weinstein monofilaments to the Weinstein Enhanced Sensory Test. *Journal of Hand Therapy, 6,* 11–22, discussion 50. http://dx.doi.org/10.1016/S0894-1130(12)80176-1

Williams, P. S., Basso, D. M., Case-Smith, J., & Nichols-Larsen, D. S. (2006). Development of the Hand Active Sensation Test: Reliability and validity. *Archives of Physical Medicine and Rehabilitation, 87,* 1471–1477. http://dx.doi.org/10.1016/j.apmr.2006.08.019

Winward, C. E., Halligan, P. W., & Wade, D. T. (1999). Somatosensory assessment after central nerve damage: The need for standardized clinical measures. *Physical Therapy Review, 4,* 21–28. http://dx.doi.org/10.1179/ptr.1999.4.1.21

Winward, C. E., Halligan, P. W., & Wade, D. T. (2002). The Rivermead Assessment of Somatosensory Performance (RASP): Standardization and reliability data. *Clinical Rehabilitation, 16,* 523–533. http://dx.doi.org/10.1191/0269215502cr522oa

Winward, C. E., Halligan, P. W., & Wade, D. T. (2007). Somatosensory recovery: A longitudinal study of the first 6 months after unilateral stroke. *Disability and Rehabilitation, 29,* 293–299. http://dx.doi.org/10.1080/09638280600756489

Yekutiel, M., & Guttman, E. (1993). A controlled trial of the retraining of the sensory function of the hand in stroke patients. *Journal of Neurology, Neurosurgery, and Psychiatry, 56,* 241–244. http://dx.doi.org/10.1136/jnnp.56.3.241

CHAPTER 6

Core Concepts in Motor Recovery and Rehabilitation After Stroke

Rebecca L. Birkenmeier, OTD, OTR/L

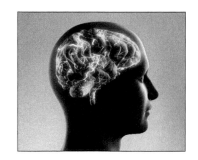

Learning Objectives

After completion of this chapter, readers will be able to

- Recognize key components of the motor system;
- Identify the most common motor impairments to occur after stroke;
- Delineate the mechanisms underlying hemiparesis, abnormal movement, and fractionation of movement deficits;
- Identify fractionation of movement and its effect on occupational performance;
- Identify assessments used for impairments versus assessments to evaluate function;
- Identify how to select appropriate assessments to evaluate at the impairment and functional levels; and
- Identify evidence-based motor intervention approaches after stroke.

Introduction

Therapists who work with people who have had **a stroke** are concerned with motor control. Therefore, therapists who work with people poststroke are responsible for understanding how movement occurs and the neural mechanisms that underlie movement. Human bodies consist of muscles (skeletal, smooth, and cardiac). The brain communicates with muscles and vice versa via descending and ascending pathways to execute movements to perform the activities people do in their daily lives. *Motor control* is the ability to regulate and direct movements in daily life (Schumway-Cook & Woollacott, 2012). The motor system is made up of many structures within the brain, including the **premotor cortex,** primary motor cortex, and supplemental motor cortex. Each area has a role that influences how a person executes a movement, and damage from a stroke can interfere with the ability to carry out the movements the person wants to make.

Key Words

- **corticospinal tract**
- **fractionation of movement**
- **hemiparesis**
- **motor assessment**
- **motor intervention**
- **motor learning**
- **spasticity**

The motor system is made up of many structures within the brain, including the **premotor cortex,** primary motor cortex, and supplemental motor cortex. Each area has a role that influences how a person executes a movement, and damage from a stroke can interfere with the ability to carry out the movements the person wants to make.

Movement is controlled at both the spinal cord and the brain by four separate subsystems (Purves, 2012). Each subsystem interacts with the other subsystems, and each subsystem helps to control movement in a different way. Damage to each subsystem can result in a different quality of motor impairment. The first subsystem includes the spinal cord and the tegmentum of the **brainstem.** The spinal cord contains lower motor **neurons** that send **axons** out from the spinal cord to innervate the muscles of the body (Purves, 2012).

The second motor subsystem consists of the upper motor neurons in the brainstem or the **cerebral cortex.** Axons from cells in the cerebral cortex or the brainstem descend to synapse with local circuit neurons that interact with spinal motor neurons and spinal interneurons of the spinal cord to cause movement to occur.

The third subsystem is the **cerebellum.** The cerebellum influences movement by regulating the movement of upper motor neurons. The cerebellum does not interact at all with local circuit neurons or lower motor neurons. A lesion in the cerebellum results in decreased coordination and impaired correction of movements (Purves, 2012). Therapists most often see **ataxia** as the primary deficit of a cerebellar stroke. People with cerebellar damage frequently experience minimal loss of strength but have profound functional problems because they are unable to perform coordinated movements.

The fourth and final subsystem consists of the **basal nuclei,** which are located deep in the cerebral cortex. The basal nuclei prevent unwanted movements from occurring and assist the upper motor neuron circuits with movement initiation (Purves, 2012). Parkinson's disease and Huntington's disease are the most common diagnoses associated with damage to the basal nuclei.

Lower Motor Neuron Circuits: Reflex Control of Movement

Execution of coordinated movement involves the integration of reflexes that are present at birth (i.e., primitive reflexes). *Primitive reflexes* are reflexes that people are born with and that integrate with age; they can reemerge in an adult with a severe stroke, leading to difficulty performing volitional movements or tasks (Botvin, Keith, & Johnston, 1978; Gutman & Schonfeld, 2009). Reflexes can be divided into four categories: (1) spinal-level reflexes, (2) brainstem reflexes, (3) midbrain reactions, and (4) equilibrium reactions. A *spinal-level reflex* is a reflex mediated by the spinal cord. Spinal reflexes are responsible for basic mobility patterns (Gutman & Schonfeld, 2009). *Brainstem reflexes* are responses to stimuli controlled by the brainstem and directly affect postural tone (Gutman & Schonfeld, 2009). *Midbrain reactions* help to facilitate **spatial orientation** during activities, and *equilibrium reactions* help the person adapt to changes in center of gravity (Gutman & Schonfeld, 2009). Integration of these reflexes allows for accurate movement execution. Therapists are concerned with the reemergence of primitive reflexes because people who experience the reemergence of reflexes after stroke can expect to have difficulty performing daily activities. Specific tests exist to determine the presence of reflexes (Gutman & Schonfeld, 2009).

Upper Motor Neuron Circuits

Cortical Control of Movement

The primary motor area is the area of the brain in which voluntary or conscious movement is initiated (Purves, 2012), and it is here that the corticospinal tracts begin. The primary motor area is also home to the motor homunculus (Purves, 2012). The *motor homunculus* is the map that describes how each body part is represented in the brain (Purves, 2012). The face, mouth, and hands all have large cortical representations. The size of the cortical representations in the motor homunculus is based on the amount of use of a particular body part. For example, the hands have a large representation because people are constantly using their hands to explore their environment.

Cortical representations can change in the context of stroke. Areas affected by stroke lose cortical representation when a lesion occurs (Kleim & Jones, 2008). Those cortical representations may have the ability to move to adjacent areas of the brain by re-creating them through new experiences (Kleim & Jones, 2008).

Table 6.1. Descending Motor Tracts Responsible for the Control of Movement

Tract Name	Responsible for
Upper Motor Neuron Circuits Originating in the Cortex	
Corticospinal tract	Movements of hand and finger
Corticobulbar tract	Movements of face, neck, tongue, and eye
Upper Motor Neuron Circuits Originating in the Brainstem	
Vestibulospinal tract	Control of posture
Tectospinal tract	Coordination of eye and head–trunk movements
Reticulospinal tract	Walking, sneezing, muscle tone
Rubrospinal tract	Facilitation of the antagonist of antigravity muscles in the limbs, causing facilitation of flexor muscle groups
Ventral corticospinal tract	Muscles of upper leg–trunk

Two descending motor tracts are responsible for the control of movement throughout the body (Purves, 2012). Upper motor neuron circuits that originate in the cortex include the corticospinal tract and the corticobulbar tract. Upper motor neuron circuits that originate in the brainstem include the vestibulospinal tract, the tectospinal tract, the reticulospinal tract, and the rubrospinal tract (Gutman, 2008; Purves, 2012). The first part of the name indicates where the tract begins and the second part indicates where the tract terminates (Purves, 2012). Each tract is responsible for movements of different muscle groups and functions but is not distinctly responsible for specific muscle groups and functions. Many of the tracts overlap, which is ultimately good for the recovery of function after stroke. Table 6.1 identifies the specific tracts and also describes some of the types of movement for which each tract is responsible (Purves, 2012).

Planning and Initiating Movement

Both the supplementary motor area (SMA) and the premotor cortex are integral to planning movement (Purves, 2012). The planned movements are then executed via the neural connections in the primary motor cortex. Damage to the SMA leads to decreased ability to perform sequences of actions that are already learned. More specifically, the SMA facilitates the performance of the upcoming, but not yet performed, parts of a sequence of actions that are familiar to the person. Learning and executing movement involves the premotor cortex. The premotor cortex filters information in the environment to decide what type of movement to make in a certain context. A lesion in this area of the brain may lead to **apraxia,** in which a person has difficulty accessing the appropriate plan to make a movement.

Common Motor Deficits After Stroke

A person with stroke may experience several common motor impairments. These impairments can include *paresis* (i.e., muscle weakness), abnormal muscle tone, ataxia, and fractionated movement deficits. A *fractionated movement deficit* is an inability to move a joint by itself. Clinically, it is also called *synergistic movement.* Impairments such as these stem from damage to the primary motor cortex, secondary sensorimotor cortical areas, **subcortical** structures, or the corticospinal tract.

Each of these motor impairments can lead to impairment in activity and participation. For example, paresis can cause problems with the ability to perform typical daily activities such as bathing, dressing, preparing meals, and doing laundry (Faria-Fortini, Michaelsen, Cassiano, & Teixeira-Salmela, 2011; Harris & Eng, 2007; Patten, Lexell, & Brown, 2004). In addition to impairment with **activities of daily living** (ADLs) after stroke, people have reported a lack of meaningful activity, which has the potential to lead to depression, a decrease in function, and a decrease in affect, health status, and quality of life (Mayo, Wood-Dauphinee, Côté, Durcan, & Carlton, 2002). An occupational therapist can expect to spend a great deal of time during therapy sessions helping the client either improve or compensate for these common motor deficits after stroke.

Paresis

Paresis is defined as an inability to volitionally activate motor neurons and is the most common movement deficit associated with stroke (Sathian et al., 2011). In the clinic, paresis is measured as weakness. This motor weakness can range from total or significant loss of muscle movement, called *plegia,* or partial loss of muscle movement, called *paresis*. With paresis, it is difficult to selectively activate motor units (Gracies, 2005a, 2005b). Paresis mostly results from damage to the corticospinal system, which includes the primary motor cortex, the corticospinal tract, and the spinal cord (Figure 6.1). With a reduced or impaired ability to recruit muscle fibers, a person is unable to execute movement in an appropriate and coordinated way (Lang, DeJong, & Beebe, 2009). The person with paresis lacks the force to produce that coordinated movement (Gracies, 2005a, 2005b). In the clinic, weakness is most often observed during evaluations such as manual muscle testing and functional tasks and when uncoordinated movements are present and the person is unable to achieve full **range of motion.**

Upper-extremity paresis results in much slower, less precise, and less efficient movements (Lang et al., 2005; Lang, Wagner, Edwards, Sahrmann, & Dromerick, 2006). For example, when reaching for a glass of water, the person may need to lean more with the trunk, may have difficulty extending the arm the appropriate distance to reach the cup, and may be unable to open the hand entirely to complete the activity. The severity of paresis will vary from person to person. People with mild paresis may appear unimpaired in performing functional tasks, and people with severe paresis or flaccidity may not be able to move at all (Lang, 2012). Paresis has been shown to be consistent across joint segments (Lang & Beebe, 2007). Allocated **active range of motion** values, as measured with a **goniometer,** are likely to be comparable across joints (Lang & Beebe, 2007). Thus, the amount of weakness in the shoulder joint will likely be comparable to the amount of weakness at the elbow and hand.

People experiencing paresis will likely have difficulty performing ADLs and **instrumental activities of daily living** (IADLs) (Faria-Fortini et al., 2011; Harris & Eng, 2007). Paresis can cause difficulty with most daily activities and can cause people to give up preferred activities because they are unable to initiate the desired movement to perform them. Occupational therapists who work with patients with stroke spend a majority of their time working on movement abilities and reducing movement

The severity of paresis will vary from person to person. People with mild paresis may appear unimpaired in performing functional tasks, and people with severe paresis or flaccidity may not be able to move at all.

Points to Ponder: Measuring Weakness in a Clinically Relevant Manner

If weakness is comparable across joints, how will this change how you evaluate your client who experienced a stroke? How can you decrease the amount of time it takes for you to perform the evaluation with this knowledge?

Core Concepts in Motor Recovery and Rehabilitation After Stroke

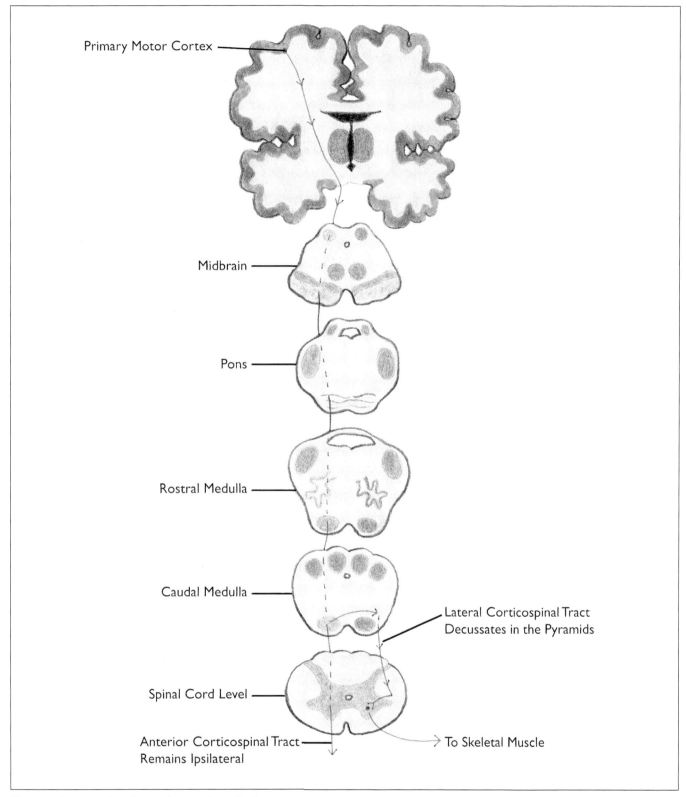

Figure 6.1. Lateral and anterior corticospinal tracts.

Source. From *Quick Reference Neuroscience for Rehabilitation Professionals: The Essential Neurologic Principles Underlying Rehabilitation Practice* (p. 151), by S. A. Gutman, 2008, Thorofare, NJ: Slack. Copyright © 2008 by Slack, Inc. Reprinted with permission.

problems associated with paresis (Latham et al., 2006). In acute and inpatient rehabilitation settings, therapists focus on the upper-extremity movement associated with performing ADLs and IADLS to help the client become independent enough to return home. In outpatient and community rehabilitation settings, therapists divide their time between working on specific functional goals of IADL and **leisure** skills and working on movement-focused retraining with the ultimate goal of facilitating movement skills so that the client can return to activities that were performed before the stroke.

To address paresis, occupational therapists typically work to remediate or compensate for upper-extremity movement limitations. For example, a treatment plan for a person experiencing flaccidity or very little muscle strength would focus on compensation and incorporating the arm into as many functional tasks as possible by having the person use the affected upper extremity as a gross assist, whereas a person who experienced a milder stroke and has good but weakened movement would benefit from a treatment plan designed to remediate movement.

Pusher syndrome is a newly categorized neurological deficit also associated with paresis in which the person experiences an altered perception of the body's orientation in relation to gravity (Karnath, Ferber, & Dichgans, 2000). Evidence has suggested that damage to the posterolateral **thalamus** is the underlying cause of pusher syndrome (Karnath & Ferber, 2000). Patients actively push their weight away from the stronger side to the weaker side, resulting in significant balance issues (Davies, 1985). In most cases of stroke, patients prefer to place all of their weight on their stronger side and lean toward the hemiparetic side without any compensation for balance (Davies, 1985).

Pusher syndrome is identified by means of three important observations: (1) The patient will regularly tilt the torso toward the paretic side of the body, (2) the patient will abduct and extend the extremities of the stronger side of the body to help push toward the weaker side, and (3) the patient will resist any attempts by the therapist to correct the posture (Davies, 1985). Treatment is typically addressed by both a physical therapist and an occupational therapist. People with pusher syndrome have worse initial function than those without the syndrome (Pedersen et al., 1996). However, by 6 months poststroke, the brain usually compensates for this deficit, and people with the syndrome reach the same functional outcome as those without it (Pedersen et al., 1996). The occupational therapist should be prepared to implement strategies to improve the performance of those with pusher syndrome because it will likely affect their ability to perform ADLs and IADLs. The Burke Lateropulsion Scale is a common outcome measure to assess whether a patient is experiencing pusher syndrome (D'Aquila, Smith, Organ, Lichtman, & Reding, 2004).

Abnormal Muscle Tone

Another common motor deficit seen after stroke is abnormal muscle tone. *Muscle tone* can be described as the resistance of muscle to passive elongation or stretch (Bohannon, Larkin, Smith, & Horton, 1987; Bohannon & Smith, 1987). Normal muscle tone can vary among healthy people. Abnormal muscle tone is most often subdivided into two categories, (1) **hypotonicity** and (2) **hypertonicity.** It is common for hypotonicity to appear first, early after stroke, with hypertonicity developing in the first few weeks (Lang, 2012). Not everyone who has a stroke will develop hypertonicity, but many times people with more severe paresis deficits are unable to overcome the pull of opposing muscle groups because of the severe weakness.

Hypotonicity is a decrease in muscle tone and occurs after damage to the corticospinal system (Fredericks & Saladin, 1996). Flaccidity is a prominent example of hypotonicity in which a complete loss of muscle tone occurs. Hypotonic limbs are easily moved, and joints are highly mobile. Flaccid paresis is most commonly seen immediately after stroke.

Spasticity is a type of hypertonicity and can be defined clinically as a velocity-dependent resistance to passive stretch (Bohannon & Smith, 1987). It results from a loss of supraspinal inhibition to the spinal cord, causing the response from the muscles to be abnormally large (Sathian et al., 2011). Spasticity is called *synergistic movement and associated reactions* in the clinic but is also described as hyperactive stretch reflexes, abnormal posturing of the extremities, and excessive coactivation of antagonist muscles, associated movements, and stereotyped movement synergies (Schumway-Cook & Woollacott, 2012). Greater resistance is felt when moving toward elbow extension (Lang, 2012). Spasticity makes movement more difficult and can limit range of motion, leading to abnormal posturing and movement execution. Clinically, spasticity feels like a tightness or stiffness of the muscles and, in cases of severe spasticity, makes it difficult for the therapist to perform **passive range of motion** with the client.

Because spasticity is prevalent in people with stroke, occupational therapists are frequently required to address its impact on daily performance. The cause of spasticity is not well understood, and it is currently not feasible to remediate or eliminate spasticity entirely. Spasticity fluctuates daily and is difficult to control. Occupational therapists can alter spasticity during a specific treatment session through the use of facilitation and inhibition techniques. Therapeutic exercise will briefly decrease the spasticity during treatment to maximize function. Once it has been performed, the treatment activity that follows should be functional in nature (Levit, 2008; Schultz-Krohn, Pope-Davis, Jourdan, & McLaughlin-Gray, 2013). This decrease in spasticity will, however, not last beyond the treatment session. For this reason, entire treatment sessions should not be spent solely on treating spasticity. The patient can also be given a home exercise program to perform outside of the clinic that includes passive stretching exercises to maintain joint mobility and stability.

Spasticity reduction methods such as medication and Botox are often prescribed by physicians in severe cases of spasticity to decrease its functional effects. Occupational therapists often identify clients who may benefit from this course of treatment. Occupational therapy after Botox therapy involves performing therapeutic exercises with the patient to maximize function. Although Botox is effective at temporarily (for about 3 months) decreasing spasticity and pain, it should not be considered as a way to increase functional use of the arm (Cardoso et al., 2005; van Kuijk, Geurts, Bevaart, & van Limbeek, 2002). Underlying muscle weakness is the likely cause of any limitation in function seen with spasticity (Francis et al., 2004).

Splinting is another treatment technique frequently prescribed to decrease spasticity in the hand. The theory underlying this intervention is that prolonged stretching of the hand muscles will lead to a decrease in spasticity. Strong evidence has suggested that this is not the case and that splinting does not reduce **contracture** or improve spasticity long term (Gracies et al., 2000; Langlois, Pederson, & Mackinnon, 1991; McPherson, Kreimeyer, Aalderks, & Gallagher, 1982; Poole, Whitney, Hangeland, & Baker, 1990; Rose & Shah, 1987; Tyson & Kent, 2011).

Ataxia

The cerebellum is situated at the base of the brain and contributes to the coordination of movement in conjunction with the motor cortex and basal nuclei. Damage to the cerebellum can result in coordination deficits between body parts. This incoordination is referred to as *ataxia*.

It is possible to experience a stroke in the cerebellum. People with cerebellar stroke do not generally have hemiparesis or sensory loss but are instead left with profound changes in the ability to execute smooth, coordinated movements (Gutman & Schonfeld, 2009). *Ataxia* is defined as the lack of voluntary coordination of muscle movements and can be observed when the person overshoots or undershoots the projected target (Gutman & Schonfeld, 2009). Special tests should be performed to determine whether a client is experiencing ataxia or weakness associated with hemiparesis (Sathian et al., 2011). Two common tests used in the clinic are (1) the finger–nose–finger test, in which the client moves his or her forefinger back and forth between his or her nose and the therapist's forefinger and (2) the finger chase. In the finger chase, the client must hold the forefinger in front of and near the therapist's forefinger. The therapist rapidly moves his or her forefinger up, down, and sideways, and the client must follow the movement with his or her own forefinger.

Ataxia should be differentiated from muscle weakness, spasticity, and other motor impairments (Sathian et al., 2011). For example, people with ataxia are generally considered to have few strength deficits and are able to execute movements quickly, but they have more pronounced deficits when moving faster and frequently overshoot the movement target. Ataxia rarely resolves; however, people with ataxia can make improvements using a compensatory approach by performing slow, controlled movements; decreasing the number of joints moving at one time; and instituting proximal stabilization (Bastian, 2002).

Fractionated Movement Deficits

Fractionation of movement refers to a person's ability move a joint segment while keeping other adjoining joints steady. Similar to paresis, fractionated movement deficits are observed after stroke damages the corticospinal system. The degree of deficit is related to the severity of paresis. An inability to isolate a particular joint affects the ability to perform daily tasks. Fractionation is most often observed at the fingers but can also be seen in other joints. Stroke movement synergies are the best observed examples of the inability to fractionate movement. Synergistic movements do not allow the client's joints to work individually. An example of synergistic movement is the flexing of the shoulder, arm, and hand while walking after stroke.

Balance Deficits

Balance is another impairment that may affect function and participation after stroke. *Balance* can be described as the ability to control the center of mass over the base of support (Donato & Pulaski, 2010). It involves the integration of many systems, and decreased balance may lead to poor ADL recovery, mobility deficits, and increased falls (Kwakkel, Wagenaar, Kollen, & Lankhorst, 1996; Lamb, Ferrucci, Volapto, Fried, & Guralnik, 2003; Loewen & Anderson, 1990; Tyson, Hanley, Chillala, Selley, & Tallis, 2006). Occupational therapists are concerned with balance in relation to how it affects a person's ability to perform functional activities.

A thorough observation of balance during functional tasks should be performed, and the specific tasks observed should be determined by client goals at the time of evaluation (Donato & Pulaski, 2010). Occupational therapists should determine whether balance can be remediated using assessment results. If it is determined that balance can be remediated, balance retraining techniques may be used during functional ADL and IADL retraining. In some cases, remediation may not be possible, and compensatory strategies may be implemented (Donato & Pulaski, 2010). Balance is an important consideration during the treatment planning process and should be addressed to maximize independence.

Evaluation of Motor Deficits After Stroke

Good clinical practice includes the evaluation of the effectiveness of treatment interventions. So with any intervention approach attempted, evaluation should be included in the treatment planning process. The reason for this is that stroke results in generalized deficits (paresis, abnormal tone, and the inability to fractionate movement) that can potentially have a profound impact on everyday life activities and quality of life. Even though it is possible for each of these impairments to occur independently of each other, they most commonly occur in some sort of combination with other impairments. This also means that the severity of impairments is generally highly correlated. For instance, the severity of paresis is highly correlated with the ability to perform fractionated movement in the upper extremity (Lang & Beebe, 2007). Likewise, the severity of spasticity is comparable to the amount of paresis (Lang & Beebe, 2007). People with pronounced paresis will likely also have a significant amount of spasticity and limited ability to fractionate movement.

> Stroke results in generalized deficits . . . that can potentially have a profound impact on everyday life activities and quality of life.

Management of a person's care after stroke in a rehabilitation setting should include minimizing impairments but also maximizing function (Duncan et al., 2005). To achieve this, early standardized assessment and intervention are critical components of a comprehensive treatment plan (Duncan et al., 2005). Clinicians can use both observation and formal evaluation to target goals that will, it is hoped, lead to the desired results (MacKenzie & Westwood, 2013; Sabari & Lieberman, 2008). Thus, selected interventions should be evidence based and be based on functional goals (Duncan et al., 2005). Standardized assessment helps the therapist develop functional goals.

Evaluation of Impairments

Occupational therapists are concerned with how the existence of impairments leads to a decrease in function. Research has demonstrated that paresis is the principal reason for loss of function after a stroke (Beebe & Lang, 2008, 2009a; Lang & Beebe, 2007; Lang et al., 2009; Prager & Lang, 2012). Evaluating impairments individually identifies which impairments are present and how those impairments may play a role in the loss of movement (Scheets, Sahrmann, & Norton, 2007).

Several assessments are commonly used to evaluate motor skill impairments after stroke. Manual muscle testing (MMT) and **dynamometry,** a pinch gauge, or both can be used to quantify the severity of paresis. MMT tests the strength of the muscle and is typically performed on patients who have experienced a stroke. An MMT score is given for shoulder abduction, elbow flexion, pinch grip, hip flexion, knee extension, and ankle dorsiflexion. Together, these scores are converted to a total force production score for both the upper extremity and the lower extremity (scored separately), ranging from 0 *(no strength)* to 100 *(full strength)*.

The Motricity Index can also be a helpful, quick assessment to gauge the severity of paresis (Collin & Wade, 1990; Demeurisse, Demol, & Robaye, 1980). Range of motion limitations occurring from paresis can be evaluated with a goniometer, and hand–finger strength can be tested using a dynamometer or pinch gauge (Mathiowetz, Kashman, et al., 1985). Spasticity can be evaluated using the Modified Ashworth Scale (Bohannon & Smith, 1987), which measures the amount of resistance during passive stretching of individual joints, rated on a 5-point scale ranging from 0 *(no increase in muscle tone)* to 4 *(affected part is rigid)*.

Therapists looking for a comprehensive measure of upper-extremity impairment might consider the Fugl-Meyer Assessment (Fugl-Meyer, Jääskö, Leyman, Olsson, & Steglind, 1975). The Fugl-Meyer Assessment has been used as an impairment measure in many research studies. This assessment includes the evaluation of range of motion, sensation, balance, and upper-extremity and lower-extremity function. No functional tasks are actually included in the administration of the Fugl-Meyer, which can take as long as 30 minutes to administer and is graded on a scale ranging from 0 to 2, where 0 = *cannot perform,* 1 = *performs task partially,* and 2 = *performs task fully.*

It is equally important to devote time to observing the client perform functional movements. During observation, the presence or absence of movement fractionation deficits can be determined, and the clinician can make note of any substitutions or associated reactions that may be occurring. Observation of function will also assist the clinician with how a specific impairment may limit performance.

Evaluation of Function in the Hospital or Clinic

Achieving functional use of affected extremities is an important goal for most people who have had a stroke (Lang, Bland, Bailey, Schaefer, & Birkenmeier, 2013). Initial evaluations performed by clinicians should include two key components: (1) identifying impairments present (discussed earlier) and (2) identifying activity and participation deficits (Duncan et al., 2005). As described, impairments lead to the inability to perform desired activities and limit participation in activities deemed important to the person with stroke (Faria-Fortini et al., 2011; Harris & Eng, 2007; Patten et al., 2004; Sveen, Bautz-Holter, Sødring, Wyller, & Laake, 1999). To satisfactorily address these limitations, it is necessary to effectively measure these types of deficits (Faria-Fortini et al., 2011).

Assessments to Measure Upper-Extremity Function

Several upper-extremity functional assessments with good reliability and validity are available. Lower-extremity assessments to evaluate balance and mobility are also available. Most lower-extremity assessments are traditionally performed by a physical therapist and, if concerns regarding mobility and balance arise, occupational therapists should refer the client to a physical therapist for evaluation and treatment. Occupational therapists should nonetheless understand how balance and mobility deficits may influence function and participation.

Because occupational therapists are most frequently charged with assessment of the upper extremities, in this section we address some of the most widely used assessments of upper-extremity functional ability. The Action Research Arm Test (ARAT), the Wolf Motor Function Test (WMFT), the Box and Block (B&B) Test, the Nine-Hole Peg Test, the Chedoke Arm and Hand Activity Inventory, and the Jebsen–Taylor Hand Function Test are the performance measures of upper-extremity function that are cited most often in the literature (Barreca et al., 2004; Barreca, Stratford, Lambert, Masters, & Streiner, 2005; Barreca, Stratford, Masters, Lambert, & Griffiths, 2006; Jebsen, Taylor, Trieschmann, Trotter, & Howard, 1969; Lang et al., 2013; Lyle, 1981; Mathiowetz, Volland, Kashman, & Weber, 1985; Wolf et al., 2005; Yozbatiran, Der-Yeghiaian, & Cramer, 2008). The Stroke Impact Scale and the Motor Activity Log are the most widely used and cited self-report measures (Duncan, Lai, Bode, Perera, & DeRosa, 2003; Duncan et al., 2002; Duncan et al., 1999; Lang et al., 2013; Uswatte, Taub, Morris, Light, & Thompson, 2006; Uswatte, Taub, Morris, Vignolo, & McCulloch, 2005). Other functional upper-extremity assessments that are used clinically include the Arm Motor Ability Test, Frenchay Arm Test, the Rivermead Motor Assessment (Arm Section), and the Functional Test for the Hemiplegic Upper Extremity (Heller et al., 1987; Kopp et al., 1997; Lincoln & Leadbitter, 1979; Poole & Whitney, 2001; Wilson, Baker, & Craddock, 1984). Each assessment has a slightly different focus, so there is no one perfect scale or gold standard.

Different assessment tools are selected and used on the basis of the therapist's preference, the setting, and where the patient is in his or her recovery (Lang et al., 2013). Furthermore, no one assessment exists that captures every upper-extremity movement (Ashford, Slade, Malaprade, & Turner-Stokes, 2008). A recent review of upper-extremity measures suggested that the ARAT and the B&B Test provide the most information to the clinician (Connell & Tyson, 2012). Evaluation should not be a one-time occurrence; rather, it should occur at the first visit, periodically to assess progress during sessions, and at discharge (Lang et al., 2013). Reassessment at several time points can assist the therapist in creating appropriate treatment strategies, evaluating the effectiveness of a specific treatment, and determining when a patient has reached a plateau during treatment (Lang et al., 2013). An in-depth review of several performance and self-report tools is provided in Table 6.2.

> Reassessment at several time points can assist the therapist in creating appropriate treatment strategies, evaluating the effectiveness of a specific treatment, and determining when a patient has reached a plateau during treatment.

Choosing an Assessment

Selection of appropriate assessments involves a variety of considerations, such as how much the assessment costs, the training required, the time it takes to administer, and how the results of the assessment will guide clinical treatment sessions and clinical practice overall (Lang et al., 2013). Many of the assessments discussed in this chapter are highly correlated (Beebe & Lang, 2009b; Lin et al., 2009). Nonetheless, therapists may choose to perform more than one assessment to gather all the information that they deem necessary (Lang et al., 2013). For instance, the ARAT may be chosen to quickly measure functional movement over time and then combined with the Motor Activity Log to explore functional problems identified by the client.

Most assessments can be easily acquired either commercially or by referring to published articles that describe how to construct any equipment required for the assessment and how to administer and score it (Lang et al., 2013). The cost of each assessment can vary from $50 to several hundred dollars (Lang et al., 2013). Availability of equipment may also be a determining factor when choosing an assessment (Lang et al., 2013). Some clinics may already have a certain assessment and see no need to purchase another one. For example, one clinic may own the ARAT, and another facility may own the WMFT, but because these measures are correlated,

Table 6.2. Performance and Self-Report Measures Commonly Used to Assess Upper-Extremity Function After Stroke

Name	Time to Administer	Reliability	Relation to Other Measures (Concurrent Validity)	Estimate of MCID[a]	Strengths	Weaknesses
			Performance Assessments			
Action Research Arm Test (ARAT)	10–15 min	Intrarater $r = 0.99$; Interrater $r = 0.98$; Test–retest $r = 0.98$	$r = 0.91$–0.94 with Fugl-Meyer; $r = 0.96$ with Motor Assessment Scale; $r = 0.87$ with Motricity Index; $r = 0.93$ with CAHAI	6 points (chronic stroke); 12 points (acute stroke, dominant hand); 17 points (acute stroke, non-dominant hand)	Quick, easily administered, appropriate at all stages of recovery	Not commercially available, but can be built from published instructions
Box and Block (BB) Test	5–10 min	Intrarater ICC = no established studies; Interrater ICC = 0.99; Test–retest ICC = 0.96	$r = 0.92$ with Fugl-Meyer; $r = 0.95$ with ARAT	6 blocks with affected hand	Quick, easily administered	Requires at least minimal distal volitional control
Chedoke Arm and Hand Activity Inventory (CAHAI)	25 min	Intrarater ICC = no established studies; Interrater ICC = 0.98; Test–retest ICC = 0.96–0.97	$r = 0.93$ with ARAT	6.3 points	Easily administered, shorter versions of the test exist if time is a concern, free to use	Takes longer than other measures that capture the same information
Jebsen-Taylor Hand Function Test	15–20 min	Interrater ICC = 0.82–1.00	$r_s = 0.84$–0.97 with Nine-Hole Peg Test; $r_s = 0.87$–0.95 with ARAT	Unknown	Standardized instructions, good measure when the ceiling is achieved on other shorter measures	Requires at least minimal distal and proximal volitional control
Nine-Hole Peg Test	10 min	Interrater/test–retest: $r = 0.68$–0.99	$r_s = 0.84$–0.97 with Jebsen-Taylor; $r_s = 0.85$–0.93 with ARAT	32.8 sec with affected hand	Quick, inexpensive to purchase	Most appropriate for higher performing individuals
Wolf Motor Function Test (WMFT)	30 min	Interrater ICC = 0.85–0.97; Test–retest ICC = 0.94–0.99	$r_s = 0.86$ (FAS) with ARAT; $r_s = 0.89$ (time) with ARAT	1.5–2.0 sec (WMFT time, chronic stroke); 19 sec (WMFT time, acute stroke); 0.2–0.4 points (WMFT FAS)	Standardized instructions; appropriate at all stages of recovery	Takes longer than other measures that capture the same information

(Continued)

Table 6.2. Performance and Self-Report Measures Commonly Used to Assess Upper-Extremity Function After Stroke (cont.)

Name	Time to Administer	Reliability	Relation to Other Measures (Concurrent Validity)	Estimate of MCID[a]	Strengths	Weaknesses
			Self-Rating Assessments			
Motor Activity Log	15–20 min	Test–retest ICC = 0.79–0.82	$r_s = 0.35-0.39$ (QOM Scale) with ARAT; $r_s = 0.31-0.32$ (AOU Scale) with ARAT; $r_s = -0.26$ to -0.33 (QOM Scale) with Nine-Hole Peg Test; $r_s = -0.16$ to -0.23 (AOU Scale) with Nine-Hole Peg Test; $r_s = -0.52$ (QOM Scale) with BB; $r_s = -0.37-0.49$ (AOU Scale) with BB; $r = 0.52-0.66$ (QOM Scale) with accelerometry	1.0–1.1 points on the QOM Scale	Inexpensive, tries to capture real-world abilities, easy to administer	Takes longer than other interviews, relies on self-ratings
Stroke Impact Scale (ADL and Hand Function Subscales)	5 min each subscale	Test–retest: ICC = 0.70–0.92	$r_s = 0.57-0.73$ with ARAT; $r_s = 0.61-0.83$ with Jebsen-Taylor; $r_s = 0.53-0.66$ with Nine-Hole Peg Test	ADLs/IADLs = 5.9 points; Hand function = 17.8 points	Inexpensive, tries to capture real-world abilities, easy to administer	Relies on self-ratings

Source. "Assessment of Upper Extremity Impairment, Function, and Activity After Stroke: Foundations for Clinical Decision Making," by C. E. Lang, M. D. Bland, R. R. Bailey, S. Y. Schaefer, and R. L. Birkenmeier, 2013. Journal of Hand Therapy, 26, p. 108. Copyright © 2013 by Elsevier. Reprinted with permission.

Note. ADLs = activities of daily living; AOU Scale = Amount of Use Scale; FAS = Functional Ability Scale; IADLs = instrumental activities of daily living; ICC = intraclass correlation coefficient; min = minutes; QOM Scale = Quality of Movement Scale; sec = seconds.

[a] Minimal clinically important difference (MCID) has been defined as "the smallest difference in score in the domain of interest which patients perceive as beneficial and which would mandate, in the absence of troublesome side effects and excessive cost, a change in the patient's management" (Jaeschke, Singer, & Guyatt, 1989, p. 408). Note that these values are labeled as estimates because they are likely influenced by the time poststroke and the severity of functional loss.

it makes sense to choose the most readily available assessment for use in practice (Lang et al., 2013).

Some assessments require that the test administrator receive formal training to become certified in test administration (e.g., the Assessment of Motor and Process Skills). Additionally, it is important to be able to perform assessments that do not require formal training according to the instructions; otherwise, the test may not accurately measure what it is supposed to measure (Cronbach, 1990). The more times a therapist administers an assessment, the more efficient he or she may become (Lang et al., 2013). In addition, the test results will be more accurate because the assessment was administered in a reliable and valid way (Lang et al., 2013).

Lengthy assessments may not be favored for routine clinical use because of the limited time available to perform an evaluation (Lang et al., 2013). Because movement is not the only area assessed after a stroke, the therapist may want to choose the briefest measure available (e.g., the B&B Test or Nine-Hole Peg Test); as a result, some vital information provided by longer assessments (e.g., ARAT or Jebsen–Taylor Hand Function Test) may not be identified. For instance, both the B&B Test and the Nine-Hole Peg Test measure only one movement, as opposed to the ARAT or Jebsen–Taylor Hand Function Test, which measure several movements ranging from simple to complex.

Evaluation of Movement Outside of the Hospital or Clinic

It is commonly assumed that if improvement in movement (as measured with clinical assessments) is demonstrated, this improvement also translates into improved upper-extremity use outside of the clinic. Clinical upper-extremity assessments, as we have described, may not accurately measure a person's ability to perform movement in the real world (Bailey & Lang, 2013). However, what really matters is the ability to return to activities that are typical for a particular person in his or her community setting. Home exercise portions of therapy are designed to make the person more successful and independent at home, but it is difficult to measure whether they actually work. Therefore, a reliable and valid tool to measure upper-extremity use outside of the clinical setting would be useful to therapists.

Several ways exist to measure movement outside of the hospital or clinic environment. Self-report questionnaires and standardized assessments (discussed in the previous section) could also be used outside of the clinic. Although self-report questionnaires may be a preferred method of assessment because they are easy to administer, their use may be inappropriate for people with decreased **cognition** (Bradburn, Rips, & Shevell, 1987; Tatemichi et al., 1994). Standardized assessments, such as those mentioned in the "Evaluation of Function in the Hospital or Clinic" section, can be time consuming and may cost a lot for assessment at this stage of recovery. One tool that is gaining increased attention and may be beneficial is the accelerometer. *Accelerometers* are small wristwatch-like devices that measure movement acceleration. By having the client wear the accelerometer in therapy and on discharge, an occupational therapist may be able to determine whether the client is using his or her affected arm more after treatment than before treatment (Bailey & Lang, 2013). Data from accelerometers and real-world arm use outside of the clinic are currently being investigated, and accelerometers may prove to be a valid measure of arm use outside the clinic. Data from accelerometers would be valuable to an occupational therapist who is concerned with determining whether the treatment interventions performed in the clinic are transferring to home on discharge.

Using Evaluations to Guide Clinical Practice

Assessment results provide information regarding the severity of the person's impairment and function after stroke. People experiencing a severe stroke and limited movement return may benefit from a compensatory approach to treatment rather than a restorative approach. Administering assessment at repeated time points enables the therapist to determine whether a chosen therapeutic choice is appropriate. Occupational therapists should use results from both impairment and functional assessments to assist with treatment planning and to measure client change over the course of treatment. Assessment results can assist therapists in choosing appropriate goals for their clients. For example, say a therapist chooses to use **constraint-induced movement therapy** (CIMT) to improve upper-extremity function. The client is assessed before treatment and then weekly during treatment, and the therapist notices steady improvement. The therapist now has objective documentation that the selected intervention, in this case CIMT, is appropriate for the client. The therapist also has information to give insurance companies to get reimbursement or additional visits. If the results from the assessment show no improvement, the therapist has objective information and is able to make a decision regarding whether to continue or discontinue a specific treatment.

Motor Intervention Approaches to Guide Treatment Planning After Stroke

Selecting treatment interventions to improve motor function after stroke can be challenging. Choosing when to compensate and when to remediate are two crucial issues that a therapist must decide. Recovery of function can be considered at either a neurological level or a functional level. *Neurological recovery* occurs as a result of neural plasticity or cortical reorganization. *Functional recovery* involves compensation using adaptive strategies or adaptive equipment to perform desired tasks. An example of an adaptive strategy is the use of one-handed dressing techniques by a person who has a flaccid upper extremity. An example of adaptive equipment is a buttonhook, used to button a shirt by a person whose weakness impedes his or her ability to button. Selecting a remediation approach or a compensation approach will depend on the severity of movement deficits and should be determined for each patient individually. Common motor-treatment interventions are detailed in the following sections.

> Selecting a remediation approach or a compensation approach will depend on the severity of movement deficits and should be determined for each patient individually.

Neural Plasticity

Current research has suggested that the mechanisms that underlie neural plasticity are the same mechanisms that underlie motor learning generally (Schumway-Cook & Woollacott, 2012). After stroke, the brain continues to be able to undergo functional and structural reorganization, which is known as *neural plasticity* (Green, 2003). Neural plasticity means that neurons and neuronal connections in the brain have the ability to change (Schumway-Cook & Woollacott, 2012). Research evidence from **neuroplasticity** and motor-learning studies has shown that practice and experience can lead to improved function after stroke (Schumway-Cook & Woollacott, 2012).

Motor-Learning Theory

Motor learning refers to the acquisition or modification of motor skills resulting from practice (Schumway-Cook & Woollacott, 2012). Movements are learned (1) through repeated practice of a task or activity and (2) from feedback given during practice of that activity. Several mechanisms underlie how changes occur at the cellular and **neural networks.** *Long-term potentiation* (LTP) is the long-lasting strengthening of synapses between nerve cells. The more the synapses are activated, the stronger the neuron becomes. LTP is one of the mechanisms by which synaptic plasticity occurs (Carlson, 2010). In LTP, a neuron and its synapses receive input from repeated practice, and if that practice is repeated over days and weeks, the changes become permanent. The old adage "Practice makes perfect" applies with motor learning. The more a task is practiced, the greater the skill the person will develop in performing that specific task.

Practice can be structured in different ways:

1. *Massed practice vs. distributed practice: Massed practice* is continuous practice of a task in which no or few rest breaks are allowed; *distributed practice* is when rest breaks between task trials are longer than the actual task (Schmidt & Lee, 2005). In other words, rest is distributed across trials, and the rest periods are longer. Massed practice is considered to be most effective in motor learning, but fatigue is likely to set in during massed practice sessions. Clinicians should err on the side of caution so as not to cause so much fatigue that injury occurs.

2. *Variable practice vs. constant practice: Variable practice* is the practice of tasks in which one aspect of the task is varied each time the task is performed. *Constant practice* is the practice of a task in the same situation. In constant practice situations, no variables are changed throughout the task. Variable practice is thought to lead to a better ability to generalize learning (Schmidt & Lee, 2005).

3. *Whole-task practice vs. part-task practice: Whole-task practice* is the practice of the whole task, whereas *part-task practice* involves practicing an activity by breaking a task down into steps. Overall, practicing the whole task is generally considered to be more effective unless the task is able to be broken down into naturally occurring steps (Schmidt & Lee, 2005; Winstein, 1991).

4. *Blocked practice vs. random practice: Blocked practice* is a practice sequence in which the same task is practiced repetitively across multiple tasks, and *random practice* is a practice sequence in which task skills are performed in a random order across multiple tasks (Schmidt & Wrisberg, 2008). In the initial stages of learning a task, blocked practice yields better performance. However, in the long term, random practice is considered more effective in learning a skill because the person will have exposure to the unique differences between task skills.

Feedback given by the therapist can enhance motor learning. Feedback should not be confused with encouragement (e.g., "good job," "keep it up"). Although encouragement is essential to motivation during treatment sessions and should still be provided, feedback as described in this section is a different term, and it can enhance motor learning.

The two main types of feedback are (1) intrinsic and (2) extrinsic. *Intrinsic feedback* is feedback that the person receives internally from sensory system information

> The old adage "Practice makes perfect" applies with motor learning. The more a task is practiced, the greater the skill the person will develop in performing that specific task.

Points to Ponder: Applying Different Types of Practice During Treatment Sessions

Sally is a 44-year-old right-handed woman who had a stroke approximately 1 month ago. She requires moderate assistance with feeding, grooming, dressing, and all hygiene tasks. Sally needs minimal assistance for ambulation with a quad cane and has a standing endurance of 2 to 3 minutes. She can transfer out of bed with minimal assistance but requires moderate assistance for transferring in and out of the bathtub or shower and toilet.

How might you structure a treatment session using the various practice conditions? How might your treatment session look if you focused on using a random practice schedule? How might it look if you were using a massed practice schedule vs. a distributed practice schedule?

as a result of the actual movement being performed (Schumway-Cook & Woollacott, 2012). This information includes visual information on movement in addition to other sensory and proprioceptive feedback determining where a limb is in body space (Schmidt & Lee, 2005). *Extrinsic feedback* is the feedback that clinicians provide and is meant to supplement intrinsic feedback received by the person (Schumway-Cook & Woollacott, 2012).

Two principal forms of extrinsic feedback have been investigated: (1) knowledge of results and (2) knowledge of performance. *Knowledge of results feedback* occurs when the clinician verbally provides information to the patient at the end of a task about the outcome of the patient's task performance and the success or failure of movement during the task (Schumway-Cook & Woollacott, 2012). This does not include feedback about the actual movements that caused the task to occur. *Knowledge of performance feedback* includes information on the actual movement (velocity or limb motion). This feedback provides information on the actual quality of movement during the task.

Occupational Therapy Task-Oriented Approach

The Occupational Therapy Task-Oriented Approach incorporates ideas from both developmental and motor-learning theories (Bass-Haugen, Mathiowetz, & Flinn, 2008). The following treatment principles are used to guide effective occupation-based treatment:

- Client-centered focus
- Occupation-based focus
- Person and environment
- Practice and feedback
- General treatment goals.

In true occupational therapy fashion, this approach does not involve a cookie-cutter method for delivering treatment. Instead, it offers a guide for how to deliver client-centered care when motor impairment is present. Therapists following the principles associated with this approach will incorporate these ideas into treatment planning.

Constraint-Induced Movement Therapy

In recent years, CIMT has been considered one of the most promising treatment techniques in improving upper-extremity movement after stroke. It is also widely popular with therapists because detailed instructions on how to perform the treatment are available, unlike many more traditional occupational performance–based treatments. Additionally, a growing body of literature has supported CIMT's ability to improve upper-extremity movement after stroke (Dromerick, Edwards, & Hahn, 2000; Page, Sisto, & Levine, 2002; van der Lee et al., 1999; Wolf et al., 2006).

CIMT involves constraining the unaffected arm, usually with a mitt or sling to allow the arm most affected by the stroke to perform all functional activities without incorporating the unaffected upper extremity. While wearing the constraint mitt, the patient performs massed practice, also called *shaping,* of many tasks for as many as 6 hours per day. Originally, the thought was that improvements from CIMT resulted because the patient overcame **learned nonuse** of the affected upper extremity, which is considered to occur when a patient who has arm weakness decides to not use the affected arm because it is uncoordinated or takes too long. However, recent research has suggested that CIMT is an effective treatment because of neural plasticity, or the regrowth and regeneration of neurons with repeated practice (Hayner, Gibson, & Giles, 2010; Miltner, Bauder, Sommer, Dettmers, & Taub, 1999; Ostendorf & Wolf, 1981; Wolf, Lecraw, Barton, & Jann, 1989). This treatment is generally used at the chronic stage of stroke (3 or more months poststroke) and is considered most effective at this time point (Wolf et al., 2006). To qualify for CIMT at the chronic stage, the patient needs to have active wrist extension of no less than 10°, 10° of thumb abduction and extension, and 10° of abduction and extension in at least two digits. Downsides of the treatment include the cost (approximately $10,000 for 2 to 3 weeks of CIMT, which is not usually reimbursed by insurance) and its limited appropriateness for people with severe cognitive deficits and those with limited endurance who may not be able to tolerate the long periods of intense exercise. CIMT has been shown to be effective with people with chronic stroke (Wolf et al., 2006).

Traditional CIMT is a detailed protocol, involving a large time commitment that is not usually compatible with typical clinical settings. To make CIMT more realistic in the clinical setting, several protocol modifications have been investigated. Research completed using a modified CIMT approach has shown the approach to be effective at improving function in the upper extremity and more realistic to perform in a typical clinical setting. Modified CIMT protocols are similar to receiving outpatient treatment, in which the client comes to see the therapist 3 times per week for a 30-minute to 1-hour session. The CIMT constraint (usually a mitt) is worn for the duration of the treatment session and then for 5 hours outside of the clinic for approximately 10 weeks. Additionally, CIMT has been shown to be effective with people with acute stroke and by modifying and shortening the treatment (Dromerick et al., 2000; Nijland, Kwakkel, Bakers, & van Wegen, 2011; Page et al., 2002).

Other Occupational Therapy Movement Treatments

Bilateral arm training involves using both arms repetitively, either simultaneously or in alternating patterns, to perform functional tasks. It is thought that the bilateral movements will stimulate both hemispheres of the brain and lead to cortical reorganization and perhaps better functional movement. Some evidence has shown that it may be an effective method of treatment of the upper extremity for people with stroke at all levels of severity (McCombe Waller & Whitall, 2008; Stewart, Cauraugh, & Summers, 2006). People regularly use both arms to perform activities in daily life, and bilateral training could be used to improve or enhance the function of the affected arm so that it can be incorporated into functional tasks (McCombe Waller & Whitall, 2008).

Biofeedback is a widely used treatment in clinical settings. Damage to the main motor pathways of the brain can cause problems such as weakness and spasticity to occur. However, some motor pathways that are not frequently used may remain unaffected by stroke. A therapist may use biofeedback to help clients learn how to activate these pathways through the use of electromyographic biofeedback when they are provided with either visual or auditory feedback regarding how much they are activating a muscle (Moreland & Thomson, 1994).

Repetitive task-specific training involves repeatedly performing a task over and over to improve function of the upper extremity (Bayona, Bitensky, Salter, & Teasell, 2005; Hubbard, Parsons, Neilson, & Carey, 2009). The task may be broken down into steps so that component movements of the task are practiced. For example, if the goal is to brush teeth, the patient may repeatedly practice grasping and releasing the toothbrush to improve hand dexterity to lead to functionally performing the task. When performing task-specific practice, it is important to grade the task and gradually make it more difficult rather than have the client repeatedly do the same task in the same way. This treatment has strong evidence to support its effectiveness (Arya et al., 2012; Blennerhassett & Dite, 2004; Boyd, Vidoni, & Wessel, 2010; Cauraugh & Kim, 2003; Winstein et al., 2004).

> When performing task-specific practice, it is important to grade the task and gradually make it more difficult rather than have the client repeatedly do the same task in the same way.

In *mirror therapy*, a mirror is placed alongside the unaffected upper extremity while hiding the patient's affected upper extremity from view (Thieme, Mehrholz, Pohl, Behrens, & Dohle, 2012). The patient performs a movement task, and it appears to the patient that both extremities are performing the requested movement normally. Mirror therapy provides visual feedback to the patient that is thought to stimulate the affected limb by increasing the excitability of neurons in the ipsilateral primary motor cortex (Garry, Loftus, & Summers, 2005; Thieme et al., 2012). Limited evidence exists for the effectiveness of mirror therapy as a stroke **rehabilitation** technique (Thieme et al., 2012). It is most beneficial to the person with very little residual movement poststroke.

Mental practice involves cognitively practicing a desired task using mental imagery in the absence of actual physical movements before attempting to perform the task (Malouin & Richards, 2010). Many studies have indicated that when used as a therapeutic technique, mental practice may lead to improvement in ADLs and of upper-extremity function (Braun, Beurskens, Borm, Schack, & Wade, 2006; Nilsen, Gillen, & Gordon, 2010; Zimmermann-Schlatter, Schuster, Puhan, Siekierka, & Steurer, 2008). This is especially true when mental practice is paired with actual physical practice of tasks (Nilsen et al., 2010). Several factors make it difficult to definitively say whether mental practice should routinely be used in clinical practice. How much mental practice should be delivered, how much the benefits of mental practice are retained over time, and how much mental practice improves occupational performance still need to be investigated (Nilsen et al., 2010). However, at this time, mental practice can be considered as an appropriate intervention strategy for stroke rehabilitation.

Functional electrical stimulation (FES) is a treatment that uses neuromuscular electrical stimulation to generate electrical pulses to specific muscles to generate a muscle contraction. When performed while a client performs a functional activity,

FES can result in improved hand grasp and manipulation needed to perform daily activities (Popovic, Popovic, & Sinkjaer, 2002).

Summary

The primary goal of an occupational therapist is to assist a client to be able to do the tasks and activities he or she wants to do in everyday life. Understanding the underlying mechanisms of movement after a stroke and knowledge of both impairment-level and functional-level assessments can help the therapist develop appropriate treatment plans centered around the client's goals. Moreover, knowledge of evidence-based treatments can assist the therapist in choosing appropriate interventions to help the client meet his or her goals. Following these suggestions helps the therapist provide good client-centered care.

References

Arya, K. N., Verma, R., Garg, R. K., Sharma, V. P., Agarwal, M., & Aggarwal, G. G. (2012). Meaningful task-specific training (MTST) for stroke rehabilitation: A randomized controlled trial. *Topics in Stroke Rehabilitation, 19,* 193–211. http://dx.doi.org/10.1310/tsr1903-193

Ashford, S., Slade, M., Malaprade, F., & Turner-Stokes, L. (2008). Evaluation of functional outcome measures for the hemiparetic upper limb: A systematic review. *Journal of Rehabilitation Medicine, 40,* 787–795. http://dx.doi.org/10.2340/16501977-0276

Bailey, R. R., & Lang, C. E. (2013). Upper extremity activity in adults: Referent values using accelerometry. *Journal of Rehabilitation Research and Development, 50,* 1213–1222. http://dx.doi.org/10.1682/JRRD.2012.12.0222

Barreca, S. R., Gowland, C. K., Stratford, P., Huijbregts, M., Griffiths, J., Torresin, W., . . . Masters, L. (2004). Development of the Chedoke Arm and Hand Activity Inventory: Theoretical constructs, item generation, and selection. *Topics in Stroke Rehabilitation, 11,* 31–42. http://dx.doi.org/10.1310/JU8P-UVK6-68VW-CF3W

Barreca, S. R., Stratford, P. W., Lambert, C. L., Masters, L. M., & Streiner, D. L. (2005). Test–retest reliability, validity, and sensitivity of the Chedoke Arm and Hand Activity Inventory: A new measure of upper-limb function for survivors of stroke. *Archives of Physical Medicine and Rehabilitation, 86,* 1616–1622. http://dx.doi.org/10.1016/j.apmr.2005.03.017

Barreca, S. R., Stratford, P. W., Masters, L. M., Lambert, C. L., & Griffiths, J. (2006). Comparing 2 versions of the Chedoke Arm and Hand Activity Inventory with the Action Research Arm Test. *Physical Therapy, 86,* 245–253.

Bass-Haugen, J., Mathiowetz, V., & Flinn, N. (2008). *Optimizing motor behavior using the occupational therapy task-oriented approach* (6th ed.). Philadelphia: Lippincott Williams & Wilkins.

Bastian, A. J. (2002). Cerebellar limb ataxia: Abnormal control of self-generated and external forces. *Cerebellum: Recent Developments in Cerebellar Research, 978,* 16–27. http://dx.doi.org/10.1111/j.1749-6632.2002.tb07552.x

Bayona, N. A., Bitensky, J., Salter, K., & Teasell, R. (2005). The role of task-specific training in rehabilitation therapies. *Topics in Stroke Rehabilitation, 12,* 58–65. http://dx.doi.org/10.1310/BQM5-6YGB-MVJ5-WVCR

Beebe, J. A., & Lang, C. E. (2008). Absence of a proximal to distal gradient of motor deficits in the upper extremity early after stroke. *Clinical Neurophysiology, 119,* 2074–2085. http://dx.doi.org/10.1016/j.clinph.2008.04.293

Beebe, J. A., & Lang, C. E. (2009a). Active range of motion predicts upper extremity function 3 months after stroke. *Stroke, 40,* 1772–1779. http://dx.doi.org/10.1161/STROKEAHA.108.536763

Beebe, J. A., & Lang, C. E. (2009b). Relationships and responsiveness of six upper extremity function tests during the first six months of recovery after stroke. *Journal of Neurologic Physical Therapy, 33,* 96–103. http://dx.doi.org/10.1097/NPT.0b013e3181a33638

Blennerhassett, J., & Dite, W. (2004). Additional task-related practice improves mobility and upper limb function early after stroke: A randomised controlled trial. *Australian Journal of Physiotherapy, 50,* 219–224. http://dx.doi.org/10.1016/S0004-9514(14)60111-2

Bohannon, R. W., Larkin, P. A., Smith, M. B., & Horton, M. G. (1987). Relationship between static muscle strength deficits and spasticity in stroke patients with hemiparesis. *Physical Therapy, 67,* 1068–1071.

Bohannon, R. W., & Smith, M. B. (1987). Interrater reliability of a Modified Ashworth Scale of muscle spasticity. *Physical Therapy, 67,* 206–207.

Botvin, J. G., Keith, R. A., & Johnston, M. V. (1978). Relationship between primitive reflexes in stroke patients and rehabilitation outcome. *Stroke, 9,* 256–258. http://dx.doi.org/10.1161/01.STR.9.3.256

Boyd, L. A., Vidoni, E. D., & Wessel, B. D. (2010). Motor learning after stroke: Is skill acquisition a prerequisite for contralesional neuroplastic change? *Neuroscience Letters, 482,* 21–25. http://dx.doi.org/10.1016/j.neulet.2010.06.082

Bradburn, N. M., Rips, L. J., & Shevell, S. K. (1987). Answering autobiographical questions: The impact of memory and inference on surveys. *Science, 236,* 157–161. http://dx.doi.org/10.1126/science.3563494

Braun, S. M., Beurskens, A. J., Borm, P. J., Schack, T., & Wade, D. T. (2006). The effects of mental practice in stroke rehabilitation: A systematic review. *Archives of Physical Medicine and Rehabilitation, 87,* 842–852. http://dx.doi.org/10.1016/j.apmr.2006.02.034

Cardoso, E., Rodrigues, B., Lucena, R., Oliveira, I. R., Pedreira, G., & Melo, A. (2005). Botulinum toxin type A for the treatment of the upper limb spasticity after stroke: A meta-analysis. *Arquivos de Neuro-Psiquiatria, 63,* 30–33. http://dx.doi.org/10.1590/S0004-282X2005000100006

Carlson, N. R. (2010). *Control of movement* (10th ed.). Amherst, MA: Allyn & Bacon.

Cauraugh, J. H., & Kim, S. B. (2003). Stroke motor recovery: Active neuromuscular stimulation and repetitive practice schedules. *Journal of Neurology, Neurosurgery, and Psychiatry, 74,* 1562–1566. http://dx.doi.org/10.1136/jnnp.74.11.1562

Collin, C., & Wade, D. (1990). Assessing motor impairment after stroke: A pilot reliability study. *Journal of Neurology, Neurosurgery, and Psychiatry, 53,* 576–579. http://dx.doi.org/10.1136/jnnp.53.7.576

Connell, L. A., & Tyson, S. F. (2012). Clinical reality of measuring upper-limb ability in neurologic conditions: A systematic review. *Archives of Physical Medicine and Rehabilitation, 93,* 221–228. http://dx.doi.org/10.1016/j.apmr.2011.09.015

Cronbach, L. J. (1990). *Essentials of psychological testing* (5th ed.). New York: HarperCollins.

D'Aquila, M. A., Smith, T., Organ, D., Lichtman, S., & Reding, M. (2004). Validation of a lateropulsion scale for patients recovering from stroke. *Clinical Rehabilitation, 18,* 102–109. http://dx.doi.org/10.1191/0269215504cr709oa

Davies, P. M. (1985). *Steps to follow: A guide to the treatment of adult hemiplegia.* New York: Springer.

Demeurisse, G., Demol, O., & Robaye, E. (1980). Motor evaluation in vascular hemiplegia. *European Neurology, 19,* 382–389. http://dx.doi.org/10.1159/000115178

Donato, S. M., & Pulaski, K. H. (Eds.). (2010). *Overview of balance impairments: Functional implications* (3rd ed.). St. Louis: Elsevier/Mosby.

Dromerick, A. W., Edwards, D. F., & Hahn, M. (2000). Does the application of constraint-induced movement therapy during acute rehabilitation reduce arm impairment after ischemic stroke? *Stroke, 31,* 2984–2988. http://dx.doi.org/10.1161/01.STR.31.12.2984

Duncan, P. W., Lai, S. M., Bode, R. K., Perera, S., & DeRosa, J. (2003). Stroke Impact Scale–16: A brief assessment of physical function. *Neurology, 60,* 291–296. http://dx.doi.org/10.1212/01.WNL.0000041493.65665.D6

Duncan, P. W., Reker, D. M., Horner, R. D., Samsa, G. P., Hoenig, H., LaClair, B. J., & Dudley, T. K. (2002). Performance of a mail-administered version of a stroke-specific outcome measure, the Stroke Impact Scale. *Clinical Rehabilitation, 16,* 493–505. http://dx.doi.org/10.1191/0269215502cr510oa

Duncan, P. W., Wallace, D., Lai, S. M., Johnson, D., Embretson, S., & Laster, L. J. (1999). The Stroke Impact Scale Version 2.0: Evaluation of reliability, validity, and sensitivity to change. *Stroke, 30,* 2131–2140. http://dx.doi.org/10.1161/01.STR.30.10.2131

Duncan, P. W., Zorowitz, R., Bates, B., Choi, J. Y., Glasberg, J. J., Graham, G. D., . . . Reker, D. (2005). Management of adult stroke rehabilitation care. A clinical practice guideline. *Stroke, 36,* e100–e143. http://dx.doi.org/10.1161/01.STR.0000180861.54180.FF

Faria-Fortini, I., Michaelsen, S. M., Cassiano, J. G., & Teixeira-Salmela, L. F. (2011). Upper extremity function in stroke subjects: Relationships between the *International*

Classification of Functioning, Disability, and Health domains. *Journal of Hand Therapy, 24,* 257–264, quiz 265. http://dx.doi.org/10.1016/j.jht.2011.01.002

Francis, H. P., Wade, D. T., Turner-Stokes, L., Kingswell, R. S., Dott, C. S., & Coxon, E. A. (2004). Does reducing spasticity translate into functional benefit? An exploratory meta-analysis. *Journal of Neurology, Neurosurgery, and Psychiatry, 75,* 1547–1551. http://dx.doi.org/10.1136/jnnp.2003.025551

Fredericks, C. M., & Saladin, L. K. (1996). *Clinical presentations in disorders of motor function.* Philadelphia: F. A. Davis.

Fugl-Meyer, A. R., Jääskö, L., Leyman, I., Olsson, S., & Steglind, S. (1975). The post-stroke hemiplegic patient: 1. A method for evaluation of physical performance. *Scandinavian Journal of Rehabilitation Medicine, 7,* 13–31.

Garry, M. I., Loftus, A., & Summers, J. J. (2005). Mirror, mirror on the wall: Viewing a mirror reflection of unilateral hand movements facilitates ipsilateral M1 excitability. *Experimental Brain Research, 163,* 118–122. http://dx.doi.org/10.1007/s00221-005-2226-9

Gracies, J. M. (2005a). Pathophysiology of spastic paresis. I: Paresis and soft tissue changes. *Muscle and Nerve, 31,* 535–551. http://dx.doi.org/10.1002/mus.20284

Gracies, J. M. (2005b). Pathophysiology of spastic paresis. II: Emergence of muscle overactivity. *Muscle and Nerve, 31,* 552–571. http://dx.doi.org/10.1002/mus.20285

Gracies, J. M., Marosszeky, J. E., Renton, R., Sandanam, J., Gandevia, S. C., & Burke, D. (2000). Short-term effects of dynamic Lycra splints on upper limb in hemiplegic patients. *Archives of Physical Medicine and Rehabilitation, 81,* 1547–1555. http://dx.doi.org/10.1053/apmr.2000.16346

Green, J. B. (2003). Brain reorganization after stroke. *Topics in Stroke Rehabilitation, 10,* 1–20.

Gutman, S. A. (Ed.). (2008). *Quick reference neuroscience for rehabilitation professionals: The essential neurologic principles underlying rehabilitation practice* (2nd ed.). Thorofare, NJ: Slack.

Gutman, S. A., & Schonfeld, A. S. (2009). *Screening adult neurologic populations: A step-by-step instruction manual* (2nd ed.). Bethesda, MD: AOTA Press.

Harris, J. E., & Eng, J. J. (2007). Paretic upper-limb strength best explains arm activity in people with stroke. *Physical Therapy, 87,* 88–97. http://dx.doi.org/10.2522/ptj.20060065

Hayner, K., Gibson, G., & Giles, G. M. (2010). Comparison of constraint-induced movement therapy and bilateral treatment of equal intensity in people with chronic upper-extremity dysfunction after cerebrovascular accident. *American Journal of Occupational Therapy, 64,* 528–539. http://dx.doi.org/10.5014/ajot.2010.08027

Heller, A., Wade, D. T., Wood, V. A., Sunderland, A., Hewer, R. L., & Ward, E. (1987). Arm function after stroke: Measurement and recovery over the first three months. *Journal of Neurology, Neurosurgery, and Psychiatry, 50,* 714–719. http://dx.doi.org/10.1136/jnnp.50.6.714

Hubbard, I. J., Parsons, M. W., Neilson, C., & Carey, L. M. (2009). Task-specific training: Evidence for and translation to clinical practice. *Occupational Therapy International, 16,* 175–189. http://dx.doi.org/10.1002/oti.275

Jaeschke, R., Singer, J., & Guyatt, G. H. (1989). Measurement of health status: Ascertaining the minimal clinically important difference. *Controlled Clinical Trials, 10,* 407–415.

Jebsen, R. H., Taylor, N., Trieschmann, R. B., Trotter, M. J., & Howard, L. A. (1969). An objective and standardized test of hand function. *Archives of Physical Medicine and Rehabilitation, 50,* 311–319.

Karnath, H. O., & Ferber, S. (2000). The neural correlate of contraversive pushing. *Annals of Neurology, 48,* 444.

Karnath, H. O., Ferber, S., & Dichgans, J. (2000). The origin of contraversive pushing: Evidence for a second graviceptive system in humans. *Neurology, 55,* 1298–1304. http://dx.doi.org/10.1212/WNL.55.9.1298

Kleim, J. A., & Jones, T. A. (2008). Principles of experience-dependent neural plasticity: Implications for rehabilitation after brain damage. *Journal of Speech, Language, and Hearing Research, 51,* S225–S239. http://dx.doi.org/10.1044/1092-4388(2008/018)

Kopp, B., Kunkel, A., Flor, H., Platz, T., Rose, U., Mauritz, K. H., . . . Taub, E. (1997). The Arm Motor Ability Test: Reliability, validity, and sensitivity to change of an instrument for assessing disabilities in activities of daily living. *Archives of Physical Medicine and Rehabilitation, 78,* 615–620. http://dx.doi.org/10.1016/S0003-9993(97)90427-5

Kwakkel, G., Wagenaar, R. C., Kollen, B. J., & Lankhorst, G. J. (1996). Predicting disability in stroke—A critical review of the literature. *Age and Ageing, 25,* 479–489. http://dx.doi.org/10.1093/ageing/25.6.479

Lamb, S. E., Ferrucci, L., Volapto, S., Fried, L. P., & Guralnik, J. M.; Women's Health and Aging Study. (2003). Risk factors for falling in home-dwelling older women with stroke: The Women's Health and Aging Study. *Stroke, 34,* 494–501. http://dx.doi.org/10.1161/01. STR.0000053444.00582.B7

Lang, C. E. (2012). Impaired motor control. In A. A. Guccione, R. A. Wong, & D. Avers (Eds.), *Geriatric physical therapy* (3rd ed., pp. 272–291). St. Louis: Elsevier/Mosby.

Lang, C. E., & Beebe, J. A. (2007). Relating movement control at 9 upper extremity segments to loss of hand function in people with chronic hemiparesis. *Neurorehabilitation and Neural Repair, 21,* 279–291. http://dx.doi.org/10.1177/1545968306296964

Lang, C. E., Bland, M. D., Bailey, R. R., Schaefer, S. Y., & Birkenmeier, R. L. (2013). Assessment of upper extremity impairment, function, and activity after stroke: Foundations for clinical decision making. *Journal of Hand Therapy, 26,* 104–114, quiz 115. http://dx.doi. org/10.1016/j.jht.2012.06.005

Lang, C. E., DeJong, S. L., & Beebe, J. A. (2009). Recovery of thumb and finger extension and its relation to grasp performance after stroke. *Journal of Neurophysiology, 102,* 451–459. http://dx.doi.org/10.1152/jn.91310.2008

Lang, C. E., Wagner, J. M., Bastian, A. J., Hu, Q. L., Edwards, D. F., Sahrmann, S. A., & Dromerick, A. W. (2005). Deficits in grasp versus reach during acute hemiparesis. *Experimental Brain Research, 166,* 126–136. http://dx.doi.org/10.1007/s00221-005-2350-6

Lang, C. E., Wagner, J. M., Edwards, D. F., Sahrmann, S. A., & Dromerick, A. W. (2006). Recovery of grasp versus reach in people with hemiparesis poststroke. *Neurorehabilitation and Neural Repair, 20,* 444–454. http://dx.doi.org/10.1177/1545968306289299

Langlois, S., Pederson, L., & Mackinnon, J. R. (1991). The effects of splinting on the spastic hemiplegic hand: Report of a feasibility study. *Canadian Journal of Occupational Therapy, 58,* 17–25. http://dx.doi.org/10.1177/000841749105800105

Latham, N. K., Jette, D. U., Coster, W., Richards, L., Smout, R. J., James, R. A., . . . Horn, S. D. (2006). Occupational therapy activities and intervention techniques for clients with stroke in six rehabilitation hospitals. *American Journal of Occupational Therapy, 60,* 369–378. http://dx.doi.org/10.5014/ajot.60.4.369

Levit, K. (2008). Optimizing motor behavior using the Bobath approach. In M. V. Radomski & C. A. Trombly-Latham (Eds.), *Occupational therapy for physical dysfunction* (6th ed., pp. 642–666). Philadelphia: Lippincott Williams & Wilkins.

Lin, J. H., Hsu, M. J., Sheu, C. F., Wu, T. S., Lin, R. T., Chen, C. H., & Hsieh, C. L. (2009). Psychometric comparisons of 4 measures for assessing upper-extremity function in people with stroke. *Physical Therapy, 89,* 840–850.

Lincoln, N., & Leadbitter, D. (1979). Assessment of motor function in stroke patients. *Physiotherapy, 65,* 48–51.

Loewen, S. C., & Anderson, B. A. (1990). Predictors of stroke outcome using objective measurement scales. *Stroke, 21,* 78–81. http://dx.doi.org/10.1161/01.STR.21.1.78

Lyle, R. C. (1981). A performance test for assessment of upper limb function in physical rehabilitation treatment and research. *International Journal of Rehabilitation Research, 4,* 483–492. http://dx.doi.org/10.1097/00004356-198112000-00001

MacKenzie, D. E., & Westwood, D. A. (2013). Occupational therapists and observation: What are you looking at? *OTJR: Occupation, Participation and Health, 33,* 4–11. http://dx.doi. org/10.3928/15394492-20120928-01

Malouin, F., & Richards, C. L. (2010). Mental practice for relearning locomotor skills. *Physical Therapy, 90,* 240–251. http://dx.doi.org/10.2522/ptj.20090029

Mathiowetz, V., Kashman, N., Volland, G., Weber, K., Dowe, M., & Rogers, S. (1985). Grip and pinch strength: Normative data for adults. *Archives of Physical Medicine and Rehabilitation, 66,* 69–74.

Mathiowetz, V., Volland, G., Kashman, N., & Weber, K. (1985). Adult norms for the Box and Block Test of manual dexterity. *American Journal of Occupational Therapy, 39,* 386–391. http://dx.doi.org/10.5014/ajot.39.6.386

Mayo, N. E., Wood-Dauphinee, S., Côté, R., Durcan, L., & Carlton, J. (2002). Activity, participation, and quality of life 6 months poststroke. *Archives of Physical Medicine and Rehabilitation, 83,* 1035–1042. http://dx.doi.org/10.1053/apmr.2002.33984

McCombe Waller, S., & Whitall, J. (2008). Bilateral arm training: Why and who benefits? *NeuroRehabilitation, 23,* 29–41.

McPherson, J. J., Kreimeyer, D., Aalderks, M., & Gallagher, T. (1982). A comparison of dorsal and volar resting hand splints in the reduction of hypertonus. *American Journal of Occupational Therapy, 36,* 664–670. http://dx.doi.org/10.5014/ajot.36.10.664

Miltner, W. H. R., Bauder, H., Sommer, M., Dettmers, C., & Taub, E. (1999). Effects of constraint-induced movement therapy on patients with chronic motor deficits after stroke: A replication. *Stroke, 30,* 586–592. http://dx.doi.org/10.1161/01.STR.30.3.586

Moreland, J., & Thomson, M. A. (1994). Efficacy of electromyographic biofeedback compared with conventional physical therapy for upper-extremity function in patients following stroke: A research overview and meta-analysis. *Physical Therapy, 74,* 534–543, discussion 544–547.

Nijland, R., Kwakkel, G., Bakers, J., & van Wegen, E. (2011). Constraint-induced movement therapy for the upper paretic limb in acute or sub-acute stroke: A systematic review. *International Journal of Stroke, 6,* 425–433. http://dx.doi.org/10.1111/j.1747-4949.2011.00646.x

Nilsen, D. M., Gillen, G., & Gordon, A. M. (2010). Use of mental practice to improve upper-limb recovery after stroke: A systematic review. *American Journal of Occupational Therapy, 64,* 695–708. http://dx.doi.org/10.5014/ajot.2010.09034

Ostendorf, C. G., & Wolf, S. L. (1981). Effect of forced use of the upper extremity of a hemiplegic patient on changes in function: A single-case design. *Physical Therapy, 61,* 1022–1028.

Page, S. J., Sisto, S. A., & Levine, P. (2002). Modified constraint-induced therapy in chronic stroke. *American Journal of Physical Medicine and Rehabilitation, 81,* 870–875. http://dx.doi.org/10.1097/00002060-200211000-00013

Patten, C., Lexell, J., & Brown, H. E. (2004). Weakness and strength training in persons with poststroke hemiplegia: Rationale, method, and efficacy. *Journal of Rehabilitation Research and Development, 41,* 293–312. http://dx.doi.org/10.1682/JRRD.2004.03.0293

Pedersen, P. M., Wandel, A., Jørgensen, H. S., Nakayama, H., Raaschou, H. O., & Olsen, T. S. (1996). Ipsilateral pushing in stroke: Incidence, relation to neuropsychological symptoms, and impact on rehabilitation. The Copenhagen Stroke Study. *Archives of Physical Medicine and Rehabilitation, 77,* 25–28. http://dx.doi.org/10.1016/S0003-9993(96)90215-4

Poole, J. L., & Whitney, S. L. (2001). Assessments of motor function post stroke. *Physical and Occupational Therapy in Geriatrics, 19,* 1–22. http://dx.doi.org/10.1080/J148v19n02_01

Poole, J. L., Whitney, S. L., Hangeland, N., & Baker, C. (1990). The effectiveness of inflatable pressure splints on motor function in stroke patients. *OTJR: Occupation, Participation and Health, 10,* 360–366.

Popovic, D. B., Popovic, M. B., & Sinkjaer, T. (2002). Neurorehabilitation of upper extremities in humans with sensory–motor impairment. *Neuromodulation, 5,* 54–66. http://dx.doi.org/10.1046/j.1525-1403.2002._2009.x

Prager, E. M., & Lang, C. E. (2012). Predictive ability of 2-day measurement of active range of motion on 3-mo upper-extremity motor function in people with poststroke hemiparesis. *American Journal of Occupational Therapy, 66,* 35–41. http://dx.doi.org/10.5014/ajot.2012.002683

Purves, D. (2012). *Movement and its central control* (5th ed.). Sunderland, MA: Sinauer Associates.

Rose, V., & Shah, S. (1987). A comparative study on the immediate effects of orthoses in reduction of hypertonus. *Australian Occupational Therapy Journal, 34,* 59–64. http://dx.doi.org/10.1111/j.1440-1630.1987.tb01570.x

Sabari, J. S., & Lieberman, D. (2008). *Occupational therapy practice guidelines for adults with stroke.* Bethesda, MD: AOTA Press.

Sathian, K., Buxbaum, L. J., Cohen, L. G., Krakauer, J. W., Lang, C. E., Corbetta, M., & Fitzpatrick, S. M. (2011). Neurological principles and rehabilitation of action disorders: Common clinical deficits. *Neurorehabilitation and Neural Repair, 25*(Suppl.), 21S–32S. http://dx.doi.org/10.1177/1545968311410941

Scheets, P. L., Sahrmann, S. A., & Norton, B. J. (2007). Use of movement system diagnoses in the management of patients with neuromuscular conditions: A multiple-patient case report. *Physical Therapy, 87,* 654–669. http://dx.doi.org/10.2522/ptj.20050349

Schmidt, R. A., & Lee, T. D. (2005). *Motor control and learning: A behavioral emphasis.* Champaign, IL: Human Kinetics.

Schmidt, R. A., & Wrisberg, C. A. (2008). *Motor learning and performance: A problem-based learning approach* (4th ed.). Champaign, IL: Human Kinetics.

Schultz-Krohn, W., Pope-Davis, S. A., Jourdan, J. M., & McLaughlin-Gray, J. (2013). Traditional sensorimotor approaches to intervention. In H. M. Pendleton & W. Schultz-Krohn (Eds.), *Pedretti's occupational therapy: Practice skills for physical dysfunction* (7th ed., pp. 796–830). St. Louis: Mosby.

Schumway-Cook, A., & Woollacott, M. H. (2012). *Motor control: Translating research into clinical practice* (4th ed.). Philadelphia: Lippincott Williams & Wilkins.

Stewart, K. C., Cauraugh, J. H., & Summers, J. J. (2006). Bilateral movement training and stroke rehabilitation: A systematic review and meta-analysis. *Journal of the Neurological Sciences, 244,* 89–95. http://dx.doi.org/10.1016/j.jns.2006.01.005

Sveen, U., Bautz-Holter, E., Sødring, K. M., Wyller, T. B., & Laake, K. (1999). Association between impairments, self-care ability and social activities 1 year after stroke. *Disability and Rehabilitation, 21,* 372–377. http://dx.doi.org/10.1080/096382899297477

Tatemichi, T. K., Desmond, D. W., Stern, Y., Paik, M., Sano, M., & Bagiella, E. (1994). Cognitive impairment after stroke: Frequency, patterns, and relationship to functional abilities. *Journal of Neurology, Neurosurgery, and Psychiatry, 57,* 202–207. http://dx.doi.org/10.1136/jnnp.57.2.202

Thieme, H., Mehrholz, J., Pohl, M., Behrens, J., & Dohle, C. (2012). Mirror therapy for improving motor function after stroke. *Cochrane Database of Systematic Reviews, 2012,* CD008449.

Tyson, S. F., Hanley, M., Chillala, J., Selley, A., & Tallis, R. C. (2006). Balance disability after stroke. *Physical Therapy, 86,* 30–38.

Tyson, S. F., & Kent, R. M. (2011). The effect of upper limb orthotics after stroke: A systematic review. *NeuroRehabilitation, 28,* 29–36. http://dx.doi.org/10.3233/Nre-2011-0629

Uswatte, G., Taub, E., Morris, D., Light, K., & Thompson, P. A. (2006). The Motor Activity Log–28: Assessing daily use of the hemiparetic arm after stroke. *Neurology, 67,* 1189–1194. http://dx.doi.org/10.1212/01.wnl.0000238164.90657.c2

Uswatte, G., Taub, E., Morris, D., Vignolo, M., & McCulloch, K. (2005). Reliability and validity of the upper-extremity Motor Activity Log–14 for measuring real-world arm use. *Stroke, 36,* 2493–2496. http://dx.doi.org/10.1161/01.STR.0000185928.90848.2e

van der Lee, J. H., Wagenaar, R. C., Lankhorst, G. J., Vogelaar, T. W., Devillé, W. L., & Bouter, L. M. (1999). Forced use of the upper extremity in chronic stroke patients: Results from a single-blind randomized clinical trial. *Stroke, 30,* 2369–2375. http://dx.doi.org/10.1161/01.STR.30.11.2369

van Kuijk, A. A., Geurts, A. C. H., Bevaart, B. J. W., & van Limbeek, J. (2002). Treatment of upper extremity spasticity in stroke patients by focal neuronal or neuromuscular blockade: A systematic review of the literature. *Journal of Rehabilitation Medicine, 34,* 51–61. http://dx.doi.org/10.1080/165019702753557836

Wilson, D. J., Baker, L. L., & Craddock, J. A. (1984). Functional Test for the hemiparetic upper extremity. *American Journal of Occupational Therapy, 38,* 159–164. http://dx.doi.org/10.5014/ajot.38.3.159

Winstein, C. J. (1991). Knowledge of results and motor learning—Implications for physical therapy. *Physical Therapy, 71,* 140–149.

Winstein, C. J., Rose, D. K., Tan, S. M., Lewthwaite, R., Chui, H. C., & Azen, S. P. (2004). A randomized controlled comparison of upper-extremity rehabilitation strategies in acute stroke: A pilot study of immediate and long-term outcomes. *Archives of Physical Medicine and Rehabilitation, 85,* 620–628. http://dx.doi.org/10.1016/j.apmr.2003.06.027

Wolf, S. L., Lecraw, D. E., Barton, L. A., & Jann, B. B. (1989). Forced use of hemiplegic upper extremities to reverse the effect of learned nonuse among chronic stroke and head-injured patients. *Experimental Neurology, 104,* 125–132. http://dx.doi.org/10.1016/S0014-4886(89)80005-6

Wolf, S. L., Thompson, P. A., Morris, D. M., Rose, D. K., Winstein, C. J., Taub, E., . . . Pearson, S. L. (2005). The EXCITE trial: Attributes of the Wolf Motor Function Test in patients with subacute stroke. *Neurorehabilitation and Neural Repair, 19,* 194–205. http://dx.doi.org/10.1177/1545968305276663

Wolf, S. L., Winstein, C. J., Miller, J. P., Taub, E., Uswatte, G., Morris, D., . . . Nichols-Larsen, D.; EXCITE Investigators. (2006). Effect of constraint-induced movement therapy on upper extremity function 3 to 9 months after stroke: The EXCITE randomized clinical trial. *JAMA, 296,* 2095–2104. http://dx.doi.org/10.1001/jama.296.17.2095

Yozbatiran, N., Der-Yeghiaian, L., & Cramer, S. C. (2008). A standardized approach to performing the Action Research Arm Test. *Neurorehabilitation and Neural Repair, 22,* 78–90. http://dx.doi.org/10.1177/1545968307305353

Zimmermann-Schlatter, A., Schuster, C., Puhan, M. A., Siekierka, E., & Steurer, J. (2008). Efficacy of motor imagery in post-stroke rehabilitation: A systematic review. *Journal of Neuroengineering and Rehabilitation, 5,* 8. http://dx.doi.org/10.1186/1743-0003-5-8

CHAPTER 7

Core Concepts in Neurocognition and Stroke

Gordon Muir Giles, PhD, OTR/L, FAOTA, and M. Tracy Morrison, OTD, OTR/L

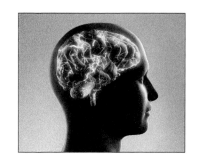

Learning Objectives

After completion of this chapter, readers will be able to

- Identify the epidemiology of cognitive disorders after stroke;
- Identify the evidence suggesting that cognitive disorders after stroke are related to outcomes in terms of activities of daily living and quality of life;
- Identify the theoretical foundations and goals of neuropsychological and occupational therapy cognitive evaluation;
- Identify different types of memory problems that may follow stroke; and
- Identify top-down and bottom-up approaches to nonspatial attention, memory, executive functioning, lateralized attention, agnosia, and apraxia poststroke.

Key Words

- agnosia
- apraxia
- Cognitive Functional Evaluation process
- errorless learning
- executive functioning
- lateralized attention
- memory
- performance-based testing
- spaced- and expanding-retrieval techniques

Introduction

Cognitive impairment after **stroke** can affect occupational performance, independence, and quality of life. Cognitive impairment may also have indirect effects on functional status and recovery after stroke through reduced engagement in **rehabilitation** and reduced community participation (Cumming, Marshall, & Lazar, 2013). In this chapter, we describe the frequency and nature of poststroke cognitive impairment. A short history of cognitive rehabilitation is followed by a discussion of cognitive rehabilitation models. The purpose of neuropsychological testing is discussed, focusing on the uses of neuropsychological testing for occupational therapists. We then discuss cognitive and performance-based testing from an occupational therapy perspective. In the remainder of the chapter, we discuss specific cognitive and perceptual functions (briefly mentioning language), focusing on those functions of particular importance to occupational therapists: nonspatial attention, **memory, executive function,** lateralized attention, **agnosia,** and **apraxia.**

Stroke and Cognitive Impairment

Cognitive impairment is common after a first stroke, with 30% to 60% of clients demonstrating poststroke cognitive impairment across studies (Barker-Collo, Feigin, Parag, Lawes, & Senior, 2010; Eskes & Salter, 2013; Feigin et al., 2010). People with hemorrhagic stroke may initially show greater cognitive impairment than people with ischemic stroke, but they may also show greater improvement (Katrak, Black, & Peeva, 2009; Kelly et al., 2003). Nys et al. (2007) tested 190 patients admitted to a specialized stroke unit 3 weeks after stroke and found that cognitive impairment was present in 74% of patients with a cortical stroke, 46% of patients with a **subcortical** stroke, and 43% of patients with an infratentorial stroke. A systematic review of studies of the cognitive sequelae of lacunar stroke found that executive functions (EFs), memory, language, attention, and visuospatial abilities were all affected, with the largest effects found for information-processing speed and for measures of global **cognition** (Edwards, Jacova, Sepehry, Pratt, & Benavente, 2013).

In patients 1 year after stroke, Sachdev, Brodaty, Valenzuela, Lorentz, and Koschera (2004) found a modest decline on the **Mini-Mental State Examination** (MMSE [Folstein, Folstein, & McHugh, 1975]; mean = 0.83, standard deviation = 2.2). Years of education was found to have a protective effect, and a further stroke during the year after the first stroke was associated with a larger decline in cognitive functioning. In a population study intended to ascertain all stroke cases (hospitalized and nonhospitalized) in Auckland, New Zealand (Barker-Collo et al., 2010; Feigin et al., 2010), 30% to 50% of patients 5 years poststroke performed below average on most neuropsychological measures, and deficits were most common in information-processing speed and EFs. Although all cognitive domains were found to be significantly related to functional outcomes, multiple regression analyses showed that only information-processing speed and visuoperceptual ability made a significant independent contribution to functional outcomes when controlling for demographics, depression, and current score on the Barthel Index (Barker-Collo et al., 2010; Feigin et al., 2010).

Performance on measures of cognition is a predictor of **functional impairment** (Walker, Sunderland, Sharma, & Walker, 2004). The presence of impaired performance on a cognitive test 3 months poststroke is significantly correlated with requiring attendant care or being discharged from the hospital to a nursing home, even after controlling for the effects of age and physical functioning (Tatemichi, Desmond, Stern, Sano, & Bagiella, 1994). Robertson, Ridgeway, Greenfield, and Parr (1997) found that functional improvement 2 years after right-hemisphere stroke was predicted by the ability to sustain attention at 2 months poststroke. EF impairment has been shown to predict participation in rehabilitation (Skidmore et al., 2010). Additionally, evidence is growing that even patients with mild stroke (defined by a **National Institutes of Health Stroke Scale** score of <6) may have EF deficits that may significantly reduce community participation (Morrison et al., 2013; Wolf, Baum, & Connor, 2009).

Individual perception of health (health-related quality of life) has increasingly been recognized as an important outcome after stroke, and several health-related quality-of-life scales have been developed, such as the Stroke Impact Scale (Carod-Artal & Egido, 2009; Duncan et al., 1999). Persistent cognitive deficits may significantly affect quality of life (Ahlsiö, Britton, Murray, & Theorell, 1984), and **poststroke depression** significantly affects cognitive functioning (Carod-Artal & Egido, 2009).

Stroke is a significant risk factor for later onset **mild** or **major neurocognitive disorder** (NCD; Ihle-Hansen et al., 2011), and NCD is a risk factor for stroke (Pasi, Poggesi, Salvadori, & Pantoni, 2012). Ihle-Hansen et al. (2011) administered neuropsychological evaluations to all patients with first transient ischemic attack or stroke who had no preexisting mild or major NCD and who were admitted to a single hospital service in Norway. A total of 184 patients completed follow-up, of whom 105 (57%) had developed cognitive impairment 1 year after the vascular event: 36 (19.6%) were diagnosed with **dementia** (major NCD) during the 1st year after the vascular event, and 69 (37.5%) were diagnosed with **mild cognitive impairment** (mild NCD). Of the 105 patients who developed NCD, 14 (13.3%) were diagnosed as having a degenerative cognitive disease (e.g., **Alzheimer's disease**); 34 (32.4%), a vascular cognitive disease; and 57 (54.3%), a mixed disease process.

Brief History of Cognitive Rehabilitation

The possibility of "reeducating" people with impaired brain function has provoked interest since the 1800s (Finger, 1994). This interest intensified after the work of Paul Broca (1824–1880), who identified cortical regions associated with speech. Broca (1861) identified the left frontal brain region as critical to speech comprehension and expression. Inspired by Broca's work, the earliest efforts to assist recovery from brain damage grew out of aphasiology (Boake, 1991; Finger, 1994). Early pioneers of cognitive rehabilitation during the 20th century included Shepherd I. Franz, Kurt Goldstein, and Alexander R. Luria. Working in the United States, Franz (1874–1933) rejected the idea that damage to a specific brain area would necessarily abolish the function related to that brain area (i.e., Franz rejected a strict localizationist position) and argued that specific functional abilities were not localized to any one brain area. His work with patients led him to emphasize the critical role of motivation in recovery of function (Finger, 1994).

Goldstein (1878–1965) made major contributions to assessment and rehabilitation (Goldstein, 1942). Goldstein described two types of assessment: One, which he termed *abstract performance testing*, used laboratory psychological tests, and the other, which he termed *concrete labor testing*, used observation of performance in a vocational work site (what occupational therapists would now call *performance-based testing*; Boake, 1991; Goldstein, 1942).

Luria (1902–1977) emphasized that patients could redevelop abilities after brain injury by using alternate strategies that relied on preserved functions. Luria believed that patients must first consciously adopt a new method of performing a previously automatic skill (i.e., a top-down approach) and then practice it until it approached **automaticity.**

The 1970s saw the introduction of the term *cognitive rehabilitation* (Boake, 1991; Gianutsos, 1980), and at the same time interest in rehabilitation after stroke was increasing (Diller et al., 1974; Gordon et al., 1985).

Cognitive Rehabilitation Models

Considerable evolution has occurred in the field of cognitive rehabilitation since the 1970s. A primary distinction in the field has been between restitution and substitution; *restitution* focuses on the recovery of lost abilities, and *substitution* relates to the development of new ways to circumvent the impaired function. Another distinction has

Whereas an *internal* strategy relates to a change in the way that the person thinks . . . an *external strategy* describes an aid . . . or an environmental modification or reduction in activity demand.

been between internal and external strategies. Whereas an *internal strategy* relates to a change in the way that the person thinks (such as the implementation of formal problem-solving routines), an *external strategy* describes an aid (such as use of a smartphone or a schedule) or an environmental modification or reduction in activity demand.

Another important distinction has been between bottom-up and top-down approaches. A *bottom-up approach* typically refers to an intervention that focuses on repetitive practice of processes that are considered fundamental cognitive processes, such as structured sensory stimulation or repetitive practice in attention skills. A *top-down approach* is one that involves higher cognitive processes to regulate lower processes, as in training in self-awareness or mental cognitive control strategies (Robertson & Murre, 1999).

Cognitive rehabilitation from the 1970s to the present has been in continuous evolution, but it can be divided into three phases: (1) general stimulation and hierarchical-based approaches, (2) targeted process-specific approaches, and (3) strategy-driven approaches targeting EF. Although to some extent all three approaches have existed in parallel, there is currently an increased research focus and a growing evidence base for the strategy-based approaches to EF retraining (Dawson et al., 2009).

General stimulation approaches attempt to stimulate the patient with the cognitive deficits or the cognitive process to enhance the function (Gianutsos, 1980; Soderback & Normell, 1986a, 1986b). By placing gradually increasing demands on the cognitive function, it is hoped that function will become more efficient. The approaches adopted have been primarily hierarchical both within and between functions so that more fundamental cognitive processes (e.g., naming ability, visual scanning) are addressed before higher order cognitive processes can be addressed (e.g., reading; Gordon & Hibbard, 1991; Whyte, 1986). This approach was often directed toward underlying cognitive skills such as attention and memory. Computers were also frequently used as an adjunct to work with the therapist (e.g., Captain's Log Mind Power Builder; BrainTrain, 2013). Little evidence has supported these approaches, and although they are still used they cannot in general be considered evidence based (das Nair & Lincoln, 2007).

Process-specific approaches are highly focused and target a specific cognitive process or skill (Gray & Robertson, 1989; Sohlberg & Mateer, 1987a, 1987b). They may also address a cognitive skill and functional skill together. So, for example, a specific attention program may be directed toward the skills required in driving or the scanning attention skill required in reading (Gray & Robertson, 1989; Robertson, Gray, & McKenzie, 1988; Robertson, Gray, Pentland, & Waite, 1990). These approaches may involve behavioral or cognitive compensatory routines and the development of self-awareness and error correction. Computers may also be used as part of the retraining program. A meta-analysis found that highly targeted cognitive retraining was a more effective model than comprehensive, but less targeted, approaches (Rohling, Faust, Beverly, & Demakis, 2009).

The third approach and the one that is currently the central focus of work by many occupational therapists is the development of programs to develop metacognitive strategies (Polatajko & Mandich, 2004, 2005; Skidmore et al., 2011; Toglia, Johnston, Goverover, & Dain, 2010). The programs involve teaching patients to identify problems, to develop their own methods to overcome them, and to implement and evaluate the solutions (Toglia et al., 2010). Strategy training can be divided into global and domain-specific strategies. Global strategies are designed to assist clients with developing a general thinking routine, which enables them to develop solutions to a wide range of novel problems that might be encountered in daily life (e.g., Cognitive Orientation to Daily Occupational Performance [CO-OP], goal plan, do, check; Polatajko & Mandich, 2005). Domain-specific cognitive strategies represent mental routines designed to gain mastery of a particular type of problem or situation. Specific strategy training is not aimed at relearning specific tasks but at teaching clients new ways of handling a narrow range of problems in an attempt to compensate for a specific compromised function.

An approach that is conceptually distinct from the cognitive rehabilitation approaches just described and one that has continued its evolution in parallel to them is the specific skill-training approach. This approach may also be considered bottom-up but rather than target cognitive skills, this approach targets functional and behavioral real-world competencies (occupations; Rotenberg-Shpigelman, Erez, Nahaloni, & Maeir, 2012). Simplifying task demands or altering the environmental affordances so that the desired behavior is elicited also has a long history in occupational therapy (see Table 7.1).

Table 7.1. Classification of Cognitive Rehabilitation Strategies

Strategy	Description
1. Global strategy learning	Global strategy learning includes approaches such as executive function retraining and interventions intended to increase self-awareness. Instead of attempting to remediate basic cognitive deficits, therapy aims at improving awareness of the impaired cognitive processes. Clients are assisted to develop top-down compensatory strategies using scripts facilitating problem solving, decision making, reasoning, and the like. These approaches may include formal training aiming to facilitate generalization, but it is assumed that clients will be able to generalize the application of these compensatory strategies to novel situations. Actual task practices are incidental: The central focus of treatment is the strategy (Guidetti & Ytterberg, 2011; Toglia et al., 2010).
2. Domain-specific strategy training	Domain-specific strategy training assists clients to manage specific perceptual, cognitive, or functional deficits. The focus is on the strategy (i.e., top-down) rather than on the task itself (e.g., an internal routine to scan the whole environment, manage interpersonal interactions, to identify things to be recorded in a personal digital assistant). Training may be provided in such a way as to attempt to maximize the chances for generalization, but generalization is assumed to occur.
3. Function-embedded cognitive retraining	Cognitive retraining is undertaken in a performance context and is specific to the task (e.g., attention retraining during driving reeducation). Although the training is context specific, some authors have proposed that generalization of skills and improved performance on other tasks will occur (e.g., Park et al., 1999), depending on the degree of overlap in processing operations between the training task and new task, that is, transfer distance (the transfer-appropriate processing hypothesis; Park et al., 1999).
4. Process-specific cognitive retraining	Interventions attempt to remediate a specific cognitive deficit via massive bottom-up stimulation of the impaired cognitive–perceptual skill such as prism adaptation training (Serino et al., 2007) or eye-patch training (Fong et al., 2013; Zoccolotti et al., 2011).
5. Task-specific training	A specific functional behavior is taught, and the therapist attempts to circumvent cognitive deficits that hamper performance by providing a routine (e.g., task-specific training; Rotenberg-Shpigelman et al., 2012) incorporating errorless learning (Giles, 2010, 2011). No assumptions are made with respect to generalization across activities. Skills trained may or may not have secondary effects on awareness, mental efficiency, and organization and influence performance in other domains. Improved self-efficacy may also positively affect engagement with rehabilitation and therefore other to-be-learned tasks (Parish & Oddy, 2007; Rotenberg-Shpigelman et al., 2012).
6. Environmental modifications and assistive technology	Environmental modifications and simplifications are included in most of the approaches described above. Part of the process of intervention is the simplification of task demands so that skills can be practiced and cueing reduced as the skills are learned. A good match between the client's abilities and environmental demands may be central to success (Evans et al., 2000; Wilson et al., 1994).

Cognitive Testing

Neuropsychological testing is the special expertise of neuropsychologists, who have a wide array of tests intended to isolate specific cognitive skills (Evans, 2010; Lezak, Howieson, Bigler, & Tranel, 2012). Testing is office based, and testing procedures are intended to allow the test taker to perform the test free of distraction; the results are intended to describe optimal performance under the best conditions. Test results are related to normative performance (scaled scores) and are intended to be directly related to the client's capacity to use cognitive functions (e.g., **short-term memory** capacity). In this section, we discuss the purposes of neuropsychological testing and the types of information occupational therapists can derive from neuropsychological test reports.

Neuropsychological assessment is concerned with the identification of the cognitive (i.e., information-processing) consequences of brain dysfunction and their behavioral manifestations (Evans, 2010; Loewenstein & Acevedo, 2010). Additional goals are as follows:

- To determine the presence of organic dysfunction and more specifically aid in diagnosis (Evans, 2010; Lezak et al., 2012). Modern imaging technologies have in many instances replaced this function, but some types of neuropathology cannot be visualized with current imaging techniques (e.g., toxic encephalopathies; Lezak et al., 2012).
- To determine the nature and severity of the cognitive impairment and whether it is a result of stroke (and not preexisting or other factors; Evans, 2010). Even when the location of a lesion is known, the specific pattern of cognitive deficits may be quite varied (Lezak et al., 2012).
- To provide realistic information to the client and family members regarding the nature and extent of cognitive impairments and to clarify issues of adjustment to disability versus personality and behavioral changes that may result from the stroke (Lezak et al., 2012). Factual information about cognitive functioning allows clients with retained self-awareness to understand what has happened to them and to set themselves realistic goals (Lezak et al., 2012).
- To provide information about the implications of the patterns of cognitive functioning (areas of cognitive strength and weakness; Evans, 2010; Lezak et al., 2012). This function of neuropsychological testing may be particularly relevant to occupational therapists because it may influence the parameters of functional retraining programs (Giles, 2011) and care planning.
- To determine whether the cognitive impairment has changed over time (Evans, 2010) and to document improvement or deterioration by comparing current test results with those obtained at an earlier time (Lezak et al., 2012). The sensitivity of neuropsychological tests makes them ideally suited for tracking the progress of recovery or deterioration after stroke, which is important in discharge planning, environmental modifications, and caregiver training.
- To use neuropsychological assessment as part of research into remediation techniques for basic cognitive functions (Evans, 2010).

Although more and more neuropsychologists are participating in the development and execution of retraining programs, most clients who work with a neuropsychologist after stroke continue to do so for neuropsychological testing. Occupational therapists can use neuropsychological test results in conjunction with their own testing to guide intervention strategies.

Performance-Based and Cognitive Testing in Occupational Therapy

Occupational therapy's focus on occupational performance provides a unique disciplinary perspective on the assessment of cognition (American Occupational Therapy Association [AOTA], 2013). When occupational therapists assess cognition, the assessment is focused on how cognitive deficits contribute to occupational performance dysfunction and more specifically on how to address cognitive deficits so as to address the occupational performance problems identified by the client as of central concern (AOTA, 2013, 2014).

Occupational therapists screen for perceptual and cognitive dysfunction when first evaluating a client and use cognitive testing to understand more about the client's performance deficits, but testing is primarily driven by performance issues (Baum & Katz, 2010; Hartman-Maeir, Katz, & Baum, 2009). Occupational therapists therefore place clients in situations (real or simulated) in which they must use skills, perform real-world tasks, and solve real-world problems that relate to the types of functions that the clients must accomplish to successfully fulfill their life roles. This assessment must by necessity also involve the emotional, personality, and behavioral consequences of the neurological dysfunction. Occupational therapists may also use performance-based testing to determine the type of performance errors that occur and the level of assistance or cueing the client requires to successfully perform the task (e.g., Executive Function Performance Test [EFPT]; see Poulin, Korner-Bitensky, & Dawson, 2013, for a review of stroke-specific executive function measures).

The central advantage of performance-based testing relates to difficulties with observing natural performance in some contexts (e.g., the acute care hospital) and the limitation of cognitive testing in the prediction of performance (Manchester, Priestley, & Jackson, 2004; Marcotte, Scott, Kamat, & Heaton, 2010; Priestley, Manchester, & Aram, 2013). Prediction problems associated with cognitive testing are bidirectional. Varying occupational histories and differences in self-awareness, capacity for behavioral self-regulation, and life experiences affect the resilience of occupational performance after stroke. This factor could be termed *functional resilience* or *functional reserve*.

Performance-based testing may be office based (e.g., EFPT; Baum et al., 2008) or occur in the real world with the unpredictable affordances and interpersonal interactions that are attendant to these settings (e.g., the Multiple Errands Test, Test of Grocery Shopping Skills; Hamera & Brown, 2000; Hamera, Rempfer, & Brown, 2005, 2009; Morrison et al., 2013). These performance-based tests may be standardized (e.g., the EFPT) or may be created by the therapist in a way that is specifically tailored to the client's performance requirements, a factor that often provides for high face validity. On one hand, clients with cognitive impairment may fail to show deficits in real-world functioning. On the other hand, office-based neuropsychological deficits may suggest an absence of impairment, but the client may nonetheless show

> When occupational therapists assess cognition, the assessment is focused on how cognitive deficits contribute to occupational performance dysfunction and more specifically on how to address cognitive deficits so as to address the occupational performance problems identified by the client as of central concern.

marked impairment in real-world functioning (Manchester et al., 2004; Priestley et al., 2013).

Process of Occupational Therapy Evaluation

People with stroke are typically referred to occupational therapy to assess for the presence of occupational performance deficits or when deficits are identified that may interfere with daily functioning or quality of life. The goal of occupational therapy is to improve or restore function or to otherwise help the client cope with impairments that result in reduced ability or participation. The initial step in the evaluation process is the *occupational profile,* which establishes the client's occupational history and experiences; daily **habits** and routines; and interests, values, and needs (AOTA, 2014). The client's concerns about performing occupations and daily life activities are identified, and his or her priorities are determined (AOTA, 2014). Tools such as the Canadian Occupational Performance Measure (COPM; Law et al., 2005) and the Activity Card Sort (Baum & Edwards, 2008) can help clinicians and clients focus on specific performance-based goals (Wolf et al., 2009).

The second step in the evaluation process is the analysis of occupational performance, during which the client's strengths and performance problems are identified (AOTA, 2014). Therapists may screen for perceptual and cognitive deficits and to provide a baseline to chart recovery. Evaluation will vary with the client's diagnosis, stage of recovery, and setting. Hartman-Maeir et al. (2009; Baum & Katz, 2010) have described the Cognitive Functional Evaluation process to be used by occupational therapists with people with suspected cognitive disabilities. They stated that the interview, cognitive screen, performance-based testing, and environmental assessment should always be performed, and that the test of specific cognitive function and specific measures of cognitive performance should be implemented when other assessments indicate that further information is necessary.

The process is intended to be customized to each person's needs but can include as many as six components:

1. The occupational therapist gathers background information from the client or the client's significant others through interview and delineates the client's occupational profile (occupational history, current status, and occupational goals) as well as the client's views regarding the nature of any deficit that he or she might have. Several standardized measures can be used in addition to an interview (e.g., the Activity Card Sort; Baum & Edwards, 2008), and use of the COPM is recommended (Law et al., 2005).

2. Cognitive screening tools are used to create a preliminary profile of the client's strengths and weaknesses using standardized methods and instruments. Appropriate screening methods depend on the client's age, diagnosis, stage of illness, and type of treatment setting (e.g., MMSE, Allen Cognitive Level Screen–5, Loewenstein Occupational Therapy Cognitive Assessment; Folstein et al., 1975; Katz, Itzkovich, Averbuch, & Elazar, 1989; Riska-Williams et al., 2007).

3. Performance-based cognitive function and EF measures are intended to capture occupational performance deficits that would be the target of occupational therapist cognitive intervention (e.g., the Routine Task

Inventory [Katz, 2006], Kitchen Task Assessment [Neistadt, 1992], the Assessment of Motor and Process Skills [Fisher & Bray Jones, 2010a, 2010b], and the EFPT [Baum et al., 2008; Morrison et al., 2013]).

4. Tests of specific cognitive functions are intended to provide an in-depth understanding of specific cognitive domains so as to better understand the client's occupational performance deficits or to help in the design of interventions to help the client overcome occupational performance deficits. Occupational therapists give preference to tests with established ecological validity (e.g., the Rivermead Behavioral Memory Test [RBMT; Wilson et al., 1999; Wilson, Cockburn, & Baddeley, 1991, 2003], Test of Everyday Attention [TEA; Robertson, Ward, Ridgeway, & Nimmo-Smith, 1994], and Behavioral Assessment of the Dysexecutive Syndrome [Wilson, Alderman, Burgess, Emslie, & Evans, 1996]).

5. Specific measures of cognitive performance in occupations determine how specific cognitive deficits manifest themselves in occupational performance (e.g., the ADL Checklist for Neglect, the Catherine Bergego Scale [CBS]; Azouvi et al., 2002; Hartman-Maeir & Katz, 1995).

6. Environmental assessment provides the therapist with information about the environment and context in which the client needs to function in his or her daily life. Although in this schematic presentation this assessment occurs last, in reality environmental affordances have a major effect on daily life activities, and so the environmental assessment is best considered an ongoing part of the evaluation.

Specific Functions

In the rest of this chapter, we focus on the types of cognitive and perceptual deficits that are of central importance to the occupational therapist's role of maximizing the client's occupational performance poststroke. We use a standard format in discussing each of these cognitive and perceptual functions (except language, which is the central focus of speech–language therapists). Each section begins with a discussion of the current understanding of the processes and subsystems involved in the cognitive function, followed by a discussion of evaluation. Evidence for the effectiveness of intervention is reviewed. Interventions are categorized as bottom-up or top-down and described. Of necessity, discussions are brief, and citations are included as a point of departure for the reader's future study.

Understanding how cognitive functions are disrupted is essential for occupational therapists to develop individualized intervention programs. Although robust evidence for some areas of intervention is lacking, the effectiveness of cognitive rehabilitation has increasingly been recognized (AOTA, 2013).

Understanding how cognitive functions are disrupted is essential for occupational therapists to develop individualized intervention programs.

Aphasia

Aphasiology is an area of special expertise of speech–language therapists. It is important, however, that occupational therapists understand the types of language disorders that may follow stroke. The work of Broca (1861), Wernicke (1874), and Lichtheim (1885) divided the **aphasias** into seven types (a typology that remains current; Caplan, 2012). Table 7.2 shows the seven language syndromes with their associated features. The left hemisphere is largely responsible for the semantic

Table 7.2. Aphasia Syndromes

Syndrome	Speech Output	Comprehension	Repetition	Naming	Paraphasia	Hemiparesis	Hemisensory	Site of Lesion
Broca (motor)	Nonfluent	Good	Poor	Poor	Uncommon	Common	Uncommon	Broca's area Area 44
Wernicke (sensory)	Fluent	Poor	Poor	Poor	Common	Uncommon	Uncommon	Wernicke's area Posterior area 22
Conduction	Fluent	Good	Poor	Poor	Common	Uncommon	Common	Left inferior parietal Supramarginal gyrus Angular gyrus
Global	Nonfluent	Poor	Poor	Poor	Common	Common	Common	Entire left perisylvian region
Transcortical								
Motor	Nonfluent	Good	Good	Poor	Uncommon	Uncommon	Uncommon	Left prefrontal
Sensory	Fluent	Poor	Good	Poor	Common	Uncommon	Common	Left posterior temporal inferior to Wernicke's area
Mixed	Nonfluent	Poor	Good	Poor	Uncommon	Common	Common	Variable
Anomic	Fluent	Good	Good	Poor	Uncommon	Uncommon	Uncommon	Left basal ganglia
Subcortical	Variable	Variable	Good	Variable	Common	Common	Common	Variable

aspects of communication; the right hemisphere is primarily responsible for **prosody,** the nonsemantic emotional aspects of communication. Prosody includes pitch, loudness, timbre, tempo, stress, accent, and intonation. Right-brain damage may impair both production and comprehension of prosody (Caplan, 2012).

Attention

The majority of the stroke literature (Norman & Shallice, 1986) on **attention** has examined lateralized attention, which we discuss later in this chapter. However, deficits in nonspatial attentional tasks have been identified in people with stroke and are related to the location of the lesion (Godefroy, Lhullier, & Rousseaux, 1996), but they are less common after stroke than after other forms of brain injury (Zoccolotti et al., 2011). Posner and Petersen (1990) described three attentional processes: (1) orienting, (2) target detection, and (3) tonic arousal (see Chapter 3). Other important theoretical models for the role of attention in human functioning have been provided by Norman and Shallice (1986), Schneider and Shiffrin (1977), and Shiffrin and Schneider (1977).

The distinction between conscious and automatic processes may reflect the participation of different neural mechanisms served by different neuroanatomical systems and reflect different rehabilitation interventions, one using conscious control (top-down) and the other involving massive practice in responding to attentional demands (bottom-up; Loetscher & Lincoln, 2013; Zoccolotti et al., 2011). Many of the cognitive processes that are disrupted after brain damage may be the result of deficits in attention. The following types of attentional processes have been described:

- *Spatial attention:* the ability to detect and allocate attention to different parts of space (see "Lateralized Attention and Related Disorders" section)
- *Selective attention:* the ability to maintain a consistent behavioral set requiring activation and inhibition of responses that are dependent on the selection of target stimuli from background stimuli
- *Sustained attention:* the ability to maintain a consistent response set during continuous or repetitive activity and over a long period of time
- *Alternating attention:* the ability to switch response sets as a response to environmental cues so that two activities with distinct response requirements can be performed in sequence
- *Divided attention:* the capacity to divide attention so as to respond to two or more tasks occurring during the same time period (*multitask;* Loetscher & Lincoln, 2013).

Evaluation

Occupational therapists typically assess attention through cancellation tasks and sustained vigilance tasks using computers. Standardized measures of complex attentional processes have been lacking, and the TEA (Robertson, Ward, et al., 1994) is the first standardized, noncomputerized test of attention for use by occupational therapists. The TEA uses relatively familiar everyday materials and is plausible and acceptable to participants (Robertson, Ward, et al., 1994). Participants are asked to imagine that they are on vacation in Philadelphia, where they are required to perform several activities. Factor analysis of the standardization sample ($N = 154$) identified four factors: (1) Visual Selective Attention and Speed, (2) Attentional Switching, (3) Sustained Attention, and (4) Auditory–Verbal Working Memory (Robertson, Ward, Ridgeway, & Nimmo-Smith, 1996).

Intervention

Recent meta-analysis and systematic reviews of attention training after stroke have found very limited support for its effectiveness (Zoccolotti et al., 2011). Neither Cicerone et al. (2011) nor Zoccolotti et al. (2011) found evidence to support strategy application or computer-based practice to improve attention in people poststroke. However, Rohling et al. (2009) found a small to medium effect size for attention retraining for people poststroke, and Loetscher and Lincoln (2013) found a statistically significant short-term effect of attentional retraining over treatment as usual for divided attention. Nonetheless, Loetscher and Lincoln concluded that the evidence was insufficient to make a judgment regarding the lasting effects of attentional retraining on either attention or functional outcomes poststroke.

The techniques most frequently used to rehabilitate nonspatial attention are bottom-up highly structured activities, usually pencil and paper or computer based, that are designed to stress specific attentional systems (Loetscher & Lincoln, 2013; Park, Proulx, & Towers, 1999; Zoccolotti et al., 2011). In these tasks, clients have to respond selectively to various stimuli with variation in cueing, distraction, stimulus complexity, or other factors. The majority of reports in the literature have used Sohlberg and Mateer's (1987a) attention process training (Zoccolotti et al., 2011). Occupational therapists may also develop specific functional tasks to stress attentional functions (e.g., graded kitchen activities requiring alternating attention; Zoltan, 2007).

Memory

Surprisingly little research has examined the frequency of memory impairment after stroke (das Nair & Lincoln, 2007). Prescott, Garraway, and Akhtar (1982) evaluated memory functioning of 149 patients 4 weeks after stroke and found that 9% had slight and 15% had moderate to severe memory disturbance. These authors, however, used measures of **orientation** and retrograde memory and did not include measures of anterograde memory. Wade, Parker, and Langton Hewer (1986) examined the memory of 138 patients 3 and 6 months after acute stroke. At 3 months, 29% of patients had significantly impaired scores on memory for a paragraph-length story, and 39% had significantly impaired visual memory, with 14% unable to reproduce a picture immediately after seeing it (Wade et al., 1986). Motor loss was not associated with memory loss, but impairment in **activities of daily living** (ADLs) was (Wade et al., 1986).

Half of the people who survive stroke note subjective memory disturbance (Sorensen, Boysen, Jensen, & Schnohr, 1982) and rate their memories as significantly worse than orthopedic control participants (Tinson & Lincoln, 1987). Nys et al. (2007) found that 3 weeks after stroke, 25.6% of patients had deficits in verbal memory, and 22% had deficits in visual memory. Hurford, Charidimou, Fox, Cipolotti, and Werring (2013) found considerable improvement in the 3 months after acute ischemic stroke in attention, perceptual skills, and EFs, but little change in verbal or visual memory. Limited data appear to have confirmed that memory impairments frequently continue into the postacute period but that increased use of compensatory strategies ameliorates the impact of memory impairment somewhat (Wilson, 1991).

Structure of Memory

Although controversy continues about how to divide the different subcomponents of memory (Cowan, 2008; Yin & Knowlton, 2006), there is general agreement that remembering and executing any skilled behavior involve conceptually distinct memory systems and that these memory systems may be differentially impaired by stroke (Baddeley, 2004; Cohen & Conway, 2008). Understanding the effects of stroke on different memory systems offers opportunities to alter the way retraining is provided so as to improve rehabilitation effectiveness and so provides an example of how cognitive testing can serve the development of skills retraining programs.

Memory systems can be conceptualized as declarative and nondeclarative; another important area of memory functioning is **prospective memory.** *Declarative memory* is available to introspection (i.e., the person knows that he or she knows something; see Chapter 3, Table 3.2). It may be divided into immediate or sensory (iconic, echoic, tactile, haptic), short-term or **working memory** (responsible for management of subspan or continually rehearsed material), and supraspan **episodic** and **semantic memory** subtypes (Cowan, 2008). The conscious awareness and recall of any supraspan material (not maintained by rehearsal) involves episodic or semantic memory. *Episodic memory* relates to discrete events that retain temporal and sensory associations, whereas *semantic memory* is organized knowledge about the world that is not context specific and includes the majority of information learned in institutional education (e.g., facts and dates; Frankland & Bontempi, 2005; Tulving, 1983). Episodic memory involves the participation of medial temporal lobe structures (hippocampus; entorhinal, perirhinal, and parahippocampal

Understanding the effects of stroke on different memory systems offers opportunities to alter the way retraining is provided so as to improve rehabilitation effectiveness and so provides an example of how cognitive testing can serve the development of skills retraining programs.

areas) in the storage process as well as other neocortical areas including **prefrontal cortex** (Eichenbaum, 2001; Frankland & Bontempi, 2005).

Nondeclarative memory can be thought of as the store of acquired patterns of behavior that are not necessarily mediated by cognitive learning. Nondeclarative knowledge is not available to introspection: Information is accessed through performance (Giles, 2011). Nondeclarative memory consists of multiple memory systems, including activity–outcome learning, stimulus–response learning, classical conditioning, various types of **priming,** habituation, sensitization, evaluative conditioning, and motor learning (Squire & Wixted, 2011).

Remembering to carry out intended actions after an activity-filled delay *(prospective memory)* is a critical component of safety and independence in the community (McDonald et al., 2011). The intended activity may be triggered by either an event (event based; e.g., mailing a letter when you see a mailbox) or a prespecified time (time based; e.g., call John at 9:30) but is absent a specific reminder to carry out the action and often involves interruption of an ongoing activity (Ellis & Kvavilashvili, 2000). Prospective memory depends on a range of cognitive functions, including forming an intention, remembering that a task needs to be performed *(retrospective memory),* maintaining and periodically monitoring that intention, interrupting ongoing activity, and initiating the action to complete the intention. Prospective memory therefore involves both memory and EFs and depends particularly on rostral prefrontal cortex (approximating **Brodmann's area** 10) but also on areas of the **parietal lobe** and the anterior cingulate (Burgess, Gonen-Yaacovi, & Volle, 2011; Volle, Gonen-Yaacovi, Costello Ade, Gilbert, & Burgess, 2011).

Kim, Craik, Luo, and Ween (2009) compared prospective memory functioning between independent community-dwelling people poststroke without self-identified cognitive impairment and age- and education-matched control participants. Relative to control participants, the participants with stroke were impaired on prospective memory tasks, particularly those tasks that were novel and required self-initiated interruption of an ongoing task and the initiation of a time-based task (i.e., one without salient environmental cues; Kim et al., 2009).

Evaluation

Screening for acute or severe memory impairment may be accomplished by assessing orientation. Remember that impaired orientation, although often a sign of ongoing memory impairment, may occur as an isolated memory impairment or as a part of a **delirium.** Although some exceptions exist, return of orientation usually occurs in the sequence of person, place, and then time (Giles & Clark-Wilson, 1999).

To assess orientation to person, the therapist asks the client for his or her name. If the client is unable to speak or write, he or she is provided with a list of names and asked to indicate which one is correct. A client is oriented to place if he or she can state his or her exact location. Clients may also be oriented, however, if they can tell you what town they are in and that they are in a hospital. Many people do not know the names or exact locations of the hospitals in their community. Clients who give a nonspecific response can be told the correct information to determine whether they can retain it.

A person is oriented to time if he or she knows the year, month, day of the week, and approximate time of day (many hospitalized people without cerebral pathology miss the number of the day of the month by one or two; Lezak et al., 2012). A person

> Remember that impaired orientation, although often a sign of ongoing memory impairment, may occur as an isolated memory impairment or as a part of a **delirium.** Although some exceptions exist, return of orientation usually occurs in the sequence of person, place, and then time.

is at least partially oriented if he or she can state the year, month, whether it is early or late in the month, and the approximate time of day. It is important, however, to assess all aspects of orientation because it is not uncommon for a person to correctly state the date, day of the week, and month but still incorrectly identify the year.

Assessing Other Aspects of Memory

A person can be fully oriented but nonetheless have memory impairment significant enough to interfere with everyday functioning. Numerous tests of memory are available, most of which are in the professional practice area of neuropsychologists (Evans, 2010). Neuropsychologists frequently assess verbal memory (including word list learning, e.g., the California Verbal Learning Test II [Delis, Kramer, Kaplan, & Ober, 2000] and story recall [Wechsler, 2009]) and visual memory (design reproduction; Corwin & Bylsma, 1993; Shin, Park, Park, Seol, & Kwon, 2006). Less frequently assessed are tactile memory, incidental learning, remote memory, prospective memory, and autobiographical memory (Lezak et al., 2012).

Adequate occupational therapy evaluation of memory functioning includes structured interview of the client and the family, standardized testing, and observation of the client in daily life. A combination of methods will allow the therapist to evaluate where real-world performance breaks down. Evaluation of memory should include the ability to recall written, visual, and verbal information at 30 seconds and 30 minutes, and it should include an examination of the client's ability to learn novel behaviors. Behavioral observation of the client performing daily activities will indicate whether his or her memory functioning is adequate for current ADLs or **instrumental activities of daily living** (IADLs). Prospective memory (remembering to do things in the future) can be assessed by setting the client future tasks and seeing whether the client remembers to perform them or setting complex functional tasks (e.g., planning a menu, shopping and cooking). However, the RBMT has several subtests that address prospective memory.

A standardized test of behavioral memory skills used by occupational therapists, the RBMT (Wilson et al., 2008) is a short (30-minute) assessment with subtests designed to assess different types of memory disorders; normative data are available for clients as old as age 90. Another test to assess memory is the Contextual Memory Test (Toglia, 1993), which has the advantage of allowing clients to predict how well they will perform on the test as a measure of self-awareness of memory functioning.

Intervention

Memory Retraining
A Cochrane Review published in 2007 (das Nair & Lincoln, 2007) identified only two randomized controlled trials of memory retraining in which participants consisted of at least 75% people with stroke; the review provided little evidence for memory retraining's effectiveness. Therapy for memory dysfunction directed at correcting the defective process or function (restitution) has been found to be largely ineffective in people with clinically significant impairment (das Nair & Lincoln, 2007; Robertson & Murre, 1999; Rohling et al., 2009; Wilson, Gracey, Malley, Bateman, & Evans, 2009). In their evidence-based recommendations for memory rehabilitation, Piras, Borella, Incoccia, and Carlesimo (2011) indicated that compensatory approaches are probably effective in addressing memory disorders (e.g.,

prospective memory dysfunction) and that there is also evidence for the use of external cueing devices and specific learning strategies to relearn material related to daily living.

External Strategies

People who are not neurologically impaired use external (top-down) strategies for remembering more often than they use internal strategies (Harris, 1980). Low-tech memory aids are most widely used among people with brain injury from various etiologies (Evans, Wilson, Needham, & Brentnall, 2003), but this may change because both potential users and clinicians are optimistic about the usability of assistive technology (de Joode, van Heugten, Verhey, & van Boxtel, 2010). Various external aids are available, and selection should depend on the client's pattern of impairment, needs, and acceptance of the aid. Because of the client's memory impairment, a structured approach to training and practice is essential, and several training systems are available in the literature (Burke, Danick, Bemis, & Durgin, 1994; Kime, 2006; Sohlberg & Mateer, 1989). External aids include passive systems such as checklists, timetables, memory books (Burke et al., 1994), and daily planners or organizers and active systems such as personal digital assistants (Gentry, Wallace, Kvarfordt, & Lynch, 2008; Kim, Burke, Dowds, Boone, & Park, 2000), mobile phones, and paging systems (Teasdale et al., 2009; Wilson, Scott, Evans, & Emslie, 2003).

Both passive and active memory aids provide scaffolding to assist with executive function deficits in that they encourage users to identify what it is they want to remember and to record the pertinent details of the activities and the date and time that they are to be accomplished (McDonald et al., 2011). However, passive external memory aids (e.g., diaries, timetables) require the user to develop a habit of frequent checking, whereas active systems (e.g., mobile phones, paging systems) reduce the demands on the person for self-initiation (Giles & Shore, 1989) by cueing attention and instructing users to carry out actions at the intended time (McDonald et al., 2011).

McDonald et al. (2011) compared the use of Google Calendar (an active system) with a standard diary (passive system) as compensatory methods in a group of 12 people with **acquired brain injury** of various etiologies (including 4 people with stroke). Google Calendar was found to be more effective than a standard diary in enhancing prospective memory performance and also proved more popular with participants. Both interventions were least effective with those with the most severe cognitive impairments; however, training in the use of the devices was limited (McDonald et al., 2011).

The external cueing system with the most data to support its use is NeuroPage, a remote paging service delivering preprogrammed reminders to people with neurological impairment via pager or smartphone (Wilson et al., 2003). This system can be used as a way to learn routines and then discontinued or used as an ongoing cueing system (Fish, Manly, Emslie, Evans, & Wilson, 2008). In comparing use patterns between people with traumatic brain injury (TBI) and stroke, participants with TBI demonstrated the ability to develop a self-sustaining routine after discontinuing use of the pager, whereas the performance of participants with stroke returned to baseline levels after discontinuing use of the pager. This difference was associated with older age, shorter time poststroke, and poorer executive functioning in the poststroke group (Fish et al., 2008).

Specific Learning Strategies

Specific techniques may be used that facilitate the learning of important information. In people with profound memory impairments, specific task routines may be overlearned to the point at which they become automatic, and introspective (declarative) remembering becomes unnecessary (Giles, 2010).

The **spaced-** and **expanding-retrieval techniques** are relatively simple strategies for maximizing the recall of limited amounts of information in people with severe memory disorder (Cermak, Verfaellie, Lanzoni, Mather, & Chase, 1996; Davis, Massman, & Doody, 2001; Schacter, Rich, & Stampp, 1985). These techniques have been used primarily with face–name recognition training because this aspect of memory impairment may be particularly disturbing to people, and improvement can have positive effects on **self-esteem** (Davis et al., 2001). The effectiveness of the techniques has been demonstrated in people with stroke (Clare et al., 2000; Davis et al., 2001; Schacter et al., 1985). The expanding-retrieval technique is essentially a spaced-retrieval technique in which the between-recall interval is gradually increased. Failure results in returning to the beginning and re-presentation of the to-be-learned material. The intervention is based on the idea that the act of recall is more powerful in encoding the information than the simple representation of the stimulus association, so the more work the client does in re-creating the memory trace, the more likely he or she is to encode it. The technique is not a way to retrain memory in the abstract sense; it is a way to memorize specific information.

The training method of **errorless learning** was first proposed by Terrace (1963) and subsequently has been used widely with clinical populations (Giles & Clark-Wilson, 1988; Giles, Ridley, Dill, & Frye, 1997; Hunkin, Squires, Parkin, & Tidy, 1998; Kern, Liberman, Kopelowicz, Mintz, & Green, 2002; Komatsu, Minimua, Kato, & Kashima, 2000; O'Carroll, Russell, Lawrie, & Johnstone, 1999; Parkin, Hunkin, & Squires, 1998). In errorless learning, the therapist provides sufficient support (i.e., cueing, implicit guidance) to prevent the propagation of errors, and support is gradually withdrawn as learning takes place. As a practical matter, it may be very difficult to completely prevent all errors; however, errors can be kept to a minimum (Giles, 2010).

Executive Functions

The term *executive functions* serves as an umbrella term to describe multiple higher order thinking processes that are needed to manage task complexity and change and to facilitate independent and purposeful participation in home, work, and community life. EFs serve to coordinate multiple behaviors, including goal setting, problem solving, inhibition, organization, planning, and multitasking, to support functional task performance (Stuss, 1991). Although distinct from metacognitive abilities, EFs work in concert with self-awareness and personal motivation and are recognized as characteristics of individual personality (Fernandez-Duque, Baird, & Posner, 2000). The **frontal lobes,** and in particular the prefrontal cortex, mediate executive processing through the coordination of cortical and subcortical brain regions (Hazy, Frank, & O'Reilly, 2007).

Executive deficits can develop after ischemic stroke or **hemorrhage** as a result of disruption in intracranial blood flow, damaging brain tissue (see Chapter 3,

EFs serve to coordinate multiple behaviors, including goal setting, problem solving, inhibition, organization, planning, and multitasking, to support functional task performance.

"Frontal Subcortical Networks" section). The size and laterality of the vascular injury directly relate to the degree of deficits experienced by the person (Lee et al., 2012).

Assessment

Because EFs coordinate multiple behaviors, they are difficult to identify through traditional measures of cognition (Manchester et al., 2004; Priestley et al., 2013). EFs are best identified through top-down assessments that require the person to establish goals and determine a course of action. Executive abilities are measurable during novel and dynamic test conditions similar to those found in the real world (Morrison et al., 2013; Shallice & Burgess, 1991). During the clinical assessment of EFs, task complexity can be determined through a person-centered perspective because task complexity and task novelty may increase in the context of cognitive and motor impairments. For example, a client with hemiparesis may experience challenge and novelty during bathing activities despite a history of independently bathing because the client now has to manage cognitive–motor interference (Petruccelli & Delenick, 2013) or perform previously bimanual tasks with one hand (Walker et al., 2004).

The assessment of EFs may include a variety of evaluation methods including self-report questionnaires, paper-and-pencil tests, or performance-based assessments. Many self-report measures of EFs ask clients to rate their ability to function in daily life. Questionnaires may also include informant forms for the purpose of response comparison (Odhuba, van den Broek, & Johns, 2005). Self-report and informant-report paper-and-pencil measures are common in the measurement of cognition; however, the ecological validity of self-report measures of EF are questionable because they may not correspond to clients' real-world functional abilities (Morrison et al., 2013).

Only a few EF measurement methods have psychometric rigor, and these tools require the client to perform single complex tasks or multiple tasks in real-world settings (Baum, Morrison, Hahn, & Edwards, 2003; Morrison et al., 2013). These top-down tests are designed to require the client to self-initiate, problem solve, organize, plan, and manage self-determined goals without prompting from the examiner (Alderman, Burgess, Knight, & Henman, 2003). Performance-based measures of EFs build on the tradition of clinical observations (Giles, 2011; Giles & Clark-Wilson, 1993) but use specific methods to support reliable scoring of task performance (Baum et al., 2008; see Poulin et al., 2013, for a review of stroke-specific EF assessments). Performance-based measures of EF create a test scenario that requires the client to initiate, plan, and execute functional tasks. Many of these measures require the examiner to allow time to pass without providing cues, even when the client makes errors or experiences task challenge (Morrison et al., 2013).

Intervention

Recent meta-analysis and systematic reviews of intervention for executive dysfunction after stroke have drawn somewhat disparate conclusions (Chung, Pollock, Campbell, Durward, & Hagen, 2013; Poulin, Korner-Bitensky, Dawson, & Bhercr, 2012), with Poulin et al. (2012) indicating that there are interventions that ameliorate executive dysfunction, and Chung et al. (2013) concluding that the evidence

Although specific tasks or behaviors that are affected by EF deficits can be practiced and thereby remediated, EF involves solving novel problems, so that interventions to remediate EF cannot be practiced to automaticity.

is insufficient to support or refute the effectiveness for interventions for poststroke executive dysfunction.

Although specific tasks or behaviors that are affected by EF deficits can be practiced and thereby remediated (i.e., a bottom-up intervention), EF involves solving novel problems, so that interventions to remediate EF cannot be practiced to automaticity. EF remediation involves learning internal thinking routines and are therefore by definition top-down. Therapeutic interventions focused on the rehabilitation of EFs build on clients' self-awareness and personal motivation to improve functional skill performance. Clients with low motivation and decreased self-awareness are unlikely to benefit from interventions targeting EF (Clark-Wilson, Baxter, & Giles, in press). EF training is best achieved through client-centered goals because of the close relationship between motivation and executive processing (Schutz & Wanlass, 2009), and selection of functional tasks for EF training should reflect these goals. Therapists can support realistic yet client-centered goal development with therapeutic feedback during the occupational interview. After testing with performance-based measures of EFs, debriefing sessions focus on the client's ability to develop plans, monitor task performance, detect errors, and generate new strategies to reduce errors. Debriefing sessions encourage problem solving while improving **self-efficacy.**

Clients with impairments of executive attention are susceptible to daily derailments that challenge their ability to complete personal and work-related goals. Goal derailments may be the result of various influences, including environmental stimuli (e.g., a social context that over- or understimulates the client); behavioral influences (e.g., **anxiety** or depression); or competing habits, tasks, and activities. A clinical intervention based on Duncan's (1986) theory of goal neglect, *goal management training* (GMT) teaches self-instructional strategies to increase mindfulness and support the client's functional task performance by increasing self-awareness of attentional drift (Levine et al., 2000, 2011; Schweizer et al., 2008). During GMT, the client is guided to use a predetermined method to review goals, identify constituent subgoals and tasks (e.g., to-do lists), consider task demands, and stay focused on task completion throughout the task performance. According to GMT principles, the client internalizes a behavioral strategy (although this may also have been externally cued) and compares current behavior and task performance with goal states. Once the GMT process is mastered, the client demonstrates treatment efficacy through self-initiated strategy application that supports task performance.

Levine et al. (2011) evaluated GMT outcomes among a cohort of clients with chronic stroke via its effects on cognitive measures. Despite promising treatment observations, Levine et al. identified no superiority of the GMT group over a control group. A systematic review of 12 studies of GMT found that effective interventions combined GMT with other interventions such as problem-solving training, but found insufficient evidence to support the use of GMT alone (Krasny-Pacini, Chevignard, & Evans, 2014).

The *CO-OP model* was developed for use with children with developmental coordination disorder but has been widely used to teach adults with executive dysfunction a strategy to overcome occupational performance deficits. CO-OP teaches a global strategy derived from the work of Meichenbaum (1977; goal, plan, do, check) and uses this global strategy in a process of guided discovery to assist clients with developing their own domain-specific strategies to solve specific performance problems that clients self-identify and choose to address. CO-OP is intended to assist the client with learning a general approach to problem solving that he or she is expected to be able to apply to novel performance problems and use to develop new domain-specific strategies independently (Polatajko & Mandich, 2011). The client is guided in dynamic performance analysis in which the client identifies the performance problems and then identifies and evaluates potential strategies to solve them. The client then implements that strategy and checks to see whether it worked. CO-OP has been applied with people with stroke, and some positive results of single cases and small series have been reported (Dawson et al., 2009; McEwen, Polatajko, Huijbregts, & Ryan, 2009).

In addition, EF interventions may take a compensatory approach through the provision of external devices, for example, a smartphone, to help clients manage their time and monitor their daily accomplishments.

Lateralized Attention and Related Disorders

Unilateral neglect is common and affects as many as 80% of clients with acute right-hemisphere stroke and 15% to 20% of clients with acute left-hemisphere stroke (Parton, Malhotra, & Husain, 2004; Stone, Patel, Greenwood, & Halligan, 1992; Zoccolotti et al., 1989). Spontaneous recovery occurs in many affected people, but in as many as one-third, problems in spatial awareness are persistent and a cause of significant handicap (Denes, Semenza, Stoppa, & Lis, 1982; Zoccolotti et al., 1989). The concept of *unilateral neglect* is complex and a focus of considerable attention in acute stroke rehabilitation (Bowen, Hazelton, Pollock, & Lincoln, 2013).

Estimates of the frequency of hemispatial neglect vary greatly on the basis of how long poststroke the assessment is performed and the sensitivity of the assessment procedures (Katz, Hartman-Maeir, Ring, & Soroker, 1999; Paolucci, Antonucci, Grasso, & Pizzamiglio, 2001). Unilateral neglect syndromes are far more common and persistent after right-hemisphere stroke; however, the negative impact on outcome has been strongly associated with the unilateral neglect and not the side of the lesion (Katz et al., 1999; Paolucci et al., 2001). Although neglect improves or resolves in most people, a history of neglect is associated with worse ADL and IADL functional outcomes (Jehkonen, Laihosalo, & Kettunen, 2006; Katz et al., 1999).

The presence of neglect is predictive of difficulties with upper-body dressing (Walker et al., 2004), self-care and transfers (Nijboer, van de Port, Schepers, Post, & Visser-Meily, 2013), outcome on the Barthel Index (Lincoln, Drummond, & Berman, 1997; Mahoney & Barthel, 1965), the need for greater amounts of occupational and physical therapy (Kalra, Perez, Gupta, & Wittink, 1997), longer hospital stays (Katz et al., 1999), and the persistence of incontinence on hospital discharge and is predictive of the need for institutional care (Paolucci et al., 2001). Neglect appears to slow the course of recovery from stroke and impedes rehabilitative efforts (Appelros, Karlsson, Seiger, & Nydevik, 2002; Lincoln et al., 1997; Sunderland, Wade, & Langton Hewer, 1987).

Varieties of Spatial Neglect

This section describes varieties of spatial neglect and methods for the evaluation of spatial neglect. Special note should be taken, however, of the absence of evidence that many of these techniques have durable or significant effects on the real-world performance of people with neglect (Bowen et al., 2013; Zoccolotti et al., 2011), such that they are best considered experimental.

Unilateral neglect is differentiated from **homonymous hemianopsia, hemi-anesthesia,** and **hemiplegia,** which are primary sensory and motor disorders. Although hemianopsia does not cause unilateral neglect, the conditions frequently co-occur, and in combination they are associated with more severe functional difficulties and worse outcomes (Luukkainen-Markkula, Tarkka, Pitkänen, Sivenius, & Hämäläinen, 2011). In the absence of basic sensory and motor deficits, a unilateral neglect syndrome is characterized by slowness or failure to orient, attend, or respond to or to describe novel stimuli presented in the hemispace **contralateral** to the lesion. People with unilateral neglect orient toward the hemispace *ipsilateral* (on the same side) as the lesion and away from the hemispace contralateral to the lesion. The bias to orient and attend away from contralateral space is not absolute, but it can be considered to be an attentional gradient (Halligan & Marshall, 1994). In severe cases, the person may fail to respond to all stimuli presented to contralateral hemispace. Many people can report stimuli on the neglected side if directed to the involved hemispace by the examiner; however, the attentional set allowing orientation to the habitually neglected hemispace shows rapid deterioration in affected people.

Detailed examinations of neglect syndromes have found complex overlapping representations of space that may be differentially affected by stroke. People may have neglect syndromes related to attending to the body (personal neglect), object-centered neglect (centered on the external object), or spatial neglect. Spatial neglect has been further divided into neglect of peripersonal space (within arm's reach), extrapersonal space (beyond arm's reach; collectively described as radial neglect), and vertical space (altitudinal neglect; Robertson, Hogg, & McMillan, 1998). Subtypes of neglect may occur in various combinations, with left-sided, lower vertical neglect and peripersonal (proximal radial) neglect frequently reported in combination (Heilman, Watson, & Valenstein, 2012) such that people may miss their left footplate and walk into low objects on the left. Spatial neglect occurs more frequently than personal neglect (Appelros et al., 2002; Appelros, Karlsson, Thorwalls, Tham, & Nydevik, 2004).

Hemispace may be defined according to eye position, head position, and trunk position. Demarcation is clearest when all the hemispaces are consistent (i.e., in the eyes-, head-, and trunk-forward position; Karnath, 1994). Forms of neglect may be dissociable, and distinctions can be made among *attending* (failing to take note of objects or events in one-half of space), *intending* or *motor neglect* (being unable to perform actions or maintain action in one hemispace), and *representation* (being unable to imagine or think about one-half of space; Bisiach, Capitani, Luzzatti, & Perani, 1981; Bisiach & Luzzatti, 1978; Denis, Beschin, Logie, & Della Sala, 2002). Additionally, these disorders appear distinct from the visuospatial or visuoconstruction disorders that are particularly associated with right parietal lesions (Kerkhoff, 1998).

The higher frequency of unilateral neglect after damage to the right side of the brain has been explained by asymmetry of brain function for the direction of attention (Sterzi et al., 1993). Various theories, however, have attempted to describe the actual mechanism that underlies the asymmetry and, hence, the more frequent occurrence of left neglect. Heilman et al. (2012) suggested that the temporoparietal region of the brain includes attentional cells, but that in the left hemisphere

Detailed examinations of neglect syndromes have found complex overlapping representations of space that may be differentially affected by stroke.

these cells have predominantly right hemispace receptive fields, whereas those in the right hemisphere have a greater number of bilateral receptive fields. As a result of this asymmetry, the right hemisphere can attend to both contralateral and ipsilateral stimuli, but when the right side is damaged, the left cannot attend to ipsilateral stimuli, resulting in left neglect (Heilman et al., 2012).

Evaluation

People with severe unilateral neglect may ignore all stimuli on the affected side. Functionally, they may have a range of deficits, such as not shaving or combing their hair on the affected side, missing food on the affected side of their plate, walking into or toward the side of doorways, failing to cross the street safely, or becoming lost in the community.

There is reason to believe that, despite the clinical and prognostic importance of neglect syndromes, neglect is often overlooked in routine clinical practice (Chen, Hreha, Fortis, Goedert, & Barrett, 2012; Menon & Korner-Bitensky, 2004). No individual test of neglect has been found to identify all clients with neglect (Parton et al., 2004; Stone et al., 1992). As noted, hemineglect is not a unitary disorder and is itself dissociable along several dimensions (Robertson, Tegnér, Goodrich, & Wilson, 1994; Zoccolotti, Antonucci, & Judica, 1992), such that a test battery addressing various forms of neglect and observation of performance across tasks and environments is preferable to any one evaluation method. Azouvi et al. (2002) found that a single observational measure of behavioral neglect (the CBS) was more sensitive to neglect than any single paper-and-pencil measure that they examined and was not significantly different than the entire battery of paper-and-pencil measures they evaluated.

Paper-and-Pencil Methods
Several paper-and-pencil methods are commonly used to evaluate unilateral neglect:

- The client is asked to bisect a horizontal line drawn on a sheet of paper. People with left neglect typically bisect the line significantly to the right of the true center point. With successive line length (shortest, 20 millimeters; longest, 200 millimeters), the extent of the displacement to the right increases. In addition to varying the length of the lines, the center points may be presented slightly to the right, to the left, or directly in front of the person.
- The client is asked to draw objects from memory (e.g., a clock, a flower, a house). People with unilateral neglect may draw only one half of the object or omit details in the neglected hemispace. Clock drawing may be particularly sensitive and was the only test that added sensitivity to the behavioral measures in the study by Azouvi et al. (2002) described earlier.
- The client is asked to perform a letter-, number-, shape-, or random line–cancellation task. Cancellation tasks vary in difficulty according to figure density, pseudorandom irregular distribution, and the presence of distractors. Both target detection and starting point should be noted (Azouvi et al., 2002) because approximately 80% of neurologically healthy people will use a left-to-right search strategy (typical of a reader of English), but most clients with left neglect will begin searching on the right (Azouvi et al., 2002) and display a search pattern that is unsystematic (Butler,

Lawrence, Eskes, & Klein, 2009). Heilman et al. (2012) described an assessment for object-centered neglect in which geometric shapes are complete or incomplete on either the left or the right side. Clients with left neglect will fail to cancel those geometric shapes with openings on the left side (Heilman et al., 2012).

Standardized Measures of Unilateral Neglect

Menon and Korner-Bitensky (2004) identified 62 measures of neglect at the impairment and activity level, of which 28 were standardized (see their article for the Unilateral Spatial Neglect Assessment Summary Guide). The most widely researched batteries with behavioral measures are the Behavioral Inattention Test (BIT; Hartman-Maeir & Katz, 1995; Wilson, Cockburn, & Halligan, 1987) and the CBS (Azouvi et al., 1996, 2002).

The *BIT* (Hartman-Maeir & Katz, 1995; Wilson et al., 1987) is intended to be an ecologically valid test of unilateral neglect. It is a battery divided into two parts. The first part, the conventional tests, consists of six paper-and-pencil tests; the second part, the behavioral tests, involves simulated everyday activities.

The *CBS* (Azouvi et al., 1996, 2002) is a reliable and valid observational behavioral assessment of unilateral (left) neglect used by occupational therapists and involving ratings of client behaviors in 10 everyday situations (e.g., grooming or shaving the left half of the face, colliding with people or objects such as doors or furniture). Although not measuring all forms of neglect, the CBS assesses personal neglect, neglect of peripersonal space (within arm's reach), and neglect of extrapersonal space (beyond arm's reach), as well as perceptual, representational, and motor neglect. Each item is rated on a 4-point scale with 0 indicating *no neglect* and 3 indicating *severe neglect*. The total score is out of 30, and various cutoff scores have been proposed. Luukkainen-Markkula et al. (2011) used a score of 0 to 4 on the CBS as indicating *no neglect*. Azouvi et al. (2002) distinguished four levels of impairment, with 0 indicating *no neglect*, 1 to 10 indicating *mild neglect*, 11 to 20 indicating *moderate neglect*, and 21 to 30 indicating *severe neglect*. Because the CBS is a rating system for client behaviors and not a test, it rates client-initiated activities that may or may not be structured by the therapist and may therefore be a more accurate representation of the client's spontaneous behaviors than structured testing situations. Therapist ratings can be compared with those of the client as a measure of **anosognosia** (Azouvi et al., 1996, 2002). The CBS was originally published in English (Azouvi et al., 1996); more recently, a detailed description of a structured method of assessing for neglect using the CBS has been reported as the Kessler Foundation Neglect Assessment Process (Chen et al., 2012).

Intervention

Interventions for neglect can use either a top-down or a bottom-up approach. In a top-down approach, interventions encourage conscious awareness of the disability and explicitly train patients to reorient toward the habitually neglected hemispace using compensatory strategies (Zoccolotti et al., 2011). In a bottom-up approach, interventions are directed at the impairment but do not require awareness or consciously driven behavioral change and consist of massively stimulating the patient with information originating in the habitually neglected hemispace (e.g., wearing prisms or patches; Bowen et al., 2013; Zoccolotti et al., 2011). A recent review has identified 18 different interventions for hemispatial neglect (Luauté, Halligan, Rode, Rossetti, & Boisson, 2006), finding support for 6 of them significant enough to justify clinical use (i.e., visual scanning training, visual scanning training plus trunk rotation, visual scanning training plus neck muscle vibration, and mental imagery [video feedback and prism adaptation]). However, studies of interventions for neglect are rife with inconsistent findings, and a meta-analysis by Bowen et al. (2013) found no statistically significant effect of intervention, compared with control, for immediate or persisting effects on ADLs or persisting effects on standardized neglect assessments. However, they did find a statistically significant immediate effect on standardized neglect assessments compared with control participants (Bowen et al., 2013). Table 7.3 provides a brief overview of some experimental interventions for hemispatial neglect.

Visual scanning training is one of the most well-established interventions for visuospatial neglect, but research has slowed from what it was in the 1980s and 1990s (Zoccolotti et al., 2011). Zoccolotti et al. concluded that even for visual scanning training, there is controversy regarding the real generalization of trained tasks to untrained tasks and to patients' everyday functioning.

Table 7.3. Interventions for Spatial Neglect

Intervention	Theoretical Rationale	Implementation and Procedures
Top-Down		
Visual scanning training (also called *visuospatial orientation training;* Antonucci et al., 1995; Paolucci et al., 1996; Pizzamiglio et al., 1992; Zoccolotti et al., 2011)	Intensive scanning training (e.g., daily training over 4–8 weeks) may result in neurological reorganization and transfer to functional skills.	• Identifying objects in a picture: The client describes a picture in detail (picture complexity is gradually increased and verbal and visual cueing are reduced) as the client's visual exploratory ability increases • Premade cancellation tasks: The client crosses out a defined target (with feedback and instruction in strategy use) • Letter- and word-cancellation tasks • Reading and copying from a newspaper • Computerized scanning tasks
Bottom-Up		
Prism adaptation (Serino et al., 2007)	Prism glasses can be used to shift the visual field to the right. Adaptation to the prisms results in a temporary effect after their removal. Clients who have accommodated to the shift to the right will, on the removal of the prisms, show a shift to the left in their midline estimation.	Client wears prismatic lenses that induce a visual field shift of 10° to the right as client points to objects in space. Prisms are worn on a sessional basis (20 minutes) for 2 weeks.
Eye-patch training (Fong et al., 2013; Zoccolotti et al., 2011)	Used to reduce the client's attentional bias toward the right.	Wearing the patch deprives the client of visual information to the right side by patching the nasal visual field of the left eye and the temporal visual field of the right eye or by occluding the right eye.
Limb activation training (Fong et al., 2013; Robertson et al., 2002)	Used to increase the client's attention to neglected hemispace by inducing the client to move in that hemispace.	Robertson et al. (2002) used an automatic device that turned off a tone that sounded whenever the client had failed to move the left side for a defined period. Limb activation training has been found to be ineffective in reducing neglect but promotes motor control of the hemiplegic upper extremity (Fong et al., 2013).
Caloric vestibular stimulation (Karnath, 1994; Sturt & Punt, 2013)	Used to increase tonic alertness.	Thirty cubic centimeters of ice water are introduced to the contralesion outer ear.
Neck vibration (Zoccolotti et al., 2011)	Used to increase tonic alertness.	A vibrator or transcutaneous electrical nerve stimulation is applied to the contralesion posterior neck muscles.

Visual Object Agnosia

Agnosia, classically defined by H.-L. Teuber as a "normal percept that has . . . been stripped of its meaning" (Milner & Teuber, 1968, p. 293), is a modality-specific failure to recognize an object (i.e., recognition of the meaning fails in one sensory system but occurs immediately using another sensory modality). An agnosic deficit can affect any sensory system, but here we limit discussion to *visual object agnosia* (Bauer, 2012), which is the inability to recognize objects visually despite apparently adequate visual acuity. Estimates of the frequency of visual object agnosia after stroke are variable, and agnosia has been found to affect 2.2% to 36.1% of people with stroke (Paolucci, McKenna, & Cooke, 2009; Rowe, 2009). Failure to name an object, even when allowed to physically manipulate the object, is usually indicative of *anomia* (a language disorder).

Following Lissauer (1889), visual object agnosia may be divided into two types: (1) apperceptive and (2) associative. *Apperceptive visual agnosia* is a deficit in the final integration of various perceptual attributes. People with this type of visual agnosia usually have widespread brain pathology, and the disorder often occurs against a background of severe cognitive impairment. *Associative agnosia* more closely fits the classic definition of agnosia. People with associative visual agnosia can see an object with sufficient clarity to match or draw it, but do not know what the object is (i.e., the object's purpose or meaning is not recognized), which has been interpreted as failure to access semantic memory (Bauer, 2012). The fact that affected people can draw the object and not recognize it indicates that the motor system does not have the ability to cue the identification process. People with agnosia find it easier to recognize real objects than photographs, and recognize photographs more easily than line drawings. This pattern of responses suggests that the fine-grained information found in real situations assists in the recognition of objects (Bauer, 2012).

Assessment

Occupational therapy assessment of visual object agnosia should exclude anomia, aphasia, inattention or perceptual disorders, or major NCD (Bauer, 2012), and therapists should remember that recognition failure is modality specific and rule out apraxia. To assess for visual object agnosia, the therapist can place an array of common objects in front of the client. The client is asked to name an object, point to an object specified by the examiner, or to specify the object's use. Toglia (1989) proposed a specific evaluation technique for the assessment of visual object agnosia. Central to Toglia's method is the idea that task conditions influence visual perception and that tasks can be graded in difficulty. Toglia proposed varying the visual integrative demands of object recognition by altering six parameters: (1) environment, (2) familiarity, (3) direction, (4) amount, (5) spatial arrangements, and (6) response rate.

- *Environment* is the context in which recognition takes place (i.e., the setting in which the object is normally used); in-context recognition is easier than out-of-context recognition.
- *Familiarity* is how frequently an object is encountered in daily life. Self-related objects, such as a toothbrush, may be easier to recognize than objects to which the client is unaccustomed.

> **People with agnosia find it easier to recognize real objects than photographs, and recognize photographs more easily than line drawings.**

- *Direction* is the verbal instructions given for the task; for example, pointing to an object and asking "What is this?" is easier than asking the client to list the items on a table.
- *Amount* is the number of objects presented at one time.
- *Spatial arrangement* is the way in which objects are presented during testing. A left-to-right arrangement (for clients who read left to right) is easier than a scattered, visually overlapping arrangement.
- *Response rate* is the speed of response demanded.

Toglia (1989) recommended beginning with an intermediate level of difficulty and varying the demands of the task according to success or failure. Of course, this type of tabletop testing is an attempt to delineate the way performance breaks down and is not a substitute for evaluation in real-life settings.

Intervention

Toglia's (1989) assessment procedures indicate a method of treating the disorder— or at least of minimizing its effect on day-to-day functioning. By limiting the task demands over the six characteristics just outlined, the difficulty of the object recognition required of the client can be reduced. For example, it is much more difficult to select the shaving cream from a toiletries bag full of toilet items than it is to select it when it is the only other item on the sink next to the razor.

Conflicting stimulus demands can reveal agnosic phenomena. For example, giving the client ice cream in a glass may lead to the client sucking on the spoon as though it were a straw. Awareness of such issues is most important for the therapist during the design and implementation of functional retraining programs (e.g., feeding, dressing).

Apraxia

Praxis is the ability to organize and skillfully execute purposive movements (Foundas, 2013). The *apraxias* are disorders of skilled, purposeful movement that cannot be accounted for by weakness, akinesia, abnormal **tone,** sensory loss, incomprehension of or inattention to commands, or noncooperation (i.e., apraxia is defined by exclusion; Buxbaum et al., 2008; Foundas, 2013).

Apraxia has been associated with left-sided lesions. Donkervoort et al. (2000), reviewing 10 published studies, reported that the prevalence of apraxia in patients with left-sided lesions ranged from 28% to 57% (median = 45%) and that the prevalence of apraxia in patients with right-sided lesions ranged from 0% to 34% (median = 8%). In their own study of patients in the Netherlands, Donkervoort et al. (2000) identified the presence of apraxia in 28% of people with left-sided lesions in rehabilitation centers and identified the presence of apraxia in 37% of nursing home residents with left-sided lesions. Prevalence was not affected by age, gender, or whether the stroke was ischemic or hemorrhagic. Studying a subset of these patients, Donkervoort, Dekker, and Deelman (2006) found that resolution of apraxia over the 5-month period of the study was uncommon (12% of the left-hemisphere stroke patients found to be apraxic at the start of the study were no longer considered apraxic at the end of the 20-week study period). Various types of apraxia have been described (Liepmann, 1900, 1920; Pearce, 2009); here, we focus on ideomotor apraxia and ideational apraxia.

In *ideomotor apraxia,* the person demonstrates variable ability to perform skilled movements. A person with ideomotor apraxia may be unable to perform a purposeful motor task on command, even though he or she understands the idea or concept of the task. The same person may be able to carry out some well-practiced motor tasks automatically. For example, if asked to brush his or her teeth, the person can clearly demonstrate understanding of what is being asked, yet be unable to pick up the toothbrush. At another time, he or she may brush his or her teeth spontaneously (i.e., an automatic–voluntary dissociation). Even when able to perform a task, people with ideomotor apraxia demonstrate systematic abnormalities of movement. They often have intact distal fine movements but have difficulty with the spatial organization of movement or with the segmental relative positioning of limbs (Clark et al., 1994). When a skilled movement requires simultaneous movement at two joints, the movement may not be adequately coordinated. The timing of movements may be impaired; for example, shaving may be difficult because the person's wrist does not move so as to keep the blade passing smoothly over the skin (Clark et al., 1994).

The term *ideational apraxia* has been variously defined and continues to cause confusion. Hecaen (1968, p. 40) described it as an "impairment of the logical and harmonious sequence of the several elementary movements that make up a complex act, though each movement by itself is executed correctly." People with ideational apraxia cannot carry out a series of actions in the sequence required to achieve the goal. The logical sequence of single movements is not respected, objects are improperly used, or movements in the sequence are skipped or repeated (Poeck & Lehmkuhl, 1980). Patients have severe difficulty using tools in real-life settings (Randerath, Goldenberg, Spijkers, Li, & Hermsdörfer, 2011).

Evaluation

Assessment of Ideomotor Apraxia

Because the presence of apraxia is, in part, established by the exclusion of other disorders that could account for the observed impairment, it is necessary to have a thorough understanding of the client's movement difficulties. Pyramidal and extrapyramidal disorders, basal ganglia or cerebellar disorders (disorders of posture and tone), tremor, **dysmetria,** and stereotypic movements should be excluded. The identification and specification of apraxic difficulties rely a great deal on the judgment of the experienced therapist. All tests of apraxia rely on observer judgment (Butler, 2002). Less experienced staff may miss the disorder entirely and attribute the client's behavior to noncooperation (this response is partly a reaction to the intermittent nature of some of the difficulties; LeClerc & Wells, 1998). Many clients with apraxia are also aphasic and have spatial neglect, so it is important to establish that the client can understand instructions and attend to the hemispace (Bickerton et al., 2012). Neurological testing for ideomotor apraxia commonly involves asking the client to pantomime actions or to use gestural communication and may include the following procedures:

- Gesture in response to the command "Wave good-bye, give a thumbs-up, or salute."
- Pantomime in response to the command "Show me how you would use a pair of scissors [or screwdriver, hammer, lock and key]." If the client uses a

body part as an object and cannot be corrected through, first, a verbal command or, second, demonstration, then he or she is making an apraxic error.

- Gesture, copying therapist's imitation.
- Pantomimed tool use, copying therapist's imitation.
- Actual tool use.

Pantomime is likely to be the most sensitive measure of ideomotor apraxia, and although problems with pantomime may not translate into problems with functional performance (Butler, 2002), pantomime failure should increase the therapist's "index of suspicion" for functional problems resulting from ideomotor apraxia. Functionally, people with ideomotor apraxia may be clumsy; have marked delay in following a command; appear to be attentive to commands but then do something else; or half-perform the asked-for task, which then turns into another action. They may have profound difficulties in using objects (e.g., in the actions required to coordinate dressing or in the skilled manipulation of tools) or may have great difficulty manipulating a key, door latch, or faucet. Clients may demonstrate marked associated behaviors or displacement activity in which the effort to engage in the behavior is displaced into other activities. They may display behavioral dysregulation related to frustration at being unable to perform the activity.

Some performance-based apraxia assessments have become available (Goldenberg & Hagmann, 1998; van Heugten et al., 2000). Van Heugten, Dekker, Deelman, Stehmann-Saris, and Kinebanian (1999) developed a method to assess apraxia by observing ADLs. Using this procedure, four activities are scored in terms of independence and deficits in initiation, execution, and control of the activities: (1) washing the face and upper body, (2) donning a shirt or blouse, (3) preparing and eating a sandwich, and (4) preparing a cup of hot chocolate. Scores range from 0 *(totally dependent)* to 3 *(totally independent),* leading to a total potential score of 16 for each activity (see the original report for the assessment itself).

Donkervoot, Dekker, and Deelman (2002) examined the characteristics of this assessment procedure by comparing the performance of 106 left-hemisphere patients with stroke-related apraxia on the ADL observations, the Barthel Index, a neuropsychological apraxia test, and other tests of motor skills. Multivariate analyses showed that the specific ADL observations designed to assess apraxia were associated with severity of apraxia, not with basic motor impairments. The Barthel Index was associated with motor impairments and not with severity of apraxia. Donkervoot et al. concluded that evaluation of disability in stroke patients with apraxia cannot rely only on general ratings of ADL independence. In addition, the specific ADL observation procedure is needed to measure disability resulting from apraxia (Donkervoort et al., 2002).

Assessment of Ideational Apraxia

Many standardized measures of ideational apraxia are available but are not widely used (see, e.g., Bickerton et al., 2012; De Renzi & Lucchelli, 1988). Clinically, ideational apraxia is evaluated by asking the client to perform serial acts that require a specific order of execution. For example, the client may be given a piece of paper, an envelope, and a stamp and asked to prepare a letter to be mailed. The task requires the client to fold the paper, place it in the envelope, and seal and place a stamp on the envelope. Clients may be asked to brush their teeth, a task that requires them to open the toothpaste, take a toothbrush from a holder, place toothpaste on the toothbrush, brush the teeth, sip from a cup of water to rinse the mouth, and spit the water into a basin or sink. In attempting to perform such tasks, the client can usually perform each step of the task but may be unable to integrate the individual actions to complete the sequence.

Intervention

Meta-analyses and systematic reviews of apraxia training after stroke have drawn somewhat disparate conclusions (Cantagallo, Maini, & Rumiati, 2012; Cicerone et al., 2011; West, Bowen, Hesketh, & Vail, 2008), with Cicerone et al. (2011) and Cantagallo et al. (2012) indicating that interventions exist that are successful in promoting recovery from apraxia, and West et al. (2008) concluding that the evidence to support or refute the effectiveness of interventions for poststroke apraxia is insufficient. Interventions for apraxia can use either a top-down or a bottom-up approach. In a top-down approach, interventions encourage conscious awareness of the disability and explicitly train patients in strategies designed to circumvent the apraxic disturbance (Cantagallo et al., 2012; Geusgens et al., 2006; Geusgens, van Heugten, Cooijmans, Jolles, & van den Heuvel, 2007). In a bottom-up approach, interventions are directed at specific apraxic performance problems in real-world activities (Cantagallo et al., 2012). Additionally, environmental modifications can reduce apraxic problems in performing functional tasks. Cantagallo et al. described several reasons that treatment for apraxia has not entered mainstream clinical practice, including the frequency of spontaneous improvement in the first few months after onset and the automatic–voluntary dissociation.

Conclusion

Progress continues to be made in understanding the nature of the cognitive deficits that may follow stroke, and models of brain function are being refined to better account for the problems demonstrated by people with stroke. This increased understanding is allowing for improved assessment and the development of theoretically driven intervention methods that have the potential to improve client functioning and quality of life. Two types of approach to cognitive rehabilitation are evident in the literature across types of impairment: (1) strategy training (a top-down approach; see Box 7.1) and (2) direct practice (a bottom-up approach; see Box 7.2). Bottom-up approaches are of two types and may either address the impaired cognitive processes (e.g., prism adaptation in spatial neglect; Zoccolotti et al., 2011) or attempt to intervene with the affected performance skills (e.g., Goldenberg & Hagmann's [1998] intervention for apraxia).

Currently, interventions often show experimental promise . . . but show little evidence of transfer to everyday occupational performance.

Currently, interventions often show experimental promise (mostly short-term effects on laboratory measures) but show little evidence of transfer to everyday occupational performance, and large-scale controlled trials of cognitive rehabilitation after stroke are largely unavailable (Bowen et al., 2013; Bowen, Knapp, Gillespie, Nicolson, & Vail, 2011). Neuropsychologists are interested in whether interventions have an effect on information processing (cognition), whereas occupational therapists are interested in whether interventions improve occupational performance and participation. Occupational therapists should therefore exercise

Box 7.1. A Top-Down Approach to Apraxia

Van Heugten et al. (1998) reported a program of compensatory training for clients with apraxia resulting from stroke. Occupational therapists provided intervention in response to performance difficulties according to a hierarchy involving provision of instructions, assistance, and feedback. Clients showed large improvements in activities of daily living (ADL) functioning on all measures and small improvements on an apraxia test and a measure of motor functioning. The effect sizes for ADL improvement were large compared with those for measures of apraxia and motor functioning.

The results suggested that the program succeeded in teaching clients compensatory strategies that enabled them to function more independently, despite the lasting presence of apraxia. Donkervoort, Dekker, Stehmann-Saris, and Deelman (2001) conducted a randomized controlled trial comparing this strategy-training approach integrated into usual occupational therapy with occupational therapy as usual. After 8 weeks of treatment, the clients who received the strategy training improved significantly more than the comparison group on ratings of ADLs (including the Barthel Index); however, the superiority of the strategy-training group was lost at 5-month follow-up assessment. Further studies of this approach have replicated its effectiveness and have demonstrated durability of the effects at 20 weeks and enhanced transfer of training effects to nontrained tasks over ADL retraining as usual at 8 weeks, although this superiority was lost at 20 weeks (Geusgens et al., 2006, 2007).

Box 7.2. A Bottom-Up Approach to Apraxia

Goldenberg and Hagmann (1998) reported a program of therapy provided to 15 patients with marked apraxia after left-hemisphere stroke. Apraxic errors were characterized as *fatal* or *reparable* errors. Each week, the participants were tested and provided with intervention for 1 of 3 activities of daily living (ADLs). In the following week, a second activity was trained, and in the 3rd week, the third activity was trained. At the end of therapy, 10 of the 15 participants could perform all three activities without fatal errors. Fatal errors were eliminated only when the activity was being trained (indicating that the improvement was dependent on the training and that there was no generalization from trained to untrained tasks). At 6 months, intervention gains were maintained only in participants who routinely engaged in the activities at home (Goldenberg, Daumüller, & Hagmann, 2001). Goldenberg et al. further compared direct training of activities with exploration training aimed at teaching the patient structure–function relationships associated with correct performance. Exploration training had no effect on performance, whereas direct training reduced errors and need for assistance. Because the improvement in functioning was limited to the activities that were trained, and even to the specific objects that were used in training, Goldenberg et al. recommended that intervention for ADLs and instrumental activities of daily living for clients with apraxia be tied to clients' specific needs and reflect the routines of clients' daily life.

caution in interpreting the research literature because of differing criteria for evaluating effectiveness.

Considering the evidence reviewed in this chapter, it is apparent how difficult it is to develop interventions addressing cognitive disorders that show robust effects on the client's long-term occupational performance and participation (Bowen et al., 2011, 2013; Giles, 2010; Zoccolotti et al., 2011). Both top-down and bottom-up approaches have shown only limited evidence of transfer, so it behooves occupational therapists to target intervention to areas of specific importance to the individual client and retain a commitment to being client centered and a focus on the remediation of occupational performance problems in everyday life (AOTA, 2013).

References

Ahlsiö, B., Britton, M., Murray, V., & Theorell, T. (1984). Disablement and quality of life after stroke. *Stroke, 15,* 886–890. http://dx.doi.org/10.1161/01.STR.15.5.886

Alderman, N., Burgess, P. W., Knight, C., & Henman, C. (2003). Ecological validity of a simplified version of the multiple errands shopping test. *Journal of the International Neuropsychological Society, 9,* 31–44. http://dx.doi.org/10.1017/S1355617703910046

American Occupational Therapy Association. (2013). Cognition, cognitive rehabilitation, and occupational performance. *American Journal of Occupational Therapy, 67*(Suppl.), S9–S31. http://dx.doi.org/10.5014/ajot.2013.67S9

American Occupational Therapy Association. (2014). Occupational therapy practice framework: Domain and process (3rd ed.). *American Journal of Occupational Therapy, 68*(Suppl. 1), S1–S48. http://dx.doi.org/10.5014/ajot.2014.682006

Antonucci, G., Guariglia, C., Judica, A., Magnotti, L., Paolucci, S., Pizzamiglio, L., & Zoccolotti, P. (1995). Effectiveness of neglect rehabilitation in a randomized group study. *Journal of Clinical and Experimental Neuropsychology, 17*, 383–389. http://dx.doi.org/10.1080/01688639508405131

Appelros, P., Karlsson, G. M., Seiger, A., & Nydevik, I. (2002). Neglect and anosognosia after first-ever stroke: Incidence and relationship to disability. *Journal of Rehabilitation Medicine, 34*, 215–220. http://dx.doi.org/10.1080/165019702760279206

Appelros, P., Karlsson, G. M., Thorwalls, A., Tham, K., & Nydevik, I. (2004). Unilateral neglect: Further validation of the Baking Tray Task. *Journal of Rehabilitation Medicine, 36*, 258–261. http://dx.doi.org/10.1080/16501970410029852

Azouvi, P., Marchal, F., Samuel, C., Morin, L., Renard, C., Louis-Dreyfus, A., . . . Bergego, C. (1996). Functional consequences and awareness of unilateral neglect: Study of an evaluation scale. *Neuropsychological Rehabilitation, 6*, 133–150. http://dx.doi.org/10.1080/713755501

Azouvi, P., Samuel, C., Louis-Dreyfus, A., Bernati, T., Bartolomeo, P., Beis, J.-M., . . . Rousseaux, M.; French Collaborative Study Group on Assessment of Unilateral Neglect. (2002). Sensitivity of clinical and behavioural tests of spatial neglect after right hemisphere stroke. *Journal of Neurology, Neurosurgery, and Psychiatry, 73*, 160–166. http://dx.doi.org/10.1136/jnnp.73.2.160

Baddeley, A. (2004). The psychology of memory. In A. D. Baddeley, M. D. Kopelman, & B. A. Wilson (Eds.), *The essential handbook of memory disorders for clinicians* (pp. 1–13). Chichester, England: Wiley.

Barker-Collo, S., Feigin, V. L., Parag, V., Lawes, C. M., & Senior, H. (2010). Auckland Stroke Outcomes Study. Part 2: Cognition and functional outcomes 5 years poststroke. *Neurology, 75*, 1608–1616. http://dx.doi.org/10.1212/WNL.0b013e3181fb44c8

Bauer, R. M. (2012). Agnosia. In K. M. Heilman & E. Valenstein (Eds.), *Clinical neuropsychology* (5th ed., pp. 238–295). New York: Oxford University Press.

Baum, C. M., Connor, L. T., Morrison, T., Hahn, M., Dromerick, A. W., & Edwards, D. F. (2008). Reliability, validity, and clinical utility of the Executive Function Performance Test: A measure of executive function in a sample of people with stroke. *American Journal of Occupational Therapy, 62*, 446–455. http://dx.doi.org/10.5014/ajot.62.4.446

Baum, C. M., & Edwards, D. (2008). *Activity Card Sort* (2nd ed.). Bethesda, MD: AOTA Press.

Baum, C. M., & Katz, N. (2010). Occupational therapy approach to assessing the relationship between cognition and function. In T. D. Marcotte & I. Grant (Eds.), *Neuropsychology of everyday functioning* (pp. 63–90). New York: Guilford Press.

Baum, C. M., Morrison, T., Hahn, M., & Edwards, D. F. (2003). *Executive Function Performance Test: Test protocol booklet.* St. Louis: Washington University School of Medicine.

Bickerton, W. L., Riddoch, M. J., Samson, D., Balani, A. B., Mistry, B., & Humphreys, G. W. (2012). Systematic assessment of apraxia and functional predictions from the Birmingham Cognitive Screen. *Journal of Neurology, Neurosurgery, and Psychiatry, 83*, 513–521. http://dx.doi.org/10.1136/jnnp-2011-300968

Bisiach, E., Capitani, E., Luzzatti, C., & Perani, D. (1981). Brain and conscious representation of outside reality. *Neuropsychologia, 19*, 543–551. http://dx.doi.org/10.1016/0028-3932(81)90020-8

Bisiach, E., & Luzzatti, C. (1978). Unilateral neglect of representational space. *Cortex, 14*, 129–133. http://dx.doi.org/10.1016/S0010-9452(78)80016-1

Boake, C. (1991). History of cognitive rehabilitation following head injury. In J. S. Kreutzer & P. H. Wehman (Eds.), *Cognitive rehabilitation for persons with traumatic brain injury: A functional approach* (pp. 3–12). Baltimore: Paul H. Brookes.

Bowen, A., Hazelton, C., Pollock, A., & Lincoln, N. B. (2013). Cognitive rehabilitation for spatial neglect following stroke. *Cochrane Database of Systematic Reviews, 2013*, CD003586. http://dx.org/10.1002/14651858.CD003586.pub3

Bowen, A., Knapp, P., Gillespie, D., Nicolson, D. J., & Vail, A. (2011). Non-pharmacological interventions for perceptual disorders following stroke and other adult-acquired, non-progressive brain injury. *Cochrane Database of Systematic Reviews, 2011*, CD007039. http://dx.doi.org/10.1002/14651858.CD007039.pub2

BrainTrain. (2013). *Captain's Log Mind Power Builder.* Retrieved from http://www.braintrain.com/captains-log-mindpower-builder

Broca, P. (1861). Remarques sur le siege de la faculte de language articule: Suivies d'une observation d'aphemie (perte de parole) [Remarks on the seat of the faculty of articulate language: Followed by an observation of aphemia (loss of speech)]. *Bulletins de la Société Anatomique de Paris, 6*, 330–357, 398–407.

Burgess, P. W., Gonen-Yaacovi, G., & Volle, E. (2011). Functional neuroimaging studies of prospective memory: What have we learnt so far? *Neuropsychologia, 49*, 2246–2257. http://dx.doi.org/10.1016/j.neuropsychologia.2011.02.014

Burke, J. M., Danick, J. A., Bemis, B., & Durgin, C. J. (1994). A process approach to memory book training for neurological patients. *Brain Injury, 8*, 71–81. http://dx.doi.org/10.3109/02699059409150960

Butler, B. C., Lawrence, M., Eskes, G. A., & Klein, R. (2009). Visual search patterns in neglect: Comparison of peripersonal and extrapersonal space. *Neuropsychologia, 47*, 869–878. http://dx.doi.org/10.1016/j.neuropsychologia.2008.12.020

Butler, J. A. (2002). How comparable are tests of apraxia? *Clinical Rehabilitation, 16*, 389–398. http://dx.doi.org/10.1191/0269215502cr493oa

Buxbaum, L. J., Haaland, K. Y., Hallett, M., Wheaton, L., Heilman, K. M., Rodriguez, A., & Gonzalez Rothi, L. J. (2008). Treatment of limb apraxia: Moving forward to improved action. *American Journal of Physical Medicine and Rehabilitation, 87*, 149–161. http://dx.doi.org/10.1097/PHM.0b013e31815e6727

Cantagallo, A., Maini, M., & Rumiati, R. I. (2012). The cognitive rehabilitation of limb apraxia in patients with stroke. *Neuropsychological Rehabilitation, 22*, 473–488. http://dx.doi.org/10.1080/09602011.2012.658317

Caplan, D. (2012). Aphasia syndromes. In K. M. Heilman & E. Valenstein (Eds.), *Clinical neuropsychology* (5th ed., pp. 22–41). New York: Oxford University Press.

Carod-Artal, F. J., & Egido, J. A. (2009). Quality of life after stroke: The importance of a good recovery. *Cardiovascular Diseases, 27*(Suppl. 1), 204–214. http://dx.doi.org/10.1159/000200461

Cermak, L. S., Verfaellie, M., Lanzoni, S., Mather, M., & Chase, K. A. (1996). Effects of spaced repetitions on amnesia patients' recall and recognition performance. *Neuropsychology, 10*, 219–227. http://dx.doi.org/10.1037/0894-4105.10.2.219

Chen, P., Hreha, K., Fortis, P., Goedert, K. M., & Barrett, A. M. (2012). Functional assessment of spatial neglect: A review of the Catherine Bergego Scale and an introduction of the Kessler Foundation Neglect Assessment Process. *Topics in Stroke Rehabilitation, 19*, 423–435. http://dx.doi.org/10.1310/tsr1905-423

Chung, C. S., Pollock, A., Campbell, T., Durward, B. R., & Hagen, S. (2013). Cognitive rehabilitation for executive dysfunction in adults with stroke or other adult non-progressive acquired brain damage. *Cochrane Database of Systematic Reviews, 2011*, CD008391. http://dx.doi.org/10.1002/14651858.CD008391.pub2

Cicerone, K. D., Langenbahn, D. M., Braden, C., Malec, J. F., Kalmar, K., Fraas, M., . . . Ashman, T. (2011). Evidence-based cognitive rehabilitation: Updated review of the literature from 2003 through 2008. *Archives of Physical Medicine and Rehabilitation, 92*, 519–530. http://dx.doi.org/10.1016/j.apmr.2010.11.015

Clare, L., Wilson, B. A., Carter, G., Breen, K., Gosses, A., & Hodges, J. R. (2000). Intervening with everyday memory problems in dementia of Alzheimer's type: An errorless learning approach. *Journal of Clinical and Experimental Neuropsychology, 22*, 132–146. http://dx.doi.org/10.1076/1380-3395(200002)22:1;1-8;FT132

Clark, M. A., Merians, A. S., Kothari, A., Poizner, H., Macauley, B., Gonzalez Rothi, L. J., & Heilman, K. M. (1994). Spatial planning deficits in limb apraxia. *Brain, 117*, 1093–1106. http://dx.doi.org/10.1093/brain/117.5.1093

Clark-Wilson, J., Baxter, D., & Giles, G. M. (In press). Revisiting the Neurofunctional Approach: Conceptualizing the core components for the rehabilitation of everyday living skills. *Brain Injury.*

Cohen, G., & Conway, M. A. (2008). *Memory in the real world* (3rd ed.). Hove, England: Psychology Press.

Corwin, J., & Bylsma, F. W. (1993). Psychological examination of traumatic encephalopathy. *Clinical Neuropsychologist, 7,* 3–21. http://dx.doi.org/10.1080/13854049308401883

Cowan, N. (2008). What are the differences between long-term, short-term, and working memory? *Progress in Brain Research, 169,* 323–338. http://dx.doi.org/10.1016/S0079-6123(07)00020-9

Cumming, T. B., Marshall, R. S., & Lazar, R. M. (2013). Stroke, cognitive deficits, and rehabilitation: Still an incomplete picture. *International Journal of Stroke, 8,* 38–45. http://dx.doi.org/10.1111/j.1747-4949.2012.00972.x

das Nair, R., & Lincoln, N. B. (2007). Cognitive rehabilitation for memory deficits following stroke. *Cochrane Database of Systematic Reviews, 2007,* CD002293. http://dx.doi.org/10.1002/14651858.CD002293.pub2

Davis, N. R., Massman, P. J., & Doody, R. S. (2001). Cognitive intervention in Alzheimer disease: A randomized placebo-controlled study. *Alzheimer Disease and Associated Disorders, 15,* 1–9. http://dx.doi.org/10.1097/00002093-200101000-00001

Dawson, D. R., Gaya, A., Hunt, A., Levine, B., Lemsky, C., & Polatajko, H. J. (2009). Using the Cognitive Orientation to Occupational Performance (CO-OP) approach with adults with executive dysfunction. *Canadian Journal of Occupational Therapy, 76,* 115–127. http://dx.doi.org/10.1177/000841740907600209

de Joode, E., van Heugten, C., Verhey, F., & van Boxtel, M. (2010). Efficacy and usability of assistive technology for patients with cognitive deficits: A systematic review. *Clinical Rehabilitation, 24,* 701–714. http://dx.doi.org/10.1177/0269215510367551

De Renzi, E., & Lucchelli, F. (1988). Ideational apraxia. *Brain, 111,* 1173–1185. http://dx.doi.org/10.1093/brain/111.5.1173

Delis, D. C., Kramer, J. H., Kaplan, E., & Ober, B. A. (2000). *California Verbal Learning Test–Second edition (CVLT–II).* San Antonio: Psychological Corporation.

Denes, G., Semenza, C., Stoppa, E., & Lis, A. (1982). Unilateral spatial neglect and recovery from hemiplegia: A follow-up study. *Brain, 105,* 543–552. http://dx.doi.org/10.1093/brain/105.3.543

Denis, M., Beschin, N., Logie, R. H., & Della Sala, S. (2002). Visual perception and verbal descriptions as sources for generating mental representations: Evidence from representational neglect. *Cognitive Neuropsychology, 19,* 97–112. http://dx.doi.org/10.1080/02643290143000105

Diller, L., Ben-Yishay, Y., Gerstman, L. J., Goodkin, R., Gordon, W., & Weinberg, J. (1974). *Studies in cognition and rehabilitation in hemiplegia* (Rehabilitation Monograph, Vol. 50). New York: Institute of Rehabilitation Medicine, New York University Medical Center.

Donkervoort, M., Dekker, J., & Deelman, B. G. (2002). Sensitivity of different ADL measures to apraxia and motor impairments. *Clinical Rehabilitation, 16,* 299–305. http://dx.doi.org/10.1191/0269215502cr492oa

Donkervoort, M., Dekker, J., & Deelman, B. G. (2006). The course of apraxia and ADL functioning in left hemisphere stroke patients treated in rehabilitation centres and nursing homes. *Clinical Rehabilitation, 20,* 1085–1093. http://dx.doi.org/10.1177/0269215506071257

Donkervoort, M., Dekker, J., Stehmann-Saris, F. C., & Deelman, B. G. (2001). Efficacy of strategy training in left hemisphere stroke patients with apraxia: A randomised clinical trial. *Neuropsychological Rehabilitation, 11,* 549–566. http://dx.doi.org/10.1080/09602010143000093

Donkervoort, M., Dekker, J., van den Ende, E., Stehmann-Saris, J. C., & Deelman, B. G. (2000). Prevalence of apraxia among patients with a first left hemisphere stroke in rehabilitation centres and nursing homes. *Clinical Rehabilitation, 14,* 130–136. http://dx.doi.org/10.1191/026921500668935800

Duncan, J. (1986). Disorganisation of behaviour after frontal lobe damage. *Cognitive Neuropsychology, 3,* 271–290. http://dx.doi.org/10.1080/02643298608253360

Duncan, P. W., Wallace, D., Lai, S. M., Johnson, D., Embretson, S., & Laster, L. J. (1999). The Stroke Impact Scale version 2.0: Evaluation of reliability, validity, and sensitivity to change. *Stroke, 30,* 2131–2140. http://dx.doi.org/10.1161/01.STR.30.10.2131

Edwards, J. D., Jacova, C., Sepehry, A. A., Pratt, B., & Benavente, O. R. (2013). A quantitative systematic review of domain-specific cognitive impairment in lacunar stroke. *Neurology, 80,* 315–322. http://dx.doi.org/10.1212/WNL.0b013e31827deb85

Eichenbaum, H. (2001). The hippocampus and declarative memory: Cognitive mechanisms and neural codes. *Behavioural Brain Research, 127*, 199–207. http://dx.doi.org/10.1016/S0166-4328(01)00365-5

Ellis, J., & Kvavilashvili, L. (2000). Prospective memory in 2000: Past, present, and future directions. *Applied Cognitive Psychology, 14*, S1–S9. http://dx.doi.org/10.1002/acp.767

Eskes, G., & Salter, K., on behalf of the Mood and Cognition in Stroke Writing Group and the Evidence-Based Review in Stroke Rehabilitation Team. (2013). Mood and cognition in stroke. In M. P. Lindsay, G. Gubitz, M. Bayley, & S. Phillips; Stroke and Best Practices and Standards Advisory Committee (Eds.), *Canadian best practice recommendations for stroke care* (4th ed., Chapter 7). Ottawa, Ontario: Canadian Stroke Network.

Evans, J. J. (2010). Basic concepts and principles of neuropsychological assessment. In J. M. Gurd, U. Kischka, & J. C. Marshall (Eds.), *The handbook of clinical neuropsychology* (2nd ed., pp. 15–27). Oxford, England: Oxford University Press.

Evans, J. J., Wilson, B. A., Needham, P., & Brentnall, S. (2003). Who makes good use of memory aids? Results of a survey of people with acquired brain injury. *Journal of the International Neuropsychological Society, 9*, 925–935. http://dx.doi.org/10.1017/S1355617703960127

Evans, J. J., Wilson, B. A., Schuri, U., Andrade, J., Baddeley, A., Bruna, O., . . . Taussik, I. (2000). A comparison of "errorless" and "trial-and-error" learning methods for teaching individuals with acquired memory deficits. *Neuropsychological Rehabilitation, 10*, 67–101. http://dx.doi.org/10.1080/096.020100389309

Feigin, V. L., Barker-Collo, S., Parag, V., Senior, H., Lawes, C. M., Ratnasabapathy, Y., & Glen, E.; ASTRO Study Group. (2010). Auckland Stroke Outcomes Study: Part 1. Gender, stroke types, ethnicity, and functional outcomes 5 years poststroke. *Neurology, 75*, 1597–1607. http://dx.doi.org/10.1212/WNL.0b013e3181fb44b3

Fernandez-Duque, D., Baird, J. A., & Posner, M. I. (2000). Awareness and metacognition. *Consciousness and Cognition, 9*, 324–326. http://dx.doi.org/10.1006/ccog.2000.0449

Finger, S. (1994). *Origins of neuroscience: A history of explorations into brain function.* New York: Oxford University Press.

Fish, J., Manly, T., Emslie, H., Evans, J. J., & Wilson, B. A. (2008). Compensatory strategies for acquired disorders of memory and planning: Differential effects of a paging system for patients with brain injury of traumatic versus cerebrovascular aetiology. *Journal of Neurology, Neurosurgery, and Psychiatry, 79*, 930–935. http://dx.doi.org/10.1136/jnnp.2007.125203

Fisher, A. G., & Bray Jones, K. (2010a). *Assessment of Motor and Process Skills: Vol. 1. Development, standardization, and administration manual* (7th ed.). Fort Collins, CO: Three Star Press.

Fisher, A. G., & Bray Jones, K. (2010b). *Assessment of Motor and Process Skills: Vol. 2. User manual* (7th ed.). Fort Collins, CO: Three Star Press.

Folstein, M. F., Folstein, S. E., & McHugh, P. R. (1975). "Mini-Mental State": A practical method for grading the cognitive state of patients for the clinician. *Journal of Psychiatric Research, 12*, 189–198. http://dx.doi.org/10.1016/0022-3956(75)90026-6

Fong, K. N., Yang, N. Y., Chan, M. K., Chan, D. Y., Lau, A. F., Chan, D. Y., . . . Chan, C. C. (2013). Combined effects of sensory cueing and limb activation on unilateral neglect in subacute left hemiplegic stroke patients: A randomized controlled pilot study. *Clinical Rehabilitation, 27*, 628–637. http://dx.doi.org/10.1177/0269215512471959

Foundas, A. L. (2013). Apraxia: Neural mechanisms and functional recovery. *Handbook of Clinical Neurology, 110*, 335–345. http://dx.doi.org/10.1016/B978-0-444-52901-5.00028-9

Frankland, P. W., & Bontempi, B. (2005). The organization of recent and remote memories. *Nature Reviews Neuroscience, 6*, 119–130. http://dx.doi.org/10.1038/nrn1607

Gentry, T., Wallace, J., Kvarfordt, C., & Lynch, K. B. (2008). Personal digital assistants as cognitive aids for individuals with severe traumatic brain injury: A community-based trial. *Brain Injury, 22*, 19–24. http://dx.doi.org/10.1080/02699050701810688

Geusgens, C., van Heugten, C. M., Cooijmans, J. P., Jolles, J., & van den Heuvel, W. J. (2007). Transfer effects of a cognitive strategy training for stroke patients with apraxia. *Journal of Clinical and Experimental Neuropsychology, 29*, 831–841. http://dx.doi.org/10.1080/13803390601125971

Geusgens, C., van Heugten, C., Donkervoort, M., van den Ende, E., Jolles, J., & van den Heuvel, W. (2006). Transfer of training effects in stroke patients with apraxia: An exploratory study. *Neuropsychological Rehabilitation, 16,* 213–229. http://dx.doi.org/10.1080/09602010500172350

Gianutsos, R. (1980). What is cognitive rehabilitation? *Journal of Rehabilitation, 46,* 36–40.

Giles, G. M. (2010). Cognitive versus functional approaches to rehabilitation after traumatic brain injury: Commentary on a randomized controlled trial. *American Journal of Occupational Therapy, 64,* 182–185. http://dx.doi.org/10.5014/ajot.64.1.182

Giles, G. M. (2011). A neurofunctional approach to rehabilitation following brain injury. In N. Katz (Ed.), *Cognition, occupation, and participation across the life span* (3rd ed., pp. 351–381). Bethesda, MD: AOTA Press.

Giles, G. M., & Clark-Wilson, J. (1988). The use of behavioral techniques in functional skills training after severe brain injury. *American Journal of Occupational Therapy, 42,* 658–665. http://dx.doi.org/10.5014/ajot.42.10.658

Giles, G. M., & Clark-Wilson, J. (Eds.). (1993). *Brain injury rehabilitation: A neurofunctional approach.* San Diego: Singular.

Giles, G. M., & Clark-Wilson, J. (Eds.). (1999). *Rehabilitation of the severely brain injured adult: A practical approach.* Cheltenham, England: Stanley Thornes.

Giles, G. M., Ridley, J. E., Dill, A., & Frye, S. (1997). A consecutive series of adults with brain injury treated with a washing and dressing retraining program. *American Journal of Occupational Therapy, 51,* 256–266. http://dx.doi.org/10.5014/ajot.51.4.256

Giles, G. M., & Shore, M. (1989). The effectiveness of an electronic memory aid for a memory-impaired adult of normal intelligence. *American Journal of Occupational Therapy, 43,* 409–411. http://dx.doi.org/10.5014/ajot.43.6.409

Godefroy, O., Lhullier, C., & Rousseaux, M. (1996). Non-spatial attention disorders in patients with frontal or posterior brain damage. *Brain, 119,* 191–202. http://dx.doi.org/10.1093/brain/119.1.191

Goldenberg, G., Daumüller, M., & Hagmann, S. (2001). Assessment and therapy of complex activities of daily living in apraxia. *Neuropsychological Rehabilitation, 11,* 147–169. http://dx.doi.org/10.1080/09602010042000204

Goldenberg, G., & Hagmann, S. (1998). Therapy of activities of daily living in patients with apraxia. *Neuropsychological Rehabilitation, 8,* 123–141. http://dx.doi.org/10.1080/713755559

Goldstein, K. (1942). *Aftereffects of brain injuries in war: Their evaluation and treatment; The application of psychologic methods in the clinic.* New York: Grune & Stratton.

Gordon, W. A., & Hibbard, M. R. (1991). The theory and practice of cognitive remediation. In J. S. Kreutzer & P. H. Wehman (Eds.), *Cognitive rehabilitation for persons with traumatic brain injury: A functional approach* (pp. 13–22). Baltimore: Paul H. Brookes.

Gordon, W. A., Hibbard, M. R., Egelko, S., Diller, L., Shaver, M. S., Lieberman, A., & Ragnarsson, K. (1985). Perceptual remediation in patients with right brain damage: A comprehensive program. *Archives of Physical Medicine and Rehabilitation, 66,* 353–359.

Gray, J. M., & Robertson, I. H. (1989). Remediation of attentional difficulties following brain injury: Three experimental single case studies. *Brain Injury, 3,* 163–170. http://dx.doi.org/10.3109/02699058909004548

Guidetti, S., & Ytterberg, C. (2011). A randomised controlled trial of a client-centred self-care intervention after stroke: A longitudinal pilot study. *Disability and Rehabilitation, 33,* 494–503. http://dx.doi.org/10.3109/09638288.2010.498553

Halligan, P. W., & Marshall, J. C. (1994). Focal and global attention modulate the expression of visuo-spatial neglect: A case study. *Neuropsychologia, 32,* 13–21. http://dx.doi.org/10.1016/0028-3932(94)90065-5

Hamera, E., & Brown, C. E. (2000). Developing a context-based performance measure for persons with schizophrenia: The Test of Grocery Shopping Skills. *American Journal of Occupational Therapy, 54,* 20–25. http://dx.doi.org/10.5014/ajot.54.1.20

Hamera, E., Rempfer, M., & Brown, C. E. (2005). Performance in the "real world": Update on Test of Grocery Shopping Skills (TOGSS). *Schizophrenia Research, 78,* 111–112, author reply 113–114. http://dx.doi.org/10.1016/j.schres.2005.04.019

Hamera, E., Rempfer, M., & Brown, C. E. (2009). *The Test of Grocery Shopping Skills.* Bethesda, MD: AOTA Press.

Harris, J. E. (1980). Memory aids people use: Two interview studies. *Memory and Cognition, 8,* 31–38. http://dx.doi.org/10.3758/BF03197549

Hartman-Maeir, A., & Katz, N. (1995). Validity of the Behavioral Inattention Test (BIT): Relationships with functional tasks. *American Journal of Occupational Therapy, 49,* 507–516. http://dx.doi.org/10.5014/ajot.49.6.507

Hartman-Maeir, A., Katz, N., & Baum, C. M. (2009). Cognitive Functional Evaluation (CFE) process for individuals with suspected cognitive disabilities. *Occupational Therapy in Health Care, 23,* 1–23. http://dx.doi.org/10.1080/07380570802455516

Hazy, T. E., Frank, M. J., & O'Reilly, R. C. (2007). Towards an executive without a homunculus: Computational models of the prefrontal cortex/basal ganglia system. *Philosophical Transactions of the Royal Society of London, Series B: Biological Sciences, 362,* 1601–1613. http://dx.doi.org/10.1098/rstb.2007.2055

Hecaen, A. (1968). Suggestions for a typology of apraxia. In M. L. Simmel (Ed.), *The reach of mind: Essays in memory of Kurt Goldstein* (pp. 37–56). New York: Springer.

Heilman, K. M., Watson, R. T., & Valenstein, E. (2012). Neglect and related disorders. In K. M. Heilman & E. Valenstein (Eds.), *Clinical neuropsychology* (5th ed., pp. 296–348). New York: Oxford University Press.

Hunkin, N. M., Squires, E. J., Parkin, A. J., & Tidy, J. A. (1998). Are the benefits of errorless learning dependent on implicit memory? *Neuropsychologia, 36,* 25–36. http://dx.doi.org/10.1016/S0028-3932(97)00106-1

Hurford, R., Charidimou, A., Fox, Z., Cipolotti, L., & Werring, D. J. (2013). Domain-specific trends in cognitive impairment after acute ischaemic stroke. *Journal of Neurology, 260,* 237–241. http://dx.doi.org/10.1007/s00415-012-6625-0

Ihle-Hansen, H., Thommessen, B., Wyller, T. B., Engedal, K., Øksengård, A. R., Stenset, V., . . . Fure, B. (2011). Incidence and subtypes of MCI and dementia 1 year after first-ever stroke in patients without pre-existing cognitive impairment. *Dementia and Geriatric Cognitive Disorders, 32,* 401–407. http://dx.doi.org/10.1159/000335361

Jehkonen, M., Laihosalo, M., & Kettunen, J. E. (2006). Impact of neglect on functional outcome after stroke: A review of methodological issues and recent research findings. *Restorative Neurology and Neuroscience, 24,* 209–215.

Kalra, L., Perez, I., Gupta, S., & Wittink, M. (1997). The influence of visual neglect on stroke rehabilitation. *Stroke, 28,* 1386–1391. http://dx.doi.org/10.1161/01.STR.28.7.1386

Karnath, H. O. (1994). Subjective body orientation in neglect and the interactive contribution of neck muscle proprioception and vestibular stimulation. *Brain, 117,* 1001–1012. http://dx.doi.org/10.1093/brain/117.5.1001

Katrak, P. H., Black, D., & Peeva, V. (2009). Do stroke patients with intracerebral hemorrhage have a better functional outcome than patients with cerebral infarction? *PM&R, 1,* 427–433. http://dx.doi.org/10.1016/j.pmrj.2009.03.002

Katz, N. (2006). *Routine Task Inventory–Expanded manual.* Retrieved from http://www.allen-cognitive-network.org

Katz, N., Hartman-Maeir, A., Ring, H., & Soroker, N. (1999). Functional disability and rehabilitation outcome in right hemisphere damaged patients with and without unilateral spatial neglect. *Archives of Physical Medicine and Rehabilitation, 80,* 379–384. http://dx.doi.org/10.1016/S0003-9993(99)90273-3

Katz, N., Itzkovich, M., Averbuch, S., & Elazar, B. (1989). Loewenstein Occupational Therapy Cognitive Assessment (LOTCA) battery for brain-injured patients: Reliability and validity. *American Journal of Occupational Therapy, 43,* 184–192. http://dx.doi.org/10.5014/ajot.43.3.184

Kelly, P. J., Furie, K. L., Shafqat, S., Rallis, N., Chang, Y., & Stein, J. (2003). Functional recovery following rehabilitation after hemorrhagic and ischemic stroke. *Archives of Physical Medicine and Rehabilitation, 84,* 968–972. http://dx.doi.org/10.1016/S0003-9993(03)00040-6

Kerkhoff, G. (1998). Rehabilitation of visuospatial cognition and visual exploration in neglect: A cross-over study. *Restorative Neurology and Neuroscience, 12,* 27–40.

Kern, R. S., Liberman, R. P., Kopelowicz, A., Mintz, J., & Green, M. F. (2002). Applications of errorless learning for improving work performance in persons with schizophrenia. *American Journal of Psychiatry, 159,* 1921–1926. http://dx.doi.org/10.1176/appi.ajp.159.11.1921

Kim, H. J., Burke, D. T., Dowds, M. M., Jr., Boone, K. A., & Park, G. J. (2000). Electronic memory aids for outpatient brain injury: Follow-up findings. *Brain Injury, 14,* 187–196. http://dx.doi.org/10.1080/026990500120844

Kim, H. J., Craik, F. I. M., Luo, L., & Ween, J. E. (2009). Impairments in prospective and retrospective memory following stroke. *Neurocase, 15,* 145–156. http://dx.doi.org/10.1080/13554790802709039

Kime, S. K. (2006). *Compensating for memory deficits using a systematic approach.* Bethesda, MD: AOTA Press.

Komatsu, S., Minimua, M., Kato, M., & Kashima, H. (2000). Errorless and effortful processes involved in the learning of face–name associations by patients with alcoholic Korsakoff's syndrome. *Neuropsychological Rehabilitation, 10,* 113–132. http://dx.doi.org/10.1080/096020100389200

Krasny-Pacini, A., Chevignard, M., & Evans, J. (2014). Goal management training for rehabilitation of executive functions: A systematic review of effectiveness in patients with acquired brain injury. *Disability and Rehabilitation, 36,* 105–116. http://dx.doi.org/10.3109/09638288.2013.777807

Law, M., Baptiste, S., Carswell, A., McColl, M. A., Polatajko, H., & Pollock, N. (2005). *The Canadian Occupational Performance Measure* (4th ed.). Ottawa, Ontario: CAOT Publications.

LeClerc, C. M., & Wells, D. L. (1998). Use of a content methodology process to enhance feeding abilities threatened by ideational apraxia in people with Alzheimer's-type dementia. *Geriatric Nursing, 19,* 261–267. http://dx.doi.org/10.1016/S0197-4572(98)90099-4

Lee, M., Saver, J. L., Alger, J. R., Hao, Q., Salamon, N., Starkman, S., . . . Liebeskind, D. S. (2012). Association of laterality and size of perfusion lesions on neurological deficit in acute supratentorial stroke. *International Journal of Stroke, 7,* 293–297. http://dx.doi.org/10.1111/j.1747-4949.2011.00726.x

Levine, B., Robertson, I. H., Clare, L., Carter, G., Hong, J., Wilson, B. A., . . . Stuss, D. T. (2000). Rehabilitation of executive functioning: An experimental–clinical validation of goal management training. *Journal of the International Neuropsychological Society, 6,* 299–312. http://dx.doi.org/10.1017/S1355617700633052

Levine, B., Schweizer, T. A., O'Connor, C., Turner, G., Gillingham, S., Stuss, D. T., . . . Robertson, I. H. (2011). Rehabilitation of executive functioning in patients with frontal lobe brain damage with goal management training. *Frontiers in Human Neuroscience, 5,* 1–9. http://dx.doi.org/10.3389/fnhum.2011.00009

Lezak, M. D., Howieson, D. B., Bigler, E. D., & Tranel, D. (2012). *Neuropsychological assessment* (5th ed.). New York: Oxford University Press.

Lichtheim, L. (1885). On aphasia. *Brain, 7,* 434–484.

Liepmann, H. (1900). Das krankheitsbild der apraxie ("motrischen asymbolie") auf Grund eines Falles von einseitiger Apraxie [The syndrome of apraxia (motor asymbolia) based on a case of unilateral apraxia] (W. H. O. Bohne, K. Liepmann, & D. A. Rottenberg, Trans.). In D. A. Rottenberg & F. H. Hochberg (Eds.), *Neurological classics in modern translation* (pp. 15–44). New York: Hafner Press.

Liepmann, H. (1920). Apraxie [Apraxia]. *Ergebnisse der Gesamten Medizin, 1,* 516–543.

Lincoln, N. B., Drummond, A. E. R., & Berman, P.; SUE Study Group. (1997). Perceptual impairment and its impact on rehabilitation outcome. *Disability and Rehabilitation, 19,* 231–234. http://dx.doi.org/10.3109/09638289709166532

Lissauer, H. (1889). Ein fall von seelenblindheit nebst conem beitrage zur theorie derselben [A case of mind-blindness together with a theory of it]. *Archive Psychiatrie, 21,* 222–270. http://dx.doi.org/10.1007/BF02226765

Loetscher, T., & Lincoln, N. B. (2013). Cognitive rehabilitation for attention deficits following stroke. *Cochrane Database of Systematic Reviews, 2013,* CD002842. http://dx.doi.org/10.1002/14651858.CD002842.pub2

Loewenstein, D., & Acevedo, A. (2010). The relationship between activities of daily living and neuropsychological performance. In T. D. Marcotte & I. Grant (Eds.), *Neuropsychology of everyday functioning* (pp. 93–112). New York: Guilford Press.

Luauté, J., Halligan, P., Rode, G., Rossetti, Y., & Boisson, D. (2006). Visuo-spatial neglect: A systematic review of current interventions and their effectiveness. *Neuroscience and Biobehavioral Reviews, 30,* 961–982. http://dx.doi.org/10.1016/j.neubiorev.2006.03.001

Luukkainen-Markkula, R., Tarkka, I. M., Pitkänen, K., Sivenius, J., & Hämäläinen, H. (2011). Comparison of the Behavioural Inattention Test and the Catherine Bergego Scale in assessment of hemispatial neglect. *Neuropsychological Rehabilitation, 21,* 103–116. http://dx.doi.org/10.1080/09602011.2010.531619

Mahoney, F. I., & Barthel, D. W. (1965). Functional evaluation: The Barthel Index. *Maryland State Medical Journal, 14,* 61–65.

Manchester, D., Priestley, N., & Jackson, H. (2004). The assessment of executive functions: Coming out of the office [Review]. *Brain Injury, 18,* 1067–1081. http://dx.doi.org/10.1080/02699050410001672387

Marcotte, T. D., Scott, J. C., Kamat, R., & Heaton, R. K. (2010). Neuropsychology and the prediction of everyday functioning. In T. D. Marcotte & I. Grant (Eds.), *Neuropsychology of everyday functioning* (pp. 5–38). New York: Guilford Press.

McDonald, A., Haslam, C., Yates, P., Gurr, B., Leeder, G., & Sayers, A. (2011). Google Calendar: A new memory aid to compensate for prospective memory deficits following acquired brain injury. *Neuropsychological Rehabilitation, 21,* 784–807. http://dx.doi.org/10.1080/09602011.2011.598405

McEwen, S. E., Polatajko, H. J., Huijbregts, M. P., & Ryan, J. D. (2009). Exploring a cognitive-based treatment approach to improve motor-based skill performance in chronic stroke: Results of three single case experiments. *Brain Injury, 23,* 1041–1053. http://dx.doi.org/10.3109/02699050903421107

Meichenbaum, D. (1977). *Cognitive–behavior modification: An integrative approach.* New York: Plenum Press.

Menon, A., & Korner-Bitensky, N. (2004). Evaluating unilateral spatial neglect post stroke: Working your way through the maze of assessment choices. *Topics in Stroke Rehabilitation, 11,* 41–66. http://dx.doi.org/10.1310/KQWL-3HQL-4KNM-5F4U

Milner, B., & Teuber, H.-L. (1968). Alteration of perception and memory in man. In L. Weiskrantz (Ed.), *Analysis of behavioral change* (pp. 268–375). New York: Harper & Row.

Morrison, M. T., Giles, G. M., Ryan, J. D., Baum, C. M., Dromerick, A. W., Polatajko, H. J., & Edwards, D. F. (2013). Multiple Errands Test–Revised (MET–R): A performance-based measure of executive function in people with mild cerebrovascular accident. *American Journal of Occupational Therapy, 67,* 460–468. http://dx.doi.org/10.5014/ajot.2013.007880

Neistadt, M. E. (1992). The Rabideau Kitchen Evaluation–Revised: An assessment of meal preparation skill. *OTJR: Occupation, Participation and Health, 12,* 242–253.

Nijboer, T., van de Port, I., Schepers, V., Post, M., & Visser-Meily, A. (2013). Predicting functional outcome after stroke: The influence of neglect on basic activities in daily living. *Frontiers in Human Neuroscience, 7,* 182. http://dx.doi.org/10.3389/fnhum.2013.00182

Norman, D. A., & Shallice, T. (1986). Attention to action: Willed and automatic control of behavior. In R. J. Davidson, G. E. Schwartz, & D. Shapiro (Eds.), *Consciousness and self-regulation: Advances in research and theory* (Vol. 4, pp. 1–18). New York: Plenum.

Nys, G. M. S., van Zandvoort, M. J. E., de Kort, P. L. M., Jansen, B. P. W., de Haan, E. H. F., & Kappelle, L. J. (2007). Cognitive disorders in acute stroke: Prevalence and clinical determinants. *Cerebrovascular Diseases, 23,* 408–416. http://dx.doi.org/10.1159/000101464

O'Carroll, R. E., Russell, H. H., Lawrie, S. M., & Johnstone, E. C. (1999). Errorless learning and the cognitive rehabilitation of memory-impaired schizophrenic patients. *Psychological Medicine, 29,* 105–112. http://dx.doi.org/10.1017/S0033291798007673

Odhuba, R. A., van den Broek, M. D., & Johns, L. C. (2005). Ecological validity of measures of executive functioning. *British Journal of Clinical Psychology, 44,* 269–278. http://dx.doi.org/10.1348/014466505X29431

Paolucci, A., McKenna, K., & Cooke, D. M. (2009). Factors affecting the number and type of impairments of visual perception and praxis following stroke. *Australian Occupational Therapy Journal, 56,* 350–360. http://dx.doi.org/10.1111/j.1440-1630.2008.00743.x

Paolucci, S., Antonucci, G., Grasso, M. G., & Pizzamiglio, L. (2001). The role of unilateral spatial neglect in rehabilitation of right brain-damaged ischemic stroke patients: A matched comparison. *Archives of Physical Medicine and Rehabilitation, 82,* 743–749. http://dx.doi.org/10.1053/apmr.2001.23191

Paolucci, S., Antonucci, G., Guariglia, C., Magnotti, L., Pizzamiglio, L., & Zoccolotti, P. (1996). Facilitatory effect of neglect rehabilitation on the recovery of left hemiplegic stroke patients: A cross-over study. *Journal of Neurology, 243,* 308–314. http://dx.doi.org/10.1007/BF00868403

Parish, L., & Oddy, M. (2007). Efficacy of rehabilitation for functional skills more than 10 years after extremely severe brain injury. *Neuropsychological Rehabilitation, 17,* 230–243. http://dx.doi.org/10.1080/09602010600750675

Park, N. W., Proulx, G., & Towers, W. M. (1999). Evaluation of the attention process training programme. *Neuropsychological Rehabilitation, 9,* 135–154. http://dx.doi.org/10.1080/713755595

Parkin, A. J., Hunkin, N. M., & Squires, E. J. (1998). Unlearning John Major: The use of errorless learning in the reacquisition of proper names following herpes simplex encephalitis. *Cognitive Neuropsychology, 15,* 361–375. http://dx.doi.org/10.1080/026432998381131

Parton, A., Malhotra, P., & Husain, M. (2004). Hemispatial neglect. *Journal of Neurology, Neurosurgery, and Psychiatry, 75,* 13–21.

Pasi, M., Poggesi, A., Salvadori, E., & Pantoni, L. (2012). Post-stroke dementia and cognitive impairment. In M. Paciaroni, G. Agnelli, V. Caso, & J. Bogousslavsky (Eds.), *Manifestations of stroke* (pp. 65–69). Basel, Switzerland: Karger.

Pearce, J. M. S. (2009). Hugo Karl Liepmann and apraxia. *Clinical Medicine, 9,* 466–470. http://dx.doi.org/10.7861/clinmedicine.9-5-466

Petruccelli, G. E., & Delenick, C. D. (2013, April). *Utilizing performance-based cognitive assessments in acute care.* Paper presented at the American Occupational Therapy Association Annual Conference and Expo, San Diego.

Piras, F., Borella, E., Incoccia, C., & Carlesimo, G. A. (2011). Evidence-based practice recommendations for memory rehabilitation. *European Journal of Physical and Rehabilitation Medicine, 47,* 149–175.

Pizzamiglio, L., Antonucci, G., Judica, A., Montenero, P., Razzano, C., & Zoccolotti, P. (1992). Cognitive rehabilitation of the hemineglect disorder in chronic patients with unilateral right brain damage. *Journal of Clinical and Experimental Neuropsychology, 14,* 901–923. http://dx.doi.org/10.1080/01688639208402543

Poeck, K., & Lehmkuhl, G. (1980). Ideatory apraxia in a left-handed patient with right-sided brain lesion. *Cortex, 16,* 273–284. http://dx.doi.org/10.1016/S0010-9452(80)80062-1

Polatajko, H. J., & Mandich, A. (2004). *Enabling occupation in children: The Cognitive Orientation to Daily Occupational Performance.* Ottawa, Ontario: CAOT Publications.

Polatajko, H. J., & Mandich, A. (2005). Cognitive Orientation to Daily Occupational Performance. In N. Katz (Ed.), *Cognition and occupation across the life span* (2nd ed., pp. 237–259). Bethesda, MD: AOTA Press.

Polatajko, H. J., & Mandich, A. (2011). Cognitive Orientation to Daily Occupational Performance (CO-OP): A cognitive-based intervention for children and adults. In N. Katz (Ed.), *Cognition, occupation, and participation across the life span* (3rd ed., pp. 299–321). Bethesda, MD: AOTA Press.

Posner, M. I., & Petersen, S. E. (1990). The attention system of the human brain. *Annual Review of Neuroscience, 13,* 25–42. http://dx.doi.org/10.1146/annurev.ne.13.030190.000325

Poulin, V., Korner-Bitensky, N., & Dawson, D. R. (2013). Stroke-specific executive function assessment: A literature review of performance-based tools. *Australian Occupational Therapy Journal, 60,* 3–19. http://dx.doi.org/10.1111/1440-1630.12024

Poulin, V., Korner-Bitensky, N., Dawson, D. R., & Bherer, L. (2012). Efficacy of executive function interventions after stroke: A systematic review. *Topics in Stroke Rehabilitation, 19,* 158–171. http://dx.doi.org/10.1310/tsr1902-158

Prescott, R. J., Garraway, W. M., & Akhtar, A. J. (1982). Predicting functional outcome following acute stroke using a standard clinical examination. *Stroke, 13,* 641–647. http://dx.doi.org/10.1161/01.STR.13.5.641

Priestley, N., Manchester, D., & Aram, R. (2013). Presenting evidence of executive functions deficit in court: Issues for the expert neuropsychologist. *Journal of Personal Injury Law, 4,* 240–247.

Randerath, J., Goldenberg, G., Spijkers, W., Li, Y., & Hermsdörfer, J. (2011). From pantomime to actual use: How affordances can facilitate actual tool-use. *Neuropsychologia, 49,* 2410–2416. http://dx.doi.org/10.1016/j.neuropsychologia.2011.04.017

Riska-Williams, L., Allen, C. A., Austin, S., David, S., Earhart, C., & McCraith, D. B. (2007). *Manual for the ACLS–5 and LACLS–5.* Camarillo, CA: ACLS & LACLS Committee.

Robertson, I. H., Gray, J. M., & McKenzie, S. (1988). Microcomputer-based cognitive rehabilitation of visual neglect: Three multiple-baseline single-case studies. *Brain Injury, 2,* 151–163. http://dx.doi.org/10.3109/02699058809150939

Robertson, I. H., Gray, J. M., Pentland, B., & Waite, L. J. (1990). Microcomputer-based rehabilitation for unilateral left visual neglect: A randomized controlled trial. *Archives of Physical Medicine and Rehabilitation, 71,* 663–668.

Robertson, I. H., Hogg, K., & McMillan, T. M. (1998). Rehabilitation of unilateral neglect: Improving function by contralesional limb activation. *Neuropsychological Rehabilitation, 8*, 19–29. http://dx.doi.org/10.1080/713755556

Robertson, I. H., McMillan, T. M., MacLeod, E., Edgeworth, J., & Brock, D. (2002). Rehabilitation by limb activation training reduces left-sided motor impairment in unilateral neglect patients: A single-blind randomized control trial. *Neuropsychological Rehabilitation, 12*, 439–454. http://dx.doi.org/10.1080/09602010244000228

Robertson, I. H., & Murre, J. M. J. (1999). Rehabilitation of brain damage: Brain plasticity and principles of guided recovery. *Psychological Bulletin, 125*, 544–575. http://dx.doi.org/10.1037/0033-2909.125.5.544

Robertson, I. H., Ridgeway, V., Greenfield, E., & Parr, A. (1997). Motor recovery after stroke depends on intact sustained attention: A 2-year follow-up study. *Neuropsychology, 11*, 290–295. http://dx.doi.org/10.1037/0894-4105.11.2.290

Robertson, I. H., Tegnér, R., Goodrich, S. J., & Wilson, C. (1994). Walking trajectory and hand movements in unilateral left neglect: A vestibular hypothesis. *Neuropsychologia, 32*, 1495–1502. http://dx.doi.org/10.1016/0028-3932(94)90121-X

Robertson, I. H., Ward, T., Ridgeway, V., & Nimmo-Smith, I. (1994). *The Test of Everyday Attention*. Bury St. Edmunds, England: Thames Valley Test Company.

Robertson, I. H., Ward, T., Ridgeway, V., & Nimmo-Smith, I. (1996). The structure of normal human attention: The Test of Everyday Attention. *Journal of the International Neuropsychological Society, 2*, 525–534. http://dx.doi.org/10.1017/S1355617700001697

Rohling, M. L., Faust, M. E., Beverly, B., & Demakis, G. (2009). Effectiveness of cognitive rehabilitation following acquired brain injury: A meta-analytic re-examination of Cicerone et al.'s (2000, 2005) systematic reviews. *Neuropsychology, 23*, 20–39. http://dx.doi.org/10.1037/a0013659

Rotenberg-Shpigelman, S., Erez, A. B., Nahaloni, I., & Maeir, A. (2012). Neurofunctional treatment targeting participation among chronic stroke survivors: A pilot randomised controlled study. *Neuropsychological Rehabilitation, 22*, 532–549. http://dx.doi.org/10.1080/09602011.2012.665610

Rowe, F.; VIS Group UK. (2009). Visual perceptual consequences of stroke. *Strabismus, 17*, 24–28. http://dx.doi:10.1080/09273970802678537

Sachdev, P. S., Brodaty, H., Valenzuela, M. J., Lorentz, L. M., & Koschera, A. (2004). Progression of cognitive impairment in stroke patients. *Neurology, 63*, 1618–1623. http://dx.doi.org/10.1212/01.WNL.0000142964.83484.DE

Schacter, D. L., Rich, S. A., & Stampp, M. S. (1985). Remediation of memory disorders: Experimental evaluation of the spaced-retrieval technique. *Journal of Clinical and Experimental Neuropsychology, 7*, 79–96. http://dx.doi.org/10.1080/01688638508401243

Schneider, W., & Shiffrin, R. M. (1977). Controlled and automatic human information processing: I. Detection, search, and attention. *Psychological Review, 84*, 1–66. http://dx.doi.org/10.1037/0033-295X.84.1.1

Schutz, L. E., & Wanlass, R. L. (2009). Interdisciplinary assessment strategies for capturing the elusive executive. *American Journal of Physical Medicine and Rehabilitation, 88*, 419–422. http://dx.doi.org/10.1097/PHM.0b013e3181a0e2d3

Schweizer, T. A., Levine, B., Rewilak, D., O'Connor, C., Turner, G., Alexander, M. P., . . . Stuss, D. T. (2008). Rehabilitation of executive functioning after focal damage to the cerebellum. *Neurorehabilitation and Neural Repair, 22*, 72–77. http://dx.doi.org/10.1177/1545968307305303

Serino, A., Bonifazi, S., Pierfederici, L., & Làdavas, E. (2007). Neglect treatment by prism adaptation: What recovers and for how long. *Neuropsychological Rehabilitation, 17*, 657–687. http://dx.doi.org/10.1080/09602010601052006

Shallice, T., & Burgess, P. W. (1991). Deficits in strategy application following frontal lobe damage in man. *Brain, 114*, 727–741. http://dx.doi.org/10.1093/brain/114.2.727

Shiffrin, R. M., & Schneider, W. (1977). Controlled and automatic information processing: II. Perceptual learning, automatic attending, and a general theory. *Psychological Review, 84*, 127–190. http://dx.doi.org/10.1037/0033-295X.84.2.127

Shin, M. S., Park, S. Y., Park, S. R., Seol, S. H., & Kwon, J. S. (2006). Clinical and empirical applications of the Rey–Osterrieth Complex Figure Test. *Nature Protocols, 1*, 892–899. http://dx.doi.org/10.1038/nprot.2006.115

Skidmore, E. R., Holm, M. B., Whyte, E. M., Dew, M. A., Dawson, D., & Becker, J. T. (2011). The feasibility of meta-cognitive strategy training in acute inpatient stroke rehabilitation:

Case report. *Neuropsychological Rehabilitation, 21,* 208–223. http://dx.doi.org/10.1080/09602011.2011.552559

Skidmore, E. R., Whyte, E. M., Holm, M. B., Becker, J. T., Butters, M. A., Dew, M. A., . . . Lenze, E. J. (2010). Cognitive and affective predictors of rehabilitation participation after stroke. *Archives of Physical Medicine and Rehabilitation, 91,* 203–207. http://dx.doi.org/10.1016/j.apmr.2009.10.026

Söderback, I., & Normell, L. A. (1986a). Intellectual Function Training in adults with acquired brain damage: An occupational therapy method. *Scandinavian Journal of Rehabilitation Medicine, 18,* 139–146.

Söderback, I., & Normell, L. A. (1986b). Intellectual Function Training in adults with acquired brain damage: Evaluation. *Scandinavian Journal of Rehabilitation Medicine, 18,* 147–153.

Sohlberg, M. M., & Mateer, C. A. (1987a). *APT: Attention Process Training manual.* Puyallup, WA: Association for Neuropsychological Research and Development.

Sohlberg, M. M., & Mateer, C. A. (1987b). Effectiveness of an attention-training program. *Journal of Clinical and Experimental Neuropsychology, 9,* 117–130. http://dx.doi.org/10.1080/01688638708405352

Sohlberg, M. M., & Mateer, C. A. (1989). Training use of compensatory memory books: A three stage behavioral approach. *Journal of Clinical and Experimental Neuropsychology, 11,* 871–891. http://dx.doi.org/10.1080/01688638908400941

Sorensen, P. S., Boysen, G., Jensen, G., & Schnohr, P. (1982). Prevalence of stroke in a district of Copenhagen: The Copenhagen City Heart Study. *Acta Neurologica Scandinavica, 66,* 68–81. http://dx.doi.org/10.1111/j.1600-0404.1982.tb03130.x

Squire, L. R., & Wixted, J. T. (2011). The cognitive neuroscience of human memory since H. M. *Annual Review of Neuroscience, 34,* 259–288. http://dx.doi.org/10.1146/annurev-neuro-061010-113720

Sterzi, R., Bottini, G., Celani, M. G., Righetti, E., Lamassa, M., Ricci, S., & Vallar, G. (1993). Hemianopia, hemianaesthesia, and hemiplegia after right and left hemisphere damage: A hemispheric difference. *Journal of Neurology, Neurosurgery, and Psychiatry, 56,* 308–310. http://dx.doi.org/10.1136/jnnp.56.3.308

Stone, S. P., Patel, P., Greenwood, R. J., & Halligan, P. W. (1992). Measuring visual neglect in acute stroke and predicting its recovery: The Visual Neglect Recovery Index. *Journal of Neurology, Neurosurgery, and Psychiatry, 55,* 431–436. http://dx.doi.org/10.1136/jnnp.55.6.431

Sturt, R., & Punt, T. D. (2013). Caloric vestibular stimulation and postural control in patients with spatial neglect following stroke. *Neuropsychological Rehabilitation, 23,* 299–316. http://dx.doi.org/10.1080/09602011.2012.755831

Stuss, D. T. (1991). Self-awareness and the frontal lobes: A neuropsychological perspective. In J. Strauss & G. R. Goethals (Eds.), *The self: Interdisciplinary approaches* (pp. 255–278). New York: Springer-Verlag.

Sunderland, A., Wade, D. T., & Langton Hewer, R. (1987). The natural history of visual neglect after stroke: Indications from two methods of assessment. *International Disability Studies, 9,* 55–59. http://dx.doi.org/10.3109/03790798709166235

Tatemichi, T. K., Desmond, D. W., Stern, Y., Sano, M., & Bagiella, E. (1994). Cognitive impairment after stroke: Frequency, patterns, and relationship to functional abilities. *Journal of Neurology, Neurosurgery, and Psychiatry, 57,* 202–207. http://dx.doi.org/10.1136/jnnp.57.2.202

Teasdale, T. W., Emslie, H., Quirk, K., Evans, J., Fish, J., & Wilson, B. A. (2009). Alleviation of carer strain during the use of the NeuroPage device by people with acquired brain injury. *Journal of Neurology, Neurosurgery, and Psychiatry, 80,* 781–783. http://dx.doi.org/10.1136/jnnp.2008.162966

Terrace, H. S. (1963). Discrimination learning with and without "errors." *Journal of the Experimental Analysis of Behavior, 6,* 1–27. http://dx.doi.org/10.1901/jeab.1963.6-1

Tinson, D. J., & Lincoln, N. B. (1987). Subjective memory impairment after stroke. *International Disability Studies, 9,* 6–9. http://dx.doi.org/10.3109/02599148709166217

Toglia, J. P. (1989). Visual perception of objects: An approach to assessment and intervention. *American Journal of Occupational Therapy, 43,* 587–595. http://dx.doi.org/10.5014/ajot.43.9.587

Toglia, J. P. (1993). *Contextual Memory Test.* Tucson, AZ: Therapy Skill Builders.

Toglia, J. P., Johnston, M. V., Góverover, Y., & Dain, B. (2010). A multicontext approach to promoting transfer of strategy use and self regulation after brain injury: An exploratory study. *Brain Injury, 24,* 664–677. http://dx.doi.org/10.3109/02699051003610474

Tulving, E. (1983). *Elements of episodic memory.* Oxford, England: Clarendon Press.

van Heugten, C. M., Dekker, J., Deelman, B. G., Stehmann-Saris, J. C., & Kinebanian, A. (1999). Assessment of disabilities in stroke patients with apraxia: Internal consistency and inter-observer reliability. *OTJR: Occupation, Participation and Health, 19,* 55–73.

van Heugten, C. M., Dekker, J., Deelman, B. G., van Dijk, A., Stehmann Saris, J. C., & Kinebanian, A. (1998). Outcome of strategy training in stroke patients with apraxia: A phase II study. *Clinical Rehabilitation, 12,* 294–303. http://dx.doi.org/10.1191/026921598674468328

van Heugten, C. M., Dekker, J., Deelman, B. G., van Dijk, A., Stehmann Saris, J. C., & Kinebanian, A. (2000). Measuring disabilities in stroke patients with apraxia: A validation of an observational method. *Neuropsychological Rehabilitation, 10,* 401–414. http://dx.doi.org/10.1080/096020100411989

Volle, E., Gonen-Yaacovi, G., Costello Ade, L., Gilbert, S. J., & Burgess, P. W. (2011). The role of rostral prefrontal cortex in prospective memory: A voxel-based lesion study. *Neuropsychologia, 49,* 2185–2198. http://dx.doi.org/10.1016/j.neuropsychologia.2011.02.045

Wade, D. T., Parker, V., & Langton Hewer, R. (1986). Memory disturbance after stroke: Frequency and associated losses. *International Rehabilitation Medicine, 8,* 60–64.

Walker, C. M., Sunderland, A., Sharma, J., & Walker, M. F. (2004). The impact of cognitive impairment on upper body dressing difficulties after stroke: A video analysis of patterns of recovery. *Journal of Neurology, Neurosurgery, and Psychiatry, 75,* 43–48. http://dx.doi.org/10.1136/jnnp.2003.035071

Wechsler, D. (2009). *Wechsler Memory Scale–Fourth Edition (WMS–IV) technical and interpretive manual.* San Antonio: Pearson.

Wernicke, C. (1874). *Der aphasische symptomenkomplex: Eine psychologische studie auf anatomisher basis* [The aphasic symptom complex: A psychological study from an anatomical basis]. Breslau, Germany: Cohn & Weigart.

West, C., Bowen, A., Hesketh, A., & Vail, A. (2008). Interventions for motor apraxia following stroke. *Cochrane Database of Systematic Reviews, 2008,* CD004132. http://dx.doi.org/10.1002/14651858.CD004132.pub2

Whyte, J. (1986). Outcome evaluation in the remediation of attention and memory deficits. *Journal of Head Trauma Rehabilitation, 1,* 64–71. http://dx.doi.org/10.1097/00001199-198609000-00010

Wilson, B. A. (1991). Long-term prognosis of patients with severe memory disorders. *Neuropsychological Rehabilitation, 1,* 117–134. http://dx.doi.org/10.1080/09602019108401386

Wilson, B. A., Alderman, N., Burgess, A. W., Emslie, H., & Evans, J. J. (1996). *Behavioral Assessment of the Dysexecutive Syndrome.* Bury St. Edmunds, England: Thames Valley Test Company.

Wilson, B. A., Baddeley, A., Evans, J. J., & Shiel, A. (1994). Errorless learning in the rehabilitation of memory impaired people. *Neuropsychological Rehabilitation, 4,* 307–326.

Wilson, B. A., Clare, E., Baddeley, A. D., Cockburn, J., Watson, P., & Tate, R. (1999). *The Rivermead Behavioural Memory Test–Extended version.* London: Pearson Assessment.

Wilson, B. A., Cockburn, J., & Baddeley, A. D. (1991). *The Rivermead Behavioral Memory Test.* Bury St. Edmunds, England: Thames Valley Test Company.

Wilson, B. A., Cockburn, J., & Baddeley, A. D. (2003). *The Rivermead Behavioural Memory Test* (2nd ed.). London: Pearson Assessment.

Wilson, B. A., Cockburn, J., & Halligan, P. W. (1987). *Behavioral Inattention Test: Manual.* London: Thames Valley Test Company.

Wilson, B. A., Gracey, F., Malley, D., Bateman, A., & Evans, J. J. (2009). The Oliver Zangwill Centre approach to neuropsychological rehabilitation. In B. A. Wilson, F. Gracey, J. J. Evans, & A. Bateman (Eds.), *Neuropsychological rehabilitation: Theory, models, therapy, and outcome* (pp. 47–67). Cambridge, England: Cambridge University Press.

Wilson, B. A., Greenfield, E., Clare, E., Baddeley, A. D., Cockburn, J., Watson, P., & Nannery, R. (2008). *The Rivermead Behavioural Memory Test* (3rd ed.). London: Pearson Assessment.

Wilson, B. A., Scott, H., Evans, J., & Emslie, H. (2003). Preliminary report of a NeuroPage service within a health care system. *NeuroRehabilitation, 18,* 3–8.

Wolf, T. J., Baum, C. M., & Connor, L. T. (2009). Changing face of stroke: Implications for occupational therapy practice. *American Journal of Occupational Therapy, 63,* 621–625. http://dx.doi.org/10.5014/ajot.63.5.621

Yin, H. H., & Knowlton, B. J. (2006). The role of the basal ganglia in habit formation. *Nature, 7,* 464–476. http://dx.doi.org/10.1038/nm1919

Zoccolotti, P., Antonucci, G., & Judica, A. (1992). Psychometric characteristics of two semi-structured scales for the functional evaluation of hemi-inattention in extra-personal space. *Neuropsychological Rehabilitation, 2,* 179–191.

Zoccolotti, P., Antonucci, G., Judica, A., Montenero, P., Pizzamiglio, L., & Razzano, C. (1989). Incidence and evolution of the hemineglect disorder in chronic patients with unilateral right brain damage. *International Journal of Neuroscience, 47,* 209–216. http://dx.doi.org/10.3109/00207458908987435

Zoccolotti, P., Cantagallo, A., De Luca, M., Guariglia, C., Serino, A., & Trojano, L. (2011). Selective and integrated rehabilitation programs for disturbances of visual/spatial attention and executive function after brain damage: A neuropsychological evidence-based review. *European Journal of Physical and Rehabilitation Medicine, 47,* 123–147.

Zoltan, B. (2007). *Vision, perception, and cognition: A manual for the evaluation and treatment of the adult with acquired brain injury* (4th ed.). Thorofare, NJ: Slack.

CHAPTER 8

Core Concepts in Emotional Regulation and Psychosocial Issues After Stroke

Ganesh Muneshwar Babulal, MOT, OTR/L, and Lisa Tabor Connor, PhD, MSOT

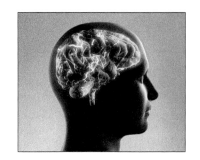

Learning Objectives

After completion of this chapter, readers will be able to

- Identify the components of emotions and how resulting common psychosocial issues are a product of the emotion process;
- Delineate the relationships among the constructs of emotion, cognition, and emotional dysregulation;
- Delineate the key features among common types of emotional consequences after stroke;
- Identify the use of specific screening instruments for clients with mood disorders; and
- Recognize the role of mediating factors and mechanisms of emotional control in clients with stroke.

Key Words

- **cognition**
- **emotion**
- **emotional consequences**
- **emotional regulation**
- **mediators**
- **screening instruments**
- **social support**

Introduction

Emotions are salient in everyday life and, at the same time, they are complex, multidimensional phenomena that elude a simple definition. Emotions are typically perceived as serving both positive and negative functions. Positive emotions may inform people that their goals are met, they are satisfied, and they have control; negative emotions may indicate that all is not well or that a disturbance needs to be addressed (Dalgleish & Bramham, 1999). Numerous psychological and cognitive theories of emotions have elucidated the purpose, function, and organization of emotions in the brain. Prominent theories have characterized emotion as biological and evolutionary, as socially constructed cues, as physiological responses, and as cognitive appraisal of events (Dalgleish, 2004; Fox, 2008). Despite differences in theoretical characterization, the ultimate goal is to understand human behavior and the role of emotions in healthy people and how they change during illness and in disease states.

Despite differences in theoretical characterization, the ultimate goal is to understand human behavior and the role of emotions in healthy people and how they change during illness and in disease states.

We do not explore these theories in detail, but we draw on common concepts found in many theories. Emotion may be conceived of and described through four pragmatic approaches: (1) general language (descriptions or phrases), (2) self-report (subjective or lived experience), (3) behavior (objective or observed), and (4) physiology (vital signs or brain imaging; Ortony, Clore, & Collins, 1988). Each approach provides a different perspective on emotions; as a result, it may be confusing to overlap two or more methods to describe and research emotion. Hence, it is important for therapists and researchers to understand which method or perspective is being used when discussing emotion.

Scientific Perspective on Emotion

A brief review of emotion from psychology and **neuroscience** perspectives follows, with information about how emotion is conceptualized from the perspective of emotion science. We present a description of the nature of interactions between emotion and cognition.

Historical Account of Emotion

Previously, emotion was not studied or researched with the scientific rigor applied to research on cognition. Concepts in cognitive neuroscience such as memories, thoughts, and opinions were conceived as clear and unequivocal, whereas emotional constituents were deemed too subjective and difficult to operationalize; thus, cognition and emotion were studied independently (Dalgleish & Power, 1999; Lane, Nadel, & Ahern, 2000). More recent paradigm shifts in cognitive neuroscience have argued that not only do emotion and cognition share some of the same circuitry in the brain, but it is difficult to fractionate and study them separately (Pessoa, 2008). For example, cognitive operations such as attention, memory, and decision making are guided and modulated by emotions during everyday activities. Conversely, how one feels about something is influenced by one's goals, focus of attention, and ability to recall facts or events; as a result of this interaction between emotion and cognition, new research is working to explore how this relationship unfolds during everyday activities (Fox, 2008). Additionally, emotional regulation is conceptualized to be dependent on overlapping emotive and cognitive processes, so it is crucial for practitioners to understand the components of each concept, its roles, and the overall impact on performance and participation (Gross, Sheppes, & Urry, 2011). We briefly look at the constituents of the emotion–cognition system and propose a theoretical framework to summarize their relationship to each other and in neurorehabilitation.

Emotion and Interrelated Constituents

The construct of emotion is often presented as vague, especially when concepts such as feelings, moods, or attitudes are used interchangeably to describe the phenomena. We briefly define each term to differentiate them and demonstrate their relationship to each other.

Emotion is a brief episode triggered by an event or object that causes global change in the brain, body, and behavior; *mood* is a general state of lesser intensity and of more prolonged duration that can be caused by an emotion; *feeling* is the internal, subjective mental representation of the emotion; and *attitude* is a pervasive affective stance or preference for an event or object (Dalgleish, 2000; Davidson, Jackson, & Kalin, 2000; Fox, 2008). To illustrate these concepts, take, for example, a 26-year-old male college student who had a hemorrhagic stroke, resulting in mild hemiparesis in the right upper extremity. The onset of the stroke immediately produced the emotions of fear and surprise, which subsided after a few hours; he experienced depressed and anxious moods several months after the stroke; he reported feeling lonely and sad about his hemiparesis and is hesitant to go out in public; finally, he reported his attitude toward personal health has changed, and he wants to exercise and eat more nutritious meals to prevent another stroke.

Although it is easy to substitute one term for another, it is important to be able to distinguish each concept and its role in the construct of emotion. Emotions and moods are commonly encountered in rehabilitation and are the most difficult to separate; emotions are the products of a process (e.g., sadness) and are short in intensity, whereas moods are the long-term representation of emotions (e.g., depression). It is critical for therapists to understand the domain they are probing in the emotive process when inquiring about how a client may feel.

Defining the process (or processes) by which emotions arise is complicated because of their varying intensity (happiness: passing a final exam vs. winning the lottery). However, the main constituents of emotion are agreed on. The emotion process can be divided into two constituents, (1) generation and (2) regulation, and the entire process is governed by five components: (1) appraisal (cognitive), (2) bodily changes (physiological), (3) preparation for action (motivational), (4) execution of action (motor expression), and (5) emotional experience (subjective). All critical elements are posited to operate independently; however, they synchronize and function concertedly for the brief episode of an emotion (Fox, 2008; Gross et al., 2011). The process of generating emotions occurs when some event or object has meaning in a specific context to a person's goals, irrespective of whether the person is consciously aware or not (Fox, 2008). Once attention is directed to an event or object, physiological changes are expressed in the body via the sympathetic and parasympathetic nervous systems. As the person continues to attend to the event or object, goals are formed either consciously or subconsciously to act in response to it. Then motoric expression occurs on the basis of the operationalized goals to interact with the event or object. Finally, the person's internal experience of the emotion and feeling occurs, and at this point, the shift from emotion generation to regulation occurs.

A common misconception is that emotion generation and regulation are two independent entities. However, they rely on interdependent processes (Gross et al., 2011). *Emotion regulation* often refers to **antecedent**-based regulation (acting before an event can trigger an emotion) or response-based regulation (acting after an event triggers an emotion). Both strategies involve attention, selection, and some behavior output (Gyurak, Goodkind, Kramer, Miller, & Levenson, 2012). Five different stages identify how a person may regulate his or her emotion (see Figure 8.1): (1) *situation selection,* choosing a situation to increase or decrease the prospect of an emotion occurring; (2) *situation modification,* changing some aspect of the situation to affect emotion; (3) *attentional deployment,* choosing to focus attention on parts of a situation; (4) *cognitive change,* changing cognitive appraisal of a situation; and (5) *response modification,* changing some aspect of the emotion response mechanism after an event has occurred (Gross et al., 2011).

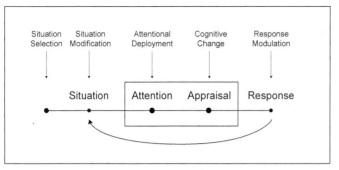

Figure 8.1. A process model of emotion regulation that highlights five families of emotional regulation strategies.

Source. From "Cognition and Emotion Lecture at the 2010 SPSP Emotion Preconference," by J. J. Gross, G. Sheppes, and H. L. Urry, 2011, *Cognition and Emotion, 25,* p. 768. Copyright © 2011 by Taylor & Francis. Reprinted with permission.

In everyday life, most people are able to maintain their emotional generation and regulation in homeostasis. However, this balance can easily become disrupted and difficult to detect by clinicians in the event of mood disorders, trauma, chronic disease, and neurological disorders such as **stroke.**

To instantiate these concepts, let's look at an example of a client who is recovering from alcohol use disorder (per the fifth edition of the *Diagnostic and Statistical Manual of Mental Disorders,* or *DSM–5;* American Psychiatric Association [APA], 2013) and using strategies to maintain sobriety when going to a restaurant with friends who do drink. She starts by avoiding triggers such as bars or liquor stores (situation selection); when eating out with friends in a restaurant where alcohol is served, she sits away from the bar (situation modification); if her friends order drinks, she attends to the conversation instead of the drinks (attentional deployment); she limits blaming herself or past choices by thinking about the positive changes sobriety will make in her life (cognitive change); and she verbally declines an alcoholic beverage when asked by the server (response modulation).

In everyday life, most people are able to maintain their emotional generation and regulation in homeostasis. However, this balance can easily become disrupted and difficult to detect by clinicians in the event of mood disorders, trauma, chronic disease, and neurological disorders such as **stroke.** So, if the client mentioned above experiences a stroke, she may have newfound difficulty controlling the cognitive and emotive components required to effectively regulate her emotions and thus may have difficulty maintaining sobriety.

Cognitive Constituents

Cognition, that is, one's set of thinking abilities and skills, is often conceptualized as including the components of memory, attention, executive functioning (planning and decision making), and language. ***Memory*** is the encoding, storing, and retrieving of information; ***attention*** involves deploying cognitive resources to something in the environment and inhibiting irrelevant information to complete a task; ***executive functions*** are the higher mental processes that serve goal formation and maintenance, planning, and decision making; and *language* consists of communication and comprehension of written and verbal information (Connor & Maeir, 2011; Radomski & Latham, 2008). A review of imaging studies argued that cortical and **subcortical** structures are integrated in both emotive and cognitive domains. The **amygdala** (responsible for fear-based processing) is involved in attention and associative learning; the ventromedial **prefrontal cortex** and anterior cingulate cortex (responsible for decision making) are involved in processing emotions; and the hypothalamus (responsible for hormone production) is involved in goal-directed behavior (Pessoa, 2008). Neural circuitry of various brain structures affects cognitive processing of attention, perception, and memory and has an integral role in the experience of emotions; it would be problematic to separate feeling and thinking without considering their dependent roles (Barrett, Mesquita, Ochsner, & Gross, 2007). As discussed, it is critical to view cognition and emotion as integrated components of a larger system rather than as two completely independent systems.

Impact of Cognition and Emotion on Participation

Participation is an important goal for rehabilitation, and understanding how emotion and cognition support participation may provide new avenues for treatment that improves the client's ability to participate in valued occupations after illness or injury. It has been reported that at least 50% of people with stroke will experience significant emotive and cognitive changes lasting a minimum of 3 to 12 months poststroke; some of these changes may persist years poststroke (Hochstenbach, Anderson, van Limbeek, & Mulder, 2001; Hochstenbach, Prigatano, & Mulder, 2005; Visser-Keizer, Meyboom-de Jong, Deelman, Berg, & Gerritsen, 2002). Additionally, clients will need to learn how to accept and adjust to these changes because of their strong influence on everyday activities. Briefly, the concept of participation has gained recognition and interest in disability advocacy, social policy, and rehabilitation and among stakeholders, including scientists, researchers, health care professionals, and educators.

The *International Classification of Functioning, Disability and Health* has defined *participation* as "involvement in a life situation" (World Health Organization [WHO], 2001, p. 10). This definition is generally accepted as encompassing, which has led to its widespread use. In rehabilitation, some consensus exists on factors that may be integral to participation. These factors include choice, control, access, meaning, inclusivity, and social connectedness (Hammel et al., 2008). In a study that assessed participation during rehabilitation, disability poststroke, presence of depression, and executive function impairments were found to be significant factors influencing participation (Skidmore et al., 2010). Participation in self-chosen meaningful activities is the driving force impelling how clients structure their lives after stroke and is the foundation of how therapists should structure therapy.

Figure 8.2 displays a theoretical framework elaborating on participation, emotion, and cognition (PEC) and the interaction among these constructs. Note the two outer circles, one labeled *environment* and one labeled *time*. Within the environment circle are three overlapping circles representing three internal factors (emotion, cognition, participation); they are in the foreground of the external factors (environment and time) because they do not exist in a vacuum. The environment includes both built and natural dimensions, social support, policy, and technology, and it influences how one feels, thinks, and acts. Additionally, everything is captured in the domain of time, which contains an infinite number of past, present, and future events.

To illustrate the utility of this framework, consider the example of two clients. Mr. Jones and Mr. Anderson each had a stroke and have similar profiles of impairment and prior occupational histories. Both are White and 56 years old, have comparable annual income as corporate executives, have a strong social support network, and are being treated by the same therapist in a rehabilitation institution. Mr. Jones presents with low

Participation is an important goal for rehabilitation, and understanding how emotion and cognition support participation may provide new avenues for treatment that improves the client's ability to participate in valued occupations after illness or injury.

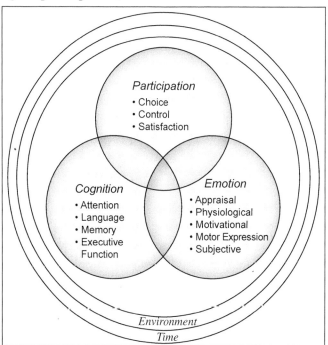

Figure 8.2. Participation–emotion–cognition theoretical framework highlighting the interaction among these internal factors.

Points to Ponder: Approaching Clients Recovering From a Stroke

On the basis of the PEC framework, how would you explain the relationships among emotion, cognition, and participation and their overall impact on recovery for Mr. Jones and Mr. Anderson? If disruption in the emotion domain continues, how should an occupational therapist address it in therapy?

motivation, continually doubts himself, ruminates on past decisions and lifestyle, and demonstrates little effort in his therapy. In contrast, Mr. Anderson is motivated, demonstrates maximal efforts in therapy despite failures and near falls, is optimistic, and wants to return to his work. As a result, Mr. Jones experiences poorer performance, a longer recovery stay in rehabilitation, and becomes very depressed and stressed. Mr. Anderson was discharged earlier to his home, reports feeling content despite the stroke, and returned to work on a gradual schedule. Occupational therapists see clients with similar conditions, age, race, ethnicity, and social class and might ponder why some do better than others. This framework is an attempt to depict and better understand the relationships among cognition, emotion, and participation.

Emotional Dysregulation: Expressing and Comprehending Emotion

In this section, we describe both common and uncommon sequelae affecting expression and comprehension of emotion, including symptomatology and prevalence. We discuss emotional lability, comprehension of emotion in others, and comprehension of emotion through speech.

Expression: Emotional Lability

Generation and regulation of emotions occur at the subjective level, often without conscious awareness. Disruptions in both processes are associated with commonly known mood disorders such as bipolar disorder. **Emotional lability,** also known as *pseudobulbar affect, labile affect,* or *emotional incontinence,* is a common disorder seen poststroke (Tang et al., 2009). It is a neurological syndrome that is characterized by uncontrollable emotional expressions of excessive or spontaneous crying or laughing. It is typically observed in neurological conditions such as stroke or traumatic brain injury (Work, Colamonico, Bradley, & Kaye, 2011). Emotional lability is a specific phenomenon that occurs after a stroke and is not typically associated with major depression, poststroke depression, or feeling sad. Rather, emotions may start or stop abruptly and may be triggered by thoughts of the stroke, the person's body, or family, and people report having no control over their expression (House, Dennis, Molyneux, Warlow, & Hawton, 1989). Clinically, people with stroke often report feeling a loss of control over their internal emotions and how they are expressed in the presence of others.

Although the specific mechanisms and lesion locations are unclear, emotional lability is deemed a natural biological consequence of stroke rather than a psychological disorder (Morris, Robinson, & Raphael, 1993). Nearly half of people with stroke will experience some form of emotional lability; 40% will experience significant interferences in social activities owing to emotional lability, and the condition may last for several weeks up to a few years (National Stroke Association [NSA], 2011; Tang et al., 2009). This form of emotional expression is often a source of embarrassment because of its unpredictable nature. It is important for therapists to recognize and address this poststroke sequela with family members to help them understand it. Typically, an experienced neurologist or physiatrist will recognize the symptoms and accurately diagnose the disorder.

Comprehension of Emotions in Others

Emotions have a variety of purposes, including serving as a biological awareness aid for survival, as internal cues for motivation, as an external window into how one feels internally, and as a means of social communication (Fox, 2008). Comprehending emotions in others is a cornerstone of social communication, building relationships, and interacting in the community. Typically, comprehension of another person's emotion may be obtained through verbal speech, facial expression, and body language. Facial expressions and body posturing provide insight into how a person might feel—a smile conveys happiness or contentment, and a frown conveys displeasure or sadness. These facial characteristics used to convey emotion are accepted as a universal norm because they are found in most cultures and races in the world (Ekman, 2003).

Deficits in emotional comprehension have been a research focus for decades because of their perplexing pathology and low prevalence. The presence of mood disorders and other emotional consequences poststroke provides a window into the disruption that occurs in the brain, resulting in emotional comprehension deficits. Less common diagnoses such as *aprosodia* (inability to express and comprehend emotional prosody in speech), *expressive **agnosia*** (inability to perceive facial expressions, body language, and vocal intonation), and *anosognosia* (diminished insight into disability or symptoms or neglecting loss of function) are some stroke sequelae that may result in comprehension disruptions (Annoni, Staub, Bruggimann, Gramigna, & Bogousslavsky, 2006). Right-hemisphere lesions have been implicated as leading to a range of misunderstood emotions and perceived indifference by the person with stroke to others (Harciarek, Heilman, & Jodzio, 2006).

Prosody: Expression and Comprehension of Emotion Through Speech

Prosody "provides the melodic contour" (Myers, 1999, p. 73) of speech, conveying the emotional intent of the message through modulations of pitch, stress, and duration of speech sounds. Particularly after right-hemisphere stroke, prosodic production can be compromised (Ross, 1981; Ross & Monnot, 2008; Wertz, Henschel, Auther, Ashford, & Kirshner, 1998). The person with a right-hemisphere stroke with a prosodic production deficit sounds flat or monotone and may be limited to increasing volume to convey that he or she is angry. Comprehension of emotional prosody, too, can be compromised after right-hemisphere stroke (Ross, 1981; Ross & Monnot, 2008; Starkstein, Fedoroff, Price, Leiguarda, & Robinson, 1994). Comprehension aprosodia puts a patient in the position of not understanding the emotional content of others' speech; the patient will particularly have difficulty with understanding a message when it is spoken in an inconsistent tone of voice or is said sarcastically.

Although the production and comprehension of prosody may be impaired, little evidence has demonstrated that those with aprosodia are unable to experience the emotions that underlie the message. An experienced speech–language pathologist will test for production and comprehension aprosodias and may help distinguish them from psychiatric sequelae of stroke.

Emotional Consequences of Stroke

The physical consequences of stroke such as **hemiplegia** or **aphasia** are more salient and treatable than the emotional consequences. Emotional consequences or sequelae or mood disorders may not be as apparent, and failure to recognize them may impede rehabilitation and cause greater problems in reintegration back into the community (Hochstenbach et al., 2005). Typically, emotional changes experienced shortly (days

The physical consequences of stroke such as **hemiplegia** or **aphasia** are more salient and treatable than the emotional consequences. Emotional consequences or sequelae or mood disorders may not be as apparent, and failure to recognize them may impede rehabilitation and cause greater problems in reintegration back into the community.

to weeks) poststroke are considered biological or organic in nature as a response to the traumatic event. These may include feeling sad, feeling hopeless or helpless, being irritable, and experiencing changes in sleeping, eating, and thinking (House, 1987; House et al., 1991). However, when commonly experienced negative emotions persist for longer durations (from weeks to months), they are classified as *mood disorders*.

Disruptions of mood are present when the person has a deficit in regulating that specific mood over time; this then impairs the mood generation process, creating an imbalance that persists over time. Depression, anxiety, anger, or apathy are the most typical disorders after a stroke and tend to interfere with daily functioning. Thus, it is crucial to understand the role and import of those emotional disorders in stroke recovery and intervene as a part of a rehabilitation team.

Additionally, it is important for therapists to consider obtaining information from a variety of sources, including a clinical interview, medical chart, family or caregivers, objective observation, and client self-report screening measures. Because of the enduring nature of mood states, it is vital to assess and evaluate how a client is feeling at different time points over the course of rehabilitation. This assessment will serve to identify and address any problems, improve the efficacy of therapy, and enable the client to better reintegrate into the community.

Depression

Poststroke depression (PSD) is the most commonly reported mood disorder experienced at some time interval after stroke; the reported prevalence ranges from 33% to 66% irrespective of ischemic or hemorrhagic stroke (Hackett, Yapa, Parag, & Anderson, 2005; House et al., 1991). The course of PSD and symptoms vary with major and minor depression diagnoses. PSD often results in poor social outcomes, decreased functional or physical recovery (delay may be 1 to 2 years), decreased rehabilitation efficacy, poor quality of life, and impaired cognitive processing (Hama, Yamashita, Yamawaki, & Kurisu, 2011; Morris et al., 1993; Robinson-Smith & Pizzi, 2003). Although depression has a high incidence in the stroke population, PSD is also difficult to diagnose reliably because of the assessment challenges associated with self-report, cognitive impairments, pain, fatigue, emotional lability, and comorbidity with other mood disorders such as apathy and anosognosia.

According to *DSM–5,* the number of symptoms present and the duration of those symptoms over time are the important factors distinguishing between major and persistent depressive disorder (*dysthymia;* APA, 2013). The criteria for a major PSD diagnosis include having five or more symptoms (e.g., fatigue or loss of energy, insomnia or hypersomnia, thoughts of death or suicide, significant weight loss or gain, reduced ability to think) in a 2-week interval and a change in function, with one required symptom being either depressed mood or loss of interest. A diagnosis of dysthymia does not require the full criteria for major PSD, but the person must have at least two symptoms that persist for most of the day (APA, 2013). Clients with major PSD have a better prognosis than clients with dysthymia, with 75% resolution of symptoms 2 years poststroke; however, they have an increased likelihood of depression in an attenuated form persisting years after stroke as a result of conversion from major PSD to a minor form of depression (Chemerinski & Robinson, 2000).

Most important, people with PSD in early recovery have been noted to have 3 times greater risk of mortality 10 years after stroke than those without PSD (Morris et al., 1993). The variation in PSD and complexity in acquiring an accurate diagnosis make this emotional consequence of stroke critical to identify early on in the recovery process. Use of reliable and free depression screens such as the Patient Health Questionnaire–9 is a quick and valid way to obtain information about the number and severity of symptoms of depression a client may have (Spitzer, Kroenke, & Williams, 1999).

Points to Ponder: Collaborating With Other Disciplines to Manage Poststroke Emotional Consequences

The nursing staff suspect that a recently admitted client with stroke is depressed, and they are unsure how to proceed. From an occupational therapy perspective, what would be an appropriate first step to investigate their concerns?

- Speak with the client about nursing's concerns.
- Use an appropriate depression screen.
- Consult a psychologist or psychiatrist.
- Approach the client's family or caregivers regarding the concerns.
- Report the concerns to the attending physician.

Anxiety

Anxiety is defined as an overwhelming sense of worry or fear that may involve physical changes such as decreased energy and **concentration,** tachycardia, nausea, tense muscles, shortness of breath, and headache (NSA, 2006). Depression and anxiety tend to occur as comorbid consequences, not as a result of their similar symptomatology but rather because their diagnostic entities are not distinct (Morrison, Pollard, Johnston, & MacWalter, 2005; NSA, 2006). Poststroke anxiety (PSA) as both a symptom and a disorder (generalized anxiety disorder) has a prevalence range of 11% to 28%. It is associated with increased dependence in **activities of daily living** (ADLs) and decreased social support, with anxiety symptomatology persisting for as long as 3 years after the initial stroke (Aström, 1996; D'Alisa, Baudo, Mauro, & Miscio, 2005). As a result of PSA's co-occurrence with depression, PSA rates are projected to be higher than the current prevalence of depression. However, it is difficult to clearly delineate anxiety from depression (Leppävuori, Pohjasvaara, Vataja, Kaste, & Erkinjuntti, 2003). Younger clients (younger than age 59) and women tend to be more susceptible to PSA (Barker-Collo, 2007).

A recent longitudinal study assessed anxiety and depression at 5 years poststroke and found that 29% of the study population had anxiety at the 5-year mark, and anxiety at 6 months significantly predicted anxiety at 5 years (Lincoln et al., 2013). People with stroke encounter numerous barriers (fatigue, sleeplessness, pain) during rehabilitation; PSA diminishes a person's ability to take an active role in his or her rehabilitation. As a result, clients with anxiety may be reluctant about or even refuse therapy. This makes it even more important for therapists to screen for symptoms of anxiety. Screens such as the State–Trait Anxiety Inventory assess two types of anxiety—state anxiety and trait anxiety—to provide information about how anxious a client is at the moment of assessment and compare it with how anxious the client feels in general daily life (Spielberger, Gorsuch, Lushene, Vagg, & Jacobs, 1983).

Anger

Anger is a sparsely researched emotional consequence of stroke and may include explosive outbursts, decreased impulse control, increased irritability, hostility, insult, derogatory remarks, and reactive aggression. An important distinction is that between *instrumental anger* (delayed response with a desired, planned goal of revenge or retaliation) and *reactive anger* (immediate response to a negative, threatening, or fearful event; Scarpa & Raine, 1997). The prevalence of people with stroke who experience reactive anger has been estimated at 35%, with 37% of those being categorized as having intense aggression (Santos, Caeiro, Ferro, Albuquerque, & Luísa Figueira, 2006). Anger has also been shown to co-occur with emotional lability and, to a smaller degree, with PSD (Kim, Choi, Kwon, & Seo, 2002).

Anger can be construed as a normative emotional reaction and a healthy coping skill when it is controlled and deemed appropriate with respect to an external event (House, 1987). It is challenging to parse out whether anger was a premorbid personality trait because stroke does not directly cause anger but may trigger it as a reaction to perceived threats in the environment or an inability to complete a task (Santos et al., 2006). Anger becomes a barrier in rehabilitation when it creates stressful dynamics among the client, family, therapists, and caregivers; it disturbs the process of functional recovery and may result in the client abandoning efforts to complete a task. It is relatively easier to discern anger and hostility in acute and postacute phases of stroke recovery; however, it is crucial for therapists to use empathy and positive guiding strategies to redirect attention and efforts to tasks that encourage functional performance. A quick and valid screen such as the Spielberger State–Trait Anger Scale is an efficient way to gather information and address the potential triggers for a client's anger (Spielberger, Jacobs, Russell, & Crane, 1983), especially if the client perceives anger as getting in the way of therapeutic progress.

> Anger becomes a barrier in rehabilitation when it creates stressful dynamics among the client, family, therapists, and caregivers; it disturbs the process of functional recovery and may result in the client abandoning efforts to complete a task.

Apathy and Consequences for Motivation

Apathy is reduction in motivation or lack of initiation (Starkstein, Fedoroff, Price, Leiguarda, & Robinson, 1993), and it often co-occurs with PSD, although it may appear alone (Caeiro, Ferro, & Figueira, 2012; Withall, Brodaty, Altendorf, & Sachdev, 2011). Apathy has a negative impact on rehabilitation because it limits the degree to which patients actively engage in therapy. Moreover, apathy is associated with poor stroke outcome (Caeiro et al., 2012). Mayo, Fellows, Scott, Cameron, and Wood-Dauphinee (2009) conducted a study with more than 400 patients with stroke and followed them at 1, 3, 6, and 12 months poststroke to determine the rate and persistence of apathy according to caregivers. Half of the patients had low apathy scores throughout the follow-up period, but 3% had high apathy scores that remained high, and 33% had elevated scores (classified as minor apathy) that remained elevated throughout the follow-up. Apathy was associated with poor cognition, low functional status, and an increased number of comorbidities. Most important, increases in apathy, even minor increases, had a negative impact on physical function, participation, and perceptions of health status (Mayo et al., 2009).

One of the challenges in measuring apathy is that many assessment tools rely on proxy respondents (see Knapp & Hewison, 1999), either family members or clinicians (such as in the Mayo et al., 2009, study). In a study by Hama et al. (2007)

with 237 patients with stroke, depression and anxiety symptoms were evaluated by both the patient (with the Zung Self-Rating Depression Scale [Zung, 1965] and the Apathy Scale [Starkstein et al., 1993]) and through a semistructured interview with a caregiver (the Neuropsychiatric Inventory; Cummings et al., 1994). Depression was observed in 31.6% of the patients using self-report but in 40.2% using the proxy report. Apathy was found in 40.1% using the self-report measure, but in only 19.2% using the proxy report.

Self-reported apathy, in fact, negatively correlated with improvement on the **FIM™** (Uniform Data System for Medical Rehabilitation, 1997), whereas self-reported depressive symptoms did not. In Hama et al.'s (2007) study, proxy reports of depression and apathy failed to predict FIM improvement. Thus, it appears that self-report measures of apathy are more tightly coupled with changes in functional recovery during rehabilitation than are proxy reports or self-reported PSD and ought to be probed by rehabilitation professionals. Accordingly, in the Mayo et al. (2009) study, apathy symptoms may have been underreported by caregivers, and the importance of apathy to functional recovery underestimated. Use of the self-report version of the Apathy Evaluation Scale may help clinicians to understand patients' apathy status better (see Marin, Biedrzycki, & Firinciogullari, 1991).

Anosognosia

Equal in impact to apathy for its devastating effect on recovery and participation in rehabilitation activities is the unawareness of one's cognitive, emotional, or physical deficits after stroke, termed ***anosognosia*** (Orfei, Caltagirone, & Spalletta, 2009; Ramachandran, 1995). Although Ramachandran (1995) restricted his definition to denial of physical deficits, we use the term more broadly. Anosognosia is more common after right-hemisphere stroke and often co-occurs with visuospatial neglect (Visser-Keizer et al., 2002). Anosognosia is not a general lack of awareness, as is commonly discussed in the traumatic brain injury literature (see Crosson et al., 1989), but rather a lack of appreciation of stroke-related deficits in cognition, emotion, or physical function.

A salient example of anosognosia is the patient who denies that his hemiparetic limb is his own, despite evidence to the contrary (Ramachandran, 1995). The patient may say that someone is in bed with him or her, may deny that the arm is his or her own, may attempt to throw it out of bed, or may claim that it belongs to the examiner. We, among others (Vuilleumier, 2004), argue, however, that anosognosia can extend beyond impaired awareness of physical deficits to cognitive and emotive consequences of stroke, that is, explicit verbal denial of the presence of impairment or disease that may extend to denial of cognitive or emotive impairment.

In fact, some have argued that distinct and dissociable forms of anosognosia exist (see Jehkonen, Ahonen, Dastidar, Laippala, & Vilkki, 2000; Spalletta et al., 2007). Visser-Keizer et al. (2002) conducted a study examining the extent to which patients and their caregivers agreed on the existence of and severity of cognitive and emotional deficits after stroke. Those with right-hemisphere lesions had significant discrepancies with their caregivers' reports of both the existence and severity of cognitive and emotional deficits 3 months after stroke compared with those with left-hemisphere lesions. A ***discrepancy score*** is the standard method of rating lack of awareness as a difference between the client and either the caregiver or the clinician. The discrepancy reported by Visser-Keizer et al. was not related to greater caregiver burden or the extent to which the patients with right-hemisphere lesions had greater cognitive deficits than those with left-hemisphere lesions. The conclusion drawn by Visser-Keizer et al. is that anosognosia was the likely source of discrepancy between patients and caregivers in their awareness of the presence and severity of cognitive and emotional impairments after stroke.

Although few treatment options for anosognosia are available, knowledge of its presence and education of family and other staff members regarding anosognosia may reduce the frustration surrounding the patient's apparent lack of participation in rehabilitation or lack of appreciation of his or her deficits. Unfortunately, a single measure of anosognosia that captures its multidimensional nature does not yet exist (see Orfei et al., 2009, for a review and discussion of this issue). Several measures tap aspects of anosognosia, for example, the Structured Awareness Interview (Marcel, Tegnér, & Nimmo-Smith, 2004), the Patient Competency Rating Scale (Prigatano et al., 1986), the Self-Awareness of Deficit Interview (Fleming, Strong, & Ashton, 1996), and the Awareness Questionnaire (Sherer, Bergloff, Boake, High, & Levin, 1998). Knowledge of the specific targets of these tools is essential when choosing the most relevant dimensions on which to measure a patient's awareness of deficit.

In terms of treatment of anosognosia, few large-scale studies have been conducted, although several studies with fewer patients have been reported. Two types of approaches have been reported: (1) vestibular stimulation (e.g., Cappa, Sterzi, Vallar, & Bisiach, 1987; Ronchi et al., 2013) and (2) awareness training (e.g., Fotopoulou, Rudd, Holmes, & Kopelman, 2009; Youngjohn & Altman, 1989). Vestibular stimulation studies have found inconsistent remission of anosognosia from patient to patient with short-term remission reported for responders.

Awareness training studies, too, have reported inconsistent results in remission of anosognosia. In an intervention in a mixed group of survivors of traumatic brain injury and stroke, Youngjohn and Altman (1989) reported that participants in an awareness group improved in their ability to make performance predictions for memory recall and the ability to do math problems both from one attempt to the next within a treatment session and from one session to the next. Limited generalization to everyday tasks, such as predictions about driving ability, was noted.

Fotopoulou et al. (2009) reported more dramatic results in a single case study of a patient with severe and long-lasting (22 days) anosognosia for hemiparesis. The patient was shown a 90-second video clip of herself answering questions about her hemiparesis and attempting to move her hemiparetic limb. Instantly and permanently, the patient regained insight into her deficit.

Although studies have been conducted on awareness training in people with traumatic brain injury, clearly more work needs to be done to examine awareness training in people with anosognosia after stroke. The Fotopoulou et al. approach may be a particularly promising one; improving awareness through video training may increase clients' ability to participate in rehabilitation and may improve long-term outcome (Hartman-Maeir, Soroker, Oman, & Katz, 2003).

Psychosocial Implications: Mediators and Modulators of Emotional Control

In this section, we provide common mediators and modulators of emotional control poststroke. These include personality, self-esteem, self-efficacy, coping, social support, and participation.

Psychological Constituents of Emotional Regulation

Psychological constituents of emotional regulation include prestroke personality, self-esteem, and self-efficacy.

Prestroke Personality

The Five-Factor Model of Personality was developed over the past 3 decades to understand questions about motivation, aging, and individual personality differences. The five domains include (1) Openness, (2) Conscientiousness, (3) Extraversion, (4) Agreeableness, and (5) Neuroticism (Costa, Fagan, Piedmont, Ponticas, & Wise, 1992). Moreover, each domain is defined by six related facets to capture and reflect the broadest dimensions of that specific trait. For example, *neuroticism* is defined by anxiety, angry hostility, depression, self-consciousness, impulsiveness, and vulnerability. A person is assessed on each of the five traits and then receives a score for each trait in an ordinal range (e.g., ranging from *very low* to *very high*) to construct a personality profile.

Several studies have investigated and determined how prestroke personality traits (neuroticism, extraversion, openness, agreeableness, and conscientiousness) play a role in the presence of mood disorders in poststroke recovery. One study found that high neuroticism and low agreeableness were significantly related to the presence of agitation and irritability in patients and distress in caregivers 3 months poststroke (Greenop, Almeida, Hankey, van Bockxmeer, & Lautenschlager, 2009). Numerous studies have concluded that high scores on the Neuroticism domain significantly correlate with the presence of depression poststroke (Janssen et al., 2010; Knaut, Subramanian, McFadyen, Bourbonnais, & Levin, 2009). Moreover, high neuroticism poststroke is also associated with 2 to 5 times the risk of depression, and the presence of depression or anxiety prestroke is associated with 8 times the risk of PSD (Storor & Byrne, 2006).

These studies illustrate that prestroke personality should be taken into account along with stroke sequelae because personality serves as an important predictor for mood disorders after stroke. Personality is a part of identity and is typically constant throughout the lifespan. However, a stroke directly affects and can alter personality as a result of the changes in emotions, cognition, and physical abilities. The use of the NEO Five-Factor Inventory, Short Form, is an efficient method to determine how a client's personality varies on each of the five scales (Costa et al., 1992). The information may be used to understand which personality scale has a stronger propensity to co-occur with other mood disorders.

> **Prestroke personality should be taken into account along with stroke sequelae because personality serves as an important predictor for mood disorders after stroke.**

Self-Esteem and Self-Efficacy

Self-esteem and **self-efficacy** are often used synonymously to explain the motivational domain of a person's life. Hence, it is important to understand the distinction between each concept as it relates to rehabilitation. *Self-esteem* is a person's appraisal of his or her self-worth and typically contains beliefs about the self; it may also consist of the need for respect from others and need for self-respect (Fox, 2008; Heatherton & Polivy, 1991). This traditional psychological concept is not static and changes throughout the lifespan. Additionally, it can be depicted on a continuum with polar opposites, where a person may be characterized as having high or low self-esteem.

Various life events, however, may have an impact on a person's self-esteem; a traumatic event such as stroke may affect a person's self-worth. People with more severe stroke and resulting **functional impairments** such as aphasia or hemiparesis typically report low self-esteem from hospital admission to as much as 3 months poststroke; level of self-esteem has been a consistent predictor of functional recovery after stroke (Chang & Mackenzie, 1998). Low self-esteem has been correlated with increased frequency of depression and anxiety, lower cognitive functioning, and poor functional mobility and self-care in clients discharged to the community (Vickery, Sepehri, Evans, & Jabeen, 2009).

Because self-esteem is intimately tied into motivation and self-appraisal, it is important to recognize its role in rehabilitation. Practitioners can gain insight into a client's self-esteem with simple questions about how the client is feeling about a specific situation and the self. This information may assist in interventions to help raise low self-esteem, empower the client, and facilitate productive therapy. A quick and free measure is the State Self-Esteem Scale, which assesses how the person is feeling at the moment and may offer insight into the impact of stroke and recovery on the person's self-esteem (Heatherton & Polivy, 1991).

Self-efficacy is a person's belief in his or her functional capabilities to perform as required to influence how events affect his or her life. Four sources support self-efficacy: (1) mastery (successful completion of a task or challenge strengthens self-efficacy, whereas failure at a task weakens it); (2) social modeling (seeing others complete a task fortifies a person's belief in his or her ability to complete a task); (3) social persuasion (verbal encouragement or discouragement has an impact on a person's belief in his or her ability to complete a task); and (4) somatic or emotional states (emotions, as do mood and feelings, and **stress** have an impact on a person's belief in his or her ability to complete a task at any time; Bandura, 1977; Bandura, Barbaranelli, Caprara, & Pastorelli, 1996).

Self-efficacy is a central concept for rehabilitation because it describes particular ways in which a person is able to self-motivate, feel, think, and interact with his or her environment. For example, a client with stroke who has low self-efficacy may doubt his or her ability to do a task in therapy, ruminate on life decisions, have low energy, and feel sad, which may result in poorer performance, longer recovery rate, and depression or stress. Contrast this with a client with high self-efficacy who may have a greater resiliency to stress and a shorter recovery period and make stronger efforts, despite failures.

In rehabilitation, studies focusing on self-efficacy have demonstrated that clients with a high sense of self-efficacy after stroke have shorter stays in therapy, have larger increases in functional recovery, and self-report higher quality of life poststroke (Korpershoek, van der Bijl, & Hafsteinsdóttir, 2011). Therapists can affect a client's self-esteem and self-efficacy by providing feedback and strong encouragement, creating opportunities to model success, setting realistic and time-sensitive goals for task completion, and mediating the emotion regulation process to reframe failures and negative emotions as modular components of the rehabilitation process (Brown, Stoffel, & Munoz, 2011).

In summary, self-efficacy and self-esteem are internal subjective processes that encompass perception, thinking, planning, and action. Both concepts are integral in emotional and cognitive domains to ultimately promote successful rehabilitation for people with stroke.

Social Support

Other potential mediators and modulators of emotional control include the person's response to loss and coping style and the extent to which family and extended network are able to support the person with stroke in his or her recovery. A key recovery outcome that depends on these personal and environmental factors is the person's ability to participate in meaningful occupations and to resume roles and responsibilities.

Loss, Grief, and Coping

A stroke is a sudden, traumatic event that often leaves physical, cognitive, and emotive consequences for the client and his or her social support network to manage. As with any traumatic event, there is a loss of self, and the situation requires the client to engage a **coping** mechanism. A radical disruption in identity occurs that may be attributed to a loss of skills, roles, or physical abilities that were core to the client's sense of self (e.g., being a writer, provider, mother). The grief accompanying the loss leaves the client vulnerable to emotional disorders (Mukherjee, Levin, & Heller, 2006).

To maximize the benefit of rehabilitation, the client needs to acknowledge the stroke, understand its repercussions, and accept at least the temporary loss of the previous abilities and occupations. Moreover, it is important for practitioners to acknowledge that a significant life event has occurred and provide assistance in the adjustment process. Because no two strokes are identical, however, the brain lesion location, extent of damage, personality, culture of the client, social support, and resulting cognitive, emotional, and physical functions poststroke all contribute to the degree of adjustment after stroke (Mukherjee et al., 2006).

Finset and Andersson (2000) examined the relationship among coping styles, depression, apathy, and brain lesion in people with brain injury, including stroke. They found that people with brain injury had two dimensions of coping, as did age-matched controls. Although healthy adults demonstrated primarily an approach-oriented coping style (actively attempting to overcome obstacles) or an avoidance-oriented coping style (ignoring or denying obstacles), people with brain injury showed a correlation between coping styles. Moreover, those whose coping style was primarily avoidant tended to be depressed. Those who lacked a specific coping style tended to be apathetic. Although coping styles were not related to lesion location, apathy was related to subcortical and right-hemisphere lesions. Rochette, Bravo, Desrosiers, St.-Cyr Tribble, and Bourget (2007) reported that coping styles measured within weeks of stroke, as assessed with a modified version of the Ways of Coping Questionnaire (Folkman & Lazarus, 1988), predicted a significant proportion of the variance in participation at 6 months poststroke.

More recently, Donnellan, Hevey, Hickey, and O'Neill (2006) reviewed the literature on coping strategies poststroke, pointing out that most studies were not firmly grounded in a theoretical model of coping, that many coping instruments without known psychometric properties are being used to study coping styles, and that results from these studies have been inconsistent. Clearly, more development work needs to be done in this area of research to help practitioners understand the mechanisms of psychological coping after stroke. The loss of identity and associated grief reaction is a complex process with continuing adjustment potentially lasting months or years poststroke. Practitioners are uniquely positioned to assist the client through this process, even though the science of coping lags behind the need for answers in clinical practice.

Social Support and Recovery

In addition to the person-centered characteristics such as coping that a client brings to bear on the recovery process, the social environment is an important contributor to emotional well-being and the extent of recovery. Friedland and McColl (1987) pointed out that social support could buffer the negative psychosocial consequences of stroke. Glass, Matchar, Belyea, and Feussner (1993) found, in fact, that social support is an important and measurable contributor to functional recovery. In their study, participants were followed 6 months after stroke and were measured in terms of their stroke severity, social support, and functional status (as measured by the Barthel Index [Mahoney & Barthel, 1965]). Participants with the most severe stroke and the greatest social support showed the most improvement over time in functional status. Specifically, those with high levels of emotional support showed the most improvement in functional status. Those with moderate levels of instrumental support, that is, physical support with chores and routines, also showed improvements in functional recovery (Glass & Maddox, 1992).

This pattern was replicated and extended in a more recent study (Tsouna-Hadjis, Vemmos, Zakopoulos, & Stamatelopoulos, 2000) that reported additionally that those with higher levels of social support were also less depressed at 6 months after onset. An interesting finding, however, is that attempts to conduct social support intervention trials targeting family members of people with stroke have been unsuccessful (Friedland & McColl, 1992).

In the larger domain of social support interventions, however, some evidence has been found for their efficacy (see review by Hogan, Linden, and Najarian, 2002), but methodological issues prevent strong statements about the best form of social support intervention (groups vs. individual approaches, professionally led vs. peer led, or social skills training vs. larger social networks). Why these methods have not been successful with people with stroke and their families remains to be understood.

Participation

The ultimate goal of stroke rehabilitation is to return people to their former lives, enabling them to participate fully in the activities that they need and want to do and to resume their roles and responsibilities.

Of course, the ultimate goal of stroke rehabilitation is to return people to their former lives, enabling them to participate fully in the activities that they need and want to do and to resume their roles and responsibilities. Regardless of whether they are able to accomplish this in precisely the same way as before the stroke, "involvement in . . . life situation[s]"—the *International Classification of Functioning, Disability and Health's* definition of *participation* (WHO, 2001, p. 10)—is, or should be, the desired outcome of rehabilitation services (e.g., Desrosiers et al., 2003). Emotional consequences of stroke—depression, anxiety, apathy, and anger—can contribute to less-than-optimal participation outcomes. Several studies have documented the negative impact that depression has on participation postrehabilitation, but very few studies have included apathy, anxiety, or anger as predictors of participation. In some of these studies, depression was examined as an outcome of stroke rather than as a predictor of participation (e.g., Rochette et al., 2007).

To document participation restrictions poststroke, Mayo, Wood-Dauphinee, Côté, Durcan, and Carlton (2002) followed more than 400 people with stroke at 6-month intervals via a telephone survey. At 6 months poststroke, more than 50% of community-dwelling people reported restrictions in accomplishing housework and shopping independently, 53% reported not having a meaningful activity to fill the day, and 65% reported restrictions in reintegrating into community activities. In a multiple regression analysis, ability to accomplish ADLs and **instrumental activities of daily living** (IADLs) and the extent to which participants were able to reintegrate into the community were all significant predictors of mental health–related quality of life.

Similarly, Hartman-Maeir, Soroker, Ring, Avni, and Katz (2007) reported that participation was quite low in an Israeli sample that was followed 1 year poststroke, with 50% of the sample requiring assistance in ADLs and more than 70% requiring assistance in IADLs. Using the Activity Card Sort (Baum & Edwards, 2001), Hartman-Maeir et al. determined that people had retained less than 43% of their prestroke activities and were generally dissatisfied with their life situation (based on the Life Satisfaction Questionnaire (Fugl-Meyer, Branholm, & Fugl-Meyer, 1991). Moreover, only 24% of participants reported no depressive symptoms, 45% scored in the suspected depression range of the Geriatric Depression Scale (Yesavage et al., 1982), and 31% were in the probable depression range. In this study, depression score was controlled to examine the impact that activity participation had on life satisfaction, but a large proportion of the variance in life satisfaction was, indeed, accounted for by depression score. Likewise, Desrosiers et al. (2006) examined predictors of long-term participation (2 to 4 years poststroke) and found that age, motor function, upper-extremity function, and depression score on the Beck Depression Inventory (Beck, Ward, Mendelson, Mock, & Erbaugh, 1961) were significant predictors of participation.

A single study (D'Alisa et al., 2005) has examined both depression and anxiety as predictors of participation. In this study, 73 participants from a community rehabilitation program were evaluated many years poststroke for depression and anxiety with the Hospital Anxiety and Depression Scale (Zigmond & Snaith, 1983), and participation was measured with the London Handicap Scale (Harwood, Roger, Dickinson, & Ebrahim, 1994). The primary result of this study was that occupation restriction (both work and **leisure** activities) was related to physical limitations and to both depression and anxiety. Moreover, depression predicted restrictions in social integration. Thus, mood symptoms have a negative relationship with participation and social functioning, even in people who are many years beyond their stroke.

Conclusion

The process of generation and regulation of emotions has significant consequences for performance and participation in daily life. This is particularly evident in stroke and recovery after stroke. We introduced a broad overview of the historical account of emotions, the relationship between emotion and cognition, and the resulting influence of emotion and cognition on participation. The main focus of this chapter was on types of emotional dysregulation and common mood disorders seen after stroke. We described several screening tools for each mood disorder; however, it is important to know that numerous other tools are available for screening and confirming diagnosis of a mood disorder. Finally, in the last portion of the chapter we

Box 8.1. Clinical Vignettes: Mr. Rodriguez and Ms. Yokahama

Mr. Rodriguez is a 63-year-old man who is an inpatient at Excellent Rehab hospital in his hometown. He had a right-hemisphere stroke 10 days earlier, and he has significant left facial droop, left arm and leg hemiparesis, and visuospatial neglect on the left.

Mr. Rodriguez is quite pleasant during the clinical evaluation but does not understand why he is in the rehabilitation hospital. He is certain that he will be just fine and reassures you that he just needs to go home because he will do much better there. When he rises from his chair, he stumbles and nearly falls. He does not comprehend what is wrong with his leg. The nurses report that he bumps into things on the left without really noticing. He is quite adamant that nothing is wrong with him. In fact, the more you press him with the evidence that he is not attending to things on the left, showing him the bumps and cuts on his left arm, the more angry and agitated he becomes.

Mr. Rodriguez's family is very upset. They cannot seem to get him to understand that he has had a stroke and has significant difficulties taking care of himself. They are worried about him returning home by himself. How will he bathe and dress himself, cook, manage his finances, take his medications, and go shopping?

Ms. Yokahama is a 75-year-old woman in the next room at Excellent Rehab hospital. She had a right-hemisphere stroke 2 weeks ago. She has significant left hemiparesis. She does not cooperate with the staff at the rehab facility. She spends a good portion of her day crying. She refuses to participate in rehabilitation. She does not want to get dressed or eat her meals. It is difficult to motivate her to do anything.

Some questions to consider are as follows: How might the staff at Excellent Rehab hospital evaluate the emotional states of these clients? How might the emotional consequences of stroke have an impact on the rehabilitation plan for these patients? What are the likely long-term outcomes of these patients in terms of their abilities to function at home and participate in their previous activities and roles?

discussed potential mediators of emotional control and regulation and additional screening tools to assess each mediator.

To provide the opportunity to reflect on how these critical concepts have an impact on caring for and supporting clients that you may see after stroke, we provide clinical vignettes with some guiding questions in Box 8.1. Research in emotional control has resulted in a better understanding of how this normal process is disrupted in stroke. Future research is needed to explore the effects of emotional control on long-term stroke recovery and participation for chronic survivors.

References

American Psychiatric Association. (2013). *Diagnostic and statistical manual of mental disorders* (5th ed.). Arlington, VA: Author.

Annoni, J.-M., Staub, F., Bruggimann, L., Gramigna, S., & Bogousslavsky, J. (2006). Emotional disturbances after stroke. *Clinical and Experimental Hypertension, 28,* 243–249. http://dx.doi.org/10.1080/10641960600549173

Aström, M. (1996). Generalized anxiety disorder in stroke patients: A 3-year longitudinal study. *Stroke, 27,* 270–275. http://dx.doi.org/10.1161/01.STR.27.2.270

Bandura, A. (1977). Self-efficacy: Toward a unifying theory of behavioral change. *Psychological Review, 84,* 191–215. http://dx.doi.org/10.1037/0033-295X.84.2.191

Bandura, A., Barbaranelli, C., Caprara, G. V., & Pastorelli, C. (1996). Multifaceted impact of self-efficacy beliefs on academic functioning. *Child Development, 67,* 1206–1222. http://dx.doi.org/10.2307/1131888

Barker-Collo, S. L. (2007). Depression and anxiety 3 months post stroke: Prevalence and correlates. *Archives of Clinical Neuropsychology, 22,* 519–531. http://dx.doi.org/10.1016/j.acn.2007.03.002

Barrett, L. F., Mesquita, B., Ochsner, K. N., & Gross, J. J. (2007). The experience of emotion. *Annual Review of Psychology, 58,* 373–403. http://dx.doi.org/10.1146/annurev.psych.58.110405.085709

Baum, C. M., & Edwards, D. (2001). *Activity Card Sort test manual.* St. Louis: Penultima Press.

Beck, A. T., Ward, C. H., Mendelson, M., Mock, J., & Erbaugh, J. (1961). An inventory for measuring depression. *Archives of General Psychiatry, 4,* 561–571. http://dx.doi.org/10.1001/archpsyc.1961.01710120031004

Brown, C., Stoffel, V., & Munoz, J. P. (2011). *Occupational therapy in mental health: A vision for participation.* Philadelphia: F. A. Davis.

Caeiro, L., Ferro, J. M., & Figueira, M. L. (2012). Apathy in acute stroke patients. *European Journal of Neurology, 19,* 291–297. http://dx.doi.org/10.1111/j.1468-1331.2011.03508.x

Cappa, S., Sterzi, R., Vallar, G., & Bisiach, E. (1987). Remission of hemineglect and anosognosia during vestibular stimulation. *Neuropsychologia, 25,* 775–782. http://dx.doi.org/10.1016/0028-3932(87)90115-1

Chang, A. M., & Mackenzie, A. E. (1998). State self-esteem following stroke. *Stroke, 29,* 2325–2328. http://dx.doi.org/10.1161/01.STR.29.11.2325

Chemerinski, E., & Robinson, R. G. (2000). The neuropsychiatry of stroke. *Psychosomatics, 41,* 5–14. http://dx.doi.org/10.1016/S0033-3182(00)71168-6

Connor, L. T., & Maeir, A. (2011). Putting executive performance in a theoretical context. *OTJR: Occupation, Participation and Health, 31,* S3–S7. http://dx.doi.org/10.3928/15394492-20101108-02

Costa, P. T., Jr., Fagan, P. J., Piedmont, R. L., Ponticas, Y., & Wise, T. N. (1992). The Five-Factor Model of Personality and Sexual Functioning in outpatient men and women. *Psychiatry in Medicine, 10,* 199–215.

Crosson, B. A., Barco, P. P., Velozo, C., Bolesta, M. M., Cooper, P. V., Werts, D., & Brobeck, T. C. (1989). Awareness and compensation in postacute head injury rehabilitation. *Journal of Head Trauma Rehabilitation, 4,* 46–54. http://dx.doi.org/10.1097/00001199-198909000-00008

Cummings, J. L., Mega, M., Gray, K., Rosenberg-Thompson, S., Carusi, D. A., & Gornbein, J. (1994). The Neuropsychiatric Inventory: Comprehensive assessment of psychopathology in dementia. *Neurology, 44,* 2308–2314. http://dx.doi.org/10.1212/WNL.44.12.2308

Dalgleish, T. (2000). Roads not taken: The case for multiple functional-level routes to emotion. *Behavioral and Brain Sciences, 23,* 196–197. http://dx.doi.org/10.1017/S0140525X00272427

Dalgleish, T. (2004). The emotional brain. *Nature Reviews Neuroscience, 5,* 583–589. http://dx.doi.org/10.1038/nrn1432

Dalgleish, T., & Bramham, J. (1999). Cognitive perspective. In D. Levinson, J. James, J. Ponzetti, & P. F. Jorgensen (Eds.), *Encyclopedia of human emotions* (pp. 118–121). New York: Macmillan.

Dalgleish, T., & Power, M. J. (1999). *Handbook of cognition and emotion* (pp. 21–45). Chichester, England: Wiley.

D'Alisa, S., Baudo, S., Mauro, A., & Miscio, G. (2005). How does stroke restrict participation in long-term post-stroke survivors? *Acta Neurologica Scandinavica, 112,* 157–162. http://dx.doi.org/10.1111/j.1600-0404.2005.00466.x

Davidson, R. J., Jackson, D. C., & Kalin, N. H. (2000). Emotion, plasticity, context, and regulation: Perspectives from affective neuroscience. *Psychological Bulletin, 126,* 890–909. http://dx.doi.org/10.1037/0033-2909.126.6.890

Desrosiers, J., Noreau, L., Rochette, A., Bourbonnais, D., Bravo, G., & Bourget, A. (2006). Predictors of long-term participation after stroke. *Disability and Rehabilitation, 28,* 221–230. http://dx.doi.org/10.1080/09638280500158372

Desrosiers, J., Rochette, A., Noreau, L., Bravo, G., Hébert, R., & Boutin, C. (2003). Comparison of two functional independence scales with a participation measure in post-stroke rehabilitation. *Archives of Gerontology and Geriatrics, 37,* 157–172. http://dx.doi.org/10.1016/S0167-4943(03)00044-X

Donnellan, C., Hevey, D., Hickey, A., & O'Neill, D. (2006). Defining and quantifying coping strategies after stroke: A review. *Journal of Neurology, Neurosurgery, and Psychiatry, 77,* 1208–1218. http://dx.doi.org/10.1136/jnnp.2005.085670

Ekman, P. (2003). *Emotions revealed: Recognizing faces and feelings to improve communication and emotional life* (pp. 17–38). New York: Henry Holt.

Finset, A., & Andersson, S. (2000). Coping strategies in patients with acquired brain injury: Relationships between coping, apathy, depression, and lesion location. *Brain Injury, 14,* 887–905. http://dx.doi.org/10.1080/026990500445718

Fleming, J. M., Strong, J., & Ashton, R. (1996). Self-awareness of deficits in adults with traumatic brain injury: How best to measure? *Brain Injury, 10,* 1–15. http://dx.doi.org/10.1080/026990596124674

Folkman, S., & Lazarus, R. S. (1988). *Manual for the Ways of Coping Questionnaire.* Mountain View, CA: Consulting Psychologists Press.

Fotopoulou, A., Rudd, A., Holmes, P., & Kopelman, M. (2009). Self-observation reinstates motor awareness in anosognosia for hemiplegia. *Neuropsychologia, 47,* 1256–1260. http://dx.doi.org/10.1016/j.neuropsychologia.2009.01.018

Fox, E. (2008). *Emotion science: Cognitive and neuroscientific approaches to understanding human emotions.* Basingstoke, England: Palgrave Macmillan.

Friedland, J. F., & McColl, M. (1987). Social support and psychosocial dysfunction after stroke: Buffering effects in a community sample. *Archives of Physical Medicine and Rehabilitation, 68,* 475–480.

Friedland, J. F., & McColl, M. (1992). Social support intervention after stroke: Results of a randomized trial. *Archives of Physical Medicine and Rehabilitation, 73,* 573–581.

Fugl-Meyer, A. R., Branholm, I. B., & Fugl-Meyer, K. S. (1991). Happiness and domain-specific life satisfaction in adult northern Swedes. *Clinical Rehabilitation, 5,* 25–33. http://dx.doi.org/10.1177/026921559100500105

Glass, T. A., & Maddox, G. L. (1992). The quality and quantity of social support: Stroke recovery as psycho-social transition. *Social Science and Medicine, 34,* 1249–1261. http://dx.doi.org/10.1016/0277-9536(92)90317-J

Glass, T. A., Matchar, D. B., Belyea, M., & Feussner, J. R. (1993). Impact of social support on outcome in first stroke. *Stroke, 24,* 64–70. http://dx.doi.org/10.1161/01.STR.24.1.64

Greenop, K. R., Almeida, O. P., Hankey, G. J., van Bockxmeer, F., & Lautenschlager, N. T. (2009). Premorbid personality traits are associated with post-stroke behavioral and psychological symptoms: A three-month follow-up study in Perth, Western Australia. *International Psychogeriatrics, 21,* 1063–1071. http://dx.doi.org/10.1017/S1041610209990457

Gross, J. J., Sheppes, G., & Urry, H. L. (2011). Cognition and Emotion Lecture at the 2010 SPSP Emotion Preconference. *Cognition and Emotion, 25,* 765–781. http://dx.doi.org/10.1080/02699931.2011.555753

Gyurak, A., Goodkind, M. S., Kramer, J. H., Miller, B. L., & Levenson, R. W. (2012). Executive functions and the down-regulation and up-regulation of emotion. *Cognition and Emotion, 26,* 103–118. http://dx.doi.org/10.1080/02699931.2011.557291

Hackett, M. L., Yapa, C., Parag, V., & Anderson, C. S. (2005). Frequency of depression after stroke: A systematic review of observational studies. *Stroke, 36,* 1330–1340. http://dx.doi.org/10.1161/01.STR.0000165928.19135.35

Hama, S., Yamashita, H., Shigenobu, M., Watanabe, A., Hiramoto, K., Kurisu, K., . . . Kitaoka, T. (2007). Depression or apathy and functional recovery after stroke. *International Journal of Geriatric Psychiatry, 22,* 1046–1051. http://dx.doi.org/10.1002/gps.1866

Hama, S., Yamashita, H., Yamawaki, S., & Kurisu, K. (2011). Post-stroke depression and apathy: Interactions between functional recovery, lesion location, and emotional response. *Psychogeriatrics, 11,* 68–76. http://dx.doi.org/10.1111/j.1479-8301.2011.00358.x

Hammel, J., Magasi, S., Heinemann, A., Whiteneck, G., Bogner, J., & Rodriguez, E. (2008). What does participation mean? An insider perspective from people with disabilities. *Disability and Rehabilitation, 30,* 1445–1460. http://dx.doi.org/10.1080/09638280701625534

Harciarek, M., Heilman, K. M., & Jodzio, K. (2006). Defective comprehension of emotional faces and prosody as a result of right hemisphere stroke: Modality versus emotion-type specificity. *Journal of the International Neuropsychological Society, 12,* 774–781. http://dx.doi.org/10.1017/S1355617706061121

Hartman-Maeir, A., Soroker, N., Oman, S. D., & Katz, N. (2003). Awareness of disabilities in stroke rehabilitation—A clinical trial. *Disability and Rehabilitation, 25,* 35–44. http://dx.doi.org/10.1080/0963828021000007897

Hartman-Maeir, A., Soroker, N., Ring, H., Avni, N., & Katz, N. (2007). Activities, participation and satisfaction one-year post stroke. *Disability and Rehabilitation, 29,* 559–566. http://dx.doi.org/10.1080/09638280600924996

Harwood, R. H., Roger, A., Dickinson, E., & Ebrahim, S. (1994). Measuring handicap: The London Handicap Scale, a new outcome measure for chronic disease. *Quality and Safety in Health Care, 3,* 11–16. http://dx.doi.org/10.1136/qshc.3.1.11

Heatherton, T., & Polivy, J. (1991). Development and validation of a scale for measuring state self-esteem. *Journal of Personality and Social Psychology, 60,* 895–910. http://dx.doi.org/10.1037/0022-3514.60.6.895

Hochstenbach, J., Anderson, P. G., van Limbeek, J., & Mulder, T. T. (2001). Is there a relation between neuropsychologic variables and quality of life after stroke? *Archives of Physical Medicine and Rehabilitation, 82,* 1360–1366. http://dx.doi.org/10.1053/apmr.2001.25970

Hochstenbach, J., Prigatano, G., & Mulder, T. (2005). Patients' and relatives' reports of disturbances 9 months after stroke: Subjective changes in physical functioning, cognition, emotion, and behavior. *Archives of Physical Medicine and Rehabilitation, 86,* 1587–1593. http://dx.doi.org/10.1016/j.apmr.2004.11.050

Hogan, B. E., Linden, W., & Najarian, B. (2002). Social support interventions: Do they work? *Clinical Psychology Review, 22,* 381–442. http://dx.doi.org/10.1016/S0272-7358(01)00102-7

House, A. (1987). Mood disorders after stroke: A review of the evidence. *International Journal of Geriatric Psychiatry, 2,* 211–221. http://dx.doi.org/10.1002/gps.930020403

House, A., Dennis, M., Mogridge, L., Warlow, C., Hawton, K., & Jones, L. (1991). Mood disorders in the year after first stroke. *British Journal of Psychiatry, 158,* 83–92. http://dx.doi.org/10.1192/bjp.158.1.83

House, A., Dennis, M., Molyneux, A., Warlow, C., & Hawton, K. (1989). Emotionalism after stroke. *BMJ, 298,* 991–994. http://dx.doi.org/10.1136/bmj.298.6679.991

Janssen, H., Bernhardt, J., Collier, J. M., Sena, E. S., McElduff, P., Attia, J., . . . Spratt, N. J. (2010). An enriched environment improves sensorimotor function post-ischemic stroke. *Neurorehabilitation and Neural Repair, 24,* 802–813. http://dx.doi.org/10.1177/1545968310372092

Jehkonen, M., Ahonen, J.-P., Dastidar, P., Laippala, P., & Vilkki, J. (2000). Unawareness of deficits after right hemisphere stroke: Double-dissociations of anosognosias. *Acta Neurologica Scandinavica, 102,* 378–384. http://dx.doi.org/10.1034/j.1600-0404.2000.102006378.x

Kim, J. S., Choi, S., Kwon, S. U., & Seo, Y. S. (2002). Inability to control anger or aggression after stroke. *Neurology, 58,* 1106–1108. http://dx.doi.org/10.1212/WNL.58.7.1106

Knapp, P., & Hewison, J. (1999). Disagreement in patient and carer assessment of functional abilities after stroke. *Stroke, 30,* 934–938. http://dx.doi.org/10.1161/01.STR.30.5.934

Knaut, L. A., Subramanian, S. K., McFadyen, B. J., Bourbonnais, D., & Levin, M. F. (2009). Kinematics of pointing movements made in a virtual versus a physical 3-dimensional environment in healthy and stroke subjects. *Archives of Physical Medicine and Rehabilitation, 90,* 793–802. http://dx.doi.org/10.1016/j.apmr.2008.10.030

Korpershoek, C., van der Bijl, J., & Hafsteinsdóttir, T. B. (2011). Self-efficacy and its influence on recovery of patients with stroke: A systematic review. *Journal of Advanced Nursing, 67,* 1876–1894. http://dx.doi.org/10.1111/j.1365-2648.2011.05659.x

Lane, R. D., Nadel, L., & Ahern, G. (2000). *Cognitive neuroscience of emotion.* New York: Oxford University Press.

Leppävuori, A., Pohjasvaara, T., Vataja, R., Kaste, M., & Erkinjuntti, T. (2003). Generalized anxiety disorders three to four months after ischemic stroke. *Cerebrovascular Diseases, 16,* 257–264. http://dx.doi.org/10.1159/000071125

Lincoln, N. B., Brinkmann, N., Cunningham, S., Dejaeger, E., De Weerdt, W., Jenni, W., & De Wit, L. (2013). Anxiety and depression after stroke: A 5 year follow-up. *Disability and Rehabilitation, 35,* 140–145. http://dx.doi.org/10.3109/09638288.2012.691939

Mahoney, F. I., & Barthel, D. W. (1965). Functional evaluation: The Barthel Index. *Maryland State Medical Journal, 14,* 61–65.

Marcel, A. J., Tegnér, R., & Nimmo-Smith, I. (2004). Anosognosia for plegia: Specificity, extension, partiality and disunity of bodily unawareness. *Cortex, 40,* 19–40. http://dx.doi.org/10.1016/S0010-9452(08)70919-5

Marin, R. S., Biedrzycki, R. C., & Firinciogullari, S. (1991). Reliability and validity of the Apathy Evaluation Scale. *Psychiatry Research, 38,* 143–162. http://dx.doi.org/10.1016/0165-1781(91)90040-V

Mayo, N. E., Fellows, L. K., Scott, S. C., Cameron, J., & Wood-Dauphinee, S. (2009). A longitudinal view of apathy and its impact after stroke. *Stroke, 40,* 3299–3307. http://dx.doi.org/10.1161/STROKEAHA.109.554410

Mayo, N. E., Wood-Dauphinee, S., Côté, R., Durcan, L., & Carlton, J. (2002). Activity, participation, and quality of life 6 months poststroke. *Archives of Physical Medicine and Rehabilitation, 83,* 1035–1042. http://dx.doi.org/10.1053/apmr.2002.33984

Morris, P. L., Robinson, R. G., & Raphael, B. (1993). Emotional lability after stroke. *Australian and New Zealand Journal of Psychiatry, 27,* 601–605. http://dx.doi.org/10.3109/00048679309075822

Morrison, V., Pollard, B., Johnston, M., & MacWalter, R. (2005). Anxiety and depression 3 years following stroke: Demographic, clinical, and psychological predictors. *Journal of Psychosomatic Research, 59,* 209–213. http://dx.doi.org/10.1016/j.jpsychores.2005.02.019

Mukherjee, D., Levin, R. L., & Heller, W. (2006). The cognitive, emotional, and social sequelae of stroke: Psychological and ethical concerns in post-stroke adaptation. *Topics in Stroke Rehabilitation, 13,* 26–35. http://dx.doi.org/10.1310/tsr1304-26

Myers, P. S. (1999). *Right hemisphere damage: Disorders of communication and cognition.* San Diego: Singular.

National Stroke Association. (2006). *Recovery after stroke: Coping with emotions.* Retrieved from http://www.stroke.org/site/DocServer/NSAFactSheet_Emotions.pdf?docID=990

National Stroke Association. (2011). *Pseudobulbar affect.* Retrieved from http://www.stroke.org/site/PageServer?pagename=PBA

Orfei, M. D., Caltagirone, C., & Spalletta, G. (2009). The evaluation of anosognosia in stroke patients. *Cerebrovascular Diseases, 27,* 280–289. http://dx.doi.org/10.1159/000199466

Ortony, A., Clore, G. L., & Collins, A. (1988). *The cognitive structure of emotions.* Cambridge, England: Cambridge University Press.

Pessoa, L. (2008). On the relationship between emotion and cognition. *Nature Reviews Neuroscience, 9,* 148–158. http://dx.doi.org/10.1038/nrn2317

Prigatano, G. P., Fordyce, D. J., Zeiner, H. K., Roueche, J. R., Pepping, M., & Wood, B. C. (1986). *Neuropsychological rehabilitation after brain injury.* Baltimore: Johns Hopkins University Press.

Radomski, M. V., & Latham, T. C. (Eds.). (2008). *Occupational therapy for physical dysfunction* (6th ed.). Philadelphia: Lippincott Williams & Wilkins.

Ramachandran, V. S. (1995). Anosognosia in parietal lobe syndrome. *Consciousness and Cognition, 4,* 22–51. http://dx.doi.org/10.1006/ccog.1995.1002

Robinson-Smith, G., & Pizzi, E. R. (2003). Maximizing stroke recovery using patient self-care self-efficacy. *Rehabilitation Nursing, 28,* 48–51. http://dx.doi.org/10.1002/j.2048-7940.2003.tb02028.x

Rochette, A., Bravo, G., Desrosiers, J., St.-Cyr Tribble, D., & Bourget, A. (2007). Adaptation process, participation and depression over six months in first-stroke individuals and spouses. *Clinical Rehabilitation, 21,* 554–562. http://dx.doi.org/10.1177/0269215507073490

Ronchi, R., Rode, G., Cotton, F., Farnè, A., Rossetti, Y., & Jacquin-Courtois, S. (2013). Remission of anosognosia for right hemiplegia and neglect after caloric vestibular stimulation. *Restorative Neurology and Neuroscience, 31,* 19–24. http://dx.doi.org/10.3233/RNN-120236

Ross, E. D. (1981). The aprosodias: Functional–anatomic organization of the affective components of language in the right hemisphere. *Archives of Neurology, 38,* 561–569. http://dx.doi.org/10.1001/archneur.1981.00510090055006

Ross, E. D., & Monnot, M. (2008). Neurology of affective prosody and its functional–anatomic organization in right hemisphere. *Brain and Language, 104,* 51–74. http://dx.doi.org/10.1016/j.bandl.2007.04.007

Santos, C. O., Caeiro, L., Ferro, J. M., Albuquerque, R., & Luísa Figueira, M. (2006). Anger, hostility, and aggression in the first days of acute stroke. *European Journal of Neurology, 13,* 351–358. http://dx.doi.org/10.1111/j.1468-1331.2006.01242.x

Scarpa, A., & Raine, A. (1997). Psychophysiology of anger and violent behavior. *Psychiatric Clinics of North America, 20,* 375–394. http://dx.doi.org/10.1016/S0193-953X(05)70318-X

Sherer, M., Bergloff, P., Boake, C., High, W., Jr., & Levin, E. (1998). The Awareness Questionnaire: Factor structure and internal consistency. *Brain Injury, 12,* 63–68. http://dx.doi.org/10.1080/026990598122863

Skidmore, E. R., Whyte, E. M., Holm, M. B., Becker, J. T., Butters, M. A., Dew, M. A., . . . Lenze, E. J. (2010). Cognitive and affective predictors of rehabilitation participation after stroke. *Archives of Physical Medicine and Rehabilitation, 91,* 203–207. http://dx.doi.org/10.1016/j.apmr.2009.10.026

Spalletta, G., Serra, L., Fadda, L., Ripa, A., Bria, P., & Caltagirone, C. (2007). Unawareness of motor impairment and emotions in right hemispheric stroke: A preliminary investigation. *International Journal of Geriatric Psychiatry, 22,* 1241–1246. http://dx.doi.org/10.1002/gps.1822

Spielberger, C. D., Gorsuch, R. L., Lushene, R., Vagg, P. R., & Jacobs, G. A. (1983). *Manual for the State–Trait Anxiety Inventory.* Palo Alto, CA: Consulting Psychologists Press.

Spielberger, C. D., Jacobs, G., Russell, S., & Crane, R. S. (1983). Assessment of anger: The State–Trait Anger Scale. In J. N. Butcher & C. Spielberger (Eds.), *Advances in personality assessment* (Vol. 2, pp. 161–189). Hillsdale, NJ: Erlbaum.

Spitzer, R. L., Kroenke, K., & Williams, J. B. (1999). Validation and utility of a self-report version of PRIME–MD: The PHQ primary care study. Primary Care Evaluation of Mental Disorders. Patient Health Questionnaire. *JAMA, 282,* 1737–1744. http://dx.doi.org/10.1001/jama.282.18.1737

Starkstein, S. E., Fedoroff, J. P., Price, T. R., Leiguarda, R. C., & Robinson, R. G. (1993). Apathy following cerebrovascular lesions. *Stroke, 24,* 1625–1630. http://dx.doi.org/10.1161/01.STR.24.11.1625

Starkstein, S. E., Fedoroff, J. P., Price, T. R., Leiguarda, R. C., & Robinson, R. G. (1994). Neuropsychological and neuroradiologic correlates of emotional prosody comprehension. *Neurology, 44,* 515–522. http://dx.doi.org/10.1212/WNL.44.3_Part_1.515

Storor, D. L., & Byrne, G. J. (2006). Pre-morbid personality and depression following stroke. *International Psychogeriatrics, 18,* 457–469. http://dx.doi.org/10.1017/S1041610206003188

Tang, W. K., Chen, Y. K., Lu, J. Y., Mok, V. C., Xiang, Y. T., Ungvari, G. S., . . . Wong, K. S. (2009). Microbleeds and post-stroke emotional lability. *Journal of Neurology, Neurosurgery, and Psychiatry, 80,* 1082–1086. http://dx.doi.org/10.1136/jnnp.2009.175372

Tsouna-Hadjis, E., Vemmos, K. N., Zakopoulos, N., & Stamatelopoulos, S. (2000). First-stroke recovery process: The role of family social support. *Archives of Physical Medicine and Rehabilitation, 81,* 881–887. http://dx.doi.org/10.1053/apmr.2000.4435

Uniform Data System for Medical Rehabilitation. (1997). *Guide for the Uniform Data Set for Medical Rehabilitation (including the FIM™ instrument), version 5.1.* Buffalo, NY: Author.

Vickery, C. D., Sepehri, A., Evans, C. C., & Jabeen, L. N. (2009). Self-esteem level and stability, admission functional status, and depressive symptoms in acute inpatient stroke rehabilitation. *Rehabilitation Psychology, 54,* 432–439. http://dx.doi.org/10.1037/a0017752

Visser-Keizer, A. C., Meyboom-de Jong, B., Deelman, B. G., Berg, I. J., & Gerritsen, M. J. (2002). Subjective changes in emotion, cognition and behaviour after stroke: Factors affecting the perception of patients and partners. *Journal of Clinical and Experimental Neuropsychology, 24,* 1032–1045. http://dx.doi.org/10.1076/jcen.24.8.1032.8383

Vuilleumier, P. (2004). Anosognosia: The neurology of beliefs and uncertainties. *Cortex, 40,* 9–17. http://dx.doi.org/10.1016/S0010-9452(08)70918-3

Wertz, R. T., Henschel, C. R., Auther, L. L., Ashford, J. R., & Kirshner, H. S. (1998). Affective prosodic disturbance subsequent to right hemisphere stroke: A clinical application. *Journal of Neurolinguistics, 11,* 89–102. http://dx.doi.org/10.1016/S0911-6044(98)00007-4

Withall, A., Brodaty, H., Altendorf, A., & Sachdev, P. S. (2011). A longitudinal study examining the independence of apathy and depression after stroke: The Sydney Stroke Study. *International Psychogeriatrics, 23,* 264–273. http://dx.doi.org/10.1017/S1041610209991116

Work, S. S., Colamonico, J. A., Bradley, W. G., & Kaye, R. E. (2011). Pseudobulbar affect: An under-recognized and under-treated neurological disorder. *Advances in Therapy, 28,* 586–601. http://dx.doi.org/10.1007/s12325-011-0031-3

World Health Organization. (2001). *International classification of functioning, disability and health.* Geneva: Author.

Yesavage, J. A., Brink, T. L., Rose, T. L., Lum, O., Huang, V., Adey, M. B., & Leirer, V. O. (1982). Development and validation of a geriatric depression screening scale: A preliminary report. *Journal of Psychiatric Research, 17,* 37–49. http://dx.doi.org/10.1016/0022-3956(82)90033-4

Youngjohn, J. R., & Altman, I. M. (1989). A performance-based group approach to the treatment of anosognosia and denial. *Rehabilitation Psychology, 34,* 217–222.

Zigmond, A. S., & Snaith, R. P. (1983). The Hospital Anxiety and Depression Scale. *Acta Psychiatrica Scandinavica, 67,* 361–370. http://dx.doi.org/10.1111/j.1600-0447.1983.tb09716.x

Zung, W. W. (1965). A self-rating depression scale. *Archives of General Psychiatry, 12,* 63–70. http://dx.doi.org/10.1001/archpsyc.1965.01720310065008

CHAPTER 9

Stroke Rehabilitation Across the Continuum of Care: Introduction of the Cases

Timothy J. Wolf, OTD, MSCI, OTR/L

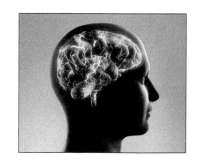

Learning Objectives

After completion of this chapter, readers will be able to

- Recognize how to use the *Occupational Therapy Practice Framework: Domain and Process* (3rd ed.; American Occupational Therapy Association [AOTA], 2014) with three case studies involving clients with stroke;
- Identify the National Institutes of Health Stroke Scale classifications of stroke severity;
- Identify the relevant information from client backgrounds, occupational histories, and symptoms presented in the case studies;
- Identify the neurological symptoms and impairments presented in the case studies; and
- Identify potential intervention priorities for the patients presented in the case studies.

Key Words

- case study
- National Institutes of Health Stroke Scale
- neurological impairment
- occupational history
- *Occupational Therapy Practice Framework*
- Person–Environment–Occupation–Performance model
- stroke symptoms

Introduction

In this chapter, I describe three case studies of hypothetical clients as each progresses through the continuum of care and **rehabilitation** after **stroke.** As opposed to the chapters in the first, core concepts section of this text, the chapters in this section do not focus exclusively on content knowledge but rather use the information that was covered in that section and apply it to the case studies. The chapters that follow all use the *Occupational Therapy Practice Framework: Domain and Process* (3rd ed.; AOTA, 2014) as a guide to the case discussion. The *Framework* is not a theory or model of practice but rather a guide to occupational therapy practice that is used to describe the process of occupational therapy services across the continuum of care. The *Framework* is meant to be used in conjunction with the theoretical models of practice and intervention approaches that guide treatment. With this in mind, all the authors of the chapters in the core concepts section used the

The *Framework* is not a theory or model of practice but rather a guide to occupational therapy practice that is used to describe the process of occupational therapy services across the continuum of care.

Person–Environment–Occupation–Performance model of practice (Baum & Christiansen, 2005) as their guiding theory. Specific information related to assessments and intervention approaches or frames of reference are provided as appropriate to the client in the given area of practice.

Occupational Therapy Practice Framework: Domain and Process (3rd Ed.)

As a quick orientation to how the *Framework* is used in this text, Exhibit 9.1 describes the process of service delivery from the *Framework*. The specific concepts and definitions that support this process can be found in the original document; however, this process is used in each of the chapters that follow.

It is important to reiterate that the *Framework* describes an iterative process in which the client's progress is continually being monitored and the assessment, development of goals, and selection of intervention approaches are continually updated. Continuous assessment and monitoring are particularly important when working with people after a neurological injury such as stroke, when symptoms resolve and functional performance can change very rapidly, especially in the early stages of recovery. The considerable variation seen in the stroke population (principally related to the extent of neurological damage) and the consequent variability seen in the course of recovery led to the inclusion of multiple cases discussed in this text.

Introduction of the Cases

As discussed in the core concepts section of the text, the **National Institutes of Health Stroke Scale** (NIHSS; Brott et al., 1989) is considered one of the gold-standard measurements of neurological impairment after stroke. The NIHSS is used to quantify the neurological symptoms present in the acute phase of stroke on a scale ranging from 0 to 42. It is apparent from this measure alone that clinical presentation varies greatly in the stroke population. A person with a stroke scale score of 5 and a person with a score of 24 will differ in the level of neurological impairment they present and in their anticipated recovery from stroke.

Given the heterogeneity of the stroke population, different classification schemes have been used in the literature as inclusion criteria in studies to define subsets of the population and also to develop new assessments and interventions that may be appropriate only for a specific subset of this population. A classification scheme that is increasingly used in the literature, and more specifically the occupational therapy literature, is based on the NIHSS and classifies patients with stroke into groups on the basis of their overall level of neurological impairment as measured by the NIHSS. The severity of stroke is stratified by NIHSS score: A score of less than 6 is classified as *mild;* 6 to 16, as *moderate;* and more than 16, as *severe* (Wolf, Baum, & Connor, 2009). Although there is a lot of variation within these groupings, they provide a framework within which to conduct research and discuss cases.

Patients with a mild stroke are typically fluent in speech and close to independent in **activities of daily living** (ADLs) by the time of discharge from the acute care setting. However, they often experience higher-level cognitive, motor, and sensory impairments; demonstrate decreased participation in home, work, community, and **leisure** activities; and are prone to develop depressive symptoms similar

Exhibit 9.1. Operationalizing the Occupational Therapy Process

Evaluation		Intervention			Targeting of Outcomes
Occupational Profile ⟷	Analysis of Occupational Performance	Intervention Plan	Intervention Implementation	Intervention Review	Outcomes
Identify the following: • Why is the client seeking service, and what are the client's current concerns relative to engaging in activities and occupations? • In what occupations does the client feel successful, and what barriers are affecting his or her success? • What aspects of the contexts or environments does the client see as supporting and as inhibiting engagement in desired occupations? • What is the client's occupational history? • What are the client's values and interests? • What are the client's daily life roles? • What are the client's patterns of engagement in occupations, and how have they changed over time? • What are the client's priorities and desired targeted outcomes related to occupational performance, prevention, participation, role competence, health and wellness, quality of life, well-being, and occupational justice?	• Synthesize information from the occupational profile to focus on specific occupations and contexts. • Observe the client's performance during activities relevant to desired occupations. • Select and use specific assessments to identify and measure contexts or environments, activity and occupational demands, client factors, and performance skills and patterns. • Select outcome measures. • Interpret assessment data to identify supports for and hindrances to performance. • Develop and refine hypotheses about the client's occupational performance strengths and limitations. • Create goals in collaboration with the client that address desired outcomes. • Determine procedures to measure the outcomes of intervention. • Delineate a potential intervention based on best practices and available evidence.	1. Develop the plan, which involves selecting • Objective and measurable occupation-focused goals and related time frames; • Occupational therapy intervention approach or approaches, such as create or promote, establish or restore, maintain, modify, or prevent; and • Methods for service delivery, including who will provide the intervention, types of intervention, and service delivery models. 2. Consider potential discharge needs and plans. 3. Recommend or refer to other professionals as needed.	1. Determine and carry out occupational therapy intervention or interventions, which may include the following: • Therapeutic use of occupations and activities • Preparatory methods and tasks • Education and training • Advocacy • Group interventions. 2. Monitor the client's response through ongoing evaluation and reevaluation.	1. Reevaluate the plan and implementation relative to achieving outcomes. 2. Modify the plan as needed. 3. Determine the need for continuation or discontinuation of occupational therapy services and for referral.	1. Early in the intervention process, select outcomes and measures that are • Valid, reliable, sensitive to change, and consistent with outcomes • Congruent with client goals • Based on their actual or purported ability to predict future outcomes. 2. Apply outcomes to measure progress and adjust goals and interventions. • Compare progress toward goal achievement to outcomes throughout the intervention process. • Assess outcome use and results to make decisions about the future direction of intervention.
		←———————Continue to renegotiate intervention plans and targeted outcomes.———————→			
		←———Ongoing interaction among evaluation, intervention, and outcomes occurs throughout the process.———→			

to the rest of the stroke population (Edwards, Hahn, Baum, & Dromerick, 2006; Hildebrand, Brewer, & Wolf, 2012; Rochette, Desrosiers, Bravo, St.-Cyr-Tribble, & Bourget, 2007; Wolf, Barbee, & White, 2011; Wolf, Stift, Connor, & Baum, 2010; Wolf et al., 2009). People with mild stroke often receive little to no rehabilitation, and the majority are discharged home from the acute setting (Rochette et al., 2007; Wolf et al., 2009). People with moderate stroke exhibit more of the classic symptoms of stroke, such as hemiparesis, speech impairment, and neglect and are most often discharged from the acute setting to an inpatient rehabilitation facility or with home health services (Wolf et al., 2009). People with severe stroke typically have a high level of impairment and are often discharged to inpatient rehabilitation facilities or skilled nursing facilities. For the purposes of this text, I discuss three cases: (1) a person with mild stroke, (2) a person with moderate stroke, and (3) a person with severe stroke.

Case 1: Steve (NIHSS Score of <6: Mild Stroke)

Steve is a 43-year-old White man who is a managing partner in a large plaintiff law firm. He has worked for the same firm since he graduated from law school 17 years ago. Steve has been very successful at this job and has progressed through the promotion chain extremely quickly compared with his peers, in large part because of his work ethic and dedication to his job. He typically starts his day at 4:30 a.m. and works until 6:00–7:00 p.m. He travels approximately 20% of his time. Although Steve admits that he loves his job, he also states that it is very stressful and can be overwhelming.

Steve has been married to his second wife, Elizabeth, for 5 years. He married his first wife during law school, but the marriage was short lived, and they divorced 7 years ago. He has one child from his first marriage, Michael (age 9). Steve shares custody with his ex-wife, and Michael lives with him part-time. He has another child with Elizabeth, Sylvia (age 3), who lives with them full-time. Steve also has medical and legal power of attorney for his only surviving parent, his mother, Cynthia (age 70). Cynthia has **major neurocognitive disorder** of the Alzheimer's type and lives in a skilled nursing facility near his home. Steve lives in an upscale gated suburban neighborhood in a three-story house with a walk-out basement.

After he married Elizabeth, Steve started attending a local contemporary Christian church with his wife and daughter. Steve shares that, up to that point, he held no particular religious beliefs and never attended church. He considers himself spiritual but is not particularly tied to Christianity. Rather, he believes in a greater power at work in his life. He places extremely high value on hard work and discipline, a value that has been instilled in him from a young age. He describes his parents as tough but fair and says they were very strict with him. He worked every summer on his grandparents' farm from the time he was old enough to walk and was expected to participate in all household chores throughout his childhood until he left home to go to college at age 18. Steve has taken the same approach with his two children and tends to be very strict with them; however, he states that Elizabeth is the primary caregiver for their daughter and his ex-wife is the primary caregiver for their son simply because Steve is gone so much. He wants to play a more active role in their lives, but his work schedule does not permit it. Steve also has two younger brothers, Chris (age 41) and Eric (age 36), who live in the area.

Medical History

Steve has an unremarkable medical history. At the time of his stroke, he was not on any medications other than multivitamins and had no current medical diagnoses. He admits, however, that he also did not go to the doctor for regular checkups and was not sure whether he had any medical conditions. His father, Steven Sr., died from cardiac arrest at age 56 when Steve was 29. In addition to **Alzheimer's disease,** Steve's mother is also being treated for **hypertension.** He has no other remarkable family medical history. Steve considers himself somewhat active and states that he tries to get to the gym 3 times a week but most weeks does not make it that often. He states that in reality he gets to the gym probably once a week for an hour. Other than that, his job is very sedentary. Steve also states that his diet is very poor and he eats out (fast food) more often than he eats at home.

Occupational History

At the time of his stroke, Steve was completely independent in all ADLs and the **instrumental activities of daily living** (IADLs) in which he participated. As previously mentioned, he was a caregiver for both of his children and his mother, although he was not very active in these roles. His wife handled all the cooking and shopping in the household, but Steve managed all the finances (monthly bills, investments, and financial planning). He only slept 3 to 4 hours a night most nights because he typically took care of his household responsibilities after work and needed to be up again by 3:30–4:00 a.m. to get ready to go to work.

In addition to his job as an attorney, Steve volunteered some weekends with Habitat for Humanity, the charity his firm had primarily chosen to support. Steve loves cars and has a small collection of classic cars that he restored in his downtime and showed at local car shows. In conjunction with this hobby, Steve loved to drive and loved that he was able to drive to most of his destinations for work. Recently, he had become a little more active in his church by volunteering as a greeter one Sunday a month. Steve has a very strong local network of friends and relatives, due to the fact that he lives in close proximity to where he was born and, with the exception of when he went away to college, has lived there his whole life. Although he does not spend a lot of time with them, he considers his friends to be his extended family and says he would feel comfortable calling on them anytime for help.

Presenting Symptoms

Steve presented to the hospital with facial numbness and weakness, facial droop on the left side, slurred speech, left-sided weakness, and extreme confusion. He walked into the emergency department with help from his wife and his brother Chris, who drove him there. The initial computerized tomography (CT) scan did not reveal an active bleed, but a follow-up magnetic resonance imaging (MRI) scan revealed a small infarct in his right **frontal lobe.** Steve was admitted to the acute stroke service and was later diagnosed with hypertension. His blood pressure was averaging close to 190/120.

Case 2: Mary (NIHSS Score of 6 to 16: Moderate Stroke)

Mary is a 62-year-old African-American woman who is a human resources (HR) manager for a local durable medical equipment company. Mary has been with the company for 12 years, first as an assistant HR manager and in her present position as manager for 5 years. Mary went into personnel management after she completed her bachelor's degree in business administration and worked in HR for a large hospital system in a variety of roles for 25 years before going to work for her current company. She states that although she has been looking forward to retirement, she really enjoys her job and says that for financial security she needs to work another 5 years.

Mary is divorced, and the only family who live near her are two grown children: David (age 32), who lives with his wife and two children several hours away, and Sarah (age 34), who lives with her boyfriend within a 15-minute drive from Mary's home. Mary lives alone in a small two-story house in an urban neighborhood. Her house is more than 100 years old and is in constant need of repair. There are nine steps into the house, the only bathroom and both bedrooms are on the second level, and her laundry room is in the basement. She has a small yard that she maintains.

Mary is a devout Christian and is very active in her childhood church, where she was baptized, raised, married, and attended with her own children. She has a very strong work ethic and desire to be independent—traits instilled in her by her mother. Her father left her mother when Mary was 12 years old and her two sisters were 10 and 8. Her mother cared for the three children by herself while working two jobs. Although her mother did not finish high school, she continually emphasized the value of education and the importance of independence to her three daughters. All three siblings ultimately obtained college degrees. Mary was the breadwinner in her household even during the 27 years she was married. After her mother had a stroke 10 years ago, Mary was her caregiver until she passed away last year. Both of Mary's sisters had moved away and were not available to provide caregiving help.

Medical History

Mary has been significantly overweight for much of her adult life. Twelve years ago, she was diagnosed with Type 2 diabetes and was prescribed metformin by her physician to help control it. She reported being compliant with medication management, but she admitted to being noncompliant with the physician's recommendations for diet and lifestyle changes and reported missing scheduled physician and diabetes clinic appointments. Ten years ago, Mary had a mild stroke and at that time was diagnosed with hyperlipidemia and hypertension. Her blood glucose levels were uncontrolled at the time of her first stroke. Mary returned home after a short acute care inpatient hospital stay, attended a few weeks of outpatient rehabilitation services, and then returned to work. She started exercising, taking her medications, lost some weight, and gained control of her blood glucose levels. At the time of the current stroke, she has a **body mass index** of 34 and is considered obese. Although her hyperlipidemia and hypertension have improved with medication since the time of her first mild stroke, she has continued to struggle to keep them under control. Currently, Mary states that she walks around her neighborhood every evening after work and considers her diet to be fairly healthy.

Occupational History

At the time of her current stroke, Mary was completely independent in ADLs and IADLs. She stated that since her first stroke she has had slight **memory** and planning problems, but has compensated by keeping a detailed calendar or journal. Living by herself, she is responsible for all of her own household management, maintenance, and financial management. She is not currently a caregiver for a family member and does not have any pets. She owns a car and drives to church, to her daughter's home, and to stores for shopping. She uses public transportation to get to work. She states that she always gets 7 to 8 hours of sleep a night. In addition to her full-time job, Mary volunteers extensively at her church. She sings in the choir every Sunday, volunteers in a ministry to drive older people to and from the store and medical appointments, and organizes a monthly potluck lunch at the church for all the members. She states that she is often called on to do other church-related work as needed. She says that she has a strong network of friends through her church whom she considers family. Most of her social activities involve friends from church or are organized through the church, such as group outings to the local theater and sporting events. Her grandchildren (her son David's children) live several hours' drive away and she sees them only 5 to 6 times a year, but she says that she considers being a grandmother to be a central role in her life.

Presenting Symptoms

While at work, Mary tried to explain to a coworker that she was losing feeling in her left arm and leg; however, her coworker was unable to understand what Mary was saying. Shortly thereafter, Mary fell and was not able to get up. Her coworker called 911, and emergency medical technicians transported Mary to the hospital via ambulance. The initial neurological evaluation at the hospital found that she had profound left-sided weakness, visual disruption, slurred speech, and sensory loss on the left side of her body. MRI confirmed a right **parietal lobe** infarct. Mary was admitted to the acute stroke service.

Case 3: Walter (NIHSS Score of >16: Severe Stroke)

Walter is a 67-year-old White retired mechanic. He lives in a condo in a suburban neighborhood with Adele, his wife of 40 years. Walter and Adele do not have children and have no family in the area. He has an older brother who lives several states away and who is in poor health. Adele does not have siblings, and both Walter's and Adele's parents are deceased.

Walter worked as a mechanic throughout his adult life and, according to Adele, was very passionate about his profession. He began working in his father's garage as a child and later owned his own shop. His declining health led him to sell the shop for a considerable profit that he used to purchase the condo in the retirement community. Because of his health problems, Walter chose to live where he did not have to perform home or yard maintenance. Adele also has chronic health conditions that limited her ability to maintain the home and garden. She has low-back pain, osteoarthritis in the knees and hands, and hypertension. Walter and Adele wanted to live in a community where they would have opportunities for socializing with people their own age. They are Jewish but state that they are not practicing. They do not go to temple often and do not celebrate many religious holidays. However, they both consider themselves to be spiritual and connected to their faith.

Medical History

Walter has several health conditions that limited his independence. While working as a mechanic, Walter sustained numerous injuries, ranging from broken fingers to a severe vertebral fracture that affected his mobility and restricted his activity level. His limited activity level was compounded by osteoarthritis in his hands, shoulders, and knees. Before his stroke, he used a rollator walker for mobility around his condo and a wheelchair for longer distances. Walter had also been diagnosed with arteriosclerosis and coronary artery disease. Seven years before his stroke, Walter had a myocardial infarction with subsequent triple-bypass surgery. At the time of his stroke, he was on beta blockers, aspirin, and a statin to help control his hypertension and hyperlipidemia and to protect his heart.

Occupational History

Before his stroke, Walter was independent or modified independent in all ADLs. He required more time and struggled with fine motor tasks, such as buttoning small buttons. However, he avoided fine motor tasks when possible (e.g., by not wearing clothing with small buttons). His participation in IADLs was limited by choice and by his health conditions. He no longer participated in household maintenance, shopping, or meal preparation. Walter and Adele did not own a pet or provide caregiving help for friends. Walter slept poorly at night as a result of constant pain and took naps throughout the day because of fatigue. At the time of his stroke, Adele was doing all the driving. Ten years ago, Walter enjoyed volunteering with students at a local trade school who were interested in auto mechanics. Occasionally, he and Adele went fishing at a local catch-and-release pond. Both Walter and Adele had an extensive network of friends in their condominium complex and spent a lot of time with them. The group organized various events throughout the week such as dinners and game nights. Adele frequently went on outings with the ladies' group, and Walter spent a lot of time watching sports with the men's group.

Presenting Symptoms

While socializing with friends at his condo, Walter mentioned that he had a bad headache that quickly worsened. Walter's friends said that he appeared very confused, began to vomit, and fell to the floor. At that time, they called 911. In the emergency department, Walter was unable to respond to simple commands and was barely responsive to neurological testing by the physician. His blood pressure was very high, 220/130. A CT scan confirmed an active bleed or ruptured aneurysm in the left hemisphere of Walter's brain with temporal, frontal, and parietal involvement. He was immediately scheduled for surgical clipping.

Conclusion

The following chapters will follow Steve, Mary, and Walter as they progress through the continuum of rehabilitation care after stroke. Each chapter begins with general information about stroke rehabilitation in that practice setting followed by a case

Table 9.1. Overview of the Three Cases

	Steve (Mild Stroke), Age 43	Mary (Moderate Stroke), Age 62	Walter (Severe Stroke), Age 67
Background	• White • Partner in a law firm • Divorced and remarried • Two kids • Legal responsibility for his mother, who has dementia • Christian	• African-American • HR manager in a DME company • Divorced with 2 grown children • Lives alone • Devout Christian • Enjoys work and must continue for 5 years for financial security • Independent woman, strong work ethic	• White • Retired mechanic • Married with no children and no nearby family • Lives in a retirement community • Both he and his wife have a history of chronic health conditions • Spiritually Jewish
Medical history	• No current medical diagnoses • Did not get regular checkups • Father died of cardiac arrest • Mother has history of dementia and hypertension • Exercises at least 1 hr/wk • Poor diet	• Obese (BMI of 34) • Diagnoses of hyperlipidemia, hypertension, and Type 2 diabetes (takes metformin) • Noncompliant with diet and lifestyle changes • Mild stroke 10 years earlier • Walks every evening, fairly healthy diet	• Diagnoses of arteriosclerosis, hypertension, hyperlipidemia, and coronary artery disease • Prior history of myocardial infarction with subsequent triple-bypass surgery • Medications: beta blockers and statins • Work injuries: broken fingers, severe vertebral fracture; osteoarthritis in hands, shoulders, and knees • Used rollator walker around condo and wheelchair for longer distances before stroke
Occupational history	• Prior independence in ADLs/IADLs • Caregiver to children and mother • Manages household finances • Poor sleep habits • Volunteers for Habitat for Humanity and at church • Collects cars and loves driving • Strong friend and family support network	• Prior independence in ADLs/IADLs • Compensates for her slight memory and planning problems after first stroke • Responsible for managing finances and household • Drives own car and uses public transportation • Church volunteer • Belongs to church choir • Strong friend network • Grandmother	• Prior independence or modified independence in all ADLs • Limited independence in IADLs (no household maintenance, shopping, or meal preparation) • Avoids fine motor tasks • Poor sleep habits; fatigue • Does not drive • Volunteered in past at mechanic trade schools • Past hobby of fishing • Strong network of friends in retirement community
Presenting symptoms	• Facial numbness and weakness, facial droop on left side, slurred speech, left-sided weakness, extreme confusion • No active bleed on CT scan, small infarct on right frontal lobe on MRI	• Left-sided weakness and sensory loss; slurred speech, visual disruption • Right parietal lobe infarct on MRI	• Worsening headache, confusion, vomiting; fell to floor; unresponsive to simple commands; very high BP • Active bleed or ruptured aneurysm in left hemisphere with temporal, frontal, and parietal involvement on CT scan

Note. ADLs = activities of daily living; BMI = body mass index; BP = blood pressure; CT = computerized tomography; DME = durable medical equipment; hr = hour; HR = human resources; IADLs = instrumental activities of daily living; MRI = magnetic resonance imaging; wk = week.

review for Steve, Mary, and Walter in that practice setting. Table 9.1 presents a quick overview of the three cases for your reference as you progress through the next chapters of this text.

References

American Occupational Therapy Association. (2014). Occupational therapy practice framework: Domain and process (3rd ed.). *American Journal of Occupational Therapy, 68*(Suppl. 1), S1–S48. http://dx.doi.org/10.5014/ajot.2014.682006

Baum, C. M., & Christiansen, C. H. (2005). Person–Environment–Occupation–Performance: An occupation-based framework for practice. In C. H. Christiansen, C. M. Baum, &

J. Bass-Haugen (Eds.), *Occupational therapy: Performance, participation, and well-being* (pp. 242–267). Thorofare, NJ: Slack.

Brott, T., Adams, H. P., Jr., Olinger, C. P., Marler, J. R., Barsan, W. G., Biller, J., . . . Hertzberg, V. (1989). Measurements of acute cerebral infarction: A clinical examination scale. *Stroke, 20,* 864–870. http://dx.doi.org/10.1161/01.STR.20.7.864

Edwards, D. F., Hahn, M., Baum, C., & Dromerick, A. W. (2006). The impact of mild stroke on meaningful activity and life satisfaction. *Journal of Stroke and Cerebrovascular Diseases, 15,* 151–157. http://dx.doi.org/10.1016/j.jstrokecerebrovasdis.2006.04.001

Hildebrand, M., Brewer, M., & Wolf, T. (2012). The impact of mild stroke on participation in physical fitness activities. *Stroke Research and Treatment, 2012,* 548682. http://dx.doi.org/10.1155/2012/548682

Rochette, A., Desrosiers, J., Bravo, G., St.-Cyr-Tribble, D., & Bourget, A. (2007). Changes in participation after a mild stroke: Quantitative and qualitative perspectives. *Topics in Stroke Rehabilitation, 14,* 59–68. http://dx.doi.org/10.1310/tsr1403-59

Wolf, T. J., Barbee, A., & White, D. (2011). Executive dysfunction immediately post-mild stroke. *OTJR: Occupation, Participation and Health, 31*(Suppl.), S23–S29. http://dx.doi.org/10.3928/15394492-20101108-05

Wolf, T. J., Baum, C., & Connor, L. T. (2009). Changing face of stroke: Implications for occupational therapy practice. *American Journal of Occupational Therapy, 63,* 621–625. http://dx.doi.org/10.5014/ajot.63.5.621

Wolf, T. J., Stift, S., Connor, L., & Baum, C. (2010). Feasibility of the EFPT at the acute stage of stroke to detect executive function deficits that impact return to work. *Work, 36,* 405–412.

CHAPTER 10

Occupational Therapy for People With Stroke in the Acute Care Setting

Becky L. Russell, OTR/L, and
Timothy J. Wolf, OTD, MSCI, OTR/L

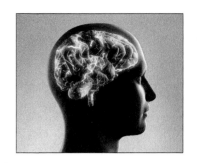

Learning Objectives

After completion of this chapter, readers will be able to

- Identify four dimensions used to guide clinical decision making when developing an appropriate occupational therapy discharge recommendation in an acute care hospital;
- Identify appropriate and relevant information from the patient's medical record that is necessary to inform occupational therapy treatment planning in the acute care setting;
- Delineate methods to develop the occupational profile in the acute care setting;
- Identify commonly used medical tests and equipment used in the acute care setting; and
- Identify appropriate occupational therapy assessment methods in the acute care setting.

Key Words

- acute care
- ADL training
- caregiver education
- cognitive remediation
- contraindications
- discharge recommendations
- Health Belief Model
- intervention planning
- medical testing
- motor function

Introduction

For a person experiencing the signs and symptoms of a **stroke,** the initial medical intervention is provided in an acute inpatient hospital setting. The main objective in the hospital setting, traditionally using the medical model, is to stabilize the patient's medical status by performing necessary diagnostics and treatments (see Chapter 1). Practicing occupational therapy in an acute care hospital has the unique challenge of merging the medical model with the *Occupational Therapy Practice Framework: Domain and Process* (3rd ed.; American Occupational Therapy Association [AOTA], 2014).

Occupational therapists practicing in the acute care hospital are at the front end of the continuum of care and initiate services that will be continued after discharge at another level of care (Table 10.1). In this scenario, the occupational therapist

Occupational therapists practicing in the acute care hospital are at the front end of the continuum of care and initiate services that will be continued after discharge at another level of care.

Table 10.1. Discharge Recommendation Options for Continued Occupational Therapy

Discharge Location	Indications
Long-term acute care	Recommend when patient requires continued specialized intensive nursing care and is progressing toward or is tolerating 3 hr/day of therapy.
Inpatient rehabilitation facility	Recommend when patient can tolerate 3 hr/day of therapy and can benefit from intensive therapy. Typically need to require 25% or greater physical assist to complete tasks.
Skilled nursing facility	Recommend when patient can tolerate 1.5 to 2 hr/day of therapy; would benefit from slower paced rehabilitation and longer length of stay.
Outpatient day treatment	Recommend when patient requires daily therapy but does not meet the requirements for inpatient rehabilitation.
Outpatient occupational therapy	Recommend when patient does not require inpatient care but is able and would benefit from further occupational therapy outside the home.
Home health occupational therapy	Recommend when a home safety evaluation is required, if the patient is unable to reasonably attend outpatient therapy, or both.
No occupational therapy on discharge	Recommend no occupational therapy if the patient presents with no impairments limiting participation or if the patient is not demonstrating potential for measurable outcome from skilled intervention.

is responsible for completing the initial assessment and treatment planning that will be used to inform services that will be provided at a different facility. Conversely, patients who receive occupational therapy in the hospital setting may not receive continued occupational therapy on discharge (despite new onset of impairments that may limit performance and participation) because of reimbursement limitations or geographic location. In the latter scenario, the occupational therapist must be prepared to complete the occupational therapy process, using best available evidence and best practice, to achieve maximum measureable outcome within the short length of stay and the limitations of the institutional setting.

Evaluation in the Acute Care Setting

In the acute care setting, the occupational therapy practitioner evaluates a wide range of people who experienced a neurological event, ranging from a transient ischemic attack to a severe stroke (**National Institutes of Health Stroke Scale** score >16; see Chapter 9). Patients may have no significant medical history, or they may have multiple comorbidities. They may have an uncomplicated medical course poststroke or require critical care for life-threatening sequelae. All of these factors need to be taken into account when performing an evaluation in the acute care setting after stroke.

The initial evaluation in this setting begins before the therapist enters the room. First, the occupational therapist completes a thorough and accurate medical record review. The occupational therapy practitioner in the acute care setting must develop the skill of reading the medical record to determine salient information to (1) safely engage the patient in the occupational therapy process and (2) prepare appropriately for the evaluation.

The occupational therapy practitioner will read and interpret information from the history and physical report from the neurologist or the emergency department physician. Of special interest are the reason for admission, results of the neurological examination and diagnostic tests, the medical assessment (with diagnosis, differential diagnosis, or both), past medical history, and the medical plan. Some common medical tests are as follows:

Table 10.2. Examples of Precautions and Contraindications to Participation in Occupational Therapy

Medical Order or Issue	Precaution or Contraindication
Tissue plasminogen activator (t-PA)	24-hr bedrest or as per physician order.
Angiogram	6-hr bedrest with extremity straight or as per physician order.
Lumbar puncture	Only mobilize with order from MD.
Seizure precautions	Follow hospital guidelines.
Fall risk	Follow hospital guidelines.
Bedrest or no-activity orders	Medical orders must be clear that the patient is stable for out-of-bed activity to proceed with testing in positions at edge of bed, in chair, or in the room.
Vital signs in abnormal range	Heart rate, blood pressure, respiration rate, and oxygen saturation are within the guidelines of the facility for rehabilitation.
Craniectomy (bone flap removal)	Consider use of helmet; follow MD orders.
External ventricular drain (EVD)	Activity only as ordered by MD. EVD clamped (by nursing) as ordered by MD. EVD must be monitored at all times for safety.

- Carotid Doppler ultrasound
- Carotid arteriography
- Cerebral angiography
- Magnetic resonance angiogram (MRA) or functional magnetic resonance imaging (fMRI)
- Transcranial Doppler
- Electrocardiogram (EKG)
- Echocardiogram
- Lumbar puncture
- Electroencephalography (EEG).

Additionally, the occupational therapist is looking for medical orders for occupational therapy and for specific orders related to activity status (e.g., if the patient is on bedrest, then evaluation of transfers and **activities of daily living** [ADLs] at chair or standing level cannot be performed). It is critical that the therapist be aware of and knowledgeable about any precautions that should be taken and contraindications to participation in occupational therapy (Table 10.2).

The therapist must be knowledgeable about the patient's health condition and plan an initial evaluation that is appropriate for the anticipated areas of strength and limitations. The therapist should select appropriate evaluation tools on the basis of the patient's possible **functional impairments** and prognostic indicators related to the review of the patient's medical record.

According to the *Occupational Therapy Practice Guidelines for Adults With Stroke* (Sabari & Lieberman, 2008), the occupational therapist should consider that the patient in this setting is often being evaluated within 24 hours of his or her admission to the hospital and is still adjusting to the change in function:

> During the acute stage, a bottom-up assessment approach is advised. Because stroke survivors in the acute stage are adapting to their loss, and because it is virtually impossible to predict recovery levels, assessments of patient factors are most critical. The resulting information enables occupational therapists to target intervention toward preventing secondary

impairments, maximizing recovery, and making decisions for immediate discharge placement from the hospital setting. (p. 15)

The occupational therapy practitioner should be well oriented to and familiar with medical equipment, lines, and tubes used in hospitals, especially those in the critical care areas (Figure 10.1).

The evaluation should include components of the domain as cited in the *Framework* (AOTA, 2014), within the scope of what is appropriate given the context of the acute care hospital. Occupational therapy evaluation performed at the beginning of the continuum of care should include the breadth of the *Framework* but, given the patient's acuity level and the context of service delivery, may not have the depth of an evaluation performed later in the continuum. For example, in evaluating ADLs for a patient 1 day after moderate stroke, grooming may be performed sitting on the edge of the bed with use of an over-the-bed table.

Finally, consideration should be given to the documentation guidelines outlined by the rehabilitation department in which the therapist is employed and to the expectations of the multiple stakeholders (i.e., the payer source, rehabilitation reviewers within the continuum of care).

Occupational therapy evaluation performed at the beginning of the continuum of care should include the breadth of the *Framework* but, given the patient's acuity level and the context of service delivery, may not have the depth of an evaluation performed later in the continuum.

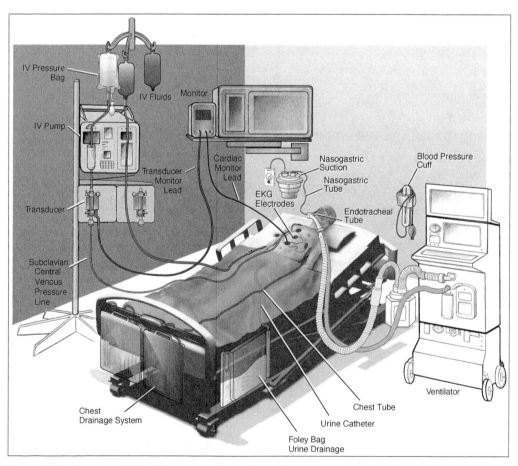

Figure 10.1. Common intensive care unit equipment.

Source. Richard Fritzler, medical illustrator, Roswell, GA.

Intervention in the Acute Care Setting

Throughout the continuum of care, including the acute care hospital, occupational therapists can draw on a variety of intervention approaches that are useful to guide clinical reasoning and intervention. A patient admitted with a transient ischemic attack or a complicated migraine who has no impairments but multiple risk factors may benefit from health promotion education framed by the occupational therapist using the Health Belief Model (Finfgeld, Wongvatunyu, Conn, Grando, & Russell, 2003). Motor-learning theory and goal-directed theory (Mastos, Miller, Eliasson, & Imms, 2007) may guide clinical thinking for the patient with **hemiplegia.** The Transtheoretical Model of Change (DiClemente, 2007) might be used with the patient with a comorbidity of addiction when patient collaboration and intentional change may result in sustainable behavior change. Each patient is unique and, with the wide variety of approaches available to draw on, the occupational therapy practitioner is in a unique position to be distinctly client centered.

Occupational Therapy Roles

The roles for occupational therapy outlined in AOTA's (2012) fact sheet, *Occupational Therapy in Acute Care,* should be considered during intervention planning: (1) facilitating early mobilization; (2) restoring function; (3) preventing further decline; and (4) coordinating care, including discharge planning. The occupational therapist should be prepared for this consultative role and be prepared by the end of the evaluation to make a recommendation regarding a safe discharge plan and whether the patient will require continued occupational therapy.

Clinical Decision Making

In developing a clinical decision regarding appropriate discharge recommendation, the occupational therapist can draw from four dimensions (Taylor, 2004):

1. The patient's current functioning and disability including level of assistance required to complete occupations (as compared with the patient's previous level of function)
2. The patient's wants and needs (including caregiver's contribution), considering patient-centered goals
3. The patient's ability to participate and tolerate the demands of therapy
4. The context of the patient's life, including the built, natural, social, and economic environments.

Points to Ponder: Discharge Determination

John was evaluated by occupational therapy 2 days after admission to the acute care hospital. The results of the occupational therapist's evaluation indicate a distinct change in current cognitive and physical function compared with John's previous level of function and that John is motivated to set goals, was able to tolerate the full session, and lives alone. Using effective clinical decision making, can you name what the most appropriate discharge recommendation is for John?

Measuring Outcome

Measuring outcome in the acute care setting can be done using change in function and change on impairment measures; however, the short length of stay and limited number of treatments pose a challenge to the practitioner. Therefore, measuring outcome may include (1) accuracy in developing appropriate discharge recommendation; (2) quality and quantity of the patient's understanding of the education provided (i.e., activity prescription for home, prescription for durable medical equipment or adaptive equipment, energy conservation, cognitive compensatory strategies, and visual strategies); and (3) measuring change in function or impairment measures.

Case Review: Steve

Steve was referred to occupational therapy for evaluation and treatment on Day 1 of his acute hospital stay after stroke with activity orders written as "out of bed as tolerated." The occupational therapist performed a review of the medical record and noted that Steve had no significant past medical history. The medical record indicated that Steve was scheduled for more diagnostic tests, and his medical plan included management of his **hypertension.**

Evaluation

On entry into the room, the occupational therapist observed Steve to be supine in bed with an IV in place and over-the-bed table in front of him. Steve's over-the-bed table was cluttered with his opened laptop, magazines, hospital-provided hygiene supplies, his cell phone, and educational materials provided by health care staff. Steve appeared anxious and mildly irritated by the presence of the therapist in the room and immediately picked up his cell phone and checked his e-mail.

The occupational therapist performed introductions and explained the role of occupational therapy. Steve did not look up from his cell phone and stated, "I am a partner in a very successful law firm and don't need any therapy." Using a different approach, the occupational therapist motivated Steve by saying that the ultimate goal of occupational therapy would be to help him return to work, home, and **leisure** activities. Although Steve was hesitant to continue, he did consent to the occupational therapy evaluation, and through interview the occupational profile was developed (AOTA, 2014).

Occupational Profile

Steve is a 43-year-old man who before admission to the hospital was independent in ADLs and **instrumental activities of daily living** (IADLs) and driving, was a managing partner in a law firm, infrequently attended a gym, and infrequently attended church. Steve indicates he needs to be able to get back to work as quickly as he can because he is working on a big case. He states, "The only outcome I am willing to accept is to be back to 100%."

When questioned about which activities he is doing well or struggling with, Steve indicates that he has been trying to work on his laptop but cannot seem to pay attention and feels overwhelmed and frustrated. Steve indicates that all he has done is open his e-mails, but he does not seem to know how to respond to them. He is upset that he has to ask for help from the nurse to go to the bathroom because he feels he is not at risk for falling.

Steve lives with his wife and their 3-year-old daughter, Sylvia. He shares custody of his 9-year-old son with his ex-wife. Steve indicates that he has a large support network of friends he can call on. His work environment is very demanding and at times overwhelming.

Assessment

To proceed with the assessment, the occupational therapist evaluated Steve's vital signs, which were as follows: (1) respiration rate, 18 breaths per minute; (2) heart rate, 88 beats per minute; (3) blood pressure, 210/130 mm Hg; and (4) oxygen saturation, 99%.

The occupational therapist immediately explained to Steve that his blood pressure was 210/130 mm Hg and asked him to remain in the chair while the physician and nurse were notified. The physician indicated that activity orders would be changed to bedrest and that therapy would be placed on hold for the day, with updated medication orders for nursing to follow.

On Day 2, a medical record review revealed that Steve's blood pressure was trending at 125/65 mm Hg, and his vital signs were stable. Activity orders were noted to have been increased to "activity as tolerated." Notes from the social worker indicated that during rounds that morning, the team specified that, assuming Steve's blood pressure continued to be under control, he would be ready for discharge on Day 3. The attending physician was waiting for recommendations from the rehabilitation team regarding discharge planning.

Steve was sitting in a recliner chair in no acute distress. The therapist noted that the room had balloons, multiple flower arrangements, and several cards stacked on the cluttered bedside table. Steve's wife, Elizabeth, and their 3-year-old, Sylvia, were visiting. Steve recognized the therapist and indicated that he was willing to participate if it meant that he could get back to work sooner ("I don't have time for this—we are swamped at the office"). Elizabeth nodded in agreement and continued to tend to Sylvia. Vital signs were taken and found to be within acceptable parameters to complete the evaluation. The occupational therapy evaluation results follow.

Cognitive Skills

Steve's Montreal Cognitive Assessment (Nasreddine et al., 2005) score was 21 of 30, indicating **mild cognitive impairment.** Errors were noted in **executive function** skills, delayed recall, **attention,** and language.

During functional tasks, the occupational therapist observed that Steve has difficulty interpreting feedback from the environment. For example, when the water was running too quickly out of the faucet, he did not adjust the flow until cued. Given that Steve was more medically stable, it would be appropriate, when possible, to administer a performance-based assessment of executive function to detect more subtle cognitive deficits that could affect return to everyday life activities. Multiple options are available that could be appropriate on the basis of Steve's occupational history, including but not limited to the Executive Function Performance Test (Baum et al., 2008) and the Weekly Calendar Planning Activity (Toglia, 2009).

Communication and Social Skills

Steve scored 15 of 15 on the Boston Naming Test (Lansing, Ivnik, Cullum, & Randolph, 1999). Steve was noted to be **dysarthric** but was able to name all items. He was noted to have a low frustration tolerance and frequently snapped at his wife

Table 10.3. Upper-Extremity Assessment for Steve

UE	PROM	AROM	MMT	Sensation	Coordination	Tone
Left	WNL	WNL	Graded 4/5 for shoulder flexion–abduction; elbow flexion–extension; forearm supination–pronation	Decreased discrimination for light touch, 3/5; intact for pain/temperature, 5/5; and impaired proprioception, 3/5	Slowed rate and rhythm for finger to nose and serial opposition; Nine-Hole Peg Test = 28 s (below average norm of 18.49 s; Erasmus et al., 2001)	WNL
Right	WNL	WNL	WNL; graded 5/5	WNL for light touch, pain–temperature, and proprioception	WNL Nine-Hole Peg Test = 18 s	WNL

Note. AROM = active range of motion; MMT = manual muscle testing; PROM = passive range of motion; s = seconds; UE = upper extremity; WNL = within normal limits.

and his daughter when they were in the room during testing. Steve's wife reported that his personality seemed different; whereas Steve usually followed rules and social norms, he now seemed to be taking risks, challenging the nurses on hospital rules, and seemed to say the same answers over and over again.

Motor and Praxis Skills

The occupational therapist administered the Berg Balance Test (Berg, 1989), with Steve scoring 38 of 56, indicating a medium fall risk. Static sitting balance at the edge of the bed required supervision, but the therapist noted that during ADLs, Steve required minimum assistance during the dynamic sitting balance component to maintain upright posture and not lean to the left. Dynamic balance during activities and functional tasks also required minimal assistance. Upper-extremity function was assessed; the results are presented in Table 10.3.

Sensory–Perceptual Skills

Steve scored 12 on the Symbol Cancellation Test (Weintraub & Mesulam, 1988) with omission errors scattered throughout the page and in all **visual fields.** Steve was noted to start his search for symbols on the right side of the page and unsystematically scan the page. Results indicate general visual inattention.

Emotional Regulation Skills

Steve was noted to have a low frustration tolerance and had frequent verbal outbursts, especially directed at his wife and the hospital staff. ADL results were as follows:

- *Feeding:* modified independent
- *Dressing upper extremity:* supervision
- *Dressing lower extremity:* 25% assist
- *Grooming (standing at sink):* 25% assist
- *Bathing upper extremity:* supervision and set up
- *Bathing lower extremity:* 25% assist
- *Toileting:* supervision
- *Toilet transfer:* 25% assist
- *Tub transfer:* 25% assist.

Steve and his wife were informed of the occupational therapy evaluation results. Short-term goals were collaboratively established for grooming and dressing, safety awareness and insight, functional mobility for retrieval of ADL items, and therapeutic exercise for the left upper extremity. Education was provided on the role of occupational therapy within this setting and across the continuum. Steve and his wife expressed agreement with the plan.

Intervention Plan

The occupational therapist established a frequency of treatment for daily occupational therapy until discharge from the acute care hospital. Recommendations for discharge were for Steve to continue occupational therapy at an intensive inpatient rehabilitation facility. The social work notes indicated that the referral was in process for Steve to be discharged as soon as approval was received and orders written. Steve was transferred later that same day to an inpatient rehabilitation hospital located in a different building.

Case Review: Mary

Mary was referred to occupational therapy for evaluation and treatment on Day 1 of acute hospital stay after stroke with activity orders that read, "Out of bed as tolerated, with assistance." The occupational therapist performed a review of the medical record and noted that Mary's past medical history included diabetes mellitus, stroke (10 years poststroke without residual symptoms), hypertension, and obesity. Notes from the neurological exam confirmed the diagnosis of a new **parietal lobe** stroke and indicated that Mary has left hemiparesis, left homonymous quadrantanopsia, and poor hand–eye coordination.

Given that Mary had a right parietal lobe infarct (a lesion in this location may result in visuospatial problems), the occupational therapist, in addition to using the occupational therapy tools that are standard in the setting, completed the following assessments with Mary:

- Short Blessed Cognitive Screen (Katzman et al., 1983)
- Clock Drawing Test (Friedman, 1991)
- Mesulam Cancellation Test (Weintraub & Mesulam, 1988)
- Boston Naming Test (Lansing et al., 1999)
- **Apraxia** Screen of TULIA (Test for Upper-Limb Apraxia; Vanbellingen et al., 2011)
- ADL assessment.

Although a specific standardized tool for the ADL assessment is not used in this chapter, multiple standardized tools are available for use in the acute care setting, including but not limited to the AlphaFIM® (Stillman, Granger, & Niewczyk, 2009) and the Barthel Index (Mahoney & Barthel, 1965).

Evaluation

On entry into the hospital room, the occupational therapist observed Mary to be supine in bed, awake and alert. On initial introductions, Mary was able to state her name and consent to occupational therapy. An interview was performed and, in combination with the information in the medical record, the therapist developed the occupational profile.

Occupational Profile

Mary is a 62-year-old woman who, before admission to the hospital, was independent in ADLs, IADLs, and driving; was employed full-time as a human resources manager; and was an active member of her family and church. The medical record indicates that Mary lives alone in a two-story home with nine steps to enter. Mary was able to share that her daughter lives close to her and that her son and his family live far away. No family is present from whom to collect further information.

When questioned about activities that she is able to do and those that are causing problems, Mary indicated she has not been out of bed since the stroke and does not know what she is able to do. While stating this, Mary initiated trying to get out of bed despite the side rails being up and the IV lines, catheter tubing, and other hospital equipment being in the way. Mary had to be directed to remain in bed for the time being.

When asked about goals, Mary was only able to state that her grandchildren are the most important thing to her and that she has to go back to work because she is afraid she will lose her job. Mary says she wants to be independent in all aspects of her life, but given that the stroke happened in the past 24 hours and that she has not had the opportunity to attempt participation in tasks, goal development will be ongoing and collaborative.

Assessment

Cognitive Skills

The Short Blessed Cognitive Screen was completed, with Mary scoring 16 of 28 with noted areas of impairment being disorientation to time and date and impaired attention and recall of information. During tasks, she was observed to be impulsive, with poor problem solving and judgment, and was able to attend for only 3 to 4 minutes before requiring redirection.

Communication and Social Skills

The Boston Naming Test (Lansing et al., 1999) was administered, with Mary scoring 14 of 15, indicating that her ability to name common objects is intact. However, during development of the occupational profile, Mary was noted to be able to provide only basic information and could not provide a detailed history.

Motor and Praxis Skills

The environment is appropriately set up to evaluate Mary's ability to transfer from supine to sitting on the edge of the bed. Mary impulsively attempted to sit up without awareness of her left side and required moderate assistance. Once sitting at the edge of the bed, Mary was noted to sit with a **kyphotic** posture, with her head and trunk rotated to the right, and required 25% assistance to maintain balance and normal postural alignment. Upper-extremity function was assessed in this position; the results are presented in Table 10.4.

Once Mary was positioned in the chair, the occupational therapist administered the Apraxia Screen of TULIA (Vanbellingen et al., 2011), with Mary being asked to perform test items with her right upper extremity. Mary scored 4 of 12, indicating impairment, with the therapist noting that Mary was unable to complete any of the test

Table 10.4. Upper-Extremity Assessment for Mary

UE	PROM	AROM	MMT	Sensation	Hand Function	Coordination	Tone
Left	Shoulder flexion, 0°–110° Shoulder abduction, 0°–90° Elbow flexion, 0°–130° Mary was unable to follow the command for pronation–supination, wrist flexion–extension, and digit flexion–extension.	Shoulder flexion, 0°–80° Shoulder abduction, 0°–60° Elbow flexion, 0–95°	Shoulder flexion graded 2/5 Shoulder abduction graded 2/5 Elbow flexion graded 2/5	Impaired to light touch, proprioception, and deep pressure. Mary did not have awareness of where her left arm was in space.	When an object was placed in Mary's hand, she was able to grasp and release it but was unable to use it purposefully.	Left UE movements were noted to be dysmetric; poor coordination with poor motor control.	Modified Ashworth Scale (Bohannon & Smith, 1987) score = 1. Slight increase in muscle tone, manifested by a catch and release or by minimal resistance at the end of the ROM when the affected part(s) is moved in flexion or extension.
Right	WNL	WNL	WNL; graded 5/5	WNL for light touch, pain/temperature, and proprioception		WNL Nine-Hole Peg Test = 18 s.	WNL

Note. AROM = active range of motion; MMT = manual muscle testing; PROM = passive range of motion; ROM = range of motion; s = seconds; UE = upper extremity; WNL = within normal limits.

items that required imitation and performed poorly on test items that required pantomime, indicating the presence of ideomotor and ideational apraxia (see Chapter 7).

Sensory–Perceptual Skills

While Mary was seated at the edge of the bed, the over-the-bed table was positioned in front of her, with pencil and paper. The Clock Drawing Test (Friedman, 1991) was administered, with Mary demonstrating severe visuospatial errors on the left and disorganization on the right side of the clock. The Mesulam Cancellation Test (Weintraub & Mesulam, 1988) was administered, with Mary demonstrating significant impairment. Mary was noted to refer constantly to the stimulus (sample picture of the symbol she needed to find) and crossed out 10 symbols correctly on the right side of the page and none on the left.

By this point in the evaluation, Mary had been sitting on the edge of the bed for 10 minutes and was noted to be fatigued in sitting, with her sitting balance and posture requiring maximal assist to maintain. The occupational therapist decided to complete the remainder of the evaluation with Mary seated in the recliner chair at the bedside. Using safe transfer technique and leading with her right side, Mary required moderate assist in transferring from the bed to the chair.

Mary was noted to have decreased body awareness on the left and was unable to point to body parts on her left side. The therapist noted left-sided neglect and left spatial inattention, with Mary positioning herself with her body rotated to the right and an eye gaze preference to the right visual field.

Emotional Regulation Skills

Mary's overall presentation was flat, with a lack of awareness of *(anosognosia)* or concern with *(anosodiaphoria)* her deficits. She did not initiate modification of performance.

Activities of Daily Living Skills

In completing the ADL evaluation, the occupational therapist must consider the patient's position during testing.

In completing the ADL evaluation, the occupational therapist must consider the patient's position during testing. Optimally, the patient completes the activity in the position in which it is normally performed. In the event that the patient is unable or is unsafe to complete the activity in that position, then task modification can occur but needs to be clearly documented.

The occupational therapist used critical thinking to decide that, because of the extent of Mary's impairments, the ADL assessment would be completed in sitting with transfers to standing as needed for task completion. Results were as follows:

- *Feeding:* 75% assist, with Mary being able to use feeding utensil; Mary was noted to not eat food on the left side of the plate
- *Dressing:* 75% for both upper extremity and lower extremity, with Mary requiring constant cues to include her left side in the activity
- *Grooming (in sitting):* 75% assist because of left hemiparesis, left spatial and visual impairment, decreased organization and attention, and apraxia
- *Bathing:* 75% for both upper extremity and lower extremity
- *Toileting:* Mary had an indwelling catheter; transfer to the bedside commode required moderate assistance, toileting hygiene required 75% assistance.

At the completion of the evaluation, Mary was positioned safely in the bedside chair. The results of the occupational therapy evaluation were explained to Mary with the recommendation that Mary would benefit from further services at intensive inpatient rehabilitation. Mary was offered choices of priority areas that could be addressed in occupational therapy, and mutual goals were agreed on.

Intervention Plan

Given the anticipated 4-day length of stay in the acute care hospital, the occupational therapist established a frequency of treatment that included daily occupational therapy while in the hospital with priorities including interventions for left upper-extremity motor relearning, sitting balance in preparation for ADLs, visuospatial and cognitive remediation and compensation, ADL training, and family education (if family was available). Recommendations for referrals for physical therapy and speech–language pathology were made. Further occupational therapy services were recommended in an intensive inpatient rehabilitation facility. Potential goals are outlined in Table 10.5.

Intervention Implementation

In preparation for the treatment session, the occupational therapist reviewed the medical record. The neurologist's notes indicate that Mary is medically stable and has been started on new medication for hypertension. Notes from the social worker

Table 10.5. Mary's Intervention Planning and Implementation Outline

Occupational Therapy Intervention Priority	Goals (to Be Achieved by Discharge)	Preparatory Methods and Tasks	Occupation and Activity	Education and Training
Motor function (UE and sitting balance)	• Mary will demonstrate ability to complete a self-ROM program for LUE with 75% assist. • Mary will incorporate her LUE during ADLs 5× per task with 75% verbal cues. • Mary will demonstrate sitting balance with good postural alignment with 25% assist, in preparation for ADL tasks.	• Perform PROM and AAROM repetitions. • Body awareness activities—have Mary find her left hand, elbow, or shoulder. • Have Mary use a warm washcloth to rub her LUE. • Facilitate postural alignment in sitting using tactile cues. • Using hand-over-hand technique, facilitate Mary's performance of self-ROM for shoulder, elbow, and hand (fade assistance as able).	• Have Mary apply lotion to her LUE. • Use LUE to anchor paper during writing tasks. • Encourage use of LUE during ADLs with bilateral task demands (e.g., holding toothpaste tube while unscrewing the cap). • Complete ADL tasks sitting EOB while providing tactile cues to maintain alignment.	• Incorporate LUE into dressing or bathing task, and supine-to-sit transfer.
ADL training: self-feeding	• Mary will demonstrate self-feeding with 50% assist through use of compensatory strategies.	• Place 5 ADL utensils to the left of midline and have Mary retrieve them.	• Use strategies during meal time with meal tray.	• Use systematic scanning training with pencil-and-paper cancellation activities. • Provide and instruct Mary in use of visual strategy with tape or colored stimuli to the left.
ADL training: UE dressing	• Mary will don hospital gown while in supported sitting with 50% assist using 2 adaptive strategies.	• Do self-ROM exercise. • Do body awareness activities. • Use color contrast on left sleeve.	• Use strategies during ADL task of UE dressing.	• Teach Mary to put clothing at midline or in right visual field. • Teach Mary how to position clothing. • Teach Mary to dress her left side first.
Perceptual training	• Mary will demonstrate use of 3 compensatory strategies to increase scanning into her left visual field with 50% verbal cues. • Mary will demonstrate ability to identify 5 body parts on the left side of her body with 100% accuracy.	• Use pencil-and-paper activities that require a systematic left-to-right scan path. • Place cotton balls on Mary's left arm and have her remove them.	• Place Mary's toiletries bag to the left of midline with her toiletries to the right, and have her put them away. • Have Mary don and doff bracelet from her left arm. • Read Mary the hospital menu; with use of visual cues assist Mary in circling her menu selections.	• Instruct Mary in use of visual cue (e.g., tape, bookmark, ruler) for anchoring. • Instruct Mary's family to sit at midline or slightly to the left of Mary and teach family the value of encouraging incorporation of the LUE into daily activities.
Cognitive training	• Mary will attend to functional task for 5 min within a controlled environment.	• Have Mary name family members or activities in a photo album provided by family. • Do a simple word search placed in Mary's right visual field.	• Participate in an ADL with the just-right challenge in a quiet, controlled environment.	• Instruct family in methods to support Mary in successful task completion: quiet room, simple tasks, no distractions, perform when rested.

Note. AAROM = active assistive range of motion; ADL/ADLs = activity/activities of daily living; EOB = edge of bed; LUE = left upper extremity; min = minutes; PROM = passive range of motion; ROM = range of motion; UE = upper extremity.

state that a referral has been made to a rehabilitation hospital close to Mary's home, and discharge is pending for the following day.

The occupational therapist reviewed the goals and collected the necessary supplies to complete the activities outlined in Table 10.5. When the therapist entered her room, Mary was sitting in the recliner chair, the IV and the catheter having been discontinued. The session started with a review of the role of occupational therapy and the goals that were established in the previous session. Mary was asked to select which goals she would like to work on this session. Mary decided that she wants to be able to see better and wants to work on her perceptual goal and that she needs to be able to take care of herself to go home and wants to work on her dressing and bathing goals. Mary continued to be unaware of the deficits in her left upper extremity, so the occupational therapist used clinical reasoning to also include left upper-extremity motor relearning and awareness into the preparatory methods and task training in the session. Mary was discharged the following day to intensive inpatient **rehabilitation.**

Case Review: Walter

Postoperatively, Walter was transferred to the neurological intensive care unit (ICU). Initially, he required ventilator support because of pulmonary complications but was weaned to **continuous positive airway pressure** by Postoperative Day 2. Walter required an external ventricular drain (EVD) to decrease intracranial pressure and required close observation by the ICU staff because of concern about vasospasm. Oral food and fluids were withheld until a **dysphagia** screen could be completed.

Walter was referred to occupational therapy for evaluation and treatment on Postoperative Day 3 with activity orders that read, "Out of bed as tolerated, with assistance." The occupational therapist performed a review of the medical record and noted that Walter's past medical history included osteoarthritis, coronary artery disease, myocardial infarction status post–coronary artery bypass graft, hypertension, and multiple traumatic vertebral fractures. The medical record indicated that Walter continued to require the EVD but was tolerating it being clamped for periods of time, was experiencing intermittent cardiac **arrhythmia,** and was hyponatremic. The notes from the medical team rounds from earlier in the day indicated that Walter was neurologically stable.

Evaluation

On entry into the room, the occupational therapist observed Walter to be supine in bed with multiple lines and tubes including EVD, **nasogastric (NG) tube,** urinary catheter, 4 liters of oxygen via nasal prongs, two IV sites, and sequential compression pumps. He was connected to a vital signs monitor. Walter appeared to be asleep and in no acute distress. Walter's vital signs were as follows: (1) respiration rate, 22 breaths per minute; (2) heart rate, 88 beats per minute; (3) blood pressure, 129/78 mm Hg; and (4) intracranial pressure, 5 mm Hg.

The ICU room was observed to be orderly with a bedside recliner chair and an over-the-bed table. The television was turned off, and the lights were dimmed. A few get-well cards and a picture of Walter and Adele (his wife) standing in front of their condo were posted on the bulletin board. The nurse was just finishing flushing

Walter's NG tube and indicated that he was appropriate for therapy and that the plan for the day included getting Walter out of bed. The nurse clamped the EVD and indicated that Walter was tolerating it being clamped for approximately 45 minutes. Adele was sitting in a visitor's chair holding Walter's hand.

The occupational therapist introduced himself to Adele and explained the role of occupational therapy. Adele agreed to being interviewed before waking Walter. Through use of structured interview technique (Kielhofner & Henry, 1988), the therapist developed the occupational profile.

Occupational Profile

Walter is a 67-year-old man who before admission to the hospital was able to complete his ADLs with modifications and with the use of his walker. Adele was responsible for the cooking, cleaning, and grocery shopping. Walter has not driven for several years. He is retired from his job as a mechanic.

Walter lives with his wife in a one-level condo in a retirement community. There are no stairs to enter. Walter has a walker and a wheelchair at home and no other durable medical equipment. Adele indicates that she is in good health but becomes teary when explaining that although they have many friends with whom they socialize, they have no family who can help them.

When questioned about activities that he is able to do and those that are causing problems, Walter is unable to answer, and Adele again becomes teary and states, "I am not even sure he knows who I am, but he is calm when I hold his hand." In discussing goals, Adele indicates that for her to be able to take Walter home, he would have to be able to go to the bathroom by himself and get out of bed by himself.

Assessment

Cognitive Skills

An initial attempt using auditory stimuli resulted in a slight increase in Walter's heart and respiration rate, and Walter opened his eyes briefly but was unable to sustain wakefulness. By increasing the lighting in the room, bringing the head of the bed upright, removing the bed covers and sequential compression pumps, and having Adele participate by verbally waking Walter, he was able to open his eyes and look toward his wife on the left side of the bed.

Once positioned in the chair, with all the lines and monitoring equipment safely placed, the occupational therapist proceeded with standardized cognitive assessment. Sitting on Walter's left side, the therapist initiated the Short Blessed Cognitive Screen (Katzman et al., 1983), with Walter making eye contact with the therapist but unable to respond to the verbal questions. The test was discontinued.

Sensory–Perceptual Skills

Despite multiple trials and having Adele move to the right side of the bed, Walter was not able to shift his gaze to the right. An initial attempt at a pain assessment was made with the Analogue Pain Scale (McCormack, 1988), but Walter was unable to verbalize. Using the Checklist of Nonverbal Pain Indicators (Feldt, 2000), Walter was assessed to have no pain behaviors present.

Motor and Praxis Skills

Upper-extremity assessment was performed, with Walter having full **passive range of motion** (PROM) bilaterally. Walter was noted to have normal **tone** in the right upper extremity and was hypotonic (flaccid) throughout the left upper extremity. Walter was able to sustain wakefulness without stimuli, and although Walter was not able to follow commands for **active range of motion** and manual muscle testing, he was observed to frequently reach toward the NG tube with his right hand. His left hand was noted to be in a dependent position at the side of his body, slightly edematous with no active movement noted. Walter withdrew from noxious stimuli on the right side but not the left.

The recliner chair was positioned appropriately beside the bed considering the location of all the lines and tubes to ensure safe patient transfer (Arias & Smith, 2007; Cumming, Collier, Thrift, & Bernhardt, 2008). A rehabilitation therapy aide was called to assist with the transfer, and the nurse was asked to be present to manage the EVD and the other lines.

The Trunk Control Test (Collin & Wade, 1990) was administered. Walter was first assessed rolling from supine to his left side (weak side), for which he required 100% assist. He was then assessed in rolling from supine to his right, for which he also required 100% assist. With the occupational therapist in front and the therapy aide behind, Walter required 100% assist to transfer from side lying to sitting. Once sitting, Walter required 75% assist for static sitting balance. Walter scored 12 of 100 on the Trunk Control Test. He was noted to have poor trunk control, poor postural alignment, and inability to self-correct when leaning to the left, but he was able to initiate self-correction when he leaned to the right. Vital signs remained within normal parameters. A gait belt was securely positioned around Walter's waist. A side-by-side transfer from bed to chair required 75% assist by two people, with it being noted that Walter was able to bear weight through his right lower extremity during the transfer and attempted to reach for the chair with his right hand to help lower himself.

Communication and Social Skills

The Boston Naming Test (Lansing et al., 1999) was administered; initially, Walter attended to the stimulus when presented on the left, but as the test proceeded, he demonstrated fluctuating levels of wakefulness and needed 100% verbal cues to continue. Walter scored 0 of 15, indicating significant language impairment.

Activities of Daily Living Skills

To complete the ADL assessment, Walter was provided a rest period while the occupational therapist gathered the necessary supplies to prepare for the next step in the evaluation. To allow for a continued rest period, the occupational therapist opted to proceed with caregiver training, including educating Adele on the role of occupational therapy and instructing her in how to perform PROM and proper positioning to prevent edema and protect Walter's shoulder. Adele received the education with enthusiasm and verbalized, "I will do anything I can to help Walter get better."

With the over-the-bed table positioned in front of Walter, the therapist placed a comb on it in his left visual field. Walter was verbally instructed to pick up the comb and comb his hair. Walter was not able to follow the command to complete the task. The comb was placed in Walter's left hand, and he was instructed, "Comb your hair." Walter was able to grasp the comb but was unable to complete the task. He required 100% hand-over-hand assistance to complete it. This approach was repeated using a toothbrush and a washcloth. At this time, Walter again demonstrated fluctuating levels of wakefulness, and the nurse entered the room to indicate it was time to unclamp the EVD. Walter was positioned in the chair in a reclined position, with a pillow to support his right upper extremity and all the lines and tubes in a position of safety. The lights were dimmed, and the television remained off to allow Walter to rest. Vital signs were documented and were again noted to be within acceptable limits.

At the time of evaluation, Walter still had an NG tube and was therefore receiving no oral food and fluids, so feeding was not addressed; however, a dysphagia screen can also be part of the evaluation for a patient like Walter if the NG tube is removed. This screening is at times completed by an occupational therapist or by a speech–language pathologist; however, this is an advanced skill that would require the occupational therapist to obtain specialized training to complete. (AOTA has published a Self-Paced Clinical Course specific to this topic, *Dysphagia Care and Related Feeding Concerns for Adults* [2nd ed.; Avery, 2010].)

Intervention Plan

In developing a clinical decision regarding recommendation for discharge for Walter, the occupational therapist drew from four dimensions: (1) Walter's current functioning and disability, (2) his wants and needs (including Adele's contribution), (3) his ability to participate, and (4) his life context (meaning the environment in which he lives; Taylor, 2004).

To summarize Walter's current level of functioning, on the first dimension, he requires stimulation to maintain wakefulness but is able to sustain wakefulness for 3 to 5 minutes. Walter presents with language impairments for both receptive and expressive language, and he demonstrates the ability to track and regard in his left visual field but not in his right. Dense right hemiplegia is noted, which results in Walter requiring maximum assist for ADL tasks.

In considering Walter's wants and needs, he is unable to express his current goals. During interview with Adele, it is clear that she identifies the goals for Walter to be as independent as possible and to be able to go home. Adele conceded that, given her own age and abilities, Walter would have to be able to go to the bathroom by himself and be able to get out of bed by himself for her to be able to take care of him.

The third dimension is examining Walter's ability to participate. Medically, he continues to require ICU level of care and has an EVD in place, but he is neurologically stable with the ability to maintain acceptable vital signs during the evaluation process. He responded to therapeutic approaches during the evaluation and clearly could benefit from further occupational therapy. However, Walter presents with limited activity tolerance with fatigue and fluctuating levels of wakefulness during

Points to Ponder: Environmental Influences on Performance

The characteristics of the environment can influence the ability of the patient with cognitive impairments to perform and participate in tasks and activities. What are some environmental characteristics of the hospital room that may be appropriate for the occupational therapist to modify to maximize a patient's performance level?

the assessment and an inability to maintain wakefulness after completion of the 40-minute session.

The context of Walter's life before the **subarachnoid hemorrhage** is the fourth dimension used to determine appropriate discharge recommendations. Walter had made modifications to his daily life because of declining health, preexisting comorbidities, and previous injuries but was enjoying an active social life with Adele in their condo.

In synthesizing all dimensions of decision making as related to discharge planning, the occupational therapist is aware that Walter requires continued occupational therapy. Discharge home with community-based services of either home health occupational therapy or outpatient occupational therapy is not an option because of Walter's low level of functioning. The occupational therapist then considers the options of intensive inpatient rehabilitation (which typically requires the patient to be able to participate 3 hours per day and has a shorter length of stay); a skilled nursing facility (SNF; which typically requires participation 1.5 to 2 hours per day and has a longer length of stay); or long-term acute care (for which the patient must need specialized nursing care in addition to therapy). Currently, Walter's level of functioning, wants and needs, ability to participate, and the context of his environment lead the occupational therapist to recommend to Adele that Walter receive continued occupational therapy services in a SNF.

With an estimated length of stay of 10 days, the occupational therapist established a frequency of treatment that included occupational therapy 3 to 4 times per week while in the acute care hospital with occupational therapy priorities including interventions for upper-extremity motor relearning, sitting balance in preparation for ADLs, cognitive and perceptual remediation and compensation, ADL training, therapeutic activity (Eyres & Unsworth, 2005), and family education. Recommendations for referrals for physical therapy and speech–language pathology were made. Further occupational therapy services in the SNF were recommended (see Table 10.6).

Intervention Implementation

In preparation for the first treatment session, the occupational therapist reviewed the medical record. Neurologist notes indicate that Walter is medically stable, the EVD has been removed, and Walter has been transferred from the ICU to a neurosurgical unit. Notes from the social worker state that a referral has been made to a SNF close to Walter's home, and discharge is pending in 4 days.

The occupational therapist reviewed the goals and collected the necessary supplies to complete the activities outlined in Table 10.6. Over the course of the next three treatment sessions, the occupational therapist works toward the goals outlined. Each treatment session begins with a brief screening of Walter's impairments and functional status to note changes in status, which may occur rapidly during the acute care stage of recovery. Treatment plans follow an outline of preparatory activities, followed by purposeful and occupation-based activities, and are graded to Walter's abilities that day.

Table 10.6. Walter's Intervention Planning and Implementation Outline

Occupational Therapy Intervention Priority	Goals (to Be Achieved by Discharge)	Preparatory Methods and Tasks	Occupation and Activity	Education and Training
ADL training	• Walter will demonstrate appropriate use of 3 ADL utensils. • Walter will perform grooming task in supported sitting with 75% assist.	• Transfer Walter to bedside chair to increase alertness before training. • AROM for RUE; PROM and facilitation of AAROM for LUE. • Demonstration followed by return demonstration of utensil use. • Set up task components for grooming (on the OTB table with Walter in sitting) and provide expectation for partial task completion.	• Hand-over-hand training with each ADL utensil (e.g., toothbrush, comb, razor).	• Use mirror during training.
Motor function (UE and sitting)	• Walter will demonstrate static sitting balance on EOB with good postural alignment with 75% assist in preparation for ADL tasks. • Walter will initiate grasp–release of ADL utensil 3× with LUE.	• Rolling from supine to side lying (right and left side). • Transition movement from side lying to sitting. • Facilitation of movement in LUE through weight bearing, vibration, ROM. • Facilitation of sitting balance with good postural alignment using tactile and verbal cues. • Hand-over-hand assistance to encourage grasp–release of built-up utensils. • Have Walter pass the utensil from his right into his left hand. • While seated EOB, present ADL task (e.g., basin with water and washcloth) and have Walter initiate portions of the task.		
Visuoperceptual training	• Walter will demonstrate ability to track objects from right to left visual field with 50% verbal cues.	• Occulomotor exercises. • Tracking horizontally and vertically. • Have Walter's wife move within the room and ask Walter to track her movement. • Have Walter track a photograph that is moved horizontally within his visual field. • Because Walter previously enjoyed watching sports, place images of baseball and football on OTB table and have him shift his gaze from one to the other. • Place hospital TV within range and provide stimulus for Walter to track to find the TV.		

(Continued)

Table 10.6. Walter's Intervention Planning and Implementation Outline *(cont.)*

Occupational Therapy Intervention Priority	Goals (to Be Achieved by Discharge)	Preparatory Methods and Tasks	Occupation and Activity	Education and Training
Cognitive remediation	• Walter will attend to task for 5 min with 75% verbal cues in a controlled environment.	• Set up environment so it is free of distractions (TV turned off, door closed, lights on). • Transfer Walter to EOB or to an upright position in chair to facilitate wakefulness and attention.	• Because Walter previously enjoyed game night with his friends, have Adele bring in one of the games and have Walter take game pieces out of the box and set up a portion of the game. • Grade activity to a just-right challenge to allow for longer periods of attention. • Play a portion of the game.	
Caregiver education	• Walter's vital signs will remain stable during PROM and AAROM exercises when completed by Walter's wife.	• Perform PROM, AAROM, and AROM for Walter's UE.		• Instruct Adele in proper technique and provide written directions. • Observe Adele performing ROM and provide necessary feedback.

Note. AAROM = active assistive range of motion; ADL = activity of daily living; AROM = active range of motion; EOB = edge of bed; LUE = left upper extremity; min = minutes; OTB = over the bed; PROM = passive range of motion; ROM = range of motion; RUE = right upper extremity; UE = upper extremity.

Outcomes and Special Considerations

After a week in acute care, Walter achieved medical stability and demonstrated appropriate participation to continue occupational therapy in a SNF.

References

American Occupational Therapy Association. (2012). *AOTA Fact Sheet—Occupational therapy in acute care*. Retrieved September 1, 2012, from http://www.aota.org/404.aspx?item=%2f consumers%2fprofessionals%2fwhatisot%2frdp%2ffacts%2f43243&user=extranet%5c Anonymous&site=Corporate

American Occupational Therapy Association. (2014). Occupational therapy practice framework: Domain and process (3rd ed.). *American Journal of Occupational Therapy, 68*(Suppl. 1), S1–S48. http://dx.doi.org/10.5014/ajot.2014.682006

Arias, M., & Smith, L. N. (2007). Early mobilization of acute stroke patients. *Journal of Clinical Nursing, 16*, 282–288. http://dx.doi.org/10.1111/j.1365-2702.2005.01488.x

Avery, W. (Ed.). (2010). *Dysphagia care and related feeding concerns for adults* (2nd ed.). Bethesda, MD: American Occupational Therapy Association.

Baum, C. M., Connor, L. T., Morrison, T., Hahn, M., Dromerick, A. W., & Edwards, D. F. (2008). Reliability, validity, and clinical utility of the Executive Function Performance Test: A measure of executive function in a sample of people with stroke. *American Journal of Occupational Therapy, 62*, 446–455. http://dx.doi.org/10.5014/ajot.62.4.446

Berg, K. (1989). Measuring balance in the elderly: Preliminary development of an instrument. *Physiotherapy Canada, 41*, 304–311. http://dx.doi.org/10.3138/ptc.41.6.304

Bohannon, R. W., & Smith, M. B. (1987). Interrater reliability of a modified Ashworth Scale of muscle spasticity. *Physical Therapy, 67*, 206–207.

Collin, C., & Wade, D. T. (1990). Assessing motor impairment after stroke: A pilot reliability study. *Journal of Neurology, Neurosurgery, and Psychiatry, 53*, 576–579. http://dx.doi.org/10.1136/jnnp.53.7.576

Cumming, T. B., Collier, J., Thrift, A. G., & Bernhardt, J. (2008). The effect of very early mobilisation after stroke on psychological well-being. *Journal of Rehabilitation Medicine, 40*, 609–614. http://dx.doi.org/10.2340/16501977-0226

DiClemente, C. C. (2007). The Transtheoretical Model of Intentional Behaviour Change. *Drugs and Alcohol Today, 7,* 29–33. http://dx.doi.org/10.1108/17459265200700007

Erasmus, L.-P., Sarno, S., Albrecht, H., Schwecht, M., Pöllmann, W., & König, N. (2001). Measurement of ataxic symptoms with a graphic tablet: Standard values in controls and validity in multiple sclerosis patients. *Journal of Neuroscience Methods, 108,* 25–37. http://dx.doi.org/10.1016/S0165-0270(01)00373-9

Eyres, L., & Unsworth, C. (2005). Occupational therapy in acute hospitals: The effectiveness of a pilot program to maintain occupational performance in older clients. *Australian Occupational Therapy Journal, 52,* 218–224. http://dx.doi.org/10.1111/j.1440-1630.2005.00498.x

Feldt, K. S. (2000). The Checklist of Nonverbal Pain Indicators (CNPI). *Pain Management Nursing, 1,* 13–21. http://dx.doi.org/10.1053/jpmn.2000.5831

Finfgeld, D. L., Wongvatunyu, S., Conn, V. S., Grando, V. T., & Russell, C. L. (2003). Health Belief Model and Reversal Theory: A comparative analysis. *Journal of Advanced Nursing, 43,* 288–297. http://dx.doi.org/10.1046/j.1365-2648.2003.02712.x

Friedman, P. J. (1991). Clock drawing in acute stroke. *Age and Ageing, 20,* 140–145. http://dx.doi.org/10.1093/ageing/20.2.140

Katzman, R., Brown, T., Fuld, P., Peck, A., Schechter, R., & Schimmel, H. (1983). Validation of a short orientation–memory–concentration test of cognitive impairment. *American Journal of Psychiatry, 140,* 734–739.

Kielhofner, G., & Henry, A. D. (1988). Development and investigation of the occupational performance history interview. *American Journal of Occupational Therapy, 42,* 489–498. http://dx.doi.org/10.5014/ajot.42.8.489

Lansing, A. E., Ivnik, R. J., Cullum, C. M., & Randolph, C. (1999). An empirically derived short form of the Boston Naming Test. *Archives of Clinical Neuropsychology, 14,* 481–487. http://dx.doi.org/10.1093/arclin/14.6.481

Mahoney, F. I., & Barthel, D. W. (1965). Functional evaluation: The Barthel Index. *Maryland State Medical Journal, 14,* 61–65.

Mastos, M., Miller, K., Eliasson, A. C., & Imms, C. (2007). Goal-directed training: Linking theories of treatment to clinical practice for improved functional activities in daily life. *Clinical Rehabilitation, 21,* 47–55. http://dx.doi.org/10.1177/0269215506073494

McCormack, G. L. (1988). Pain management by occupational therapists. *American Journal of Occupational Therapy, 42,* 582–590. http://dx.doi.org/10.5014/ajot.42.9.582

Nasreddine, Z. S., Phillips, N. A., Bedirian, V., Charbonneau, S., Whitehead, V., Collin, I., . . . Chertkow, H. (2005). The Montreal Cognitive Assessment, MoCA: A brief screening tool for mild cognitive impairment. *Journal of the American Geriatrics Society, 53,* 695–699. http://dx.doi.org/10.1111/j.1532-5415.2005.53221.x

Sabari, J., & Lieberman, D. (2008). *Occupational therapy practice guidelines for adults with stroke.* Bethesda, MD: AOTA Press.

Stillman, G., Granger, C., & Niewczyk, P. (2009). Projecting function of stroke patients in rehabilitation using the AlphaFIM instrument in acute care. *PM&R, 1,* 234–239. http://dx.doi.org/10.1016/j.pmrj.2008.10.014

Taylor, M. C. (2004). A model to illustrate the process of decision making in acute care discharge planning. *Australian Occupational Therapy Journal, 51,* 213–215. http://dx.doi.org/10.1111/j.1440-1630.2004.00457.x

Toglia, J. (2009). *Weekly Calendar Planning Activity.* Dobbs Ferry, NY: Mercy College.

Vanbellingen, T., Kersten, B., Van de Winckel, A., Bellion, M., Baronti, F., Müri, R., & Bohlhalter, S. (2011). A new bedside test of gestures in stroke: The Apraxia Screen of TULIA (AST). *Journal of Neurology, Neurosurgery, and Psychiatry, 82,* 389–392. http://dx.doi.org/10.1136/jnnp.2010.213371

Weintraub, S., & Mesulam, M. M. (1988). Visual hemispatial inattention: Stimulus parameters and exploratory strategies. *Journal of Neurology, Neurosurgery, and Psychiatry, 51,* 1481–1488. http://dx.doi.org/10.1136/jnnp.51.12.1481

CHAPTER 11

Occupational Therapy for People With Stroke in the Inpatient Rehabilitation Setting

*Keri DeGroot, OTD, OTR/L, and
Mary W. Hildebrand, OTD, OTR/L*

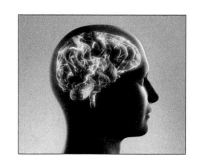

Learning Objectives

After completion of this chapter, readers will be able to

- Identify similarities and differences between an inpatient rehabilitation facility and a skilled nursing facility for providing rehabilitation services after stroke;
- Identify important factors to consider when determining discharge placement from an inpatient rehabilitation setting for mild, moderate, or severe stroke;
- Identify appropriate assessments in an inpatient rehabilitation setting for people with mild, moderate, or severe stroke;
- Differentiate among preparatory methods and tasks, activities, and occupations as interventions for people after stroke in an inpatient rehabilitation setting; and
- Recognize differences between intervention approaches (create or promote, establish or restore, maintain, modify, prevent) when treating people with stroke in an inpatient rehabilitation setting.

Introduction

Once patients with **stroke** have achieved medical stability in the acute setting, many are discharged to an inpatient **rehabilitation** setting, which may include an inpatient rehabilitation facility (IRF), a skilled nursing facility (SNF), or other settings (see Chapter 10, Table 10.1, for indications for discharge from acute care). For the purposes of this chapter, we focus only on IRFs and SNFs and their admission requirements, typical discharge dispositions, lengths of stay, and occupational therapy service delivery and roles.

Key Words

- aphasia
- discharge disposition
- dysphagia
- executive function
- hemiparesis
- inpatient rehabilitation facility
- intervention approach
- intervention implementation
- intervention plan
- mild stroke
- moderate stroke
- sensation deficits
- severe stroke
- skilled nursing facility
- unilateral left neglect

Inpatient Rehabilitation Facility

An *IRF* is defined as a facility that provides intensive therapies in an inpatient hospital environment for patients who require nursing, medical management, and an interdisciplinary approach to delivery of rehabilitation care (Centers for Medicare and Medicaid Services [CMS], 2012). It may be a free-standing rehabilitation center, a unit within a hospital, or a Veterans Health Administration rehabilitation unit (Roberts & Evenson, 2014). Admission to an IRF requires that the patient be able to tolerate 3 or more hours of therapy per day for a minimum of 5 days per week from at least two therapy modalities, one of which must be either physical therapy or occupational therapy. The patient must be medically stable, fully able to participate in and benefit from therapy, motivated to participate in intensive rehabilitation, and demonstrate potential for functional improvement in a reasonable time frame. At least 60% of patients in an IRF must have a diagnosis of 1 of the 13 CMS diagnostic groups; stroke is an included diagnosis. The overarching therapy goal for a patient admitted to an IRF is that the patient return safely to his or her home or community on discharge (CMS, 2012). Therefore, if a patient will be discharged to a nursing home for long-term care, he or she would not be suitable for an IRF (Hamby, 2011).

Most IRF patients are admitted directly from an acute care hospital, with a small percentage coming from the community, other health care settings, or SNFs (Medicare Payment Advisory Commission [MedPAC], 2013). In an IRF, a rehabilitation physician must see the patient at least 3 times per week and lead an interdisciplinary team conference 1 time per week to reassess the client's established goals and monitor and revise the treatment plan as needed (CMS, 2012; Roberts & Evenson, 2014). In 2010, the average length of stay in an IRF for a person poststroke was reported to be 16 days (MedPAC, 2011). Payment or funding sources for a client's stay in an IRF may include private insurance or self-pay, managed care, indemnity, workers' compensation, Medicare, or Medicaid (Roberts & Evenson, 2014).

In an IRF, occupational therapists provide direct treatment through one-to-one services and some group therapy as an adjunct method (Roberts & Evenson, 2014). Roberts and Evenson (2014) listed the roles of the occupational therapist in an IRF as involving the following:

- Comprehensive evaluation
- Participation in functional outcomes such as the Inpatient Rehabilitation Facility–Patient Assessment Instrument (IRF–PAI)
- Self-care skills
- Functional mobility
- Functional communication
- Social cognition
- IADLs [instrumental activities of daily living]
- Community reintegration
- Discharge planning
- Recommendations for continued services at the next level of care. (pp. 903–904)

Skilled Nursing Facility

A *SNF* is a provider that meets Medicare requirements for Part A coverage (MedPAC, 2013). In addition, the majority of SNFs are dually certified as nursing homes for long-term care residents and are free-standing and for-profit facilities (MedPAC, 2013). SNFs provide short-term skilled nursing care and therapy services such as occupational therapy, physical therapy, and speech–language pathology therapy for people who require 24-hour care or who may need to bridge the gap between an acute care hospital and an IRF with another level of care. SNFs may also admit patients who require intravenous medication or wound care or who have a disability with a new functional deficit.

Medicare Part A requirements for admission to a SNF include patients having had a 3-day medically necessary inpatient acute care hospitalization within the past 30 days; a reasonable and necessary need for skilled nursing care, therapy, or both; and being unable to participate in the 3 hours of therapy per day necessary to be admitted to an IRF; typically, 1.5 hours is expected. A Minimum Data Set (MDS) screen is completed on each qualified Medicare patient that divides him or her into one of six resource utilization groups (RUGs) and determines the total number of minutes of therapy he or she receives and the disciplines that may treat him or her (Lohman, 2014). A SNF allows for a slower progression toward functional improvement and, unlike an IRF, discharge disposition from a SNF may include a nursing home (Hamby, 2011). Medicare recipients have a maximum length of stay in a SNF of 100 days with other criteria or terms as required by Medicare (Hamby, 2011). For patients in SNF short-term rehabilitation, occupational therapy is provided as a direct one-to-one service. Payment or funding sources for clients' stay in a SNF are the same as those for IRF clients (Roberts & Evenson, 2014).

Roberts and Evenson (2014, p. 904) and the American Occupational Therapy Association's (AOTA; 2013) fact sheet titled *Occupational Therapy's Role in Skilled Nursing Facilities* provide lists with the following roles for occupational therapists working with short-term rehabilitation patients in a SNF:

> A SNF allows for a slower progression toward functional improvement and, unlike an IRF, discharge disposition from a SNF may include a nursing home.

- Teaching self-care skills
- Teaching mobility skills during **activities of daily living** (ADLs), such as bed, chair, and wheelchair transfers; toilet and tub–shower transfers; and locomotor activities
- Teaching IADL and community skills, such as car transfers, homemaking activities, public dining, care of pets, and so forth
- Providing training in the use of adaptive equipment, compensatory techniques, and environmental modifications to increase safety and independence
- Addressing behavioral health needs of clients, such as depression or **anxiety**
- Preparing the client for community reintegration, such as dining in public or emergency response
- Assessing the need for home modifications and safety equipment to increase safety on discharge
- Exploring adaptations and compensatory strategies for return to volunteer or paid employment
- Educating clients on community resources to support needs after discharge
- Assessing current **leisure** skills for modification or compensatory strategies to continue participation or pursuit of new leisure activities.

Table 11.1. Discharge Disposition Recommendation Options

Options	Indications
Home with no supervision	Recommend when patient is independent in ADL or IADL tasks and has adequate safety awareness to be without supervision. Patient may continue with outpatient therapy.
Home with intermittent supervision	Recommend when patient can be safe alone for short periods of time but still needs help with some ADL or IADL tasks.
Home with 24-hour supervision	Recommend when patient is safe to go home but requires assistance or supervision 24 hours a day for safety or ADL or IADL tasks.
Assisted living facility	Recommend when a patient is safe with intermittent supervision, but family or others are unable to provide this support at home.
Skilled nursing facility	Recommend when a patient could continue to benefit from therapy at a less intense rate and requires 24-hour nursing care.
Long-term care facility	Recommend when a patient is no longer making progress in therapy but requires 24-hour care that family or others are unable to provide.
Outpatient day treatment	Recommend when a patient requires daily therapy but no longer meets the requirements for inpatient rehabilitation.
Outpatient occupational therapy	Recommend when a patient no longer requires 24-hour nursing care but is able and would benefit from further occupational therapy outside the home.
Home health occupational therapy	Recommend when a home safety evaluation is required and if the patient is homebound.

Source. Adapted from "Discharge Planning: A Consultative Partnership," by J. Hamby, in *Occupational Therapy in Acute Care* (pp. 687–698), by H. Smith-Gabai (Ed.), 2011, Bethesda, MD: AOTA Press.

Note. ADLs = activities of daily living; IADLs = instrumental activities of daily living.

For both IRFs and SNFs, the occupational therapy process as outlined in the *Occupational Therapy Practice Framework: Domain and Process* (3rd ed.; AOTA, 2014) includes completion of an initial evaluation with an occupational profile and analysis of occupational performance, establishment of long- and short-term goals, development and implementation of a treatment plan, review of intervention and modification of the plan as needed, and tracking of outcomes with a discharge evaluation.

As in the acute care setting, occupational therapists are essential team members in deciding the patient's discharge destination and recommending what level of therapy should follow discharge (see Table 11.1).

Evaluation in the Inpatient Rehabilitation Setting

The occupational therapy initial evaluation in the inpatient rehabilitation setting begins with a thorough medical chart review before meeting the patient. Important information gleaned from the chart that may inform the evaluation process includes (1) transfer status and functional activity assistance levels from the acute care hospital therapist and (2) orders for physical activity and precautions from the inpatient rehabilitation physician. Possible areas for precautions for patients with stroke are as follows:

- Fall
- Swallowing
- Physical activity restrictions
- Blood pressure
- Intracranial pressure
- Glucose levels (with history of diabetes)
- Precautions from recent surgical procedures (hip, sternal, spinal).

Occupational therapy assessment of the client with stroke in a rehabilitation setting is more client centered, holistic, and comprehensive than in the acute care hospital. According to the *Occupational Therapy Practice Guidelines for Adults With Stroke* (Sabari & Lieberman, 2008), in acute care it is more appropriate for the occupational therapist to perform a bottom-up assessment because stroke survivors are adapting to their loss, and recovery is unpredictable in the early stages. Occupational therapists in the rehabilitation setting, however, must determine the needs and personal interests of the stroke survivor and family to assess performance in valued activities and the client factors that affect performance (Sabari & Lieberman, 2008). Occupational therapists in the inpatient rehabilitation setting, therefore, must dynamically move between top-down and bottom-up approaches as they monitor progress and recovery (Sabari & Lieberman, 2008). The top-down approach in the inpatient rehabilitation setting begins with conducting an occupational profile with assessments such as the Activity Card Sort (ACS; Baum & Edwards, 2008) or the Canadian Occupational Performance Measure (COPM; Law et al., 2005). After determining the occupations that the patient wants to do, the occupational therapist assesses the patient's performance in those activities. However, note that reimbursement mechanisms in the United States require that occupational therapists in inpatient rehabilitation settings focus on ADLs and IADLs (Bonder, 2014; Sabari & Lieberman, 2008). Typically, occupational therapists in the inpatient rehabilitation setting use assessments of ADLs and IADLs such as the **FIM™** (Uniform Data System for Medical Rehabilitation, 1997) or the Assessment of Motor and Process Skills (AMPS; Fisher, 1993).

Finally, the occupational therapist will assess the client's body functions, body structures, performance skills, and the elements of the environment and context that can support or be barriers to the client's ability to participate in his or her high-priority activities. In an inpatient rehabilitation setting, this may include assessments of strength (manual muscle testing [MMT]), **cognition** (Executive Function Performance Test [EFPT]; Baum et al., 2008), or depression (Beck Depression Inventory [BDI®] Fast-Screen for Medical Patients; Beck, Steer, & Brown, 2000). Standardized assessments are routinely used in the inpatient rehabilitation setting because of the need for therapists to establish a baseline, reevaluate to determine progress for treatment and discharge, and provide data for program evaluation (Sabari & Lieberman, 2008).

Intervention in the Inpatient Rehabilitation Setting

Intervention in the inpatient rehabilitation phase is governed by a focus on "restoration of client factors, adaptation of contexts, and reintegration of the client and family into the home and community" (Rybski, 2006, p. 69). Thus, the medical model is less evident in an IRF and SNF than in the acute care hospital. Because rehabilitation settings use a more client-centered approach, the client is expected to participate in setting goals and assume responsibility for his or her therapies (Rybski, 2006).

Intervention Approaches and Models

The *Framework* (AOTA, 2014) defines five intervention approaches: (1) create or promote (health promotion); (2) establish or restore (remediation, restoration); (3) maintain; (4) modify (compensation, adaptation); and (5) prevent (disability prevention). Each approach is important to use in treatment with stroke survivors in an inpatient rehabilitation setting. Many models of practice or frames of reference

Occupational therapy assessment of the client with stroke in a rehabilitation setting is more client centered, holistic, and comprehensive than in the acute care hospital.

fit within the *Framework* intervention approaches, and often multiple models will influence a client's plan of care.

The create-or-promote approach is vital to incorporate in intervention with stroke survivors to establish performance patterns for healthy lifestyle behaviors such as healthy diet or physical activity. The establish-or-restore approach focuses on restoring performance skills and will guide treatment of deficits resulting from stroke such as weakness, decreased balance, or **unilateral neglect.** Concepts from the Dynamic Interactional Model (DIM; Toglia, 2011) focus on training new cognitive skills that can be transferred to other situations and fit under the *Framework* intervention approaches of maintain and modify. In addition, training in and use of adaptive equipment uses the modify approach. Preventing disability or secondary conditions is crucial at all stages of rehabilitation, for example, to prevent **learned nonuse,** pain, **contracture,** or depression (see Tables 11.3, 11.7, and 11.12 later in the chapter for further designation of *Framework* intervention approaches used in each case).

Measuring Outcomes

Rybski (2006, p. 70) stated that the rehabilitation phase for stroke survivors should help the client to "engage in daily life activities, increase occupational performance, resume roles, increase quality of life, and promote a healthy lifestyle." Therefore, occupational therapy outcomes from the inpatient setting should focus on these areas. However, with the required emphasis in inpatient rehabilitation on ADLs and IADLs, occupational therapy outcomes are most frequently measured by determining change in ADL and IADL assessment scores from admission to discharge. In addition, change on impairment measures is often measured and used to track improvement. An occupational therapist may also measure outcomes by assessing the degree to which a client and family understand and apply education received on discharge, including recommendations for home modifications, durable medical equipment, further occupational therapy services, community resources, or support groups (Roberts & Evenson, 2014).

Although Rybski (2006, p. 70) stated that improvement in quality of life should be considered after this phase as well, many facilities fail to measure this in a standardized, systematic way. Occupational therapists need to broaden the scope of typically measured outcomes by evaluating occupations beyond ADLs and IADLs and attending to these other important constructs.

> The rehabilitation phase for stroke survivors should help the client to "engage in daily life activities, increase occupational performance, resume roles, increase quality of life, and promote a healthy lifestyle." (Rybski, 2006, p. 70)

Case Review: Steve

Steve was referred to an IRF for evaluation from occupational therapy, physical therapy, and speech therapy. Evaluations began on Day 2 of his stay (i.e., the day after his admission). Occupational therapy was the first to see Steve in the morning for an evaluation of bathing and dressing. The occupational therapist reviewed Steve's medical chart, paying particular attention to the physician's orders of fall precautions and activity as tolerated. Nursing notes also indicated that during the previous evening, Steve had been irritable and had three emotional outbursts at staff.

Evaluation

When the occupational therapist entered Steve's room, Steve was observed to be sitting at the edge of the bed eating his breakfast from the tray on the over-the-bed table in front of him. He was wearing a hospital gown and grip socks and had his laptop computer and cell phone on the tray next to his breakfast. The occupational therapist explained the rehabilitation process and the role of occupational therapy in the inpatient stroke unit. Steve was oriented to self but had inconsistencies in **orientation** to place and situation. He said, "I'm not sure why I had to go to another hospital; I just need to get home and all of this will be fine."

Occupational Profile

The ACS (Baum & Edwards, 2008) was used to enhance the initial interview and gain more insight into Steve's occupational profile and activities that are important to him. The ACS is a measure of occupation that enables occupational therapists to help clients describe their instrumental, leisure, and social activities. Steve was first asked to divide the cards into activities he did and did not do before the stroke. The occupational therapist and Steve then discussed which of the activities he did before were important for him to continue doing. Through this assessment and further discussion, the therapist determined that Steve's main goals were returning to work, bathing and dressing independently, and being able to manage his family's finances. This type of assessment was chosen because it did not require that Steve perform activities he had done previous to the stroke. It also provided information about Steve's insight into his deficits. He demonstrated decreased insight by inaccurately stating which activities would or would not be difficult for him as a result of his stroke. While performing the ACS, Steve stated that although he was fine after this first stroke, he was anxious about having another stroke, becoming disabled, and being unable to work in the future. The occupational therapist provided education about the psychological consequences of stroke and assured Steve that having anxiety or depression was common after such a serious event. The occupational therapist stated that she would recommend a psychiatric referral to the rehabilitation team to help Steve contend with possible anxiety and depression.

Self-Care

The initial evaluation included the FIM (Uniform Data System for Medical Rehabilitation, 1997), a measure of impairment in self-care, mobility, and cognition, to assess ADL performance. The FIM was selected because it is standard for many inpatient rehabilitation settings in the United States, and its 7-point scale allows for sensitivity to change during an inpatient stay. The FIM measures the level of a patient's disability and indicates how much assistance is required for the patient to carry out ADLs. See Table 11.2 for Steve's initial FIM scores.

> **The FIM . . . is standard for many inpatient rehabilitation settings in the United States, and its 7-point scale allows for sensitivity to change during an inpatient stay.**

Throughout the bathing and dressing session, Steve was impulsive during standing and transfers and needed physical intervention to recover from three loss-of-balance incidents. He expressed annoyance at the therapist's close physical proximity when standing to perform activities, saying, "I can do it, you don't need to be right there." He fatigued easily and required two rest breaks in the ADL session.

Balance

The physical therapist evaluated Steve's balance using the *Berg Balance Scale,* the most widely used balance assessment of static and dynamic balance abilities (Berg,

Table 11.2. Steve's Admission FIM™ Scores and Barriers to Performance

FIM Category (ADL)	FIM Score	Barriers to Performance
Eating	6	Required increased time to manage containers due to decreased left fine motor control.
Grooming	4	Assessed standing at sink. Required set up of items and minimum assistance to maintain balance.
Bathing	4	Assessed seated and standing in the shower. Required assistance for washing the left lower leg and steadying assistance when standing to wash buttocks.
Upper-body dressing	5	Required the therapist to retrieve the shirt; was able to don shirt without physical intervention but required minimum verbal cues for technique.
Lower-body dressing	4	Assistance required for balance when standing to pull up pants and for donning left shoe.
Toileting	4	Required contact guard assist for balance during clothing management.
Bladder management	7	As reported by nursing.
Bowel management	7	As reported by nursing.
Transfers: bed, chair, w/c, toilet (tub, shower NT)	4	Required minimum assistance for balance during all transfers and used grab bars when available. All transfers were either stand pivot or stand step.
Locomotion	4	As reported by physical therapist: minimum assistance of 1 required secondary to decreased dynamic balance and endurance without a device.

Note. ADL = activity of daily living; NT = not tested; w/c = wheelchair.

Maki, Williams, Holliday, & Wood-Dauphinee, 1992; Donato & Halliday Pulaski, 2011). The physical therapist scored Steve's balance as 40 of a possible 56, indicating a moderate risk for falls. In addition to requiring assistance for balance during standing activities, Steve showed decreased dynamic sitting balance when dressing at the edge of bed and required supervision and minimum verbal cues to correct sitting posture from leaning to the left.

Motor Skills

Steve's **active range of motion** (AROM) and MMT were measured, with full AROM and strength (5 of 5) found in the right upper extremity. Steve was able to move the left upper extremity through full **range of motion** (ROM) with increased time and effort and had 4 of 5 strength throughout the left upper extremity. Steve had a slight decrease in **proprioception** and light touch discrimination in the left hand. The *Action Research Arm Test* (ARAT; Nijland et al., 2010), a measure of upper-limb functioning, showed some decreased fine motor control (FMC) in the left hand, with a score of 49 for the left and 57 for the right.

Process Skills

Steve's **executive functioning** skills were assessed with the *EFPT,* an assessment of cognitive integration and functioning that uses four basic tasks (Baum et al., 2008). The EFPT was selected because of its wide availability, brief training time, and low cost. Steve's score on the EFPT was 27 of 100, an indication of executive function deficits. He struggled on the bill paying portion of the test and became upset that he could not problem solve which bill to pay first. He required direct verbal instruction to complete the task. Steve also had difficulty with attention to task, pausing often to talk to the occupational therapist about unrelated topics. During the cooking task in the ADL suite kitchen, he forgot to turn off the burner on the stove, left a potholder near the burner, and required physical intervention from the therapist to prevent the potholder from catching fire.

Assessment

The occupational therapist formulated the following problem statements to support treatment planning:

- Due to decreased balance and impulsivity, Steve has difficulty completing ADL and IADL tasks safely.
- Due to decreased left upper-extremity strength and FMC, Steve has difficulty performing several ADL and IADL tasks.
- Steve's decreased insight into his deficits reduces safety in performing activities and prevents incorporation of compensatory strategies.
- Due to decreased executive functioning, **attention,** and problem solving, Steve has difficulty performing cognitive IADL tasks such as paying bills.

Steve's strengths included his ability to move his left upper extremity throughout the full ROM, good family support, and good economic status. His weaknesses included decreased balance, endurance, left upper-extremity strength, and FMC. Weaknesses also included executive function deficits, divided attention, and poor awareness or insight.

After all evaluations, the occupational therapist, Steve, and Steve's wife set goals of modified independence in all ADLs, increased strength and FMC in the left upper extremity, and minimum assistance in paying bills. Owing to the short length of stay, Steve's desire to return to work would be further addressed in outpatient therapy.

Intervention Plan

Because of Steve's relatively high level of functioning during the initial evaluation, his private insurance company initially approved only 7 days of inpatient rehabilitation. However, after the first team conference, at the request of the case manager, the insurance company approved an additional 3 days because of Steve's decreased safety awareness and balance. Steve would participate in 60 minutes of occupational therapy for 6 days per week in the IRF. Goals and treatment planning for Steve are outlined in Table 11.3.

Intervention Implementation

Steve chose which goals to work on in each therapy session (see Table 11.3). He was also given homework each day to increase repetitions of functional left upper-extremity movements and activities. Steve progressed through the free-weight home exercise program beginning with only a 1-pound weight for two sets of 10 repetitions to using a 2-pound weight for four sets of 10 to 15 repetitions per set with his left upper extremity.

Using concepts from the DIM (Toglia, 2011), both the task and the environment were manipulated to provide a continued level of challenge for Steve during cognitive tasks. Steve progressed from being unable to perform these activities in a noisy

Points to Ponder: Case Study—Steve

In light of the discovery of Steve's decreased left fine motor control during his upper-extremity evaluation, what are a few of the functional activities you would want to assess in addition to basic ADLs on the basis of his occupational history?

Table 11.3. Steve's Intervention Planning Outline

Occupational Therapy Intervention Priority	Intervention Approach (*Framework* [AOTA, 2014])	Goals (to Be Achieved by Discharge)	Preparatory Methods and Tasks	Occupation and Activity	Education and Training
UE strength and coordination	Establish or restore	• Steve will perform LUE FMC and strengthening home exercise program with modified independence. • Steve will incorporate L hand into all functional activities with fewer than 2 verbal cues.	• Wrist cuff weights added to L wrist during activities to increase LUE strength • LUE exercise program using free weights, starting with 10 repetitions of each exercise and 1-lb weights • Practicing screwing and unscrewing jar lids • Counting out coins from L hand • Practicing opening envelopes	• Two-handed typing on laptop with therapist instruction for adaptive strategies • Incorporating L hand into ADLs such as buttoning shirt, donning socks and shoes, shaving, and pulling up pants	• Educating Steve on home exercise program for LUE strengthening and FMC
Standing balance	Establish or restore	• Steve will complete ADL routine standing with occasional seated rest breaks with supervision only for balance.	• Practicing standing and reaching for ball, cones, etc., by mat in therapy gym • Reaching for and folding laundry in the therapy gym • Reaching for items on therapy kitchen shelves • Filing folders at various heights in therapy office	• Completing morning self-care routine in standing (to challenge standing balance)	• Educating Steve and family on fall prevention at home
Cognition	Establish or restore Modify	• Steve will complete complex bill-paying task in distracting environment with minimum verbal cues using adaptive strategies.	• Counting out simple sums of play money • Doing money management task worksheets developed by therapy department	• Money management tasks using Steve's own bills and checkbook brought in by his wife	• Educating Steve on strategies to compensate for decreased attention
ADL training	Establish or restore Modify	• Steve will complete morning ADL routine with modified independence using adaptive equipment as needed.		• Full bathing and dressing sessions using Steve's own clothes and adaptive equipment	• Educating Steve on adaptive equipment options for the home • Issuing and practicing with adaptive equipment and strategies for dressing outside of actual dressing sessions (e.g., long-handled shoehorn for L shoe)

Note. ADL/ADLs = activity/activities of daily living; FMC = fine motor control; L = left; LUE = left upper extremity; UE = upper extremity.

or stimulating environment to being able to complete increasingly complex tasks in the therapy gym with only minimum verbal cues to focus. Steve was encouraged to approach new cognitive tasks using the same strategies he had developed for others. For instance, after being taught cognitive strategies for money management, he practiced making himself a daily schedule using the same strategies.

Discharge Outcomes

Steve's left upper-extremity AROM and MMT were reassessed near discharge and were found to be full AROM and 4+/5 strength. His left FMC had improved as indicated by his ability to use his left upper extremity to assist in all ADLs. Steve's Berg Balance Scale score had improved to 54 of 56, indicating he was at low risk for falls. He continued to have problems with higher-level cognitive tasks that required organization, planning, or divided attention with distractions present.

Steve's discharge plan was to go home with his wife and son and with his brother, Chris, available to help some days of the week. The day before discharge, Steve's wife, Elizabeth, and Chris were present in therapy for family training. The occupational therapist explained that although Steve was doing much better physically, they should be aware of some remaining cognitive deficits. The family was encouraged to keep a quiet environment if Steve was completing a task for which he needed a lot of **concentration.** They were also educated on the dangers of driving immediately after stroke and were told that Steve's ability to drive would be evaluated further in outpatient therapy. Steve's family was encouraged to let him do as much as he could safely do for himself. Information was also given to them on preventing falls in the home. Steve's discharge FIM scores are presented in Table 11.4.

Steve was referred to a neuropsychologist for testing to gain further insight into cognitive deficits before he was discharged from inpatient therapy. He was referred to outpatient therapy for continued treatment. Results of neuropsychological testing were sent to the outpatient therapy team. Steve was also referred to the local

Table 11.4. Steve's Discharge FIM™ Scores and Barriers to Performance

FIM Category (ADL)	FIM Score	Barriers to Performance
Eating	7	Independent including container management
Grooming	7	Independent standing at sink
Bathing	6	Modified independent due to use of long-handled bath sponge to wash feet from a seated position
Upper-body dressing	7	Independent in gathering and donning shirt
Lower-body dressing	6	Modified independent due to taking increased time to don left shoe and sock. Performed all lower-body dressing in a seated position except for pulling up pants
Toileting	7	Independent without the use of grab bars
Bladder management	7	As reported by nursing
Bowel management	7	As reported by nursing
Transfers: bed, chair, w/c, toilet (tub, shower NT)	6	Modified independent due to occasional slight LOB but able to self-correct
Locomotion	6	Modified independent without a device due to occasional slight LOB but able to self-correct

Note. ADL = activity of daily living; LOB = loss of balance; NT = not tested; w/c = wheelchair.

stroke support group associated with the hospital system and given access information for online stroke support groups.

Case Review: Mary

Mary was discharged from acute care to an IRF for intensive occupational, physical, and speech therapy 1 week after her stroke. On the 2nd day, the occupational therapist began an initial evaluation. A chart review revealed Mary's history of diabetes, a previous stroke, **hypertension,** and obesity. The acute care hospital report stated that Mary had a right **parietal lobe cerebrovascular accident** with resulting left hemiparesis, left neglect, and lack of awareness of her deficits. Precautions noted in the chart review were "fall precautions," "activity as tolerated," and "left neglect."

Evaluation

The occupational therapist found Mary supine in bed with the head of the bed raised and the over-the-bed table with her breakfast tray in front of her. The occupational therapist observed that the food on the left side of the tray was untouched. Mary's daughter, Sarah, was seated on the right side of the bed and was encouraging Mary to eat all her breakfast. The occupational therapist began the interview with a rapport-building discussion about the role of occupational therapy in rehabilitation and of Mary's stroke and past medical history. Sarah acted as historian when Mary was unable to answer questions about former occupations or past medical history. Mary was oriented to self and place. A cognitive screening with the *Short Blessed Memory Test,* a cognitive screening tool (Katzman et al., 1983), indicated that Mary had difficulty with memory items and attention. Her total score was 12/28, indicating moderate impairment.

A simple auditory screening was performed with no indication of hearing loss. Mary wore her prescription bifocals for a functional screening of reading. She was unable to scan to the left of each line and stated that her eyes were bothering her. She said, "I must need a new prescription." The occupational therapist performed a pursuit–tracking screening and noted that Mary did not scan to the left side.

Occupational Profile

Results of the *COPM,* a subjective measure of a person's occupational performance in self-care, productivity, and leisure (Law et al., 2005), showed that Mary's five most important priorities and targeted outcomes were as follows:

1. Attending church services and activities
2. Taking care of herself (i.e., toileting, bathing, grooming, dressing, managing medications)
3. Reading to her grandchildren
4. Preparing meals and cooking
5. Returning to work.

However, when asked on the COPM which of these activities were now difficult for her to do to her satisfaction, Mary was unable to identify problems she would have because of impairments from her stroke. She stated that she felt she could perform her previous activities, including work and social activities, "as soon as I get some rest and get back home."

Self-Care

The occupational therapist assessed self-care activities, scored them on the FIM (Uniform Data System for Medical Rehabilitation, 1997), and reported observations of barriers to Mary's performance (see Table 11.5).

During observation of functional activities, the occupational therapist scored the *Catherine Bergego Scale* (CBS), a standardized assessment for unilateral left neglect using 10 functional activities (Azouvi et al., 1996). Mary's total CBS score on the 10 items was 21 of 30, indicating a moderate level of left neglect. When administered the CBS questions for self-evaluation of left neglect (measuring **anosognosia**), Mary scored 5 of 30, indicating that she had decreased awareness of her left neglect.

Table 11.5. Mary's Admission FIM™ Scores and Barriers to Performance

FIM Category (ADL)	FIM Score	Barriers to Performance
Eating	3	Assessed sitting at bed level with tray at midline on an OTB table. Verbal and physical cueing required secondary to not eating food on left side of tray; LUE hemiparesis; food pocketing in left cheek.
Grooming	3	Assessed at w/c level at bathroom sink. Verbal and physical cueing required to initiate, sequence, and attend to grooming tasks (brushing teeth and hair). Required verbal cues to brush teeth, comb hair, and wash left side. Required moderate assistance for all tasks secondary to left hemiparesis.
Bathing	0 (NT)	Unable to test secondary to fatigue. Performed bed bath with washcloth and basin while sitting in bed with basin at midline on OTB table. Required cues to attend to task; was distracted by roommate. Required moderate assistance to wash left side of body; moderate to maximum assistance with perineum and lower body.
Upper-body dressing	3	Assessed at EOB with moderate assistance secondary to fair dynamic sitting balance. Verbal and physical cueing required to dress LUE; unable to identify front or back of pullover shirt and position to don; moderate assistance required to don shirt and bra.
Lower-body dressing	2	Assessed at w/c level secondary to fair dynamic sitting balance. Verbal and physical cueing required to properly sequence donning undergarments, sweatpants, socks, and shoes; appeared unaware of LLE; moderate to maximum assistance to don sweatpants with elastic waistband secondary to hemiparesis and fair dynamic sitting balance.
Toileting	3	Moderate assistance secondary to fair+ static sitting balance; moderate assistance for toileting hygiene secondary to fair dynamic sitting balance and left hemiparesis; moderate assistance for clothing management.
Bladder management	6	As reported by nursing.
Bowel management	6	As reported by nursing.
Transfers: bed, chair, w/c, toilet (tub, shower NT)	3	Transfers assessed: stand pivot transfers. Moderate assistance required secondary to fair– (fair minus) dynamic standing balance, left hemiparesis, poor safety awareness secondary to being unaware of left-side weakness or paralysis; does not look to left to transfer to left; fatigue; fear of falling.
Locomotion	2	Reported by physical therapist: moderate assistance of 1 required secondary to left hemiparesis with wheeled walker and walker splint for left hand, fair– (fair minus) dynamic standing balance, and fatigue. Physical therapist reported patient unaware of wall on left.

Note. ADL = activity of daily living; EOB = edge of bed; LLE = left lower extremity; LUE = left upper extremity; NT = not tested; OTB = over the bed; w/c = wheelchair.

Table 11.6. Mary's Initial Upper-Extremity Evaluation Results

Movement	LUE		RUE	
	MMT	PROM	MMT	PROM
Shoulder flexion	2/5	WNL	5/5	WNL
Shoulder abduction	2/5	WNL	5/5	WNL
Shoulder external rotation	2/5	WNL	4+/5	WNL
Shoulder internal rotation	2/5	WNL	4+/5	WNL
Elbow flexion	2+/5	WNL	5/5	WNL
Elbow extension	2+/5	WNL	5/5	WNL
Pronation	3/5	WNL	5/5	WNL
Supination	3/5	WNL	4+/5	WNL
Wrist flexion	3/5	WNL	5/5	WNL
Wrist extension	2+/5	WNL	5/5	WNL
Finger flexion	2+/5	WNL	5/5	WNL
Finger extension	2/5	WNL	4+/5	WNL

Note. LUE = left upper extremity; MMT = manual muscle testing; PROM = passive range of motion; RUE = right upper extremity; WNL = within normal limits.

Motor Skills

After observing significant hemiparesis of the left during functional activities, the occupational therapist performed an upper-extremity **passive range of motion** (PROM), AROM, MMT, and sensory screen (see Table 11.6). The ARAT was also used to further assess overall upper-extremity function during tasks (Nijland et al., 2010). This test was selected because of its high sensitivity with this population, as well as its superior responsiveness over other measures in some subsets of the stroke population (Rabadi & Rabadi, 2006; van der Lee, Beckerman, Lankhorst, & Bouter, 2001). Mary scored a 57 on the right hand and a 15 on the left hand.

Assessment

Sensation screening found that Mary had decreased light touch, tactile localization, proprioception, and **stereognosis** of the left upper extremity and normal sensation of the right upper extremity. After completing the initial assessment, the occupational therapist analyzed the data to develop problem statements and list Mary's strengths and weaknesses (AOTA, 2013):

- Mary requires verbal and physical cues to attend to the left side to perform ADLs and IADLs because of unilateral left neglect.
- Mary's decreased awareness of deficits; decreased left upper-extremity AROM, strength, and endurance; decreased balance; and decreased left upper-extremity sensation limit her ability to perform ADLs and IADLs safely and independently.
- Cognitive deficits in initiation, attention, and **short-term memory** require verbal and physical cues to begin and complete ADLs and IADLs safely and independently.

Mary's strengths included movement in the left upper extremity, a high level of family and community support, economic status, and motivation to return to her home, community, and work. Her weaknesses included comorbid conditions (diabetes mellitus, hypertension, and obesity), previous history of stroke, decreased left upper-extremity AROM and strength, and decreased sitting and standing balance. Weaknesses in cognitive function included left neglect and decreased initiation, attention, and short-term memory.

Points to Ponder: Case Study—Mary

The occupational therapist chose to assess Mary's suspected unilateral left neglect with the Catherine Bergego Scale (CBS; Azouvi et al, 1996). The *CBS* assesses personal or body neglect, near extrapersonal neglect, and far extrapersonal neglect. Give an example of a behavior that Mary has exhibited for each type of neglect.

Name 3 paper-and-pencil assessments of unilateral left neglect often used in rehabilitation settings. Discuss which type of neglect these paper-and-pencil assessments are measuring and why.

Intervention Plan

The occupational therapist created a treatment plan for 60 minutes per day, 5 days per week, for 3 weeks and consultation with and caregiver training for Sarah. The occupational therapist collaborated with Mary and Sarah to create goals to increase participation in Mary's desired occupations and roles: attending church, taking care of herself, reading to her grandchildren, and cooking. They agreed that working on ADLs and IADLs, being aware of and using her left side, performing cognitive intervention activities, and increasing her left upper-extremity ROM and strength would help her to achieve her goals. They also agreed that these activities would facilitate her return to work but that she would address her work role extensively in outpatient therapy after discharge from the IRF. Discharge planning was discussed with Mary and her daughter with a goal to return to her home with her daughter as caregiver for a few weeks and receive outpatient occupational therapy to address barriers to participation in ADLs, IADLs, work, leisure, and social activities in the home and community environment. Goals and treatment plan for occupational therapy in the IRF are outlined in Table 11.7.

Intervention Implementation

Toglia's (2011) DIM is the theoretical basis for the cognitive interventions described in this section. In keeping with the model's principles, the occupational therapist emphasized increasing Mary's self-awareness of her functional capacity, using appropriate processing strategies to compensate for cognitive deficits, grading activity complexity, and adjusting environmental factors to meet and present a just-right challenge for her ability.

Awareness

Mary's lack of awareness of her hemiparesis and unilateral left neglect was vitally important to address in each session because of concerns about safety and to address an initial lack of motivation to participate in therapy. After evaluating Mary's level of awareness, the occupational therapist determined that Mary understood at a low level that her functioning was impaired (i.e., she had an intellectual level of awareness, Crosson et al., 1989). The occupational therapist used a hierarchy of cues and prompts in functional tasks to promote Mary's awareness of errors. For example, when Mary did not put her left arm in the sleeve of her shirt, the occupational therapist would begin cueing by saying, "How do you know that you put your shirt on correctly?" If Mary was unable to problem solve, the occupational therapist might

Table 11.7. Mary's Intervention Planning Outline

Occupational Therapy Intervention Priority	Intervention Approach (*Framework* [AOTA, 2014])	Goals (to Be Achieved by Discharge)	Preparatory Methods and Tasks	Occupation and Activity	Education and Training
ADL training	Establish or restore Modify	• Mary will perform dressing, grooming, bathing, and toileting with modified independence using adaptive equipment and strategies as needed.	• Practicing with a reacher by picking up lightweight items placed on the floor	• Putting on shirt using adaptive strategy (e.g., put on LUE first) • Putting on her own clothing using adaptive strategies in the morning in preparation to attend IRF church services	• Educating and instructing Mary on ADLs with 1-handed techniques
IADLs	Establish or restore Modify	• Mary will prepare a simple meal with SBA using 1 verbal cue for safety and adaptive equipment or strategies as needed.		• Making a cup of coffee or tea in therapy gym kitchen • Making a low-calorie healthy treat to serve to her grandchildren when they visit	• Educating Mary on use of 1-handed adaptive equipment such as rocker knife and cutting board with nails to hold fruit
Awareness and use of L side	Establish or restore Modify	• Mary will perform ADLs with SBA with 1 verbal cue from caregiver to attend to the L side of her body. • Mary will use LUE in simple meal preparation with SBA with 1 verbal cue from caregiver to use LUE.	• Using tactile cues to L side of face and mouth to get Mary to wash face and brush teeth on L • Placing red tape on L side of lunch tray and cueing Mary to scan to the L to find the red tape • Bearing weight through LUE while standing at kitchen counter	• Placing grooming items on L side of sink and asking Mary to scan to the L to find them while performing morning grooming routine • Stabilizing bowl with LUE while mixing ingredients	• Educating Mary, her daughter, and staff on L neglect and compensatory strategies to improve awareness • Instructing Mary to perform LUE massage with RUE
Cognition	Establish or restore Modify Create or promote	• Mary will complete a grocery list for diabetic healthy diet meals for 3 days with minimum assistance from caregiver while using cognitive strategies.		• Copying ingredients for a healthy recipe from a diabetic diet cookbook while in her room with the TV and radio turned off • Making a weekly menu of diabetic healthy meals that Mary would typically prepare to control her glucose levels • Making a grocery list of healthy foods for Sarah to buy to stock refrigerator and pantry in preparation for discharge	• Educating Mary on strategies to compensate for decreased attention
Motor function (UE and balance)	Establish or restore Modify Create or promote	• Mary will increase independence in ADLs and IADLs by performing LUE PROM home exercise program with SBA and caregiver cues as needed. • Mary will increase standing endurance while performing a homemaking task to 12 min while using a mobility aid, kitchen counter, or table for stability.	• Practicing sit-to-stand transfers and standing while playing a board game with OTB table for stability • Performing LUE PROM home exercise program in her room 2×/day while watching TV • Reaching for items in kitchen cabinets while standing	• Reaching for clothing hanging in closet during morning ADL routine and for items in kitchen cabinets to prepare snack by using her RUE to lift or guide her LUE • Standing to place clothing in washer, take out of dryer, and fold at a table in the therapy gym for increasing lengths of time without rest breaks	• Instructing Mary in performing LUE PROM exercises and proper position of the LUE

Note. ADL/ADLs = activity/activities of daily living; IADLs = instrumental activities of daily living; IRF = inpatient rehabilitation facility; L = left; LUE = left upper extremity; min = minutes; OTB = over the bed; PROM = passive range of motion; RUE = right upper extremity; SBA = standby assist.

say, "You didn't put your shirt on correctly. Can you see what you did wrong?" The occupational therapist would continue to offer more specific cues if Mary was unable to evaluate her performance (Gillen & Rubio, 2011).

Another intervention the occupational therapist used to increase awareness of Mary's performance was to compare how Mary performed a functional task before her stroke with how she was doing it in therapy. For example, the occupational therapist would ask, "How long did it take you to put on your makeup for work before your stroke?" or "How long do you think it will take you to put on your makeup now?" After timing the task in therapy, the occupational therapist would compare the time with Mary's estimate. As Mary's awareness of her impairments increased, the occupational therapist administered a depression screening, the BDI FastScreen for Medical Patients (Beck et al., 2000), and was careful to monitor Mary for signs of depression and communicate this to all team members working with Mary.

Unilateral Left Neglect

The occupational therapist addressed unilateral left neglect in most intervention activities. She and Mary would discuss the therapy activity and any difficulties they might expect Mary to have because of neglect. Mary would then perform the activity, and the occupational therapist would elicit feedback from her about how she performed. The occupational therapist would then provide feedback (verbal, visual, and physical) about performance. If problems occurred, then Mary and the occupational therapist brainstormed compensatory techniques and performed the task again using the compensatory techniques (Gillen & Rubio, 2011).

Environmental interventions for unilateral left neglect included placing items on the left side of the room, table, or sink; providing verbal or tactile cues on the left; and putting perceptual anchors on the left such as bright red tape or a marker line on the left side of Mary's tray or reading material. However, for safety, the occupational therapist and staff always placed the nurse call button on her right within easy reach. In all activities, the occupational therapist encouraged Mary to find and move or use her left upper extremity.

Attention, Initiation, Memory

To increase Mary's ability to attend to tasks, the occupational therapist avoided having Mary in overstimulating environments such as the busy therapy gym and turned off the television or radio in her hospital room when doing morning ADLs. The occupational therapist reduced the numbers of items in each activity or the clutter in the environment and graded the number of steps or directions for an activity. The occupational therapist also developed checklists to help Mary remember, attend to, and complete tasks. Mary had used memory strategies after her first stroke and was familiar with using a memory notebook with sections for a daily log, a calendar, names of hospital staff, and personal notes (Gillen & Rubio, 2011).

Motor Function (Upper Extremity, Balance, Endurance)

The occupational therapist began working with Mary's dynamic sitting balance during activities such as bathing and dressing that required reaching and weight shifting to the left while seated. She graded these activities by using adaptive equipment in the beginning such as a long-handled shoehorn, shower chair, and reacher and decreasing their use as Mary's balance improved. To increase standing endurance and balance, the occupational therapist included standing in retrieving clothes from the closet, dressing, and preparing meals. The occupational therapist placed many items to the left to encourage weight shifting toward the left.

Because Mary had significant left hemiparesis, the occupational therapist provided education on shoulder management to Mary and Sarah shortly after admission. The information included positioning the left upper extremity with pillows in bed or when sitting or on a wheelchair lap tray. She emphasized not pulling on Mary's left arm, posted tips on shoulder management on the wall, and provided an appropriate sling for wear during transfers and gait training.

Mary performed left upper-extremity weight bearing during activities such as using her left upper extremity to push up in transfers, stabilizing on the grab bar when performing toilet hygiene, stabilizing the toothbrush when putting toothpaste on it, or holding a bowl when preparing a simple recipe.

The occupational therapist also taught Mary adaptive strategies for using the right upper extremity to help the left upper extremity (e.g., dressing the left upper extremity and left lower extremity first) and emphasized bilateral tasks as much as possible using both arms simultaneously in activities such as wiping off a counter, using a washcloth, and using the walker with a walker splint for the left hand. In many activities, the occupational therapist encouraged Mary to perform frequent repetitions of upper-extremity movements to increase strength.

In the 3rd week of her IRF stay, Mary began to develop increased **tone** in the left upper extremity. The occupational therapist rated Mary's tone in elbow, wrist, and finger flexion on the Modified Ashworth Scale (Naghdi, Ansari, Azarnia, & Kazemnejad, 2008) as 2—more marked increase in tone through most of the ROM but easily moved. The occupational therapist encouraged self-PROM exercises to maintain left upper-extremity PROM.

Sensation Deficits in the Left Upper Extremity

The occupational therapist performed sensory reeducation of the left hand by encouraging Mary to explore a variety of tools, utensils, and products with different tactile characteristics in a graded progression from textures or surfaces with distinctive features to more difficult-to-distinguish objects. Mary was asked to imagine objects and think about their features before and after stimulation with them. She was also asked to feel the object with the left hand and then with the right, unaffected hand while looking at them and with vision occluded (Carey, 2012). As Mary improved in touch discrimination and stereognosis, the occupational therapist increased the difficulty of discrimination tasks.

Discharge Outcomes

In Week 3 of Mary's IRF stay, the occupational therapist arranged several sessions of family training with Mary's daughter, Sarah, and friends from church. The day before discharge, the occupational therapist evaluated self-care skills and upper-extremity ROM, MMT, and sensation in a morning session and IADL skills in the afternoon session (see Tables 11.8 and 11.9).

Rescreening of Mary's left upper-extremity sensation found that she had improved in light touch, tactile localization, proprioception, and stereognosis of the left upper extremity compared with her initial evaluation results. Mary was also able to prepare a simple meal with contact guard assistance in the therapy kitchen.

Table 11.8. Mary's Discharge FIM™ Scores and Barriers to Performance

FIM Category (ADL)	FIM Score	Barriers to Performance
Eating	5	Assessed while seated in bedside chair with tray at midline on an OTB table. One verbal cue required to scan to eat food on left side of tray; used brightly colored tape as anchor for scanning on left side; used rocker knife to cut meat.
Grooming	5	Assessed standing at bathroom sink. Required 2 verbal cues to use strategies to complete all grooming tasks. One rest break in 15 minutes.
Bathing	5	Assessed while seated on a shower chair with back using hand-held showerhead, long-handled sponge.
Upper-body dressing	6	Assessed at EOB; increased time required to put on bra and shirt.
Lower-body dressing	4	Assessed at EOB; CGA for pulling up pants in standing.
Toileting	4	Used grab bars and raised toilet seat; CGA for clothing management.
Bladder management	7	As reported by nursing.
Bowel management	7	As reported by nursing.
Transfers: bed, chair, w/c, toilet (tub, shower NT)	4	Transfers assessed: stand–step transfers. One verbal cue required to look to left when transferring to left. CGA for safety.
Locomotion	4	Reported by physical therapist: CGA for safety; 1–2 verbal cues to look to left while ambulating with wheeled walker with LUE walker splint.

Note. ADL = activity of daily living; CGA = contact guard assistance; EOB = edge of bed; LUE = left upper extremity; NT = not tested; OTB = over the bed; w/c = wheelchair.

Discharge recommendations included the following: Mary was to be discharged to home with supervision or minimum assistance from Sarah and friends for ADLs, IADLs, and social and leisure activities. A shower chair, hand-held showerhead, long-handled sponge, and grab bars in the shower and around the toilet were recommended. Continued use of a memory notebook or diary was recommended because of decreased attention and memory for daily tasks such as medication management. Mary and Sarah were given exercises to increase Mary's strength, endurance, and balance as well as a list of community resources for stroke support, diabetes education, and exercise opportunities. Outpatient occupational therapy was recommended for Mary to continue to address cognitive deficits and IADL, work, leisure, and social pursuits.

Table 11.9. Mary's Discharge Upper-Extremity Evaluation Results

Movement	LUE		RUE	
	MMT	PROM	MMT	PROM
Shoulder flexion	3+/5	WNL	5/5	WNL
Shoulder abduction	3+/5	WNL	5/5	WNL
Shoulder external rotation	4–/5	WNL	4+/5	WNL
Shoulder internal rotation	4–/5	WNL	4+/5	WNL
Elbow flexion	4+/5	WNL	5/5	WNL
Elbow extension	4/5	WNL	5/5	WNL
Pronation	4/5	WNL	5/5	WNL
Supination	4/5	WNL	4+/5	WNL
Wrist flexion	4/5	WNL	5/5	WNL
Wrist extension	4/5	WNL	5/5	WNL
Finger flexion	4/5	WNL	5/5	WNL
Finger extension	4–/5	WNL	4+/5	WNL

Note. LUE = left upper extremity; MMT = manual muscle testing; PROM = passive range of motion; RUE = right upper extremity; WNL = within normal limits.

Case Review: Walter

Walter was discharged from acute care to a SNF 3 weeks after his stroke. A review of his medical chart showed that Walter had fall precautions and an order for a low bed and chair and bed alarm. Walter was to engage in activity as tolerated and sit up in a chair at 90° for all meals because of **aspiration** precautions. The National Dysphagia Diet–2 (Avery, 2011) with honey-thick liquids was prescribed for Walter.

Evaluation

The occupational therapist performed an initial evaluation on the morning of Walter's 2nd day in the SNF. Walter's wife, Adele, was present and acted as historian because Walter was unable to answer many questions. The initial evaluation began with a discussion of Walter's stroke and past medical history and what to expect in occupational therapy sessions in a SNF.

Occupational Profile

Information was gathered from Adele about Walter's previous level of functioning and social support available (see Chapter 9). Walter was unable to understand COPM interview questions (Law et al., 2005). The occupational therapist led a discussion with Adele, with some input from Walter, to determine what his five most important priorities might be. The collaboration resulted in the following priorities:

1. Taking care of himself (i.e., toileting, bathing, grooming, dressing)
2. Spending time with Adele
3. Watching sports on TV with his friends
4. Eating out with friends
5. Fishing.

Process Skills

Walter was alert throughout the 60-minute evaluation but required more verbal cueing to attend at the end of the session. Walter indicated that he needed to rest by nodding when asked. He was oriented to self through pointing at three written choices but not to place, time, or situation. He was unable to perform other cognitive screenings because of global aphasia.

A simple auditory screening was performed, indicating apparent mild to moderate hearing loss. Adele confirmed that Walter had a mild hearing loss before the stroke. Walter was unable to perform a vision screening because of decreased ability to understand and follow directions. Adele stated that he had received new prescription trifocals within the past 3 months. The occupational therapist performed a pursuit–tracking screening and noted that Walter did not scan to the right upper and lower **visual field** quadrants.

The occupational therapist was unable to perform standard upper-extremity sensation screenings, but Walter appeared to respond equally to physical cues to his right hand and forearm and his left hand and forearm.

Social Interaction Skills

Responses to yes-or-no questions during the occupational therapy evaluation appeared to be 75% accurate. This was later confirmed by the speech–language pathologist. Walter's highest rate of success in responding to questions was with verbal, written, and gestural cues. Both the speech–language pathologist and the occupational therapist worked with Adele on how best to communicate with Walter.

Activities of Daily Living Skills

The occupational therapist assessed self-care activities, scored them on the FIM, and reported observations of barriers to Walter's performance (see Table 11.10).

Motor Skills

After observing dense **hemiplegia** of the right upper extremity during activities, the occupational therapist performed upper-extremity ROM and MMT with demonstration and simple one-step commands. The occupational therapist noted that Walter's bilateral upper-extremity PROM was affected in some joints by his osteoarthritis. No voluntary movement was noted in the right upper extremity. When performing upper-extremity PROM, the occupational therapist noted a small amount of **hypertonicity** in flexor synergy and rated it on the Modified Ashworth Scale (Naghdi et al., 2008). The occupational therapist also noticed that Walter grimaced

Table 11.10. Walter's Admission FIM™ Scores and Barriers to Performance

FIM Category (ADL)	FIM Score	Barriers to Performance
Feeding	2	Assessed sitting at bed level with tray at midline on an OTB table. Required physical cueing to retrieve food on right side of tray; Walter did not appear to understand verbal cueing. Unable to use RUE secondary to hemiplegia.
Eating	5	NDD–2 with honey-thick-consistency liquids secondary to aspiration of thin liquids and modified barium swallow study in acute hospital. Required supervision to follow swallowing precautions.
Grooming	2	Assessed sitting at bed level with tray at midline on an OTB table. Required physical cueing to initiate, sequence, and attend to grooming tasks—brushing teeth and hair. Required hand-over-hand assistance to brush teeth, comb hair, and wash face. Required maximum assistance for all items secondary to right hemiplegia; did not scan to right side of table for grooming items.
Bathing	0 (NT)	Unable to test secondary to decreased ability to follow directions; decreased strength; poor dynamic sitting balance; right hemiplegia. Performed bed bath with washcloth and basin while sitting in bed with basin at midline on OTB table. Required cues to initiate and attend to task. Required maximum assist to wash chest, RUE, and right lower body; required total assistance with perineum and back.
Upper-body dressing	2	Assessed while seated in w/c with maximum assistance secondary to poor dynamic sitting balance. Required physical cueing and maximum assistance to dress RUE and to don large pullover knit T-shirt secondary to right hemiplegia, receptive aphasia, lack of visual scanning to right side.
Lower-body dressing	1	Assessed at bed level. Physical assistance required to perform bed mobility (rolling to left side, bridging to pull up undergarments and sweatpants); socks and shoes required total assistance; maximum assistance required to don sweatpants with elastic waistband secondary to hemiplegia and decreased ability to perform bed mobility and bridging; total assistance required for pulling up clothing.
Toileting	1	Total assistance required secondary to Foley catheter and bedpan.
Bladder management	1	Total assistance required secondary to Foley catheter.
Bowel management	0 (NT)	Nursing has not reported.
Transfers: bed to w/c (chair, tub, shower NT)	2	Transfer assessed: bent pivot transfers. Maximum assistance of 1 required secondary to decreased ability to understand and follow directions, right hemiplegia, inability to scan or look to the right when transferring to right; poor safety awareness; fatigue.
Locomotion	1	Reported by physical therapist: maximum assistance of 2 required secondary to right hemiplegia, poor dynamic standing balance, and fatigue. Physical therapy reported Walter appeared unable to see items on the right.

Note. ADL = activity of daily living; NDD–2 = National Dysphagia Diet–2; NT = not tested; OTB = over the bed; RUE = right upper extremity; w/c = wheelchair.

Table 11.11. Walter's Initial Upper-Extremity Evaluation Results

Movement	LUE		RUE		Modified Ashworth Scale
	MMT	PROM	MMT	PROM	
Shoulder flexion	3+/5	BFL	0/5	BFL	1
Shoulder abduction	3+/5	BFL	0/5	BFL	1
Shoulder external rotation	3/5	BFL	0/5	BFL	1+
Shoulder internal rotation	4/5	BFL	0/5	BFL	1
Elbow flexion	5/5	WNL	0/5	WNL	1+
Elbow extension	5/5	WNL	0/5	WNL	0
Pronation	4+/5	WNL	0/5	WNL	1
Supination	4/5	WFL	0/5	WFL	1+
Wrist flexion	4/5	WNL	0/5	WNL	1+
Wrist extension	4/5	WNL	0/5	BFL	0
Finger flexion	4/5	WNL	0/5	WNL	1+
Finger extension	4+/5	WNL	0/5	WFL	1

Note. BFL = below functional limits; LUE = left upper extremity; MMT = manual muscle testing; PROM = passive range of motion; RUE = right upper extremity; WFL = within functional limits; WNL = within normal limits.

when she moved the right shoulder during PROM and found that it had a one-finger-width **subluxation** (see Table 11.11).

Assessment

After completing the initial evaluation, the occupational therapist analyzed the data to identify barriers to performance. She developed the following problem statements:

- Walter requires physical cues to scan to the right side to perform ADLs and IADLs because of **homonymous hemianopsia.**
- Global aphasia results in difficulty in understanding and participating in conversations or understanding directions, limiting performance in social and leisure activities.
- Right hemiplegia results in maximum assistance in ADL performance.
- Decreased strength and endurance results in fair to poor static and dynamic sitting balance and decreased safety in performing ADLs.
- Right shoulder pain and subluxation limit performance in ADL, IADL, and social and leisure activities.

The occupational therapist noted that Walter's strengths included a supportive spouse, a network of friends, relatively good economic status, and a strong work ethic. The occupational therapist rated Walter's rehabilitation potential as fair to poor because of the severity of his stroke; age; prior conditions; lack of extended family in the community; and Adele's age and chronic conditions, which limited her caregiving abilities.

Intervention Plan

The occupational therapist created a treatment plan that included direct occupational therapy for 50 minutes per day, 5 days per week, for 4 weeks and consultation and caregiver training with Adele. The occupational therapist collaborated with Walter and Adele to create goals to increase participation in Walter's desired occupations. Discharge planning was discussed with Walter and Adele with a tentative plan for Adele to work with the case manager to find a placement in a long-term care facility near their condominium.

In the weekly utilization review meeting, the therapy team recommended that Walter receive the "ultrahigh" RUG level because of his diagnosis of acute stroke. At this level, he would receive 50 minutes with the physical therapist, 50 minutes with the occupational therapist, and 45 minutes with a speech–language pathologist per day, 5 days per week, totaling 725 minutes of therapy per week. The team requested this level of therapy for Walter for 4 weeks. Goals and treatment plan for Walter are outlined in Table 11.12.

Intervention Implementation

Although the occupational therapist used the establish-or-restore intervention approach with Walter's balance and strength deficits, the severity of Walter's hemiparesis and his cognitive and language impairments required the modify intervention approach for a majority of the time (AOTA, 2014).

Global Aphasia

The speech–language pathologist is a key member of the therapy team in treating **aphasia** after stroke. Although no specific goals to address global aphasia are made through occupational therapy, the entire SNF rehabilitation team is responsible for addressing these deficits in a compassionate and effective way. Education was immediately provided by all disciplines to Adele on how to effectively communicate with Walter, including tips such as being patient and giving Walter time to talk, encouraging him to attempt conversation, writing down choices and key words, using and accepting gestures and facial expressions as communication, and talking about things that were personally relevant to Walter (Stewart & Riedel, 2011). The occupational therapist used all of these strategies during therapy sessions. In addition, all directions during therapy were concise, used simple words, and were often accompanied by tactile cues or gestures. Individual therapy sessions also had only a few treatment activities per session to avoid confusion with switching topics or activities (Stewart & Riedel, 2011). Walter's receptive communication improved significantly throughout the course of his 4-week SNF stay. Compensatory strategies were still used, but he demonstrated greater understanding of activities and directions.

> Although no specific goals to address global aphasia are made through occupational therapy, the entire SNF rehabilitation team is responsible for addressing these deficits in a compassionate and effective way.

Cognition

Each morning, Walter was asked orientation questions with written cues and was asked to point to the correct answer out of three or to give head nods once his yes-or-no responses were determined to be accurate. He was taught the compensatory method of looking at visual cues placed around his room and the calendar for assistance with orientation questions. Attention was addressed in each session with verbal and tactile cues to stay on task. Varied environments and levels of distraction present were also used to grade activities. Walter's initiation was addressed by giving him time to respond to cues and by gradually decreasing the amount and type of cues (e.g., verbal, tactile, hand over hand) required to initiate an activity. By the end

Table 11.12. Walter's Intervention Planning Outline

Occupational Therapy Intervention Priority	Intervention Approach (*Framework* [AOTA, 2014])	Goals (to Be Achieved by Discharge)	Preparatory Methods and Tasks	Occupation and Activity	Education and Training
Cognition	Establish or restore Modify	• Walter will be alert and oriented to person, place, and time using visual cues and no more than minimum verbal cues. • Walter will attend to 20 min of therapy session with minimum verbal cues in moderately distracting environment.	• Wearing earplugs, facing away from distracting environment, reducing clutter (i.e., grade environmental distractions) while performing training to use adaptive strategies for dressing • Asking Walter what month, year, etc., it is and cueing him to use environmental cues • Using a written checklist for practicing steps of adaptive strategies for putting on clothing in correct sequence	• Preparing greeting cards, appropriate decorations, or traditions for current holiday or birthday for family or friends • Using motivating activities for Walter, such as fishing game, card games, etc., to promote attention to task	• Educating Walter on visual cues inside of room for orientation
Visual perception	Modify	• Walter will locate 3 ADL items in right visual field during functional activity with minimum tactile and verbal cueing.	• Training Walter to look to right for various items using tactile head-turning cues • Practicing turning head to locate various items or signs in room and rehab unit	• Placing grooming supplies on right side of sink during morning routine grooming activity	• Training Adele to use tactile cues for finding items on the right
UE strength and tone	Establish or restore	• Walter will tolerate 5 min weight bearing through RUE during functional activity with minimum verbal cues to initiate and position. • Walter will use LUE in all functional activities with minimum verbal cues to initiate.	• Performing PROM and eventually AAROM to RUE • Performing LUE AROM exercise with free weights • Practicing weight bearing on RUE while reaching for items on therapy gym table	• Grooming while standing at sink while weight bearing through RUE • Using RUE to stabilize food tray during cutting and eating tasks • Using LUE to help push up during transfers • Using LUE to help roll in bed with bed rails	• Educating Walter to use RUE as postural support during weight-bearing activities (Gillen, 2011b)
Right shoulder pain and subluxation	Establish or restore Modify Prevent	• Walter will demonstrate decreased pain in his right shoulder when performing ADLs or leisure activities.	• Wearing GivMohr® sling when transferring or gait training • Using w/c lap tray to position RUE while being transported to therapy gym or cafeteria for meals	• Using pursed-lip breathing and relaxation techniques during dressing and bathing activities	• Educating Walter, Adele, and staff on positioning to protect right shoulder while supine in bed, transferring, or performing bed mobility • Educating Adele and staff to perform right shoulder PROM up to 90° only

(Continued)

Table 11.12. Walter's Intervention Planning Outline (*cont.*)

Occupational Therapy Intervention Priority	Intervention Approach (*Framework* [AOTA, 2014])	Goals (to Be Achieved by Discharge)	Preparatory Methods and Tasks	Occupation and Activity	Education and Training
Balance	Establish or restore	• Walter will sit EOB for donning shirt with CGA. • Walter will stand with moderate assistance during functional ADLs for 5 min.	• Sitting EOM with therapist assistance and cues to toss a ball • Practicing sit-to-stand at EOM and standing in parallel bars for short periods of time	• Participating in fly-fishing videogame seated EOM to increase sitting balance • Playing game while standing for short periods at therapy table • Performing ADLs while seated EOB • Grooming at sink in standing • Standing to pull up pants in toileting and LE dressing	
ADL retraining	Establish or restore Modify	• Walter will perform bathing and dressing in seated or standing with moderate assistance.	• Issuing elastic laces, long-handled bath sponge, plate guard, rocker knife, and straw mug	• Practicing dressing with larger, easier therapy clothes • Conducting bathing and dressing sessions using Walter's own clothes • Eating with adaptive equipment	• Training in 1-handed techniques for bathing, dressing, and grooming • Training in use of adaptive equipment
Caregiver education	Prevent Modify	• Adele will perform RUE PROM and stretch safely and independently by discharge. • Adele will assist with bathing and dressing using adaptive equipment and techniques with supervision.			• Watching Adele performing RUE PROM safely and independently • Conducting bathing and dressing sessions with Adele present • Demonstrating PROM to RUE to Adele • Demonstrating use of adaptive equipment and strategies to Adele • Educating Adele on PROM with handouts • Educating Adele on adaptive equipment and strategies for bathing and dressing

Note. AAROM = active assistive range of motion; ADL/ADLs = activity/activities of daily living; AROM = active range of motion; CGA = contact guard assistance; EOB = edge of bed; EOM = edge of mat; LE = lower extremity; LUE = left upper extremity; min = minutes; PROM = passive range of motion; RUE = right upper extremity; UE = upper extremity; w/c = wheelchair.

of his stay, Walter was consistently alert and oriented times 4 (person, place, time, and situation; A&O × 4) with written choices and visual cues.

Homonymous Hemianopsia

Because self-awareness is critical in compensating for visual–perceptual deficits, Walter's global aphasia and decreased awareness made addressing this deficit very difficult during his SNF stay. Although the use of prism glasses for rehabilitation of visual deficits after stroke has shown some promise in the literature (Gillen, 2011a), this approach was not chosen because of Walter's receptive aphasia and difficulty in new situations with complicated instructions. Although Walter made minor improvements in compensating for his visual field cut during his SNF stay (he required fewer verbal and tactile cues to use compensatory strategies), he continued to frequently miss things on the right side.

Right Shoulder Pain and Subluxation

Education on positioning and protecting the right shoulder was immediately provided to Walter, his wife, and the nursing staff (Duffy & Beland, 2011; Jenkins, 2004). See Table 11.12 for goals and activities to address shoulder pain and subluxation. Two additional preparatory methods were used to reduce Walter's right shoulder subluxation and pain. Electrical stimulation therapy was applied to his right shoulder 3 times per week for 20 minutes each session with electrodes placed on the right supraspinatus and posterior deltoid muscles. Used in conjunction with other therapies, electrical stimulation has support in the literature for effectiveness in reducing subluxation (Handy, Salinas, Blanchard, & Aitken, 2004; Koyuncu, Nakipoğlu-Yüzer, Doğan, & Özgirgin, 2010).

Walter's right shoulder was also taped to help with pain; he indicated that it felt more stable and hurt less when taped. Therefore, taping was continued within the parameters for skin protection throughout the SNF stay. Further research is warranted into the effectiveness of taping to assist with shoulder stability during the flaccid stage (Gillen, 2011b). The occupational therapist ensured scapular mobility and alignment during PROM and upper-extremity activities to reduce the risk of further pain or injury (Gillen, 2011b).

Strength and Tone

Walter progressed in his left upper-extremity free-weight exercises to doing them daily with a 2-pound weight for 2 sets of 15 repetitions each. Walter was discharged with a home exercise program for PROM to his right upper extremity for him and Adele to perform daily.

Balance and Endurance

Seated at the edge of the bed, Walter initially required maximum assistance to retain sitting balance with upper-body dressing and progressed to needing moderate tactile cues to remain in midline while he attempted to don a shirt. He progressed to requiring moderate assistance to play a fly-fishing game in standing while using a hemi-aid walker on the left side. Walter required frequent rest breaks throughout functional activity sessions at the beginning but improved to requiring only one seated rest break during a bathing and dressing session.

Activities of Daily Living

Walter was instructed in using simple one-handed techniques for ADLs. Because of Walter's general decreased cognition and aphasia, adaptive equipment was not introduced unless its use was apparent (e.g., elastic shoelaces, rocker knife, bath mitt, grab bars). Adaptive equipment for bathing and eating with his left hand gave Walter some increased independence. He was encouraged to use a grab bar with his left upper extremity to help with forward weight shifting and standing balance for toileting and toilet transfers (Kane & Buckley, 2011). Decreased balance, aphasia, and visual deficits continued to make ADLs difficult throughout his stay.

Caregiver Training

Adele was often present in occupational therapy sessions throughout the SNF stay. In addition to the education provided to her on handling aphasia, cognitive deficits, and protecting Walter's right shoulder, Adele was educated on techniques for bathing, dressing, and transfers. Unfortunately, she was unable to safely perform transfers with Walter because of her previous back condition and osteoarthritis. No family was available to stay with Walter and Adele to assist with heavier caregiving tasks.

Discharge Outcomes

Walter's progress stalled even though he and Adele were motivated to work during the SNF stay. Because he continued to have difficulty with transfers and ADLs, the decision to discharge to a long-term care facility was confirmed with all team members. It was an emotional decision for both Walter and Adele, but Adele realized through education and training from the therapy team that she could not safely provide the amount of support with ADLs that Walter required in their home. The day before discharge, the occupational therapist evaluated ADLs and upper-extremity function in a morning session. See Tables 11.13 and Table 11.14 for results.

Conclusion

Clients with stroke have an extraordinarily complex condition with many levels of strength and disability, as demonstrated by the three case studies presented in this chapter. Because of this complexity, acute care therapists must understand the criteria for admission to IRFs and SNFs to obtain optimal rehabilitation for the client with stroke and to meet funding source requirements.

Although the length of stay is shorter than in the past, the inpatient rehabilitation setting provides more time for in-depth assessment and intervention than the acute care setting. It is imperative that inpatient rehabilitation occupational therapists collaborate with the client and family to establish goals in a top-down evaluation process. Only by addressing the client's own goals will he or she be motivated to participate in and receive maximum benefit from the interventions.

The evidence-based occupational therapist in the inpatient rehabilitation setting may use preparatory methods and tasks and activities, but always with engagement in occupations as the ultimate goal of each session. The creative therapist will also plan interventions to reflect multiple treatment approaches for each client while trying to get the most bang for the buck with each activity.

It is imperative that inpatient rehabilitation occupational therapists collaborate with the client and family to establish goals in a top-down evaluation process.

Table 11.13. Walter's Discharge FIM™ Scores and Barriers to Performance

FIM Category (ADL)	FIM Score	Barriers to Performance
Feeding	4	Assessed sitting w/c level with tray in front. Occasional physical cueing required to retrieve food on right side of tray; used plate guard.
Eating	5	NDD–2 diet with thin liquids (Avery, 2011). Occasional verbal cueing still required to use swallowing strategies when eating to avoid coughing.
Grooming	4	Assessed w/c level at sink. Set-up required for brushing teeth with visual cues to sequence; minimum assistance required to comb hair thoroughly.
Bathing	3	Assessed seated in shower on transfer bench. Used long-handled bath sponge; required assistance to wash LUE, buttocks, and RLE; occasional physical cues required to sequence.
Upper-body dressing	4	Assessed while seated in w/c or EOB. Verbal or visual cueing required for sequencing; assistance required to pull shirt down once over head.
Lower-body dressing	2	Assessed at bed level or w/c level. Physical assistance required to thread RLE into pants and underwear, verbal cues to thread LLE; total assistance with pulling up clothing. Set-up to don left sock, assistance required with right sock and both shoes even with elastic shoelaces.
Toileting	1	Physical assistance required for hygiene and clothing management.
Bladder management	2	As reported by nursing.
Bowel management	2	As reported by nursing.
Transfers: bed, chair, w/c, toilet (tub, shower NT)	2	Transfer assessed: stand pivot transfers. Maximum assistance of 1 required secondary to aphasia, right hemiplegia; poor safety awareness; fatigue.
Locomotion	2	Reported by physical therapist: maximum assistance of 1 with hemi-walker required secondary to right hemiplegia, poor dynamic standing balance, and fatigue. W/c follow required during walking.

Note. ADL = activity of daily living; EOB = edge of bed; LLE = left lower extremity; LUE = left upper extremity; NDD–2 = National Dysphagia Diet–2; NT = not tested; RLE = right lower extremity; w/c = wheelchair.

Table 11.14. Walter's Discharge Upper-Extremity Evaluation Results

Movement	LUE		RUE		Modified Ashworth Scale
	MMT	PROM	MMT	PROM	
Shoulder flexion	4/5	BFL	2/5	BFL	2
Shoulder abduction	4/5	BFL	1/5	BFL	2
Shoulder external rotation	4/5	BFL	1/5	BFL	2
Shoulder internal rotation	4/5	BFL	2/5	BFL	1
Elbow flexion	5/5	WNL	2/5	WNL	3
Elbow extension	5/5	WNL	1/5	WNL	0
Pronation	4+/5	WNL	1/5	WNL	1
Supination	4/5	WFL	1/5	WFL	2
Wrist flexion	4/5	WNL	1/5	WNL	3
Wrist extension	4/5	WNL	1/5	BFL	0
Finger flexion	4/5	WNL	1/5	WNL	3
Finger extension	4+/5	WNL	0/5	WFL	1

Note. BFL = below functional limits; LUE = left upper extremity; MMT = manual muscle testing; PROM = passive range of motion; RUE = right upper extremity; WFL = within functional limits; WNL = within normal limits.

However, because length of stay is shorter than in the past, the inpatient rehabilitation occupational therapist must provide the best evidence-based intervention
techniques to maximize the benefit of participation in daily rehabilitation sessions.
Depending on circumstances such as payment source, support system, or discharge
disposition, the client with stroke may not have another opportunity to receive
such comprehensive or intensive intervention.

References

American Occupational Therapy Association. (2013). *Occupational therapy's role in skilled nurs-ing facilities.* Retrieved July 20, 2013, from http://www.aota.org/~/media/Corporate/Files/AboutOT/Professionals/WhatIsOT/RDP/Facts/FactSheet_SkilledNursingFacilities.ashx

American Occupational Therapy Association. (2014). Occupational therapy practice framework: Domain and process (3rd ed.). *American Journal of Occupational Therapy, 68*(Suppl. 1), S1–S48. http://dx.doi.org/10.5014/ajot.2014.682006

Avery, W. (2011). Dysphasia management. In G. Gillen (Ed.), *Stroke rehabilitation: A function-based approach* (3rd ed., pp. 629–645). St. Louis: Mosby.

Azouvi, P., Marchal, F., Samuel, C., Morin, L., Renard, C., Louis-Dreyfus, A., . . . Bergego, C. (1996). Functional consequences and awareness of unilateral neglect: Study of an evaluation scale. *Neuropsychological Rehabilitation, 6,* 133–150. http://dx.doi.org/10.1080/713755501

Baum, C. M., Connor, L. T., Morrison, T., Hahn, M., Dromerick, A. W., & Edwards, D. F. (2008). Reliability, validity, and clinical utility of the Executive Function Performance Test: A measure of executive function in a sample of people with stroke. *American Journal of Occupational Therapy, 62,* 446–455. http://dx.doi.org/10.5014/ajot.62.4.446

Baum, C. M., & Edwards, D. (2008). *Activity Card Sort* (2nd ed.). Bethesda, MD: AOTA Press.

Beck, A. T., Steer, R. A., & Brown, G. K. (2000). *BDI®–FastScreen for Medical Patients: Manual.* New York: Psychological Corporation.

Berg, K. O., Maki, B. E., Williams, J. I., Holliday, P. J., & Wood-Dauphinee, S. L. (1992). Clini-cal and laboratory measures of postural balance in an elderly population. *Archives of Physical Medicine and Rehabilitation, 73,* 1073–1080.

Bonder, B. (2014). Providing occupational therapy for older adults with changing needs. In B. A. Boyt Schell, G. Gillen, & M. E. Scaffa (Eds.), *Willard and Spackman's occupational therapy* (12th ed., pp. 896–910). Philadelphia: Lippincott Williams & Wilkins.

Carey, L. M. (2012). Touch and body sensations. In L. M. Carey (Ed.), *Stroke rehabilitation: Insights from neuroscience and imaging* (pp. 157–172). New York: Oxford University Press.

Centers for Medicare and Medicaid Services. (2012). *Medicare benefit policy manual.* Retrieved July 21, 2013, from http://www.cms.gov/Regulations-and-Guidance/Guidance/Manuals/downloads/bp102c01.pdf

Crosson, B., Barco, P. P., Velozo, C. A., Bolesta, M. M., Cooper, P. V., Werts, D., . . . Brobeck, T. C. (1989). Awareness and compensation in postacute head injury rehabilitation. *Journal of Head Trauma Rehabilitation, 4,* 46–54. http://dx.doi.org/10.1097/00001199-198909000-00008

Donato, S., & Halliday Pulaski, K. (2011). Overview of balance impairments: Functional implications. In G. Gillen (Ed.), *Stroke rehabilitation: A function-based approach* (3rd ed., pp. 80–99). St. Louis: Mosby.

Duffy, C., & Beland, H. E. (2011). Part two: Introduction to acute stroke rehabilitation. In G. Gillen (Ed.), *Stroke rehabilitation: A function-based approach* (3rd ed., pp. 26–42). St. Louis: Mosby.

Fisher, A. (1993). *Assessment of Motor and Process Skills* (4th ed.). Fort Collins, CO: Three Star Press.

Gillen, G. (2011a). Managing visual and visuospatial impairments to optimize function. In G. Gillen (Ed.), *Stroke rehabilitation: A function-based approach* (3rd ed., pp. 417–437). St. Louis: Mosby.

Gillen, G. (2011b). Upper extremity function and management. In G. Gillen (Ed.), *Stroke reha-bilitation: A function-based approach* (3rd ed., pp. 218–279). St. Louis: Mosby.

Gillen, G., & Rubio, K. B. (2011). Treatment of cognitive–perceptual deficits: A function-based approach. In G. Gillen (Ed.), *Stroke rehabilitation: A function-based approach* (3rd ed., pp. 501–533). St. Louis: Mosby.

Hamby, J. (2011). Discharge planning: A consultative partnership. In H. Smith-Gabai (Ed.), *Occupational therapy in acute care* (pp. 687–698). Bethesda, MD: AOTA Press.

Handy, J., Salinas, S., Blanchard, S., & Aitken, M. (2004). Meta-analysis examining the effectiveness of electrical stimulation in improving functional use of the upper limb in stroke patients. *Physical and Occupational Therapy in Geriatrics, 21,* 67–78. http://dx.doi.org/10.1080/J148v21n04_05

Jenkins, J. (2004). Adaptive strategies following stroke. In C. Christiansen & K. Matuska (Eds.), *Ways of living: Adaptive strategies for special needs* (pp. 241–255). Bethesda, MD: AOTA Press.

Kane, L., & Buckley, K. (2011). Functional mobility. In G. Gillen (Ed.), *Stroke rehabilitation: A function-based approach* (3rd ed., pp. 350–387). St. Louis: Mosby.

Katzman, R., Brown, T., Fuld, P., Peck, A., Schechter, R., & Schimmel, H. (1983). Validation of a short Orientation–Memory–Concentration Test of cognitive impairment. *American Journal of Psychiatry, 140,* 734–739.

Koyuncu, E., Nakipoğlu-Yüzer, G. F., Doğan, A., & Özgirgin, N. (2010). The effectiveness of functional electrical stimulation for the treatment of shoulder subluxation and shoulder pain in hemiplegic patients: A randomized controlled trial. *Disability and Rehabilitation, 32,* 560–566. http://dx.doi.org/10.3109/09638280903183811

Law, M., Baptiste, S., Carswell, A., McColl, M. A., Polatajko, H., & Pollock, N. (2005). *The Canadian Occupational Performance Measure* (4th ed.). Ottawa, Ontario: CAOT Publications.

Lohman, H. (2014). Payment for services in the United States. In B. A. Boyt Schell, G. Gillen, & M. E. Scaffa (Eds.), *Willard and Spackman's occupational therapy* (12th ed., pp. 896–910). Philadelphia: Lippincott Williams & Wilkins.

Medicare Payment Advisory Commission. (2011). Chapter 9: Inpatient rehabilitation facility services. In *Report to the Congress: Medicare payment policy.* Washington, DC: MedPAC. Retrieved July 20, 2013, from http://www.medpac.gov/documents/Mar11_EntireReport.pdf

Medicare Payment Advisory Commission. (2013). Chapter 10: Inpatient rehabilitation facility services. In *Report to the Congress: Medicare payment policy.* Washington, DC: MedPAC. Retrieved July 20, 2013, from http://www.medpac.gov/documents/Mar13_EntireReport.pdf

Naghdi, S., Ansari, N. N., Azarnia, S., & Kazemnejad, A. (2008). Interrater reliability of the Modified Modified Ashworth Scale (MMAS) for patients with wrist flexor muscle spasticity. *Physiotherapy Theory and Practice, 24,* 372–379. http://dx.doi.org/10.1080/09593980802278959

Nijland, R., van Wegen, E., Verbunt, J., van Wijk, R., van Kordelaar, J., & Kwakkel, G. (2010). A comparison of two validated tests for upper limb function after stroke: The Wolf Motor Function Test and the Action Research Arm Test. *Journal of Rehabilitation Medicine, 42,* 694–696. http://dx.doi.org/10.2340/16501977-0560

Rabadi, M. H., & Rabadi, F. M. (2006). Comparison of the Action Research Arm Test and the Fugl-Meyer Assessment as measures of upper-extremity motor weakness after stroke. *Archives of Physical Medicine and Rehabilitation, 87,* 962–966. http://dx.doi.org/10.1016/j.apmr.2006.02.036

Roberts, P., & Evenson, M. E. (2014). Continuum of care. In B. A. Boyt Schell, G. Gillen, & M. E. Scaffa (Eds.), *Willard and Spackman's occupational therapy* (12th ed., pp. 896–910). Philadelphia: Lippincott Williams & Wilkins.

Rybski, M. F. (2006). The client in rehabilitation and skilled-care environments. In M. N. Beckley & G. M. Giles (Eds.), *Neurorehabilitation for stroke* (Neurorehabilitation Self-Paced Clinical Course Series, pp. 67–112). Bethesda, MD: American Occupational Therapy Association.

Sabari, J. S., & Lieberman, D. (2008). *Occupational therapy practice guidelines for adults with stroke.* Bethesda, MD: AOTA Press.

Stewart, C., & Riedel, K. (2011). Managing speech and language deficits after stroke. In G. Gillen (Ed.), *Stroke rehabilitation: A function-based approach* (3rd ed., pp. 534–551). St. Louis: Mosby.

Toglia, J. P. (2011). The Dynamic Interactional Model of cognition in cognitive rehabilitation. In N. Katz (Ed.), *Cognition, occupation, and participation across the life span: Neuroscience, neurorehabilitation, and models of intervention in occupational therapy* (3rd ed., pp. 161–202). Bethesda, MD: AOTA Press.

Uniform Data System for Medical Rehabilitation. (1997). *Guide for the Uniform Data Set for Medical Rehabilitation (including the FIM™ instrument), version 5.1.* Buffalo, NY: Author.

van der Lee, J. H., Beckerman, H., Lankhorst, G. J., & Bouter, L. M. (2001). The responsiveness of the Action Research Arm Test and the Fugl-Meyer Assessment Scale in chronic stroke patients. *Journal of Rehabilitation Medicine, 33,* 110–113. http://dx.doi.org/10.1080/165019701750165916

Occupational Therapy for People With Stroke in the Outpatient Rehabilitation Setting

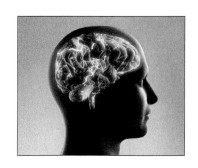

Peggy P. Barco, OTD, OTR/L, SCDCM, and
Melissa S. Dappen, MS, OTR/L

Learning Objectives

After completion of this chapter, readers will be able to

- Identify the important components of an outpatient occupational therapy treatment plan for people with stroke;
- Recognize how limitations in awareness of and insight into cognitive deficits can affect people after stroke and techniques that can be used to facilitate insight and awareness in an outpatient occupational therapy setting;
- Identify the key factors in cognitive treatment models of practice (e.g., the Dynamic Interactional Model) that can be incorporated into the outpatient treatment plan for stroke;
- Recognize what factors influence when a person poststroke may be appropriate for a referral for a comprehensive driver assessment and why a job analysis can be beneficial in outpatient occupational therapy;
- Recognize key factors that may influence a patient's rehabilitation and recovery after discharge from the hospital;
- Identify the occupational therapy process (prioritization of assessment tools, treatment planning and activity gradation, and discharge planning) in the outpatient occupational therapy setting; and
- Identify how task-oriented, occupation-based intervention can be applied in the outpatient occupational therapy setting.

Key Words

- cognitive intervention
- community reintegration
- intervention
- motor
- occupational therapy
- outpatient
- outpatient stroke rehabilitation
- sensory

Introduction

Patients who have had **strokes** enter outpatient **rehabilitation** with various levels of **functional impairment.** The commonality is that these patients have usually completed some form of acute or inpatient medical care, are living in the community, and require further occupational therapy. They vary in the type and level of severity of impairment in outpatient occupational therapy, so outpatient therapists need to be qualified to address all types of deficits that can affect function, including, but not limited to, sensory impairments, motor impairments, and cognitive impairments. The focus is community reintegration and helping the person achieve the greatest independence possible in functioning at home, in **leisure** or community activities, and at work or school.

Community reintegration is one of the most important aspects of the treatment plan and begins once the client is discharged to home (Fleming & Nalder, 2011). Key community reintegration issues reported by clients with **acquired brain injury** and their families include having to move to a more restricted living situation, regaining independence in the home, being able to independently access the community and return to driving, returning to work or study, dealing with financial strain and the breaking down of relationships, and difficulty accessing or the cessation of therapy services (Turner et al., 2007; Turner, Fleming, Ownsworth, & Cornwell, 2008).

As a patient enters outpatient rehabilitation, it is important for the occupational therapist to review any available previous medical records. Record review helps conserve interview time and familiarize the occupational therapist with the specifics of the initial evaluation. For example, some patients will need more of a focus on a motor evaluation, others on a cognitive–perceptual evaluation, and still others on a combination of several areas. As illustrated in the case reviews included in this chapter, evaluations can be individualized to clients' specific needs.

Evaluation in the Outpatient Rehabilitation Setting

Interviewing and getting to know the client are very important parts of outpatient assessment and can be done formally or informally (i.e., using structured formats). One of the more common interview tools that occupational therapists use is the Canadian Occupational Performance Measure (COPM; Law et al., 2005). Often, comprehensive reports from interviews done at the inpatient level by health care professionals are included in the medical records, and they should be reviewed to provide the necessary background information. At the outpatient level, both times for evaluation and treatment visits may be limited. Therefore, in interviewing it is important not to be repetitive but instead to be very focused on areas that are crucial to the outpatient therapy process and determining the individualized treatment plan.

The occupational therapy evaluation in the outpatient setting is focused on the residual deficits from the stroke, including motor, sensory, and cognitive deficits. Individual strengths are also important to include when observed in the initial evaluation. Each evaluation is tailored to specific client factors and ultimately focuses on functional performance.

Assessment of motor and sensory performance can be a major focus in the outpatient evaluation. Most therapists in the outpatient setting working with clients after a neurological event will begin by assessing the client's motor skills. On the basis of information gathered from chart review, therapists may choose screening tools as general as **range of motion** (ROM), manual muscle testing (MMT), and assessment of **tone** or as complex as monofilament testing or determining the client's **metabolic equivalent** (a gauge of cardiovascular fitness). Screening for visuoperceptual deficits is also frequently warranted (Di Monaco et al., 2011). When choosing the appropriate assessment tool, therapists should keep in mind which tools are sensitive enough to demonstrate improvement over time to validate service (Lin et al., 2009; Toglia & Cermak, 2009). These tools should also guide what types of activities and exercises the client should be working on outside of the therapy sessions.

Assessment of cognitive performance is focused on how **cognition** influences activities in daily life. Assessment of a patient's cognitive capacity is important to determine his or her strengths, limitations, and challenges in performance as well as to help guide what environmental strategies can be beneficial to support daily life function (Hartman-Maeir, Katz, & Baum, 2009). Depending on the amount of information available in inpatient records, outpatient therapists may choose to begin assessment with cognitive screens such as the Short Blessed Memory Test (Katzman et al., 1983), the Clock Drawing Test (Lezak, Howieson, Loring, Hannay, & Fischer, 2004), the Montreal Cognitive Assessment (MoCA; Nasreddine et al., 2005), or a more lengthy assessment, such as the Behavioral Assessment of the Dysexecutive Syndrome (BADS; Wilson, Alderman, & Burgess, 1996), the Executive Function Performance Test (EFPT; Baum et al., 2008), or the Rivermead Behavioral Memory Test (Wilson, Cockburn, Baddeley, & Hiorns, 1989). A variety of cognitive screens and assessments are available to meet the unique needs of patients with a range of deficits (Gillen, 2009; Gutman & Schonfeld, 2009; Zoltan, 2007).

Some assessments are more performance based (e.g., top-down), and others are more component based (e.g., bottom-up). Additionally, cognitive assessments can be dynamic, providing more qualitative information about how a client performs functionally (e.g., what factors enhance or decrease performance), or static, providing more quantitative data on performance. The choice of what type of assessment to use depends on many factors, which include but are not limited to client factors as well as the assessment's intended purpose (Zoltan, 2007). The length of the cognitive functional assessment process will vary and can consist of multiple stages, beginning with the interview process and progressing through screening, more in-depth assessments of cognition in occupations, and environmental assessment (Katz, Baum, & Maeir, 2011).

> Assessment of a patient's cognitive capacity is important to determine his or her strengths, limitations, and challenges in performance as well as to help guide what environmental strategies can be beneficial to support daily life function.

Intervention in the Outpatient Rehabilitation Setting

In collaboration with the client and family, the therapist will need to determine what the focus of therapy should be. Choosing an intervention model is one of the most important aspects of developing the treatment plan. Intervention models can range from chronic disease management to biomechanical and rehabilitation models to various specific cognitive-based models of intervention. Choosing a model for cognitive intervention with a specific client involves consideration of a multitude of factors including, but not limited to, the stage of recovery, severity of deficits, level of insight and awareness, the client's strengths and deficits both preinjury and postinjury, and both long-term and short-term treatment goals.

Chronic disease management is an important aspect of the client's time in outpatient therapy. Therapists should keep in mind that clients who have experienced a stroke frequently have comorbidities, including high blood pressure and diabetes, as well as poor diet, history of noncompliance with medication, or a sedentary lifestyle (Dromerick & Khader, 2003; Ovbiagele et al., 2011). Education and development of strategies for managing health conditions outside of the inpatient hospital setting are essential in the prevention of another stroke (Peralta-Catipon & Hwang, 2011).

When impaired motor function is present, the focus of outpatient occupational therapy services is often guided by the biomechanical and rehabilitative model (Latham et al., 2006; Preissner, 2010; Smallfield & Karges, 2009; Thielman, Dean, & Gentile, 2004). This approach emphasizes remediating neuromusculoskeletal function while also modifying the task or the environment to enable performance. Given the variability in the motor presentation of a client poststroke, the outpatient therapist must be adept at identifying the appropriate intervention for the client, whether it be educating the caregiver on proper handling, attempting to drive **neuroplasticity** through task-related training, or implementing (modified) **constraint-induced movement therapy** (Harris, Eng, Miller, & Dawson, 2010; Preissner, 2010; Taub, Uswatte, & Morris, 2003; Thielman et al., 2004). The therapist must consistently attend to the client's motivation and application outside therapy time. Given that the time spent in outpatient therapy is limited relative to inpatient services, the responsibility of carryover rests in the hands of the client and his or her caregivers. Thorough education and repeat demonstration, as well as check-ins on the efficacy of the home program, are essential during the outpatient phase of recovery (Harris et al., 2010).

Some cognitive intervention models are strategy and learning based, and others are more functional or environmentally based. The Dynamic Interactional Model (DIM)–Multicontext Treatment Approach (Toglia, 2005, 2011) is one such strategy- and learning-based cognitive intervention model. It focuses on the interaction among the person, the activity, and the environment. A prime consideration in this model is the client's ability to learn a strategy and apply it across a variety of situations. Therapists use techniques such as verbal cueing task analysis and facilitation of awareness to facilitate improvement in strategy use and, ultimately, performance. Thus, the emphasis in this approach is clearly on learning and generalization of the strategy to overcome deficits and improve performance.

In comparison, functional and environmental models of practice are not focused on the generalization of strategies but rather on assisting clients through training protocols, repetition and practice, and specific task modification or compensation to improve task-specific functional performance. These intervention models include the Neurofunctional Model (Giles, 2011; Rotenberg-Shpigelman, Erez, Nahaloni, & Maeir, 2012) and the Cognitive Disabilities Reconsidered Model (Levy & Burns, 2011).

Clients who have experienced a stroke can commonly lack awareness of all or some of their cognitive and perceptual deficits, and this lack of awareness has been well established as having a significant negative impact on treatment outcomes in rehabilitation (Haskins et al., 2012). Thus, knowledge of a client's self-awareness of his or her own deficits has important implications for the therapist's choice of cognitive intervention model.

In the Model of Awareness (Barco, Crosson, Bolesta, Werts, & Stout, 1991; Crosson et al., 1989), awareness is conceptualized as having different levels, not as being an all-or-none phenomenon (Figure 12.1). This is important because it can affect the choice of treatment model used with the client. If the client is not aware of a particular cognitive deficit, then his or her willingness to use a compensation or strategy (or even to participate in therapy) is extremely limited. In such cases, an intervention model that is more functional or environmental may be most appropriate. However, if the client has some presence of or potential for higher levels

Points to Ponder: Home Exercise Compliance

What strategies could a therapist use to ensure compliance with a home exercise or activity plan?

Clients who have experienced a stroke can commonly lack awareness of all or some of their cognitive and perceptual deficits, and this lack of awareness has been well established as having a significant negative impact on treatment outcomes in rehabilitation.

of awareness, a strategy or learning model of intervention is usually preferable because the client has more control over the use of the strategy and is less dependent on others to implement or modify the environment. Throughout the process of cognitive intervention, techniques to facilitate awareness at higher levels are continually emphasized so clients will be able to use strategies as efficiently as possible to improve their daily function (Barco et al., 1991; Toglia, 2011).

Finally, each model of cognitive intervention has specific techniques, strategies, and learning approaches that the occupational therapist can use as part of the intervention plan to facilitate improved functioning. Specific guidelines for the treatment of cognitive deficits such as attention deficits, memory deficits, **executive function** deficits, and neglect and hemi-inattention have been discussed in an evidence-based decision tree framework (Haskins et al., 2012) and are further described for occupational therapists in textbooks such as Gillen (2009) and Zoltan (2007).

Interventions Related to Community Integration

Reported rates of return to work after stroke can range between 19% and 73% (Treger, Shames, Giaquinto, & Ring, 2007). If work appears to be a realistic goal for the client after stroke, the occupational therapist should help prepare the client to achieve that goal. One way is by connecting the client to community resources (such as state departments of vocational rehabilitation services). Additionally, occupational therapists play an important role by serving as a liaison with employers to facilitate clients' return to work and visiting the job site to perform job analysis. A job analysis (which is similar to task analysis) includes a complete description of the job's responsibilities; materials and tools needed; safety issues; education and training required; environmental demands; sensory, language, cognitive, physical, and interpersonal demands of the job; and possible restrictions and modifications. A job analysis benefits clients who are preparing for their first work experience or those who are returning to employment after illness or injury (King & Olson, 2009). A job analysis can help direct future therapy activities, assist in work transition, and prepare for any potential job modifications.

Returning to driving after an acquired brain injury such as a stroke is particularly important because it has been shown to be associated with greater functional independence (Rapport, Bryer, & Hanks, 2008). Factors such as injury severity and cognitive and psychosocial abilities (e.g., level of self-awareness, fatigue) have been shown to influence successful return to driving (Hawley, 2001; Lundqvist, Alinder, & Rönnberg, 2008; Poole, Chaudry, & Jay, 2008; Rapport et al., 2008), and the rate of driving cessation after stroke is high (Fisk, Owsley, & Pulley, 1997; Lafont, Laumon,

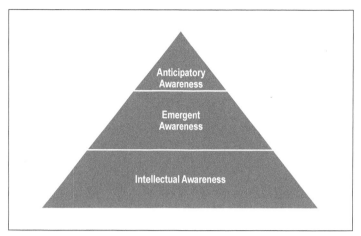

Figure 12.1. Model of Awareness. At the most basic level, *intellectual awareness* involves the client understanding the presence of a deficit area. This level supports the higher levels of awareness. Severe memory deficits, for example, may limit a client's potential for intellectual awareness because the client does not have the memory ability to integrate and profit from recent experience. If intellectual awareness is not present, clients will likely not be able or willing to use strategies independently and will need to depend on others for compensation or environmental modification. *Emergent awareness* represents the client being able to recognize a deficit area when it is actually affecting or hindering performance. Some strategy and learning intervention models may be appropriate for use in a limited manner if this level of awareness is obtained. *Anticipatory awareness* is the highest level of awareness that is achievable and consists of a client being able to anticipate that a deficit could cause a problem in a specific situation. Ideally, a client would then be able to use a strategy and learning intervention model to eventually implement compensation before the actual occurrence of the problem (because the client would have the awareness to anticipate the need to use the strategy).

Source. From "Awareness and Compensation in Postacute Head Injury Rehabilitation," by B. Crosson, P. Barco, C. A. Velozo, M. M. Bolesta, P. V. Cooper, D. Werts, and T. C. Brobeck, 1989, *Journal of Head Trauma Rehabilitation, 4*, p. 47. Copyright © 1989 by Wolters Kluwer. Reprinted with permission.

Each model of cognitive intervention has specific techniques, strategies, and learning approaches that the occupational therapist can use as part of the intervention plan to facilitate improved functioning.

Points to Ponder: Lack of Awareness and Cognitive Intervention

How would an occupational therapist's role be different if a person was not able to gain awareness of his or her cognitive deficits?

Helmer, Dartigues, & Fabrigoule, 2008; Legh-Smith, Wade, & Hewer, 1986). A meta-analysis of driving studies has shown that tests of visual perception, visual comprehension, executive functions, divided attention, and processing speed were most predictive of road performance after stroke (Devos et al., 2011). Knowing when or if a client with cognitive deficits (e.g., after a stroke) is ready to resume driving can be a difficult decision for the physician, occupational therapists, and family, and there are no clear clinical guidelines regarding when to refer a person with cognitive deficits for a comprehensive driver evaluation (Barco, Stav, Arnold, & Carr, 2012). The decision regarding when or if a driver evaluation referral is needed is often based on clinical reasoning, which includes the nature of the health condition, functional status, client's level of insight and awareness, prognosis of the health condition, progress in rehabilitation and recovery, and input from family and significant others (Barco et al., 2012). The outpatient occupational therapist plays a crucial role in knowing when a driver assessment is or is not indicated.

Measuring Outcomes

An important consideration as a client enters therapy (and according to each treatment facility's unique policies) is the number of allowable outpatient visits. Many people have limited to no outpatient visits, and others have fair to good outpatient benefits. Unfortunately, funding can dramatically affect the outcome goals that can be reasonably met. Outcome goals need to be meaningful to the client and realistic to accomplish in the amount of available time in therapy. Measuring improvement is usually based on reevaluation of key areas of function, goal status, and community reintegration.

> **Outcome goals need to be meaningful to the client and realistic to accomplish in the amount of available time in therapy.**

Case Review: Steve

Steve was referred to outpatient occupational therapy. He was found to have fairly good outpatient insurance benefits—30 visits per calendar year. Additionally, Steve was scheduled for a neuropsychological assessment. The therapist reviewed Steve's inpatient notes and proceeded to choose an assessment to further evaluate Steve. From the inpatient notes, it appeared that Steve's residual deficits were mainly cognitively based. When the occupational therapist met with Steve, Steve stated that he really was not sure that he needed therapy but that it "was what I was told to do." He told the occupational therapist that he had a stroke and had some difficulties with his left arm that had resolved. The occupational therapist scheduled Steve for 1-hour evaluation to include the interview and the assessment.

Occupational Therapy Evaluation

The therapist interviewed Steve informally before choosing which assessment to use. The records contained a fair amount of background information, so the therapist decided to focus the interview on Steve's awareness of any potential residual deficits, his current level of functioning, and his goals. Steve expressed that he was taking care of himself without any difficulties (dressing, feeding, bathing, some cooking, managing his own medications) and was very eager to resume his job and begin to drive again. He cited examples of independently making scrambled eggs, paying the bills, doing home chores, and playing with his children without any difficulty since he had been discharged from the hospital. Steve expressed a strong desire to return to driving in the near future and was very upset that his doctor and his wife would not let him drive or return to work at this time. He did not feel that he had any remaining difficulties with his cognition and stated that he was functioning at a similar level as before his stroke.

Although Steve's wife, Elizabeth, reported great improvement since inpatient therapy, she still noticed some changes in Steve. Positively, she reported that he was now able to make simple meals and take his medication independently. She stated that although he was accurate with paying bills, he needed reminders to pay the bills on time (different than before his stroke). She said he also needed reminders to do his chores. She described him as lazy and reported that he used to play creative games with his daughter and son, and now they spend most of their time together watching television. She also reported that he was recently in the garage tinkering with his cars, and she noticed that his tools were scattered all over and that he appeared to have left whatever he was doing quite a mess and incomplete. She said he used to be very organized with his tools and always put everything in its proper place. Elizabeth additionally reported that Steve's outbursts and excessive irritability seemed to have improved and were no longer a concern.

The occupational therapist wanted to have a better understanding of the types of cognitive deficits, if any, that remained from the stroke. The evaluation needed to sufficiently challenge Steve across a broad area of cognitive function. Although true performance-based evaluations are usually preferred, the therapist noticed that the EFPT was done with Steve in inpatient rehabilitation and that he appeared to have made strong gains in his functional independence since that time as he and his wife had indicated. Thus, the occupational therapist opted to use an evaluation that incorporated less routine and more novel tasks, especially because Steve's goals were very high level (wanting to return to work and drive). Although many of the cognitive-based assessment batteries for occupational therapy evaluation would have been appropriate, the therapist chose the BADS because it had novel executive function tasks, required a challenging level of function, continued to incorporate some performance-based components, and could easily be completed in the evaluation time period. Additionally, the therapist decided to do a brief motor screen (upper-extremity strength and ROM, hand grasp, and the Nine-Hole Peg Test) to verify that Steve was doing well with motor skills. Refer to the initial assessment note in Appendix 12.A.

Initial Interdisciplinary Family Conference

The interdisciplinary treatment team consisted of the physician, social worker, neuropsychologist, speech–language pathologist, physical therapist, and occupational therapist. The team met with Steve and Elizabeth to review the results of the assessments and discuss treatment recommendations. Each therapist reviewed the results of his or her assessments and discussed potential areas of intervention with Steve and his wife.

As always, it is very important that the therapist seek input as to what the client and family perceive as important areas to address in therapy. Although Steve was not sure he agreed with the findings of residual cognitive deficits, he agreed to proceed with therapy for a short period of time to prepare him for his main goals of returning to driving and work.

Points to Ponder: Cognitive Intervention Within an Interdisciplinary Team

How do various disciplines manage the overlap that may occur in the treatment of cognitive deficits?

It is very important that the therapist seek input as to what the client and family perceive as important areas to address in therapy.

Occupational Therapy Intervention Plan

The cognitive intervention approaches chosen to begin to work with Steve in outpatient therapy mainly consisted of the Model of Awareness (Barco et al., 1991; Crosson et al., 1989) and the DIM (Toglia, 2011). The reasons for using these models in combination were as follows:

- In spite of the presence of insight deficits, Steve presented at a fairly high level of functioning at initial outpatient evaluation, which showed potential for improvement in awareness and strategy use.
- Steve has high goals of returning to driving and work, so strategy and learning models have the most potential for full independence if successful.
- Steve has adequate outpatient rehabilitation benefits that allow for the extended time to facilitate awareness and work with strategies and strategy transfers to different activities and situations.
- Steve did not have any severe deficits (e.g., severe memory deficits or severe concrete thinking) that would interfere with learning ability or potential to gain awareness.

Occupational Therapy Intervention Implementation

As shown in his initial assessment, Steve presented with a lack of awareness of the existence of his cognitive deficits. The first step in the treatment approach was to facilitate awareness in hopes that Steve can increase insight into his cognitive deficits. The Model of Awareness provided an overview of the principles involved in increasing awareness. If Steve's awareness did not improve, the Model of Awareness would similarly provide guidance on how to alter the model of intervention and treatment plan accordingly. The hope was that as Steve's insight began to improve, he would begin to see the benefit of using strategies to compensate for his deficits. The therapist used the Model of Awareness in conjunction with the DIM–Multicontext Treatment Approach to help Steve learn and apply strategies for his memory and executive function deficits across a variety of functional tasks to meet his long-term goal of increasing his productivity.

Initially, the treatment focus was on increasing awareness of cognitive deficits, specifically intellectual awareness of the memory and executive function deficits. To do this, the therapist focused on building therapeutic rapport with Steve, providing education related to common deficit areas after stroke, providing gentle feedback, having Steve make a strengths and weaknesses list, and incorporating self-rating scales of performance into the therapy tasks.

A strengths and weaknesses list consists of the client's areas of strength and areas that could be worked on in therapy (e.g., weaknesses). Steve initially generated this list on his own, and the therapist slowly began to incorporate cognitive areas of concern with guided questioning. Confrontation was kept to a minimum, and items were added to the list only with Steve's permission. Moving very slowly into providing feedback and allowing Steve control of the list helped in developing trust and forming the therapeutic relationship. The list's purpose was to begin the education component of treatment regarding the existence of possible cognitive deficits.

Facilitation of awareness also included Steve rating his performance on an activity and comparing his rating with the therapist's. Steve and the occupational therapist made up a self-rating sheet together to look at areas that were deemed questionable on the strengths and weaknesses list. Again, making the list together was part of developing trust in the therapeutic relationship. Assessment of the client's self-perception of performance can be done before an activity, during an activity, and after an activity (Barco et al., 1991; Toglia, 2011). Steve rated his anticipated performance before the task and again after completion. The therapist rated the task only after completion.

Steve initially rated his performance as very good; in contrast, the therapist noted difficulties in the cognitive area and also presented observable examples to substantiate these ratings. Again, the therapist presented the examples in a minimally confrontational manner, qualifying many of the ratings with "I may be wrong, but it seemed like you might have forgotten what the instructions were at this point" (see Appendix 12.B). Over time, Steve began to become more aware of his memory deficit and difficulties with organization, and his ratings more approximated the therapist's after task completion.

As Steve's awareness increased, an updated strengths and weaknesses list was made, and Steve put on the list that he needed to work on his memory and organization skills, indicating that his intellectual awareness had improved. As Steve became more aware of the existence of these cognitive deficits, he became more receptive to what he could do to overcome or compensate for them. Although the focus on increasing his level of awareness continued throughout therapy, therapy could now begin to incorporate the use of strategies to compensate for the deficits.

First, the therapist explored compensatory strategies for memory deficits with Steve. Steve stated that in his position as an attorney, he often had to take notes during meetings with clients. He stated that he would be very willing to incorporate more note taking into his daily life to avoid gaps in his memory. He was also very comfortable with using verbal rehearsal of the information to help with memory retention. Steve agreed to try out his skill at note taking and verbal rehearsal in a variety of simulated tasks that the therapist would provide to him to challenge him in this area. As Steve progressed in his use of compensatory strategies in a therapy task, the therapist used the DIM–Multicontext Treatment Approach to generalize the strategies to different tasks, but at a similar or slightly higher level of complexity. These strategies were then eventually applied to the home environment and simulated work situations.

As tasks with memory began to become more challenging, more executive function skills were needed in the planning and organizing of different activities and compensations. Thus, Steve's difficulties in these areas became a focus of therapy.

The initial focus was on reestablishing Steve's awareness of these executive function deficits. Because Steve was previously aware of the executive function studies during his self-ratings, he was receptive to and trusted the therapist's feedback and education about the nature of the difficulties with problem solving and organization, indicating a willingness to use strategies. A common approach to executive function deficits is the use of formal problem-solving strategies (Haskins et al., 2012), which include but are not limited to approaches such as Goal Management Training (Levine et al., 2000) and Cognitive Orientation to Daily Occupational Performance (Dawson et al., 2009). These problem-solving strategies or frameworks each proceed through common steps, which can include identifying the problem and alternatives or solutions to the problem, implementing a plan for a solution, executing the solution, and self-evaluating the effectiveness of the solution.

Steve was introduced to a problem-solving organizational framework, and he provided input into modifying the framework to best meet his individual needs. The first focus was practicing the use of this framework in basic simulated problem situations to understand how to use the strategy (e.g., Steve was given problems such as "What would you do if your neighbor's dog was barking all night?"). On the basis of these simulated situations, Steve had to identify the problem, generate as many alternatives as he could, prioritize the alternatives, implement the plan, and determine ways to evaluate its effectiveness (Appendix 12.C). Throughout the process, Steve's therapist provided graded cueing and thought-provoking questions to stimulate Steve's executive functioning when required.

As Steve progressed in understanding the problem-solving process, the task challenges were increased using the DIM intervention approach, focusing on transferring the problem-solving organizational framework to new situations that would provide the just-right challenge for Steve. Steve continued to learn and work through the problem-solving process—with guided questions from his therapist using the worksheet framework—and was able to apply the strategy to problems in his own daily life. He did not reach full independence at this level, but he continued to benefit from guided questioning and structuring during more challenging problem-solving tasks. Steve was aware of the need for assistance, yet he was becoming increasingly more impatient to return to work and driving (Appendix 12.D).

Outpatient Occupational Therapy Discharge Outcome and Follow-Up Services

Thus far in outpatient therapy, Steve had progressed well in his awareness of his cognitive deficits as well as in his use of strategies for memory and executive function. He was independent in the use of memory strategies and required minimal to moderate assistance in using strategies in more challenging problem-solving situations. He was becoming very eager to return to his former activities, including driving and his work as an attorney.

Return to Driving

The occupational therapist, physician, and family were supportive of Steve's completing a full driver assessment. Steve had shown good improvement in his awareness of his cognitive deficits and in the use of related strategies. Additionally, his therapists noted that Steve did not have any visual–perceptual issues, neglects, or behavior deficits that would obviously impede driving safety.

Steve performed quite well on the driver assessment, which was performed by an occupational therapy certified driver rehabilitation specialist. The clinical portion of the assessment showed strengths in his visual acuity, motor skills, reaction time, and cognitive functioning. Steve took an on-the-road assessment and showed good knowledge of traffic signs and rules of the road, good scanning ability, good lane positioning, and good ability to make decisions in traffic, and he was able to self-navigate safely in an unfamiliar environment. No safety concerns were presented, and the recommendation was for Steve to return to driving.

Return to Work

The therapist worked with Steve to create a job analysis of his position as an attorney. The therapist chose to do this activity with Steve as part of a therapy experience in hopes that it would create increased awareness of the implications of residual deficits in relationship to his job functions. Steve had some difficulty seeing how the cognitive components (memory and executive function) related to being a plaintiff attorney. For example, one major aspect of his role as an attorney was preparing arguments to support clients' cases (involving extensive research, divergent reasoning—addressing different points of view—and extensive organization and planning). Steve had begun to do simulated job tasks using the various strategies for memory and executive function related to attorney work and was becoming more aware of the difficulties he might have on return.

Steve and the therapist used the problem-solving framework to develop an organized plan for what a return to his job might look like. Using this framework allowed Steve to exert decision making and control over his future return-to-work decisions. Part of the plan involved continuing to work on more advanced simulated work tasks in therapy for a few more visits with the eventual plan of phasing back into work very slowly, performing limited duties (much like those of a legal assistant) until he felt more competent. His physician concurred with the plan, and his fellow attorneys were very supportive of whatever approach was beneficial to Steve.

Case Review: Mary

On Mary's discharge from inpatient rehab, home health occupational therapy services arranged to see her in her home. Mary's daughter, Sarah, was present for the initial visit, which included obtaining an occupational profile and observing Mary's performance of **activities of daily living** (ADLs), including Mary and her daughter demonstrating a safe tub transfer with minimal assistance using the shower chair and grab bars, as well as a toilet transfer, which required more assistance because Sarah had not yet installed grab bars (Guidetti, Asaba, & Tham, 2009). The occupational therapist made recommendations based on Mary's ROM and bathroom setup (Schmid & Rittman, 2009).

Follow-up intervention included an in-home safety evaluation. The home exercise program provided by the inpatient rehabilitation occupational therapist was reviewed, and Sarah demonstrated her ability to lead her mother through it correctly (Harris et al., 2010). Throughout visits, Mary was noted to successfully use her memory notebook to record information, make appointments, and manage her medication with one verbal cue from Sarah. The use of an alarm set on a cell phone or watch was suggested, which Sarah later reported was successful in allowing Mary to manage her own medication.

Strategies for neglect were also set up in the home. Bright red tape was placed on the left side of each doorway, as well as the inside of the refrigerator and freezer and Mary's bathroom and bedroom mirrors (Toglia & Cermak, 2009; Warren, 2009).

The therapist also had Sarah demonstrate her ability to properly use Mary's new blood pressure cuff as well as administer medication. Both Sarah and Mary were able to verbalize the indications for each medication and the correct dosage (Ovbiagele et al., 2011).

Home health occupational therapy saw Mary 3 times before establishing that her needs within the home were met and that she and Sarah could safely manage her care, as well as leave the home. Mary decided that she was ready to start outpatient therapy, and the home health occupational therapist discharged her.

Occupational Therapy Evaluation

Sarah accompanied Mary to her outpatient evaluation. The notes from the home health occupational therapist had been faxed to the therapist to provide the best continuity of care. The outpatient occupational therapist also had access to Mary's neuropsychological testing, with minimal impairments noted in visuospatial relations, recall of verbal information, and processing speed. She noted feelings of guilt at relying on her daughter and friends for her daily needs. The neuropsychologist offered follow-up services, which Mary declined, reporting that she turned to faith for support.

The initial evaluation was scheduled for 90 minutes. The evaluation began with administration of the COPM (Law et al., 2005). Mary identified the following as performance areas to be addressed: spending time with her grandchildren; participating in church events; returning to work; driving; and cooking for family, friends, and herself. Compared with the COPM administered in inpatient rehabilitation, Mary was better able to identify her Performance and Satisfaction scores using a visual scorecard. She reflected that she had not been able to do so at the earlier administration because she did not yet understand how she would struggle in the home environment in which she had been so independent before onset (Ekstam, Uppgard, Kottorp, & Tham, 2007).

In addition to the COPM, the therapist performed other subjective assessments to determine Mary's current status. The Stroke Impact Scale (Duncan, Bode, Min Lai, & Perera, 2003) was administered and Mary's overall transformed score was 67.2%, with strength, ADLs and **instrumental activities of daily living** (IADLs), mobility, and hand use most strongly affected. She reported her recovery score as 60 of 100.

A depression screen was also administered because depression has been found to affect anywhere from 34% to more than 60% of stroke survivors (Dromerick & Khader, 2003) and has been shown to have negative effects on patients' participation. Mary received a total score of 3 on the Patient Health Questionnaire–9, indicating minimal depression (Löwe, Kroenke, Herzog, & Gräfe, 2004).

The therapist then evaluated Mary's client factors. An informal screen of visuoperceptual skills revealed a mild left visual inattention (Di Monaco et al., 2011). Cognition was assessed using the MoCA (Koski, Xie, & Finch, 2009; Toglia, Fitzgerald, O'Dell, Mastrogiovanni, & Lin, 2011). Mary scored 17 of 30, indicating deficits in visuospatial and executive function, naming, **attention,** language fluency, and delayed recall. Mary's ROM was assessed, and although she was able to tolerate full **passive ROM,** she demonstrated limited active ROM at shoulder, elbow, and wrist. MMT revealed right upper-extremity strength that was within functional limits. Flexor synergy tone was found throughout the left upper extremity.

Dynamometry was performed, and Mary demonstrated mean grip strength of 17 pounds with her left hand, compared with 50 pounds with her dominant right hand. She reported a pain score of 4 with passive ROM because of feelings of tightness (Dromerick & Khader, 2003; Kong, Lee, & Chua, 2012; Roosink et al., 2011; Wilkinson, Sakel, Camp, & Hammond, 2012).

Arm function was measured using the Action Research Arm Test (ARAT; Lang, Wagner, Dromerick, & Edwards, 2006; Lin et al., 2009). Mary received a score of 41 of 57, demonstrating impaired five-finger grip, cylindrical grasp, and pincer grip. She reported that she was performing the home exercises provided by the inpatient therapist, but only with the home health therapist (Harris et al., 2010). Mary and Sarah reported that they had been monitoring Mary's blood sugar and blood pressure. They presented a written journal documenting Mary's vital signs since discharge from the hospital. Mary's blood pressure at initial evaluation was 130/76 (Ovbiagele et al., 2011; Appendix 12.E).

Occupational Therapy Intervention Plan

After completion of all assessments and discussion with Mary and Sarah, the occupational therapist interpreted the data to identify facilitators and barriers to performance. Collaborating with Mary and Sarah, the therapist created both short-term and long-term goals for treatment (Appendix 12.F).

A copy of Mary's treatment goals was provided to Mary, who was encouraged to use her journal to keep track of her performance and achievements and as a means for communication among the therapist, Mary, Sarah, and Mary's friends, who occasionally accompanied Mary to therapy when Sarah was unavailable. Mary, Sarah, and the therapist then identified several strengths supporting Mary's recovery. At the time of evaluation, Sarah's employer had approved 3 months of family leave. Mary's friends from church had been very active in Mary's return home and had been able to help Mary and Sarah as needed. Finally, Mary's hardworking **attitude** and motivation were significant strengths in her recovery.

Mary initially attended outpatient therapy for 60-minute sessions 3 times per week. The intensity of therapy was determined by her progress, which was informally evaluated at each session and objectively reevaluated using objective measures each month, with the plan of care adjusted as needed. The therapist maintained a schedule of 3 times per week for 2 months, then tapered down to 2 times per week as Mary's progress allowed her to be more active in her recovery, participate more in the community, and prepare for her discharge from therapy services.

Occupational Therapy Intervention Implementation

Mary's occupational therapy interventions built on the progress that she made in inpatient rehabilitation. The theoretical basis for intervention continued to be task related, with occupation-based interventions performed in the safety of the clinical setting and with the expectation that Mary will then attempt these activities in the home with assistance as needed from Sarah and friends. Intervention was also based on the biomechanical and rehabilitative model (Latham et al., 2006; Preissner, 2010; Smallfield & Karges, 2009; Thielman et al., 2004). This approach emphasizes remediating neuromusculoskeletal function while also modifying the task or the environment to enable performance. Chronic disease management was also included in outpatient therapy, given Mary's medical history, including high risk factors and medication noncompliance (Peralta-Catipon & Hwang, 2011).

Neuromusculoskeletal and Movement-Related Functions: Left Hemiparesis and Muscle Tone, Endurance, and Balance

At evaluation, Mary was noted to have continued flexor synergy tone in her left upper extremity, which was noted to have improved since inpatient rehabilitation but was beginning to cause Mary pain. Mary and Sarah demonstrated proper passive stretches. The therapist encouraged Mary to contact her primary care physician to discuss muscle relaxers. Mary did so and reported good relief. Mary was then taught how to use her left arm to actively assist during activity while continuing to safely use her quad cane. Examples of activity included stabilizing a piece of paper while

Points to Ponder: Attendance

Outpatient therapy is unique in that the client typically begins and ends the day at home. Consider potential barriers to attendance in the outpatient therapy setting.

she wrote, pouring liquid into a glass and wiping up subsequent spills on counters, carrying clothes, and carrying household items (magazines, dishes, and other items, varying the size, shape, and weight). She also performed bimanual tasks while sitting, performing activities such as cutting food, folding clothes, stabilizing containers (again varying size, shape, and weight) while removing the top with her right hand, stabilizing dishes during cooking tasks, and picking up items from the floor using her left hand for gross grasp.

As Mary's strength improved, the therapist noted that she was demonstrating motor extinction at times; her left arm would drop off during activity. The therapist encouraged Mary to participate in tasks in which extinction would be quite evident. Some examples included holding her cell phone with her left hand during conversation and when accessing social networking and game applications, using both hands to balance a tray of cookies, and holding items using palmar grasp on both arms (Hayner, Gibson, & Giles, 2010). The therapist noted the length of time before the left arm started to lag and provided feedback and cues to Mary to increase the time.

As Mary became more able to actively use her left arm in activity, the therapist decided to initiate modified constraint-induced movement therapy (mCIMT; Page, Murray, & Hermann, 2011; Taub et al., 2003). After long and thorough discussion with Mary and Sarah, Mary agreed to attempt mCIMT in the clinic. For the first 2 weeks of mCIMT, Mary performed repetitive, task-specific activities with her right arm restrained and the therapist assisting her as she ambulated. Examples of activities performed included reaching, grasping, and placing self-care items on a low shelf; setting the table for a full meal; and participating in leisure activities such as Wii, board games, and T-ball in preparation for a visit from her grandchildren. Activities were graded to ensure best success for Mary, with the goals to provide motivation, increase tolerance, and increase likelihood of adherence to mCIMT outside of the clinical setting.

As Mary became more comfortable in the clinic, she agreed to attempt a more intense setting, and she began restraint at home at a frequency of 2 hours a day, 3 days a week (on days on which she was not attending therapy). She followed this schedule for 6 weeks and, with the assistance of her daughter, filled out a chart (provided by the therapist) listing the activities she performed and their duration. During therapy sessions, Mary was noted to have increased spontaneous use of her left arm during interventions. Objective measures (ARAT, dynamometry, and MMT and ROM) revealed increased ROM, strength, and coordination. Activities in the clinic were upgraded each session to provide just-right challenge to encourage Mary to continue to make gains. Her mCIMT schedule was increased to 3 hours per day, 5 days per week. Mary was tolerating this frequency well by discharge.

Sensory and Mental Functions: Higher-Level Cognitive, Attention, Memory, Perception, Thought, and Emotion

To gain a better understanding of the quality of Mary's current occupational performance, the occupational therapist administered the Assessment of Motor and Process Skills (AMPS; Fisher, 2003; Merritt, 2011). She offered a variety of ADL tasks from which Mary could choose. Mary selected the preparation of a peanut butter and jelly sandwich for one person and cleaning windows. Mary's overall quality of performance was found to be markedly unsafe, clumsy or physically effortful, and inefficient. ADL motor ability was ineffective or markedly deficient in terms of body positioning, obtaining and holding objects, and moving self and objects, although she scored well regarding sustaining performance for both motor and process skills. Moreover, Mary's ADL process skills were found to be ineffective or markedly deficient in organizing space and objects and adapting performance, whereas applying knowledge and temporal organization were both adequate with no apparent disruption observed.

The therapist also wanted to track Mary's participation in her home as well as in the community. Mary completed the Activity Card Sort: Recovery Version (Form B; Perlmutter, Bhorade, Gordon, Hollingsworth, & Baum, 2010). Mary's percentage of activities retained since onset was 25% (Turner et al., 2008). She reported the following five activities as most important to her: (1) work (paid), (2) walking, (3) volunteer work, (4) going to her children's or grandchildren's activities, and (5) entertaining at home or a club. Mary wrote these goals down in her journal just under the treatment goals that were established at the initial evaluation using the COPM.

Given noted deficits in visuoperceptual function at initial evaluation, the therapist used the Dynavision D2™ Light Training Board (Bioness Inc., Valencia, CA) for assessment and retraining of visuospatial and attention skills (Klavora, Heslegrave, & Young, 2000). The Dynavision apparatus can be used to evaluate and train oculomotor skills; visual attention; hand–eye coordination; upper-extremity ROM; and coordination, endurance, and motor planning. Mary initially performed tasks using only her right arm to provide a valid measure of her visuoperceptual skills. As therapy progressed, and she developed motor return, the Dynavision was used as a tool to challenge deficits in motor ROM and speed of her left arm. At her first attempt at Dynavision, Mary was able to smoothly track the light in all quadrants in Mode C (visual tracking tasks). Performing Mode A (self-paced tasks), Mary demonstrated reaction time of 2.38 seconds overall, with slower times noted for the left half of the light board. Mary participated in regular visual retraining, often starting sessions with 15 minutes of Dynavision and moving on to occupations. As her reaction speeds decreased, Mode B (apparatus-paced tasks) was introduced. Mary demonstrated initial difficulty keeping up with the buttons on the left lighting up every 2 seconds, but she was able to move on to the next button without **perseveration.** As her performance improved, challenges such as decreasing the length of time the button remained lit, incorporating digit sequences of various lengths for various times, or self-generating attention and **concentration** tasks (such as performing mathematics, listing states, holding conversation) were introduced. The Dynavision served as a good objective tool to track Mary's improvements in scanning abilities.

In preparation for discharge, the therapist and Mary began exploring Mary's potential to return to work (Wolf, Baum, & Connor, 2009). Although Mary had made great gains, she was concerned about the stressful, busy schedule of full-time work. Mary agreed to contact her direct supervisor to get a description of her job duties, which include managing a busy schedule, time on the computer, serving as a liaison between employees and management, and updating job descriptions and policies. While Mary has been out of the office, her administrative assistant and her supervisor have shared her duties, but they are struggling to cover the workload. Mary reported that her employers were very invested in her return and were willing to make any accommodations the therapist and physician recommended. In preparation for Mary's return on a part-time basis, her administrative assistant accompanied Mary to two sessions for education on how she can help with Mary's transition. Mary reported that she was willing to try the following suggestions:

- Reduce distractions and clutter in the work area.
- Prioritize work assignments to essential, familiar functions, broken down into small steps.
- Administrative assistant will help Mary set reminders, post memos or notes, and manage her calendar.
- Supervisor will provide typewritten notes after each meeting.
- Mary will meet with supervisor and personal assistant on a weekly basis to assess the effectiveness of accommodations. An open discourse between all three will be maintained.
- One-handed keyboard or voice recognition software should be considered.
- Work will be self-paced, allowing for breaks as needed (Job Accommodation Network, 2013).

Outpatient Occupational Therapy Discharge Outcome and Follow-Up Services

The final 2 weeks of Mary's attendance in outpatient occupational therapy were spent in reevaluation and review of Mary's gains, as well as recommendations to continue her recovery. Objective measures such as ROM and MMT, dynamometry, ARAT, and the Modified Ashworth Scale (Bohannon & Smith, 1987) demonstrated improvements in ROM, overall strength, grip strength, functional use, and decreased tone (see Table 12.1). ROM was found to be within functional levels, but with occasional motor lag when Mary was fatigued or distracted. MMT was 4 of 5 overall. Mary was encouraged to continue mCIMT postdischarge. The Activity Card Sort, Stroke Impact Scale, Patient Health Questionnaire–9, and MoCA were readministered (see Table 12.1).

Mary participated in the AMPS once more. Mary chose the following activities to perform: making pasta with sauce and beverages for two people and vacuuming the floor, including moving lightweight furniture. Mary's overall quality of performance, motor ability, and process skills appeared to be adequate with no apparent disruption observed.

Mary's COPM scores were reassessed. Mary reported improved performance and satisfaction in all areas with the exception of driving. Her mean performance score increased from 3 to 8, and her satisfaction increased from 2.2 to 7.2. Mary reported plans for an upcoming visit from her grandchildren. She had returned to weekly church services, including helping in the kitchen once a month. She brought in

Table 12.1. Mary's Standardized Assessment Scores

Assessment	Initial	Discharge
Dynamometry	17 pounds	42 pounds
MAS	1+	No tone
ARAT	41	53
ACS	25%	46%
SIS	67.2 (recovery score of 60)	89.2 (recovery score of 90)
PHQ–9	3 (minimal signs of depression)	0 (no signs of depression)
MoCA	17/30	28/30 (WNL)

Note. ACS = Activity Card Sort; ARAT = Action Research Arm Test; MAS = Modified Ashworth Scale; MoCA = Montreal Cognitive Assessment; PHQ–9 = Patient Health Questionnaire–9; SIS = Stroke Impact Scale; WNL = within normal limits.

baked goods, which she prepared with supervision from Sarah, to whom she was teaching family recipes. Mary reflected that although she has made good gains, she and Sarah did not yet feel she was ready to resume driving in the busy urban area in which she lives (Elgin et al., 2010). She and Sarah or friends were using public transportation, which was Mary's primary form of transportation before her hospitalization. The therapist gave her information on driver rehabilitation services in the area and encouraged her to follow up with her primary care provider if and when she decided she was ready. Mary was also concerned about finances because she was not returning to work full-time. Education was provided regarding long-term disability (which, if needed, would provide some income until Mary's age of retirement). Mary planned to return to work after discharge from therapy because she felt she could not balance both schedules.

Throughout her time in outpatient rehab (as well as inpatient rehab), Mary was provided with information on stroke prevention, recovery, and symptoms of stroke. The therapist again reviewed these symptoms and encouraged Mary to share them with loved ones. Mary reported that she was considering giving a talk at her church to educate others. Mary expressed interest in connecting with other survivors, and she was provided with information on local groups as well as online groups and references and publications available online or through the National Stroke Association.

Finally, Mary was given information on accessible housing and Aging in Place. Mary agreed that her current home is not likely the safest place for her to be, and she was looking into several garden apartments. She was also considering joining a gym that offered water aerobics.

Mary was directed to continue her medication as prescribed, continue monitoring her blood sugar and pressure, and continue her exercises, as well as carefully monitor her diet. She was encouraged to follow up with her primary care physician, neurologist, and physiatrist regularly.

References

American Occupational Therapy Association. (2014). Occupational therapy practice framework: Domain and process (3rd ed.). *American Journal of Occupational Therapy, 68*(Suppl. 1), S1–S48. http://dx.doi.org/10.5014/ajot.2014.682006

Barco, P. P., Crosson, B., Bolesta, M. M., Werts, D., & Stout, R. (1991). Training awareness and compensation in postacute head injury rehabilitation. In J. S. Kreutzer & P. H. Wheman (Eds.), *Cognitive rehabilitation for persons with traumatic brain injury* (pp. 129–146). Baltimore: Brookes.

Barco, P. P., Stav, W. B., Arnold, R., & Carr, D. B. (2012). Cognition: A vital component to driving and community mobility. In M. J. McGuire & E. Schold Davis (Eds.), *Driving and community mobility: Occupational therapy strategies across the lifespan* (pp. 137–171). Bethesda, MD: AOTA Press.

Baum, C. M., Connor, L. T., Morrison, T., Hahn, M., Dromerick, A. W., & Edwards, D. F. (2008). Reliability, validity, and clinical utility of the Executive Function Performance Test: A measure of executive function in a sample of people with stroke. *American Journal of Occupational Therapy, 62,* 446–455. http://dx.doi.org/10.5014/ajot.62.4.446

Bohannon, R., & Smith, M. (1987). Interrater reliability of a Modified Ashworth Scale of muscle spasticity. *Physical Therapy, 67,* 206.

Crosson, B., Barco, P. P., Velozo, C. A., Bolesta, M. M., Cooper, P. V., Werts, D., & Brobeck, T. C. (1989). Awareness and compensation in postacute head injury rehabilitation. *Journal of Head Trauma Rehabilitation, 4,* 46–54. http://dx.doi.org/10.1097/00001199-198909000-00008

Dawson, D. R., Gaya, A., Hunt, A., Levine, B., Lemsky, C., & Polatajko, H. J. (2009). Using the Cognitive Orientation to Occupational Performance (CO–OP) with adults with executive dysfunction following traumatic brain injury. *Canadian Journal of Occupational Therapy, 76*, 115–127. http://dx.doi.org/10.1177/000841740907600209

Devos, H., Akinwuntan, A. E., Nieuwboer, A., Truijen, S., Tant, M., & De Weerdt, W. (2011). Screening for fitness to drive after stroke: A systematic review and meta-analysis. *Neurology, 76*, 747–756. http://dx.doi.org/10.1212/WNL.0b013e31820d6300

Di Monaco, M., Schintu, S., Dotta, M., Barba, S., Tappero, R., & Gindri, P. (2011). Severity of unilateral spatial neglect is an independent predictor of functional outcome after acute inpatient rehabilitation in individuals with right hemispheric stroke. *Archives of Physical Medicine and Rehabilitation, 92*, 1250–1256. http://dx.doi.org/10.1016/j.apmr.2011.03.018

Dromerick, A. W., & Khader, S. A. (2003). Medical complications during stroke rehabilitation. *Advances in Neurology, 92*, 409–413.

Duncan, P. W., Bode, R. K., Min Lai, S., & Perera, S.; Glycine Antagonist in Neuroprotection Americans Investigators. (2003). Rasch analysis of a new stroke-specific outcome scale: The Stroke Impact Scale. *Archives of Physical Medicine and Rehabilitation, 84*, 950–963. http://dx.doi.org/10.1016/S0003-9993(03)00035-2

Ekstam, L., Uppgard, B., Kottorp, A., & Tham, K. (2007). Relationship between awareness of disability and occupational performance during the first year after a stroke. *American Journal of Occupational Therapy, 61*, 503–511. http://dx.doi.org/10.5014/ajot.61.5.503

Elgin, J., McGwin, G., Wood, J. M., Vaphiades, M. S., Braswell, R. A., DeCarlo, D. K., . . . Owsley, C. (2010). Evaluation of on-road driving in people with hemianopia and quadrantanopia. *American Journal of Occupational Therapy, 64*, 268–278. http://dx.doi.org/10.5014/ajot.64.2.268

Fisher, A. G. (2003). *Assessment of Motor and Process Skills: Vol. 2. User manual* (5th ed.). Fort Collins, CO: Three Star Press.

Fisk, G. D., Owsley, C., & Pulley, L. V. (1997). Driving after stroke: Driving exposure, advice, and evaluations. *Archives of Physical Medicine and Rehabilitation, 78*, 1338–1345. http://dx.doi.org/10.1016/S0003-9993(97)90307-5

Fleming, J., & Nalder, E. (2011). Transition to community integration for persons with acquired brain injury. In N. Katz (Ed.), *Cognition, occupation, and participation across the life span: Neuroscience, neurorehabilitation, and models of intervention in occupational therapy* (3rd ed., pp. 51–70). Bethesda, MD: AOTA Press.

Giles, G. M. (2011). A neurofunctional approach to rehabilitation after brain injury. In N. Katz (Ed.), *Cognition, occupation, and participation across the life span: Neuroscience, neurorehabilitation, and models of intervention in occupational therapy* (3rd ed., pp. 351–382). Bethesda, MD: AOTA Press.

Gillen, G. (2009). *Cognitive and perceptual rehabilitation*. St. Louis: Mosby.

Guidetti, S., Asaba, E., & Tham, K. (2009). Meaning of context in recapturing self-care after stroke or spinal cord injury. *American Journal of Occupational Therapy, 63*, 323–332. http://dx.doi.org/10.5014/ajot.63.3.323

Gutman, S. A., & Schonfeld, A. B. (2009). *Screening adult neurologic populations: A step-by-step instruction manual* (2nd ed.). Bethesda, MD: AOTA Press.

Harris, J. E., Eng, J. J., Miller, W. C., & Dawson, A. S. (2010). The role of caregiver involvement in upper-limb treatment in individuals with subacute stroke. *Physical Therapy, 90*, 1302–1310. http://dx.doi.org/10.2522/ptj.20090349

Hartman-Maeir, A., Katz, N., & Baum, C. M. (2009). Cognitive Functional Evaluation (CFE) process for individuals with suspected cognitive disabilities. *Occupational Therapy in Health Care, 23*, 1–23. http://dx.doi.org/10.1080/07380570802455516

Haskins, E. C., Cicerone, K., Dams-O'Connor, K., Eberle, R., Langenbahn, D., & Shapiro-Rosenbaum, A. (2012). *Cognitive rehabilitation manual: Translating evidence-based recommendations into practice*. Reston, VA: ACRM.

Hawley, C. A. (2001). Return to driving after head injury. *Journal of Neurology, Neurosurgery, and Psychiatry, 70*, 761–766. http://dx.doi.org/10.1136/jnnp.70.6.761

Hayner, K., Gibson, G., & Giles, G. M. (2010). Comparison of constraint-induced movement therapy and bilateral treatment of equal intensity in people with chronic upper-extremity dysfunction after cerebrovascular accident. *American Journal of Occupational Therapy, 64*, 528–539. http://dx.doi.org/10.5014/ajot.2010.08027

Job Accommodation Network. (2013). *Accommodation ideas for stroke*. Retrieved May 30, 2013, from http://askjan.org/media/stro.htm

Katz, N., Baum, C. M., & Maeir, A. (2011). Introduction to cognitive intervention and cognitive functional evaluation. In N. Katz (Ed.), *Cognition, occupation, and participation across the life span: Neuroscience, neurorehabilitation, and models of intervention in occupational therapy* (3rd ed., pp. 3–12). Bethesda, MD: AOTA Press.

Katzman, R., Brown, T., Fuld, P., Peck, A., Schechter, R., & Schimmel, H. (1983). Validation of a short Orientation–Memory–Concentration Test of cognitive impairment. *American Journal of Psychiatry, 140,* 734–739.

King, P. M., & Olson, D. L. (2009). Work. In E. B. Crepeau, E. S. Cohn, & B. A. Boyt Schell (Eds.), *Willard and Spackman's occupational therapy* (11th ed., pp. 615–632). Baltimore: Lippincott Williams & Wilkins.

Klavora, P., Heslegrave, R. J., & Young, M. (2000). Driving skills in elderly persons with stroke: Comparison of two new assessment options. *Archives of Physical Medicine and Rehabilitation, 81,* 701–705. http://dx.doi.org/10.1016/S0003-9993(00)90096-0

Kong, K. H., Lee, J., & Chua, K. S. (2012). Occurrence and temporal evolution of upper limb spasticity in stroke patients admitted to a rehabilitation unit. *Archives of Physical Medicine and Rehabilitation, 93,* 143–148. http://dx.doi.org/10.1016/j.apmr.2011.06.027

Koski, L., Xie, H., & Finch, L. (2009). Measuring cognition in a geriatric outpatient clinic: Rasch analysis of the Montreal Cognitive Assessment. *Journal of Geriatric Psychiatry and Neurology, 22,* 151–160. http://dx.doi.org/10.1177/0891988709332944

Lafont, S., Laumon, B., Helmer, C., Dartigues, J.-F., & Fabrigoule, C. (2008). Driving cessation and self-reported car crashes in older drivers: The impact of cognitive impairment and dementia in a population-based study. *Journal of Geriatric Psychiatry and Neurology, 21,* 171–182. http://dx.doi.org/10.1177/0891988708316861

Lang, C. E., Wagner, J. M., Dromerick, A. W., & Edwards, D. F. (2006). Measurement of upper-extremity function early after stroke: Properties of the Action Research Arm Test. *Archives of Physical Medicine and Rehabilitation, 87,* 1605–1610. http://dx.doi.org/10.1016/j.apmr.2006.09.003

Latham, N. K., Jette, D. U., Coster, W., Richards, L., Smout, R. J., James, R. A., . . . Horn, S. D. (2006). Occupational therapy activities and intervention techniques for clients with stroke in six rehabilitation hospitals. *American Journal of Occupational Therapy, 60,* 369–378. http://dx.doi.org/10.5014/ajot.60.4.369

Law, M., Baptiste, S., Carswell, A., McColl, M. A., Polatajko, H., & Pollock, N. (2005). *The Canadian Occupational Performance Measure* (4th ed.). Ottawa, Ontario: CAOT Publications.

Legh-Smith, J., Wade, D. T., & Hewer, R. L. (1986). Driving after a stroke. *Journal of the Royal Society of Medicine, 79,* 200–203.

Levine, B., Robertson, I. H., Clare, L., Carter, G., Hong, J., Wilson, B. A., . . . Stuss, D. T. (2000). Rehabilitation of executive functioning: An experimental–clinical validation of Goal Management Training. *Journal of the International Neuropsychological Society, 6,* 299–312. http://dx.doi.org/10.1017/S1355617700633052

Levy, L. L., & Burns, T. (2011). The Cognitive Disabilities Reconsidered Model: Rehabilitation of adults with dementia. In N. Katz (Ed.), *Cognition, occupation, and participation across the life span: Neuroscience, neurorehabilitation, and models of intervention in occupational therapy* (3rd ed., pp. 407–442). Bethesda, MD: AOTA Press.

Lezak, M. D., Howieson, D. B., Loring, D. W., Hannay, J., & Fischer, J. S. (2004). *Neuropsychological assessment* (4th ed.). New York: Oxford University Press.

Lin, J.-H., Hsu, M.-J., Sheu, C.-F., Wu, T.-S., Lin, R.-T., Chen, C.-H., & Hsieh, C.-L. (2009). Psychometric comparisons of 4 measures for assessing upper-extremity function in people with stroke. *Physical Therapy, 89,* 840–850. http://dx.doi.org/10.2522/ptj.20080285

Löwe, B., Kroenke, K., Herzog, W., & Gräfe, K. (2004). Measuring depression outcome with a brief self-report instrument: Sensitivity to change of the Patient Health Questionnaire (PHQ–9). *Journal of Affective Disorders, 81,* 61–66. http://dx.doi.org/10.1016/S0165-0327(03)00198-8

Lundqvist, A., Alinder, J., & Rönnberg, J. (2008). Factors influencing driving 10 years after brain injury. *Brain Injury, 22,* 295–304. http://dx.doi.org/10.1080/02699050801966133

Merritt, B. K. (2011). Validity of using the Assessment of Motor and Process Skills to determine the need for assistance. *American Journal of Occupational Therapy, 65,* 643–650. http://dx.doi.org/10.5014/ajot.2011.000547

Nasreddine, Z. S., Phillips, N. A., Bédirian, V., Charbonneau, S., Whitehead, V., Collin, I., . . . Chertkow, H. (2005). The Montreal Cognitive Assessment, MoCA: A brief screening tool for mild cognitive impairment. *Journal of the American Geriatrics Society, 53,* 695–699. http://dx.doi.org/10.1111/j.1532-5415.2005.53221.x

Ovbiagele, B., Diener, H. C., Yusuf, S., Martin, R. H., Cotton, D., Vinisko, R., . . . Bath, P. M.; PROFESS Investigators. (2011). Level of systolic blood pressure within the normal range and risk of recurrent stroke. *JAMA, 306,* 2137–2144. http://dx.doi.org/10.1001/jama.2011.1650

Page, S. J., Murray, C., & Hermann, V. (2011). Affected upper-extremity movement ability is retained 3 months after modified constraint-induced therapy. *American Journal of Occupational Therapy, 65,* 589–593. http://dx.doi.org/10.5014/ajot.2011.000513

Peralta-Catipon, T., & Hwang, J. E. (2011). Personal factors predictive of health-related lifestyles of community-dwelling older adults. *American Journal of Occupational Therapy, 65,* 329–337. http://dx.doi.org/10.5014/ajot.2011.000505

Perlmutter, M. S., Bhorade, A., Gordon, M., Hollingsworth, H. H., & Baum, M. C. (2010). Cognitive, visual, auditory, and emotional factors that affect participation in older adults. *American Journal of Occupational Therapy, 64,* 570–579. http://dx.doi.org/10.5014/ajot.2010.09089

Poole, D., Chaudry, F., & Jay, W. M. (2008). Stroke and driving. *Topics in Stroke Rehabilitation, 15,* 37–41. http://dx.doi.org/10.1310/tsr1501-37

Preissner, K. (2010). Use of the Occupational Therapy Task-Oriented Approach to optimize the motor performance of a client with cognitive limitations. *American Journal of Occupational Therapy, 64,* 727–734. http://dx.doi.org/10.5014/ajot.2010.08026

Rapport, L. J., Bryer, R. C., & Hanks, R. A. (2008). Driving and community integration after traumatic brain injury. *Archives of Physical Medicine and Rehabilitation, 89,* 922–930. http://dx.doi.org/10.1016/j.apmr.2008.01.009

Roosink, M., Renzenbrink, G. J., Buitenweg, J. R., Van Dongen, R. T., Geurts, A. C., & IJzerman, M. J. (2011). Persistent shoulder pain in the first 6 months after stroke: Results of a prospective cohort study. *Archives of Physical Medicine and Rehabilitation, 92,* 1139–1145. http://dx.doi.org/10.1016/j.apmr.2011.02.016

Rotenberg-Shpigelman, S., Erez, A. B., Nahaloni, I., & Maeir, A. (2012). Neurofunctional treatment targeting participation among chronic stroke survivors: A pilot randomised controlled study. *Neuropsychological Rehabilitation, 22,* 532–549. http://dx.doi.org/10.1080/09602011.2012.665610

Schmid, A. A., & Rittman, M. (2009). Consequences of poststroke falls: Activity limitation, increased dependence, and the development of fear of falling. *American Journal of Occupational Therapy, 63,* 310–316. http://dx.doi.org/10.5014/ajot.63.3.310

Smallfield, S., & Karges, J. (2009). Classification of occupational therapy intervention for inpatient stroke rehabilitation. *American Journal of Occupational Therapy, 63,* 408–413. http://dx.doi.org/10.5014/ajot.63.4.408

Taub, E., Uswatte, G., & Morris, D. M. (2003). Improved motor recovery after stroke and massive cortical reorganization following constraint-induced movement therapy. *Physical Medicine and Rehabilitation Clinics of North America, 14*(Suppl.), S77–S91. http://dx.doi.org/10.1016/S1047-9651(02)00052-9

Thielman, G. T., Dean, C. M., & Gentile, A. M. (2004). Rehabilitation of reaching after stroke: Task-related training versus progressive resistive exercise. *Archives of Physical Medicine and Rehabilitation, 85,* 1613–1618. http://dx.doi.org/10.1016/j.apmr.2004.01.028

Toglia, J. P. (2005). A dynamic interactional approach to cognitive rehabilitation. In N. Katz (Ed.), *Cognition and occupation across the life span* (2nd ed., pp. 29–72). Bethesda, MD: AOTA Press.

Toglia, J. P. (2011). The Dynamic Interactional Model of Cognition in cognitive rehabilitation. In N. Katz (Ed.), *Cognition, occupation, and participation across the life span: Neuroscience, neurorehabilitation, and models of intervention in occupational therapy* (3rd ed., pp. 161–202). Bethesda, MD: AOTA Press.

Toglia, J. P., & Cermak, S. A. (2009). Dynamic assessment and prediction of learning potential in clients with unilateral neglect. *American Journal of Occupational Therapy, 63,* 569–579. http://dx.doi.org/10.5014/ajot.63.5.569

Toglia, J. P., Fitzgerald, K. A., O'Dell, M. W., Mastrogiovanni, A. R., & Lin, C. D. (2011). The Mini-Mental State Examination and Montreal Cognitive Assessment in persons with mild subacute stroke: Relationship to functional outcome. *Archives of Physical Medicine and Rehabilitation, 92,* 792–798. http://dx.doi.org/10.1016/j.apmr.2010.12.034

Treger, I., Shames, J., Giaquinto, S., & Ring, H. (2007). Return to work in stroke patients. *Disability and Rehabilitation, 29*, 1397–1403. http://dx.doi.org/10.1080/09638280701314923

Turner, B., Fleming, J., Cornwell, P., Worrall, L., Ownsworth, T., Haines, T., . . . Chenoweth, L. (2007). A qualitative study of the transition from hospital to home for individuals with acquired brain injury and their family caregivers. *Brain Injury, 21*, 1119–1130. http://dx.doi.org/10.1080/02699050701651678

Turner, B. J., Fleming, J. M., Ownsworth, T. L., & Cornwell, P. L. (2008). The transition from hospital to home for individuals with acquired brain injury: A literature review and research recommendations. *Disability and Rehabilitation, 30*, 1153–1176. http://dx.doi.org/10.1080/09638280701532854

Warren, M. (2009). Pilot study on activities of daily living limitations in adults with hemianopsia. *American Journal of Occupational Therapy, 63*, 626–633. http://dx.doi.org/10.5014/ajot.63.5.626

Wilkinson, D., Sakel, M., Camp, S.-J., & Hammond, L. (2012). Patients with hemispatial neglect are more prone to limb spasticity, but this does not prolong their hospital stay. *Archives of Physical Medicine and Rehabilitation, 93*, 1191–1195. http://dx.doi.org/10.1016/j.apmr.2012.01.010

Wilson, B., Alderman, N., & Burgess, P. W. (1996). *Behavioural Assessment of the Dysexecutive Syndrome*. Flempton, England: Thames Valley Test Co.

Wilson, B., Cockburn, J., Baddeley, A. D., & Hiorns, R. (1989). The development and validation of a test battery for detecting and monitoring everyday memory problems. *Journal of Clinical and Experimental Neuropsychology, 11*, 855–870. http://dx.doi.org/10.1080/01688638908400940

Wolf, T. J., Baum, C. M., & Connor, L. T. (2009). Changing face of stroke: Implications for occupational therapy practice. *American Journal of Occupational Therapy, 63*, 621–625. http://dx.doi.org/10.5014/ajot.63.5.621

Zoltan, B. (2007). *Vision, perception, and cognition* (4th ed.). Thorofare, NJ: Slack.

Appendix 12.A. Initial Assessment Note: Steve

Subjective:

Client reports that he does not perceive any cognitive difficulties and states, "I think I am ready to return to work and start driving!" He reports complete independence in all activities at home. (*Note.* This is in contrast to his wife, who reports needing to remind him to do activities and notices disorganization and lack of structure to his day. His wife states, "He used to be very organized with his tools and always put everything in its proper place. I feel like Steve is another child that I have to organize all day long.")

Objective:

Client was assessed with brief upper-extremity motor evaluation and the Behavioral Assessment of the Dysexecutive Syndrome (BADS).

Upper-extremity range of motion: Both upper extremities are within normal limits (WNL).

Upper-extremity strength: Both upper extremities are WNL (4+) throughout.

Hand grasp (right-hand dominant): Right = 114 lb, left = 110 lb (WNL bilaterally).

Fine motor coordination (Nine-Hole Peg Test): Right = 19 s; left = 22 s (WNL bilaterally).

BADS (test of higher-level cognitive assessment; focused on executive function):

> *Subtest 1, Rule Shift Cards (assesses alternating attention, short-term memory):* Score = 20/20 accurate (profile score = 4).

> *Subtest 2, Action Program Test (assesses problem-solving skills during a novel performance-based task):* Score = 3 (profile score = 2).

> Client was observed to require two repetitions of instructions because he forgot the rules of the task. (*Note.* Client did not request repetition of instructions because he appeared to lack the recognition that he had forgotten the rules.) Client was observed to lack ability to develop an appropriate problem-solving approach and did not develop alternative strategies. He required moderate cueing (demonstration) to develop the problem-solving approach to complete the task appropriately.

> *Subtest 3, Key Search (assesses ability to plan and organize a search pattern):* Score = 10 (profile score = 2).

> Client had mild difficulty understanding instructions. He appeared to have some initial difficulty with abstracting the representation of a symbol (e.g., the square drawn on the paper was to represent a field). Client was observed to be mildly inefficient with planning, starting in a less efficient location, and the search pattern he chose was not deemed the most organized.

> *Subtest 4, Temporal Judgment (assesses ability to anticipate and plan regarding concept of time):* Score = 1 (profile score = 1).

> Client demonstrated difficulty being able to estimate time; however, his estimates were not subjectively deemed greatly inappropriate.

> *Subtest 5, Zoo Map Test (assesses ability to plan, organize, and remember details):* Score = 9 (profile score = 2).

Client observed to not plan ahead and therefore ended up having to complete the route inaccurately (e.g., breaking a rule). He was aware he broke the rule as he became mildly frustrated.

Subtest 6, Modified Six Elements (assesses ability to plan, organize, and track time and responsibilities): Score = 4 (profile score = 3).

Client was observed to spend excessive time on dictating; he began talking and became tangential with his own conversation. He proceeded with tasks in a somewhat disorganized (i.e., random) order without any obvious planning structure. He was observed to continue talking throughout the activity, causing self-distraction. He asked how long he had to do this (indicating that he forgot the instructions). He made two errors as a result of breaking a rule (partly related to decreased planning and self-distraction).

Observations:

Throughout cognitive assessment, the client thought he was doing well. He also became verbose and tangential between tasks and needed redirection back to the assessment by the therapist.

Total Profile Score 14/24, indicating low average performance.

Assessment:

Client was very cooperative with the assessment. He demonstrated good motor skills. His cognitive skills were limited, and he lacked insight into his cognitive deficits, resulting in impaired instrumental activities of daily living (IADLs) and decreased functional performance.

Problems:

1. Decreased memory skills limiting functional IADLs.
2. Decreased executive function skills (planning, problem solving, organizing) limiting functional performance abilities.
3. Decreased insight into cognitive deficits, resulting in limited to no use of compensatory strategies at this time.

Rehabilitation prognosis:

Good, pending improvement in insight abilities.

Plan:

Plan to see client 3× per week for 2 to 3 months with focus on increasing insight and use of compensatory strategies for cognitive deficits to improve functioning in daily life activities.

Short-term goals:

1. Steve will improve in insight into cognitive deficits (memory, executive function) as indicated by ability to verbalize the cognitive changes since the stroke.
2. Steve will begin to use compensatory strategies for memory deficits in a clinical setting during functional tasks as needed on 80% of occasions.

3. Steve will begin to use compensatory strategies for executive function deficits within structure of clinical setting during functional tasks as needed on 80% of occasions.

Long-term goals:

1. Steve will generalize use of compensatory strategies for memory to home environment so as to be independent in functional activities at home as indicated by report (both his and his wife's).
2. Steve will generalize use of compensatory strategies for executive function to home environment so as to be independent in functional activities at home as indicated by report (both his and his wife's).

Additional goals:

To be determined.

Appendix 12.B. Self-Rating Scale for Memory: Steve

Note. This scale can be adapted for other areas of cognitive deficits.

Date: Sept. XX, 20XX

1	2	3	4	5
Poor Memory Skills		**Average Memory Skills**		**Excellent Memory Skills**

Activity Task	Self-Rating	Therapist Rating	Observations/Comments
1. Bill paying	1 2 3 4 ⑤	1 2 ③ 4 5	*Therapist:* "Seems like I needed to repeat the instructions at least one time for you to remember."
2. Phone call	1 2 3 4 ⑤	1 ② 3 4 5	*Therapist:* "I think you did not remember the instructions correctly the first time, and I needed to help you."
3. Chore list	1 2 3 ④ 5	1 2 ③ 4 5	*Therapist:* "I needed to help you recall the first step of the instructions."

Appendix 12.C. Problem-Solving Worksheet: Steve

1. What is the problem?
The neighbor's dog is barking all night, and I cannot sleep.

2. What is the goal?
To have quiet so that I can sleep.

3. What are some solutions, and what are pros and cons of the solutions?

a. To go over and muzzle the dog myself   *Pro:* Dog would stop barking.
Con: I might get bit; I should not be on someone else's property without permission.

b. To call the police   *Pro:* Neighbor would quiet the dog or get a fine.
Con: Neighbor might get angry at me and seek to retaliate.

c. To call the neighbor and politely ask the neighbor to quiet their dog   *Pro:* Neighbor might be cooperative and try to quiet the dog; I am being equally cooperative.
Con: Neighbor may ignore my phone call.

d. To take strong sleep medicine so I can sleep through loud noises   *Pro:* I would not have to bother the neighbor; I would be able to get sleep.
Con: I might not hear other noises that I need to wake up to in the night; the medicine may not be safe for me to take over the long term.

Decision making: Choosing a solution

I am choosing Solution c. I chose this option because it has the least negative consequences and seems like a good first step. If this does not work, I can reevaluate for my next steps to the solution.

Execute:

I called the neighbor at night and politely explained the situation. The neighbor apologized and said that he would bring the dog inside the house earlier in the night so the barking would not keep me up.

Self-evaluate:

I am pleased with my solution, and I am able to sleep better at night.

Appendix 12.D. Summary of Intervention Plan for Steve

Occupational Therapy Intervention Priority	Intervention Approach (Framework [AOTA, 2014])	Goal	Preparatory Methods and Tasks	Occupation and Activity	Education and Training
Increase intellectual awareness of attention, memory, and executive function deficits	Establish or restore	• Steve will improve insight into cognitive deficits (memory, executive function) as indicated by ability to verbalize the cognitive changes since the stroke.	• Therapeutic rapport • Strengths and weaknesses list	• Structured IADLs and leisure activities—prevocational activities within clinical setting at a level of just-right challenge that would show difficulties (money management, bill paying, checkbook balancing, complex telephone calls, routine chores around clinic, collating and copying materials) • Acknowledge that cognitive deficits exist and could potentially have an impact on functioning at home	• Provide education • Gentle, constructive feedback
Increase emergent awareness of attention, memory, and executive function deficits	Establish or restore	• Steve will recognize the existence of cognitive difficulties during task performance as indicated by verbal report or signs of frustration.	• Constructive feedback • Guided questioning from therapist to cue client to deficits during task performance • Videotaping of task performance	• Structured IADLs and leisure activities—prevocational activities within clinical setting at a level of just-right challenge that would show difficulties • These activities can be similar to IADLs above with new situations and instructions applied • Recognize cognitive deficits in home-based IADLs while they are actually occurring	
Increase anticipatory awareness of attention, memory, and executive function deficits	Establish or restore	• Steve will recognize the existence of potential cognitive difficulties before task performance.	• Constructive feedback • Guided questioning from therapist to cue client to deficits before task performance • Focus is identifying and preparing for cognitive deficits before task performance	• Structured IADLs and leisure activities—prevocational activities within clinical setting at a level of just-right challenge that would show difficulties • Recognize potential area of cognitive difficulties before engaging in a home IADL	

(Continued)

Appendix 12.D. Summary of Intervention Plan for Steve *(cont.)*

Occupational Therapy Intervention Priority	Intervention Approach (*Framework* [AOTA, 2014])	Goal	Preparatory Methods and Tasks	Occupation and Activity	Education and Training
Memory function	Establish or restore	• Steve will begin to use compensatory strategies for memory deficits within a clinical setting during functional tasks as needed on 80% of occasions.	• Can trial these with short basic tasks (e.g., recall list of items, paragraph information) to demonstrate use and effectiveness	• Structured IADLs and leisure activities—prevocational activities within clinical setting at a level of just-right challenge that would present memory challenges to Steve (e.g., making a phone call and needing to ask certain questions and present detailed answers back to the therapist, activities that need to be completed in a specified order or by certain times) • Focus will be using compensatory strategies for memory effectively during these activities • Able to use compensatory strategies for memory in home and work environment effectively (e.g., keeping a notebook to track important conversations and appointments)	• Introduction to and education in compensatory strategies for memory (e.g., verbal rehearsal, checklists, note-taking options)

(Continued)

Appendix 12.D. Summary of Intervention Plan for Steve (cont.)

Occupational Therapy Intervention Priority	Intervention Approach (*Framework* [AOTA, 2014])	Goal	Preparatory Methods and Tasks	Occupation and Activity	Education and Training
Executive function and problem solving	Establish or restore	• Steve will begin to use compensatory strategies for executive function deficits within structure of clinical setting during functional tasks as needed on 80% of occasions.	• Can trial these on problem-solving worksheets to demonstrate use and effectiveness • Structured IADLs and leisure activities—prevocational activities at a level of just-right challenge that would present problem-solving challenges to Steve (e.g., how to decide which of 4 cars is a better purchase, organizing his toolbox, planning creative leisure activities to do with his children, planning and problem solving a vacation, problem solving what to do if a piece is missing while putting together a shelf; note that these tasks would actually be done in the clinic setting, which may involve making phone calls, doing Internet research, etc.) • Focus will be using a problem-solving worksheet guide	• Being able to use a structured guide as a compensatory strategy or framework for problem solving in daily life activities within his home and work environment	• Introduction to and education in compensatory strategies for problem-solving deficits

Note. AOTA = American Occupational Therapy Association; IADLs = instrumental activities of daily living.

Appendix 12.E. Initial Assessment Note: Mary

Subjective:

Client states, "I wish I could get to my old life, get out of the house, and do what I need to do." Client's daughter reports that the client has not been out of the home since discharge from inpatient rehabilitation for any purpose other than doctors' appointments.

Objective:

Blood pressure: 130/76.
Pain at rest: 1.
Pain with activity: 4 at shoulder at end range of passive range of motion (PROM).

Canadian Occupational Performance Measure

Performance Area	Performance Score	Satisfaction Score
Spend time with grandchildren	5	4
Participation in church events	1	1
Return to work	1	1
Driving	5	1
Cooking for family, friends, and self	3	4

Range of Motion (ROM)

Right Arm		Left Arm	
Motion	Active ROM (Degrees)	Motion	Active ROM (Degrees)
Shoulder flexion	0–176	Shoulder flexion	0–95
Shoulder abduction	0–172	Shoulder abduction	0–70
Shoulder external rotation	0–80	Shoulder external rotation	0–23
Elbow flexion–extension	0–156	Elbow extension	40–145
Forearm supination	0–75	Forearm supination	0–60
Wrist flexion	0–74	Wrist flexion	0–60
Wrist extension	0–67	Wrist extension	0–15

Manual Muscle Testing (MMT) of Left Upper Extremity (Right Upper Extremity Is Within Functional Limits) and Modified Ashworth Scale (MAS)

Movement	MMT	MAS
Shoulder flexion	3/5	2
Shoulder abduction	3/5	3
Shoulder external rotation	3–/5	3
Shoulder internal rotation	3+/5	0
Elbow flexion	3+/5	3
Elbow extension	3–/5	0
Pronation	4/5	2
Supination	3/5	0
Wrist flexion	3+/5	2
Wrist extension	3–/5	0
Finger flexion	3+/5	2
Finger extension	3–/5	0

Dynamometry and Pinch Meter

	Right Hand (lb)	Left Hand (lb)
Grip	50	17
Lateral pinch	14	5
Palmer pinch	12	4
Tip pinch	9	3

Action Research Arm Test: 41 of 57, demonstrating impaired five-finger grip, cylindrical grasp, and pincer grip.

Stroke Impact Scale, Version 3.0: Overall transformed score = 67.2%, with strength, activities of daily living and instrumental activities of daily living, mobility, and hand use most strongly affected. Recovery score = 60/100.

Patient Health Questionnaire–9: 3, indicating minimal depression. Patient denies need to address, stating that she turns to her faith to guide her.

Montreal Cognitive Assessment: 17 of 30, indicating **mild cognitive impairment,** with deficits in visuospatial and executive function, attention, language fluency, and delayed recall.

Assessment:

Client came to outpatient therapy clinic accompanied by daughter, Sarah, who is currently staying with client 24 hours a day, is on family leave, and has been primary source of support. Client also reports good support from friends from church, who are visiting regularly and pitch in as needed. Client presents with motor, perceptual, and cognitive deficits, which result in limitations in occupational performance.

Problems:

1. Increased tone in flexor synergy resulting in pain and decreased ROM
2. Weakness and impaired coordination limiting functional use of left upper extremity
3. Left visuoperceptual inattention resulting in impaired function and safety concern
4. Cognitive deficits including **working memory,** decreased divided and selective attention, problem solving, and planning limiting functional performance.

Rehabilitation prognosis:

Good, given client's motivation, social support, and knowledge about stroke and rehabilitation.

Plan:

Plan to see client 3× per week for 3 to 4 months, with focus on improving motor and process skills as well as enhancing cognitive skills while providing compensatory strategies to increase function in the following areas identified in collaboration with the client and her daughter at initial evaluation.

Short-term goals:

1. Mary will demonstrate improved strength and coordination of left upper extremity, as tested by standardized assessment, by discharge.
2. Mary will demonstrate no safety concerns (no bumps, no falls) at home or in the clinic for 2 straight weeks by discharge.
3. Mary will read full page of a book with no misses of words or letters by discharge.
4. Mary will complete financial management task in minimally distracting environment with supervision by discharge.
5. Mary will identify 2 areas of necessary home repairs and the appropriate steps for repair (i.e., identify repair service, get estimates, and plan date for service) by discharge.
6. Mary will journal blood pressure and blood sugar at least 1× per day for 2 full weeks by discharge.
7. Mary will complete medication management with 100% accuracy by discharge.
8. Mary will attend 1 stroke survivor support group before discharge.
9. Mary will spend 4 hours alone with grandchildren by discharge.
10. Mary will transfer to and from ground to engage in game with grandchild by discharge.
11. Mary will attend church weekly for 3 weeks straight by discharge.
12. Mary will participate in 2 church group outings accompanied by 2 friends by discharge.
13. Mary will identify 3 strategies for job accommodation in preparation for return to work on light duty by discharge.
14. Mary will complete 3 business forms with 100% accuracy by discharge.
15. Mary will perform 3 work-related tasks (answering phone and taking notes while preparing a cup of coffee) with 100% accuracy with supervision by discharge.
16. Mary will use public transportation, accompanied by Sarah, at least 2× before discharge.
17. Mary will complete a 3-dish meal prep with setup by discharge.

Long-term goals:

1. Mary will complete makeup application with no cues by 2 weeks.
2. Mary will identify 2 strategies and lifestyle changes to reduce risk of recurrent stroke within 2 weeks of starting outpatient therapy.
3. Mary will demonstrate 100% of left upper-extremity home exercises with supervision by 4 weeks.
4. Mary will schedule all necessary follow-up doctors' appointments and record them accurately in planner by 4 weeks.

Appendix 12.F. Summary of Intervention Plan for Mary

Occupational Therapy Intervention Priority	Intervention Approach (*Framework* [AOTA, 2014])	Goal	Preparatory Methods and Tasks	Occupation and Activity	Education and Training
UE strength and coordination	Establish or restore	• Mary will demonstrate 100% of LUE home exercises with supervision by 4 wk. • Mary will demonstrate improved strength and coordination of LUE, as tested by standardized assessment, by discharge.	• Provide activity log for Mary and Sarah to track exercise outside of therapy. • Mary will perform exercises in therapy clinic at beginning of each session as a warm-up and to demonstrate her skill level. • Mary will bring in activity log on a weekly basis to monitor carryover. • Mary will hold, reach, and place items of increasing weight in over-the-counter and under-the-counter or sink cabinets using LUE only. • Mary will maintain grasp of household items (groceries, laundry basket, garbage bag) using both UEs for increasing lengths of time.		• Provide education to Mary and Sarah on AROM exercises. Apply modalities when necessary.
Perceptual training	Establish or restore Modify	• Mary will demonstrate no safety concerns (no bumps, no falls) at home or in the clinic for 2 wk straight by discharge. • Mary will read full page of a book with no misses of words or letters by discharge. • Mary will complete makeup application with no cues by 2 wk.	• Mary will apply perceptual anchors to newspapers and magazines in the outpatient clinic and identify 3 people on the page. • Mary will complete grooming task (washing face, combing hair) in mirror of clinic bathroom.	• Mary will locate 30 of 30 grocery items from list within store. • Mary will ambulate to physiatrist's office using environmental signs with no more than 2 cues for way finding.	

(Continued)

Appendix 12.F. Summary of Intervention Plan for Mary (*cont.*)

Occupational Therapy Intervention Priority	Intervention Approach (*Framework* [AOTA, 2014])	Goal	Preparatory Methods and Tasks	Occupation and Activity	Education and Training
Higher-level cognition	Establish or restore Modify	• Mary will complete financial management task in minimally distracting environment with supervision by discharge. • Mary will schedule all necessary follow-up doctors' appointments and record accurately in planner by 4 wk. • Mary will identify 2 areas of necessary home repairs and the appropriate steps for repair (i.e., identify repair service, get estimates, and plan date for service) by discharge.	• Mary will complete money management worksheet. • List of physicians and phone numbers will be provided to Mary.	• Mary and Sarah will identify areas of concern in the home. • Mary will complete list of her personal bills and due dates. • Mary will use the Internet to identify options for repair services. • Mary will enter bills and due dates into her planner. • Mary will access accounts online. • Mary will initiate phone call to physician or repair service using her cell phone.	
Self-management	Maintain Prevent	• Mary will journal blood pressure and blood sugar at least 1×/day for 2 full wk by discharge. • Mary will complete medication management with 100% accuracy by discharge. • Mary will attend 1 stroke survivor support group before discharge. • Mary will identify 2 strategies or lifestyle changes to reduce risk of recurrent stroke within 2 wk of starting outpatient therapy.	• Example of journal entry will be provided. • Mary will identify a pillbox that suits her needs (given how many times a day medication is administered). • Mary will complete mock trial of medication, placing meds into pillbox following sample prescriptions. • Mary will bring in her medications and pillbox to demonstrate accurate management. • Mary will journal vitals taken during each therapy session. • Mary will identify the sodium, fat, and sugar content of various foods.	• Mary will make a list of her current medications, doses, and times of administration. • Mary will identify 1 support group and enter into her calendar or planner.	• Resources for local stroke support group will be issued. • Education re: controllable and uncontrollable factors that increase likelihood of stroke will be reviewed and issued. • Education re: accessible housing options will be reviewed and issued.

(Continued)

Appendix 12.F. Summary of Intervention Plan for Mary (cont.)

Occupational Therapy Intervention Priority	Intervention Approach (*Framework* [AOTA, 2014])	Goal	Preparatory Methods and Tasks	Occupation and Activity	Education and Training
IADL training (child care)	Establish or restore Modify	• Mary will spend 4 hr alone with grandchildren by discharge. • Mary will transfer to and from the ground to engage in game with grandchild by discharge.	• Mary will identify proper responses to emergency situations that may arise in the house around children. • Mary will practice transfer to and from ground.	• Mary will complete a list of emergency contact numbers and enter into her cell phone. • Mary will participate in leisure activity that can be shared with grandchildren. • Mary will identify activities that will engage grandchildren that are within her current skill level. • Mary will locate emergency contact numbers in cell phone and place call without assistance. • Mary will participate in leisure activity with grandchildren (if available).	• Mary will be educated in strategies for safe ground transfer technique.
IADL training (church member and volunteer)	Establish or restore Modify	• Mary will attend church weekly for 3 wk straight by discharge. • Mary will participate in 2 church group outings accompanied by 2 friends by discharge.	• Mary will bring in flyer of church activities. • Mary will identify 4 church activities that she is interested in. • Mary will work on putting on jewelry.	• Mary will identify a recipe for potluck and multiple ingredients to make recipe for large group. • Mary will verbally identify an accessible route into her church. • Mary will perform verbal gospel readings of increasing lengths. • Mary will practice unloading shopping bags of nonperishable items and stacking on shelves.	

(Continued)

Appendix 12.F. Summary of Intervention Plan for Mary (*cont.*)

Occupational Therapy Intervention Priority	Intervention Approach (*Framework* [AOTA, 2014])	Goal	Preparatory Methods and Tasks	Occupation and Activity	Education and Training
IADL training (return to work)	Establish or restore Modify	• Mary will identify 3 strategies for job accommodation in preparation for return to work on light duty by discharge. • Mary will complete 3 business forms with 100% accuracy by discharge. • Mary will perform 3 work-related tasks (answering phone and taking notes while preparing a cup of coffee) with 100% accuracy with supervision by discharge.	• Mary will work on typing speed. • Mary will work on handwriting speed and legibility. • Mary will complete complex functional activities following a checklist.	• Mary will review short- and long-term disability benefits with Sarah. • Mary will speak with the human resources department and identify what accommodations will be considered for her return to work. • Mary will check and reply to work e-mails. • Mary will enter pertinent work events into her planner. • Mary will complete practice forms provided by her workplace with decreasing time.	• Education on job accommodation strategies will be reviewed and provided.
IADL training (driving)	Establish or restore Modify	• Mary will use public transportation, accompanied by Sarah, at least 2× before discharge.	• Mary will complete driver's evaluation screens—Trail Making Tests A and B, Montreal Cognitive Assessment. • Mary will identify public transportation routes to church and grocery store. • Mary will use computer to order transit card.	• Mary will schedule appointment with neuro-ophthalmologist. • Mary will take public transportation to outpatient therapy clinic.	• Resources for driver's rehabilitation will be issued.
IADL training (meal preparation)	Establish or restore Modify	• Mary will complete a 3-dish meal prep with setup by discharge.	• Mary will make a list of grocery items needed. • Mary will identify 3 heart-healthy recipes from a diabetic cookbook.	• Mary will bring in ingredients and perform hot meal preparation of increasing complexity.	• Mary will be educated on what constitutes a heart-healthy, diabetic diet.

Note. AOTA = American Occupational Therapy Association; AROM = active range of motion; hr = hours; IADL = instrumental activity of daily living; LUE = left upper extremity; UE/UEs = upper extremity/extremities; wk = weeks.

CHAPTER 13

Living With Stroke: Constructing Communities to Enable Occupation, Health, and Well-Being

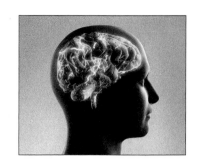

Julie D. Bass, PhD, OTR/L, FAOTA

Learning Objectives

After completion of this chapter, readers will be able to

- Identify terminology, needs, and recommendations related to staying active, fitness, self-management and chronic disease management, caregiver and family support, and community supports and resources for people living with stroke;
- Recognize features of community-based initiatives that enable occupation, health, and well-being for people living with stroke and their caregivers;
- Recognize outcomes of research on community-based programs for people living with stroke and their caregivers; and
- Identify the proposed role of rehabilitation professionals in designing community initiatives related to staying active, fitness, chronic disease management, caregiver and family support, and community supports and resources.

Key Words

- caregiver
- fitness
- formal caregiver
- informal caregiver
- objective caregiver burden
- self-efficacy
- self-management
- subjective caregiver burden

Introduction

Occupational therapy has had a long-standing involvement in providing **rehabilitation** services to people poststroke. Many of these services have focused on functional activities that are essential for self-care and discharge placements. Occupational therapy for **stroke** rehabilitation has been included in many medical reimbursement systems and, thus, the conceptualization of occupational therapy's role in stroke rehabilitation has a strong base in the medical model. Although occupational therapy will continue to have an important role in acute rehabilitation, the profession needs to become involved in the growing number of programs that address prevention and long-term needs of this population. In recent years, occupational therapists have been challenged to expand their definition of stroke rehabilitation to include the broader context of everyday life and participation in the community (American Occupational Therapy Association [AOTA], 2014a; Wolf, Baum, & Connor, 2009).

New occupational therapy interventions are needed to address stroke as a chronic rather than acute condition and promote health and well-being through occupational engagement and participation. Occupational therapists, with their unique knowledge base, have the potential to provide strong leadership in national initiatives for people living with stroke. However, occupational therapists will need to grow beyond current roles and develop skills in interprofessional teams, consultation, health education, and public health. In this chapter, I provide an overview of national priorities related to staying active, fitness, chronic disease and self-management, family and caregiver needs, and community supports and services for people poststroke; examine current interventions and programs; and propose occupational therapy roles for the future.

> Occupational therapists, with their unique knowledge base, have the potential to provide strong leadership in national initiatives for people living with stroke.

Staying Active

Overview and Recommendations

Staying active is a part of many health recommendations and applies across all age groups and most medical conditions. There is no uniform definition of *staying active* even though it is frequently included as a component of health education campaigns and research studies. Staying active is often associated with physical activity levels and physical health and has been identified as a lifestyle intervention that may contribute to improved cardiovascular health (Haskell, 2003) and a reduced risk of cognitive decline (Buchman et al., 2012).

Staying active is a challenge for many people with stroke because assistance is often required for performance of activities. In a study of 56 participants who were at least 1 year poststroke (Hartman-Maeir, Soroker, Ring, Avni, & Katz, 2007), half required some assistance in basic **activities of daily living** (ADLs; e.g., dressing, bathing), and more than 70% required full assistance in **instrumental activities of daily living** (IADLs; e.g., meal preparation, housekeeping, laundry). Decreased self-care, vocational, and **leisure** activity levels were also associated with decreased life satisfaction. Self-reported changes in work and leisure activities, especially among non-White groups, also limited social participation (McKevitt et al., 2011). In a survey of families of people living with stroke, strategies for staying active were identified as one of the five top self-care needs (Pierce, Gordon, & Steiner, 2004). Changes in activity levels have been reported across many stroke populations. People with mild stroke reported a reduction in the moderate- to high-intensity-level leisure activities that contribute to cardiovascular health (Hildebrand, Brewer, & Wolf, 2012). Even fairly young people who were many years poststroke have been found to have decreased activity levels and limitations in walking ability (Danielsson, Willén, & Sunnerhagen, 2012).

Recommendations for staying active are often noted in general health guidelines for a variety of populations, including those who are at risk for or have had strokes. Specific recommendations for staying physically active are to engage in 30 minutes of moderate-intensity exercise most days of the week and to build in opportunities for activity throughout the day (Haskell, 2003). Recommendations for staying active also include engagement in cognitive (Verghese et al., 2003) and social activities (James, Wilson, Barnes, & Bennett, 2011) for older adults. Staying active by engaging in leisure time physical activity and daily commuting has been shown to reduce the risk for stroke (Hu et al., 2005).

Staying-Active Initiatives and Outcomes

Staying-active initiatives have been developed by governmental, nonprofit, and health care organizations to increase the activity levels of individuals and communities. Most of these initiatives have been targeted toward the general or older adult populations, but some programs have been designed specifically to address the needs of people after stroke. Some of these initiatives focus on exercise as a means to increase physical activity levels, and others provide a variety of alternatives to staying active (Table 13.1).

Both exercise programs and lifestyle and activity-based programs have been shown to be effective in improving cardiovascular health. A randomized clinical trial compared structured exercise and lifestyle interventions on changes in cardiorespiratory fitness, blood pressure, and body composition for sedentary adults (Dunn et al., 1999). The lifestyle intervention group was led by health professionals and included self-assessment, education, coaching, goal setting, small-group cognitive and behavioral strategies, and recreational activities; groups initially met weekly with a gradual decrease in meeting frequency over the 24 months of the study. The lifestyle and structured exercise interventions were equally as effective in producing

Table 13.1. Staying-Active Initiatives

Agency or Organization	Program	Activities
U.S. Environmental Protection Agency (http://www.epa.gov/aging/bhc/guide.htm)	*Growing Smarter, Living Healthier: A Guide to Smart Growth and Active Aging*	Provides guidelines, examples, and resources on active aging and supportive communities.
National Council on Aging (http://www.ncoa.org/improve-health/center-for-healthy-aging/physical-activity/)	Center for Healthy Aging	Describes evidence on programs and includes resources for physical activity.
American Stroke Association (http://www.strokeassociation.org/STROKEORG/LifeAfterStroke/Life-After-Stroke_UCM_308546_SubHomePage.jsp)	Life After Stroke	Provides guidelines for physical activity and inspirational stories of people with stroke who are staying active.
National Heart, Lung, and Blood Institute (http://www.nhlbi.nih.gov/health/health-topics/topics/phys/getstarted.html)	Getting Started and Staying Active	Provides guidelines and recommendations related to physical activity and heart health.
Harvard School of Public Health (http://www.hsph.harvard.edu/nutritionsource/index.html)	The Nutrition Source	Includes information and strategies for staying active.
Washington State Department of Health (http://here.doh.wa.gov/materials/stay-active-and-independent-for-life-an-information-guide-for-adults-65/)	Stay Active and Independent for Life	Provides self-assessment, strategies, and resources for older adults.
Blue Cross Blue Shield Minnesota (http://healthandwellness.bluecrossmn.com/)	Health and Wellness Resources	Introduces a variety of health and wellness resources for everyday life.
National Institute on Aging (http://go4life.nia.nih.gov/)	Go 4 Life Initiative	Includes a variety of resources for individuals and health professionals to build activity into daily routine.
Public Broadcasting Service (http://www.pbs.org/wgbh/caringforyourparents/caregiver/gettingstarted/index.html)	Caring for Your Parents	Provides resources for staying active through physical activity, work transition, volunteering, and lifelong learning.

changes in measures of health. These findings suggest that a lifestyle intervention focusing on physical activity produces positive changes in health and is a good alternative to a structured exercise regime for some people. Whether these results generalize to the population of people with stroke is unknown; more research is needed to examine the effect of lifestyle activity interventions on health outcomes for people with stroke.

Occupational therapy practitioners may promote staying active after exploring a person's interests in an occupational profile. Assessments such as the Activity Card Sort (Baum & Edwards, 2008) provide an avenue to identify meaningful occupations and develop daily and weekly routines that include moderate-intensity activities. Public health campaigns may also benefit from an occupational therapy perspective that considers the full array of staying-active occupations for different age groups, personal capabilities, and environmental settings.

Fitness

Overview and Recommendations

Fitness has been represented as a multidimensional, hierarchical construct that addresses both physical fitness and skills (Corbin & Frank, 2012). *Physical fitness* includes physiological (e.g., metabolic, morphological, bone integrity), health-related (e.g., body composition, cardiovascular fitness, flexibility, muscular endurance, muscle strength), and skill-related (e.g., agility, balance, coordination, power, speed, reaction time) components, and *skills* consist of sports components that are important in team, individual, and lifetime fitness activities (Corbin & Frank, 2012). Physical activity is a means to acquire fitness and is one aspect of staying active. The World Health Organization (2012) provided a simple definition of physical activity as "any bodily movement produced by skeletal muscles that requires energy expenditure" (para. 1). The *McGraw-Hill Concise Dictionary of Modern Medicine* (2002) defines *physical activity* as "athletic, recreational or occupational activities that require physical skills and utilize strength, power, endurance, speed, flexibility, range of motion or agility; PA is a behavioral parameter used to evaluate a patient's cardiovascular 'reserve.'"

Physical activity and fitness are national health priorities. The U.S. Department of Health and Human Services' (DHHS) Office of Disease Prevention and Health Promotion (2008) has developed physical activity guidelines for people of all ages, including people with disabilities and chronic conditions. Major research findings on the health benefits of physical activity are summarized in these guidelines, including (1) activity reduces risk of adverse health outcomes; (2) some activity is more beneficial than none; (3) more benefits are seen with increased intensity, frequency, and duration; (4) 150 minutes per week of moderate activity shows health benefits; (5) aerobic exercise and weight training are helpful; (6) health benefits occur across the lifespan and within subgroups, including racial/ethnic groups and people with disabilities; and (7) benefits of activity outweigh the risks.

The American Heart Association (AHA) developed specific recommendations regarding physical activity and exercise for people living with stroke (Gordon et al., 2004). Similar recommendations are also presented in lay language on the AHA and American Stroke Association (ASA) website (AHA & ASA, 2012). A comparison of physical activity recommendations is summarized in Table 13.2. Although guidelines have been developed, a systematic review of studies on fitness training after stroke has suggested that task-related training to improve function is recommended, but additional research is needed to determine the optimal fitness routine and evaluate the outcomes (Brazzelli, Saunders, Greig, & Mead, 2012; Saunders, Greig, Young, & Mead, 2004).

Table 13.2. Comparison of Physical Activity Guidelines

Guideline Area	*2008 Physical Activity Guidelines for Americans* (DHHS, Office of Disease Prevention and Health Promotion, 2008)	*Physical Activity and Exercise Recommendations for Stroke Survivors* (Gordon et al., 2004)	*Healthy Living After Stroke* (AHA & ASA, 2012)
Assessment	*Disabilities and chronic medical conditions:* Consult health care professional regarding amounts and types of appropriate physical activity for abilities.	Obtain preexercise evaluation (medical history, physical examination, graded exercise testing with ECG monitoring) before starting an exercise program.	Get clearance before beginning a physical activity program.
Aerobic	*Disabilities:* 150 min/wk moderate intensity or 75 min/wk vigorous intensity or equivalent combination of moderate and vigorous intensity. *Chronic medical conditions:* Type and amount should be based on abilities and severity of condition.	*Large muscle activities:* • 40%–70% peak oxygen uptake; 40%–70% heart rate reserve; 50%–80% maximal heart rate; RPE 11–14 (6–20 scale) • 3–7 days/wk • 20–60 min/session (or multiple 10-min sessions)	*Frequency:* Be active most days of the week. *Duration:* Do what is possible and approved by physician. • 40%–70% of your maximal heart rate, which is 220 minus your age.
Muscle strengthening	*Disabilities:* Moderate or high intensity involving all major muscle groups on 2 or more days/wk. *Chronic medical conditions:* Type and amount is based on abilities and severity of condition.	*Circuit training, weight machines, free weights, isometric exercise:* • 1–3 sets of 10–15 repetitions of 8–10 exercises involving major muscle groups • 2–3 days/wk	Involve 8–10 areas of your body—arms, shoulders, chest, trunk, back, hips, legs, and ankles.
Other		*Flexibility (stretching):* • 2–3 days/wk (before or after aerobic or strength training) • Hold stretches for 10–30 s *Neuromuscular (coordination, balance):* • 2–3 days/wk	
Modifications	*Disabilities and chronic medical conditions:* Regular physical activity according to abilities; avoid inactivity.	• Testing mode should be selected or adapted to needs. • Individual approach needed for safe exercise programming. • Some people will require further evaluation and subsequent specialization. • Important component of comprehensive program.	Exercise should be individualized on the basis of interests, strengths, and current fitness level. *Severe limitations:* May perform exercises sitting in a chair and get assistance with ROM exercises for affected limbs. *Moderate limitations:* May perform physical activity in a pool or use a recumbent stationary bike with assistance. *Mild limitations:* Swimming, walking, recumbent stationary bike, stair stepper. *No functional limitations:* No modifications.

Note. AHA = American Heart Association; ASA = American Stroke Association; DHHS = U.S. Department of Health and Human Services; ECG = electrocardiogram; min = minutes; ROM = range of motion; RPE = rate of perceived exertion; s = seconds; wk = week.

Fitness Initiatives and Outcomes

In many communities, a variety of fitness options are available for people with disabilities and chronic conditions. Fitness programs may include individual fitness routines, programs offered by community organizations, and programs developed by rehabilitation professionals. Community exercise programs have been shown to be beneficial for people living with stroke. Olney et al. (2006) conducted a randomized controlled trial to compare the outcomes of supervised and unsupervised exercise programs on metabolic cost equivalents of current activities, lower-extremity strength, physical and mental health, quality of life, and speed and physiological cost index of walking. The unsupervised program consisted of 1 week of supervised instruction followed by a 9-week unsupervised home program, and the supervised program included 10 weeks (1.5 hours 3 times per week) of guided strengthening and conditioning. Both programs resulted in improved outcomes over time, but the supervised program was particularly effective in improving self-reported activity profiles and physical health components of the quality-of-life measure at Year 1. Women made greater gains in the supervised programs than men.

Community exercise programs may take a variety of forms. Water-based exercise was compared with an upper-extremity function program in a randomized controlled trial (Chu et al., 2004). Cardiovascular and functional mobility outcome measures were significantly improved in the water-based exercise group compared with the upper-extremity function program after a short 8-week program (1 hour 3 times per week). Both programs were led by rehabilitation professionals. One explanation for the better outcomes in the water-based exercise program was that water provided opportunity for increased exercise intensity and resistance.

Occupational therapy practitioners have had a long-standing involvement in fitness programs for special populations. Hippotherapy, adaptive sports and recreation programs, yoga, and water aerobics are examples of fitness programs that may be adapted to meet the needs of people with physical and cognitive challenges.

Chronic Disease Management and Self-Management

Overview and Recommendations

Chronic disease management and self-management programs have been identified as important strategies for addressing future health care needs. Preventive and wellness services and chronic disease management were specifically identified as an essential health benefit in the Patient Protection and Affordable Care Act (Pub. L. 111–148; Ulmer, Ball, McGlynn, & Bel Hamdounia, 2012). Chronic disease management and self-management programs are typically designed to maintain, manage, and improve people's health and prevent health problems.

Self-management and chronic disease management programs have been developed for a variety of conditions and are offered in a variety of formats. ***Self-management*** has been defined as a "dynamic and continuous process of self-regulation" to "manage the symptoms, treatment, physical and psychosocial consequences and life style changes inherent in living with a chronic condition" and to "monitor one's condition and to effect the cognitive, behavioral and emotional responses necessary to maintain a satisfactory quality of life" (Barlow, Wright, Sheasby, Turner, & Hainsworth, 2002, p. 178). Self-management programs work toward behavior change by increasing knowledge and addressing confidence, motivation, and **attitudes** and are often user led, meaning they are facilitated by people who have a chronic disease (Department of Health, 2001). Although self-management programs are typically offered by community and governmental agencies, chronic disease management programs are more often associated with continuing care programs offered by health care organizations. *Chronic disease management* has been defined as an "integrated care approach to managing illness which includes screenings, check-ups, monitoring and coordinating treatment, and patient education"; the outcomes are focused on improved quality of life and decreased health care costs (DHHS, 2012).

User-led self-management programs for chronic disease have received growing recognition as being cost-effective and providing people with chronic conditions with greater control over the management of their health (Department of Health, 2001). The Chronic Disease Self-Management Program (CDSMP) was developed at Stanford University and serves as a predominant model for user-led self-management programs (Department of Health, 2001). In this program, health professionals with expertise in a chronic condition provide volunteers with training to lead self-management groups for their peers. A typical self-management program may be offered in 6-week sessions for about 2.5 hours per week. The CDSMP emphasizes five core skills: (1) problem solving, (2) decision making, (3) resource utilization, (4) formation of a patient–professional partnership, and (5) taking action (Department of Health, 2001, p. 25), with benefits of "reduced severity of symptoms, significant decrease in pain, improved life control and activity, improved resourcefulness and life satisfaction" (p. 26).

Bandura's social cognitive theory provides the framework for many self-management programs (Joice, 2012). In this theory, ***self-efficacy*** (i.e., a person's perception of his or her ability to be successful in a behavior) influences actions. Self-management programs that emphasize self-efficacy aim to promote confidence in managing chronic conditions by providing people with opportunities to achieve mastery, share experiences, communicate positivism, receive feedback, and obtain support (Joice, 2012). The five core components emphasized in the CDSMP are based on social cognitive theory. Although studies on self-management programs for people with stroke are limited, preliminary support has been found that self-management programs for stroke improve self-efficacy, ability levels, and emotional status (Joice, 2012).

> Self-management programs that emphasize self-efficacy aim to promote confidence in managing chronic conditions by providing people with opportunities to achieve mastery, share experiences, communicate positivism, receive feedback, and obtain support.

Chronic Disease Management and Self-Management Initiatives and Outcomes

Various types of self-management programs for chronic conditions have been described in the literature (Barlow et al., 2002). Programs may be provided online or in the home, clinic, or community and structured for use by individuals or small groups. Many programs incorporate two or more of these formats. The content addressed in programs may include general health information, medication and symptom management, behavioral conditioning, psychosocial adjustment, lifestyle issues, social support, communication, and goal setting. The effectiveness of programs is measured in terms of changes in the participant (physical, psychological, and social health; knowledge; medication use; self-efficacy and self-management behaviors) and the demands on the health system (use of health resources, health costs; Barlow et al., 2002).

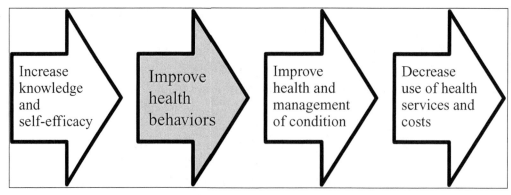

Figure 13.1. Proposed effects of self-management programs.

Source. From *Patient Self-Management Support Programs: An Evaluation* (No. 08-0011, pp. 1–43), by M. L. Pearson, S. Mattke, R. Shaw, M. S. Ridgely, and S. H. Wiseman, 2007, Washington, DC: Agency for Healthcare Research and Quality. In the public domain.

Governmental agencies and health care organizations have growing interest in self-management programs as an important strategy to improve patient outcomes and develop efficient health care delivery methods. A report on self-management programs was prepared for the Agency for Healthcare Research and Quality (Pearson, Mattke, Shaw, Ridgely, & Wiseman, 2007) and described goals, models, outcomes, content, and supportive interventions. The overall goal of self-management programs is to improve health behaviors (see Figure 13.1), which should in turn influence outcomes and costs. Different models may be used to achieve this goal, including primary care, external in-person, external call center, and remote technology. Each model has advantages and disadvantages; the recommendation of a specific model depends on the needs of the individual. All self-management programs should include both coaching and education, require that staff have core competencies (Table 13.3), and use measures to evaluate the program's outcomes (Pearson et al., 2007).

Additional research is needed to determine the outcomes of self-management programs for people poststroke. Preliminary evidence (Kendall et al., 2007) has shown that participation in a structured self-management program may prevent a decline in quality-of-life domains (family roles, ADLs, self-care, work productivity). The changes in self-efficacy for this population were limited.

Table 13.3. Knowledge and Coaching Components and Core Competencies for Staff in Self-Management Programs

Knowledge Components	Coaching Components	Core Competencies for Staff
Disease or condition	Self-assessment	Knowledge of disease or condition
Symptoms	Motivation	condition
Medications	Confidence	Interpersonal skills
Side effects	Self-efficacy	Educational skills
Self-management philosophy	Collaborative problem solving	Care management
Self-management process	Goal setting	Motivational skills
Focus areas for self-management	Emotional support	Empathy
Resources	Stress management	Compassion
	Reevaluation	

Source. Adapted from *Patient Self-Management Support Programs: An Evaluation* (No. 08-0011, pp. 1–43), by M. L. Pearson, S. Mattke, R. Shaw, M. S. Ridgely, and S. H. Wiseman, 2007, Washington, DC: Agency for Healthcare Research and Quality. In the public domain.

Self-management and chronic disease management programs have been proposed as an important strategy to improve health and quality of life for people after stroke. Rogers (1984) recognized the potential contributions of occupations in these management programs long ago: "Knowing the role occupation plays in self-development, self-management, and self-fulfillment provides a basis for understanding why occupational therapy strives to engage persons with **functional impairments** in occupational endeavors" (p. 47). The American Medical Association's (2008) *Health Care Careers Directory 2008–2009* identified training in self-management as an intervention provided by occupational therapy. Self-management has also been identified as an opportunity for patient- and family-centered care in the National Quality Strategy of the Affordable Care Act (DHHS, 2011). The number of examples of self-management programs that include occupation-based components is growing. The September/October 2011 issue of *Occupational Therapy Now* (Packer, 2011), a publication of the Canadian Association of Occupational Therapists, profiled self-management programs for a variety of chronic conditions.

Points to Ponder: Self-Management Program Activities

The Chronic Disease Self-Management Program emphasizes five core skills in self-management programs:
1. Problem solving
2. Decision making
3. Resource utilization
4. Formation of a patient–professional partnership
5. Taking action.

Brainstorm some individual or group activities for each skill that you would envision in a self-management program for people with stroke.

Caregiver and Family Support

Overview and Recommendations

Many people who have had a stroke will need support from their families for the rest of their lives. Caregivers provide assistance to people who have activity and participation limitations in a variety of ways. *Mosby's Medical Dictionary* (2009) defines a *caregiver* as "one who contributes the benefits of medical, social, economic, or environmental resources to a dependent or partially dependent individual, such as a critically ill person." Some support may be provided by professionals (formal caregivers), but more often family members serve as the primary caregivers (informal caregivers). *Informal caregiving* has been defined as "task-oriented assistance provided by individuals, usually family or friends, that is not a part of formal community support services" (Dewey et al., 2002, p. 1028).

The National Alliance for Caregiving and AARP (2009) conducted a study of general caregiving trends in the United States. This study's purpose was to examine the prevalence of caregiving, demographic characteristics of caregivers, nature and effects of caregiving, needs for information and sources, and role of the Internet and technology in caregiving and to provide recommendations for public policies. A sample of 1,480 family caregivers completed a quantitative interview; 5% of the sample identified stroke as the main reason for caregiving needs. This study estimated that almost 66 million U.S. citizens provide unpaid caregiving; about two-thirds of caregivers are female, 73% are employed, and the average age of caregivers is 49.2 years. Caregivers provide an average of 20.4 hours per week of unpaid care for 4.6 years. The greatest needs for caregiving were in the areas of transportation (83%), housework (75%), grocery shopping (75%), meal preparation (65%), finances (64%), and ADLs (56%).

Care provided to people poststroke may be substantial and differs from caregiving for people with other conditions. In a study of 340 Australians poststroke, 74% needed assistance with ADLs, with women being the majority of the informal caregivers (Dewey et al., 2002). The cost of providing this informal care was estimated to be one-third of the average weekly wage in Australia. In a study comparing caregiving for people poststroke with caregiving for people with rheumatoid arthritis (van Exel, Brouwer, van den Berg, Koopmanschap, & van den Bos, 2004), caregivers for people poststroke were more likely to be female, were less likely to be spouses or to be living with the care recipients, and had more travel expenses and demands on their time; the people with stroke were also more likely than those with rheumatoid arthritis to have serious health problems and mobility issues.

Although serving as a caregiver has many rewards, it also has enormous demands that may contribute to caregiver problems. Caregiver burden, strain, and stress are constructs commonly used to describe the negative impact of caregiving. Although caregiver burden is a multidimensional, complex construct, objective burden and subjective burden are commonly differentiated (Carretero, Garcés, Ródenas, & Sanjosé, 2009). *Subjective burden* is identified as the perceptions, attitudes, **feelings,** self-concept, and **emotions** associated with caregiving. *Objective burden* typically refers to the life demands and changes that may be documented as a by-product of caregiving (e.g., time use, economic cost, employment, physical and mental health, sociodemographic changes).

Multiple studies over the past 2 decades have examined the factors associated with caregiving burden. A review of the literature identified some trends regarding burden and strain for caregivers of people poststroke and also proposed questions for future research (Rombough, Howse, & Bartfay, 2006). Findings suggested that burden and strain, as measured by psychological, economic, physical, and social characteristics of caregivers, are related to level of social support, caregiver health, socioeconomic status, time demands, and level of disability. In a study of 110 individuals 1, 3, and 6 months poststroke and their caregivers (Bugge, Alexander, & Hagen, 1999), more than one-third of caregivers reported excessive strain. Caregivers who were spending the most time caring, helping people with the most severe strokes, or dealing with health problems of their own had higher levels of caregiver strain as measured by the Caregiver Strain Index. Of the 13 factors measured by this index, 3 were frequently identified as problems: (1) confining aspects of caregiving, (2) changes in personal plans, and (3) changes in family life.

Caregiving for people poststroke has been found to influence emotional well-being and quality of life. In a review of 20 studies on caregiving for people poststroke, Han and Haley (1999) reported increased depression in caregivers in both the acute and the chronic stroke phases. These findings suggested that failure to address caregiver needs has the potential to influence psychological outcomes for caregivers.

Although serving as a caregiver has many rewards, it also has enormous demands that may contribute to caregiver problems.

Points to Ponder: Objective and Subjective Caregiver Burden

Can you differentiate between objective and subjective caregiver burden? Review each of the following caregiver problems and label each one as objective (O) or subjective (S):

• Absences from work or school

• Loss of friendships

• Depletion of savings to purchase needed equipment

• Frustration with health care system

• Back injury associated with providing physical assistance

• Grief related to unrealized dreams and goals.

How would you obtain information related to subjective caregiving burden?

In a prospective study of 232 people 3 and 12 months poststroke and their caregivers, quality of life for caregivers was found to be associated with the level of caregiving burden (McCullagh, Brigstocke, Donaldson, & Kalra, 2005). At 3 months poststroke, the strongest predictors of quality of life and caregiver burden were emotional status of the individual and caregiver, age and gender of caregiver, and caregiving training status. At 1 year poststroke, the individual's level of dependence poststroke and family support also predicted burden and quality of life. In a study of 115 caregivers of partners who were 3 years poststroke, the greatest level of perceived burden was associated with the impact on the caregiver's personal life in terms of "feelings of heavy responsibility, uncertainty about patients' care needs, constant worries, restraints in social life, and feelings that patients rely on only their care" (Scholte op Reimer, de Haan, Rijnders, Limburg, & van den Bos, 1998, p. 1607).

Although these studies have suggested that specific factors may influence the level of caregiving burden, there are problems in making definitive conclusions. In systematic reviews of 20 studies (Han & Haley, 1999) and 39 studies (Greenwood, Mackenzie, Cloud, & Wilson, 2008) of informal caregivers of stroke survivors, definitive conclusions across studies were not possible because characteristics of people poststroke and their caregivers were not clearly described, concepts were not uniformly defined, important variables were missing, and theoretical foundations were not proposed.

Caregiving burden, caregiving needs, and quality of life of caregivers have been measured by a variety of instruments (Deeken, Taylor, Mangan, Yabroff, & Ingham, 2003). A comprehensive review of instruments measuring caregiver characteristics identified 17 measures of burden, 8 measures of needs, and 3 measures of quality of life. These different measures address many domains, including caregiver activity; family and interpersonal relations; support; social life; physical health; emotional and psychological health; finances, work, and legal matters; spiritual needs; respite, leisure, and privacy; information needs; time; relationship with the individual; and other. Studying caregiver burden is challenging because there are no consistent domains included in measures of this construct, and there is overlap in supposedly unique constructs related to caregiver burden.

Caregiver Initiatives and Outcomes

A growing number of interventions are targeted toward caregivers and are designed to improve outcomes for both the caregiver and the person with stroke. Caregiver

> A growing number of interventions are targeted toward caregivers and are designed to improve outcomes for both the caregiver and the person with stroke.

Table 13.4. Caregiver Assessment: Domains and Measures

Domains[a]	General Measures[a]	Occupational Therapy Measures
• *Person:* Health; coping skills; values and beliefs; confidence; strengths; knowledge, skills, and competence; rewards from caregiving • *Environment:* Context, social support, finances, legal factors • *Occupational performance:* Employment, caregiver tasks, functional level of recipient	• Bakas Caregiving Outcomes Scale (Bakas & Champion, 1999) • Burden Interview/Index (Visser-Meily et al., 2005) • Caregiving Appraisal Scale (Struchen et al., 2002) • Patient–Caregiver Functional Unit Scale (Fredman & Daly, 1997) • Sense of Competence Questionnaire (Scholte op Reimer et al., 1998) • Zarit Burden Interview (Zarit et al., 1985)	• Activity Card Sort (Baum & Edwards, 2008) • Canadian Occupational Performance Measure (Law et al., 2005) • Life Balance Inventory (Matuska, 2012) • Role Checklist (Oakley et al., 1986)

[a]From Lutz and Young (2010).

interventions may incorporate education, skill development, social support, counseling, and technology (Brereton, Carroll, & Barnston, 2007). Assessment of caregiver needs, areas of competence, and challenges may provide valuable information to guide recommendations for interventions. An overview of general assessment domains and measures related to caregiving (Lutz & Young, 2010) has suggested that occupational therapists should consider aspects of the person, environment, and occupational performance when evaluating caregivers (see Table 13.4). Feinberg (2003) suggested that caregiver assessments include components that are relevant to occupational therapy: inventory of caregiving activities besides ADLs; caregiver skills, quality of care, values, and priorities; and the rewards of caregiving. Occupational therapy assessments are not specifically designed for the caregiver population but still may be appropriate to use while exploring caregiver goals (see examples in Table 13.4).

A review of the literature on caregiving interventions identified important qualities for designing programs (Zarit & Femia, 2008). The content should include both education and psychological support to address the different aspects of caregiver burden. Programs should be multidimensional and responsive to people's unique needs. The length and frequency of the intervention (dosage) must be adequate to address the complex needs of caregivers at different stages. The outcomes of caregiver interventions are measured in terms of both objective and subjective burden, including mental health (e.g., depression, **anxiety**), quality of life and well-being, **coping** skills, and self-efficacy (Brereton et al., 2007; Eldred & Sykes, 2008).

Research on the effectiveness of intervention programs designed to decrease caregiver burden is limited. Very few interventions are based on theoretical models that are described in the literature. However, one study (Bakas et al., 2009) described the Telephone Assessment and Skill-Building Kit (TASK) intervention to address caregiver needs for locating information, handling recipients' emotions and behaviors, providing assistance with ADLs and IADLs, and managing personal feelings about caregiving. The outcome of this clinical trial indicated that care-givers who participated in the TASK intervention described more optimism, fewer challenges in providing care, and reduced anticipation of negative outcomes from providing care.

Community Supports and Resources

Overview and Recommendations

Life after stroke often has challenges that go beyond the issues that are addressed in acute rehabilitation programs. Inpatient programs often are limited to interventions that meet medical practice guidelines for acute care and are selected by profession-als to address short-term goals related to self-care, basic functional activities, and discharge planning (Cott, Wiles, & Devitt, 2007). Although programs that address these acute poststroke issues are undoubtedly important, perhaps even more critical needs in the community are currently unmet.

The number of people who return to their homes and communities poststroke is growing. Changes in the stroke population have been noted, with more strokes occurring at a younger age and classified as mild to moderate (Wolf et al., 2009). For people who return home poststroke, occupations of importance go beyond the self-care and basic functional activities addressed in acute rehabilitation. After discharge, these people want to get on with their lives and resume roles that are important to their identity and bring meaning to their lives (Cott et al., 2007; Robison et al., 2009; Wolf et al., 2009): social, vocational, domestic, community, and leisure. How-ever, in the United States, community rehabilitation programs that address needs in these areas are limited.

Growing research has highlighted the barriers to participation for people post-stroke and the broader population of Americans with disabilities. A 2003 NOD/Har-ris Survey found that people with disabilities report disadvantages related to overall satisfaction with life, income, community mobility, health care, and limitations to participation in work, education, civic, social, and recreational activities and religious events (National Organization on Disability, 2004). Qualitative research (White, Mackenzie, Magin, & Pollack, 2008) has provided a window into the daily experiences of living with stroke and the emotional impact of these life changes on occupational engagement.

The longer term barriers to meaningful participation after stroke may be classi-fied as person factors, environmental factors, and occupational factors. The physi-cal, cognitive, and communication changes associated with stroke have been well documented; other studies have identified specific issues for some people related to confidence, self-concept, fear of falling, fatigue, dizziness, mood changes, and bal-ance that may also influence occupational performance (Robison et al., 2009). For people poststroke, some of the occupations that pose the greatest difficulties include work and education, family, and social, mobility, and financial occupations (Ham-mel, Jones, Gossett, & Morgan, 2006).

Although the changes in person factors poststroke are often very real, the dis-ability rights community has emphasized environmental barriers that limit partic-ipation because of "economic, political, social, and cultural issues" and have an impact on "freedom, control, societal inclusion, community membership, and civil rights" (Hammel et al., 2006, pp. 45–46). In a participatory action research study of participation experienced by people poststroke (Hammel et al., 2006), barriers were identified as individual, environmental, and system or policy.

Regardless of personal, environmental, or occupational barriers, many people are successful in adapting and creating new meaning in life poststroke. Interest is growing in understanding the attributes of successful adaptation after stroke. In a qualitative study of 19 participants who were at least 12 months poststroke and 8 informal caregivers, several characteristics emerged as possible factors that contribute to better outcomes (Robison et al., 2009): personality traits associated with adaptability to change (e.g., optimistic, determined, persevering, accepting help, inventive, adjusting priorities and expectations); adoption of technology to address limitations; commitment to staying active; and social support. Interventions that reduce the impact of these barriers and support attributes to successful adaptation have been incorporated in many community rehabilitation programs.

Several characteristics emerged as possible factors that contribute to better outcomes: personality traits associated with adaptability to change; adoption of technology to address limitations; commitment to staying active; and social support.

Community Initiatives and Outcomes

Several opportunities are available for occupational therapists who are interested in community initiatives for preventing stroke or addressing long-term needs of people and their families poststroke. An ASA task force (Schwamm et al., 2005) identified recommendations for creating an integrated system of care that addresses prevention, treatment, and rehabilitation. The knowledge and skills of occupational therapists would be valuable on interprofessional teams that are working to improve programs and address the three critical functions described by the task force: (1) collaboration and communication among people and organizations; (2) coordinated and standardized procedures; and (3) evaluation of programs and services through process and outcome measures. The Canadian best practice recommendations for stroke care also address needs that are relevant to occupational therapy (Lindsay et al., 2008), including prevention through lifestyle management, stroke rehabilitation, and community follow-up and reintegration.

Prevention programs are also needed to address the behavioral factors that contribute to increased risk for stroke. Occupational therapists understand the importance of occupations in establishing healthy habits, routines, and lifestyles for people and communities. Current involvement in falls prevention programs, back injury prevention, and wellness programs provides a foundation for interventions that focus on education, consultation, and advocacy.

Additional community supports, services, and resources are needed by people with stroke and their caregivers. The types of community programs that are needed depend in part on the severity of stroke, but all programs should increase participation and community integration in home and family, work and productivity, and social and leisure occupations (Cott et al., 2007). For people with moderate to severe stroke, extended stroke community-based programs have been recommended to build in continuity and transition from acute care rehabilitation programs to the home environment (Cott et al., 2007).

Although remediation of client factors may be a focus in the acute rehabilitation stage, addressing environmental and system and policy barriers to participation are more important in the community (Hammel et al., 2006). For example, although substantial progress has been made in improving the physical accessibility of public environments, there are still barriers to participation, especially for people with cognitive impairments, because of poor signage, limited social assistance, and policies denying advanced access to venues. Occupational therapists may assist in dismantling environmental barriers by conducting environmental assessments, engaging in public awareness campaigns, and coaching clients to use strategies as they try new activities.

General Opportunities for Rehabilitation Professionals

The *Occupational Therapy Practice Framework: Domain and Process* (3rd ed.; AOTA, 2014a) describes the occupational therapy interventions and approaches that are used across different areas of practice and practice settings. In traditional rehabilitation programs for stroke, the nature of occupational therapy typically emphasizes a service delivery model that involves one occupational therapist working with one individual (at a time) who has had a stroke.

Although interventions provided in this way are very important, in this chapter I have highlighted the need for prevention programs and community-based services for people with stroke and their families. The target audiences of these programs are communities and populations; thus, the professional skills needed by occupational therapists go beyond the individual approaches typically used in acute rehabilitation programs. Education and advocacy are important types of interventions in community settings because they are cost-effective and affect the lives of more people. Similarly, the occupational therapy approaches used in community settings will likely vary from the primary focus in acute rehabilitation settings of establish or restore (remediation). Intervention approaches that create or promote; maintain; modify, compensate, or adapt; and prevent are consistent with programs for staying active, fitness, chronic disease and self-management, family and caregiver issues, and community resources and services. Table 13.5 summarizes evidence related to interventions that support occupational therapy practice in these areas. The number of opportunities is growing for occupational therapists who would like to work in these emerging settings, but job titles and job descriptions will usually not include the term *occupational therapy*. Eligibility criteria for these positions typically require a graduate degree in a health or social services field but often do not list specific health professions. Table 13.6 provides examples of occupational therapy initiatives and employment opportunities that relate to the focus areas in this chapter.

Three Case Studies: Living With Stroke in the Community

The three case studies in this text may illustrate new opportunities for occupational therapy to serve the needs of people with stroke and their families in the community. An example for each case is provided to imagine and explore new roles for occupational therapy.

Steve: Fitness and Staying Active

After his discharge, Steve had a follow-up appointment with his primary care provider, who discussed her concern for Steve and his risk for a debilitating stroke in the future. She emphasized the importance of changing his **habits** and routines and recommended that Steve obtain a lifestyle coach (who could be an occupational therapist; AOTA, 2014b) who could help him through this process. Steve reported that this stroke was an important wake-up call given that his own father died at

(text continues on page 335)

Table 13.5. Evidence That Provides Direction for Occupational Therapy Practice

Purpose and Reference	Type of Study and Publication	Method	Results	Conclusions and Recommendations
To determine the relationships among activities participation, and life satisfaction after stroke (Hartman-Maeir et al., 2007)	Staying active Cross-sectional study of participants 1 yr poststroke Published in peer-reviewed journal	56 participants 1 yr poststroke and rehabilitation evaluated in their home using the **FIM™**, Instrumental Activities of Daily Living Questionnaire, Activity Card Sort, a work questionnaire, Life Satisfaction Questionnaire, and Geriatric Depression Scale	• 50% of sample still required assistance in some ADLs. • >70% of sample required full assistance in some IADLs. • Mean leisure activity level retained was 43%. • 1 person returned to work. • 39% were satisfied with life as a whole. • Activity level was a significant predictor of life satisfaction.	There is a need for community rehabilitation services to address long-term activity and participation limitations for people with stroke.
To determine the effect of fitness training on death, dependence, disability, physical fitness, mobility, physical function, health and quality of life, mood, and incidence of adverse events (Saunders et al., 2004)	Fitness Systematic review of 12 studies with a total of 289 participants Published in peer-reviewed journal and Cochrane Collaboration	Search of the Cochrane Stroke Group Trials Register and 10 other electronic databases. Hand search of journal and reference lists Select RCT that had an intervention to improve muscle strength or cardiorespiratory fitness	• 3 studies started within 1 mo of stroke. • 2 studies examined effect of strength training. • 2 studies provided no evidence of benefit for disability. • Few common outcome measures. • Significant improvements shown in ambulation scores and maximal walking speed scores. • Other observed physical benefits were associated with tasks.	Inadequate studies. Functional benefits are related to task-specific training. Studies are needed on efficacy and feasibility soon after stroke, strength training, dose and type of training.

(Continued)

Table 13.5. Evidence That Provides Direction for Occupational Therapy Practice *(cont.)*

Purpose and Reference	Type of Study and Publication	Method	Results	Conclusions and Recommendations
To determine the effect of supervised versus unsupervised community exercise programs for people poststroke (Olney et al., 2006)	Fitness RCT Published in peer-reviewed journal	*Location:* Ontario, Canada *Participants:* Ages ≥20 yr, poststroke, able to walk 15 min with or without ambulatory devices, tolerate 45 min of activity, no contraindications for exercise *Sample size: n* = 37 per group *Interventions:* Warm-up, aerobic, strength, cool-down *Group 1:* 1.5-hr supervised exercise, 3 days/wk for 10 wk *Group 2:* 1.5-hr supervised exercise, 3 days/wk, 1 wk followed by 9-wk home program *Outcomes:* 6-min walking speed, Human Activity Profile, SF–36 Physical, SF–36 Mental, LE strength, physiological cost index *Frequency of outcome measures:* Baseline, 10 wk, 6 mo, 1 yr	• 6-min walking speed significantly increased in both groups with no significant differences at 1 yr. • *Human Activity Profile:* Supervised group increased activities over time and was statistically significant at 1 yr. Unsupervised group showed nonsignificant increase until 10 wk and then declined. • *SF–36 Physical:* Supervised group increased significantly from baseline to 1 yr. Unsupervised group showed no significant improvements until last assessment. • *SF–36 Mental:* Supervised group increased significantly from baseline to 10 wk. Unsupervised group showed no significant improvements until last assessment. • *LE strength:* No significant difference shown in either group. • *Physiological cost index:* Supervised group showed no significant change. Unsupervised group was significantly improved at 1 yr. • Some interaction effects by gender.	People poststroke living in the community who engage in supervised or unsupervised exercise programs may make improvements in physical ability that are maintained after 1 yr. Supervised programs may provide a supportive role that addresses the physical component of quality-of-life and activity profiles. Economical home-based programs that include exercise may produce improvements in physical function that are maintained at 1 yr.

(Continued)

Table 13.5. Evidence That Provides Direction for Occupational Therapy Practice (cont.)

Purpose and Reference	Type of Study and Publication	Method	Results	Conclusions and Recommendations
To determine the effectiveness of water-based exercise on cardiovascular fitness and functional mobility (Chu et al., 2004)	Fitness Single-blind RCT Peer-reviewed journal	*Location*: Public community center in Canada *Participants*: Community-dwelling people with unilateral weakness poststroke, only 1 CVA, >1 yr poststroke, independent in walking, medically stable, no previous MCI, no significant musculoskeletal problems *Sample size*: N = 12, voluntary sample *Interventions*: Water-based exercise program (*n* = 7), 8 wk, 3 days/wk, 1 hr/session; UE program (*n* = 6), 8 wk, 3 days/wk, 1 hr/session *Outcome*: VO2 max, maximal workload, gait speed, Berg Balance Scale, muscle strength	• Water-based exercise group showed greater improvements in VO2 max, gait speed, and muscle strength. • Control group's improvement in Berg Balance Score approached significance.	Water-based exercise programs may improve cardiovascular fitness, LE strength, and functional mobility. Water-based programs in the community may be a cost-effective way to improve fitness in people poststroke.
To determine the effect of a community-based fitness program for participants with stroke on their cardiorespiratory fitness, mobility, LE strength, balance, activity, participation, and UE function (Pang et al., 2005; Pang et al., 2006)	Fitness Prospective, single-blind RCT Peer-reviewed journals (reported in 2 different journals)	*Participants*: 63 people who were >1 yr poststroke and living in the community *Interventions*: FAME program, compared with seated UE program (19 wk, 1 hr/session, 3×/wk) *Outcomes*: Maximal oxygen consumption, 6-min walk test, Berg Balance Scale, Physical Activity Scale, leg strength, Wolf Motor Function Test, Fugl–Meyer Assessment, grip strength, Motor Activity Log	• Participants in the fitness group had significantly better cardiovascular fitness, mobility, LE strength, balance, activity, and participation outcomes than UE group. • Participants in the UE group had significantly more improvement in UE function than the fitness group.	Community-based programs should be targeted to the needs of people with stroke. Fitness may improve mobility and physical activity levels for people with stroke, and UE groups may improve arm function.

(Continued)

Table 13.5. Evidence That Provides Direction for Occupational Therapy Practice *(cont.)*

Purpose and Reference	Type of Study and Publication	Method	Results	Conclusions and Recommendations
To determine whether an individualized self-management program for people with stroke changed self-efficacy, locus of control, mobility, ADLs, subjective outcomes, anxiety, and depression (Jones et al., 2009)	Self-management Chronic disease management Single-subject design Peer-reviewed journal	*Participants:* 10 people poststroke *Intervention:* Self-management workbook focused on self-efficacy *Outcomes:* Stroke Self-Efficacy Questionnaire, Rivermead Mobility Index, Activities of Daily Living Scale, Subjective Index of Physical and Social Outcome, Hospital Anxiety and Depression Scale	• All 10 participants improved on most of the outcome measures. There was statistically significant change in self-efficacy and locus of control.	Individualized self-management programs should be studied further for their impact on self-efficacy.
To determine whether self-management interventions for stroke are effective in influencing self-efficacy for people poststroke (Jones & Riazi, 2011)	Self-management Chronic disease management Systematic review Peer-reviewed journal	Databases were searched for articles published between 2000 and 2009. 22 articles met the criteria and were reviewed	• There is beginning evidence that self-management programs based on self-efficacy principles have benefits for people poststroke.	Further research is needed.
To determine whether a self-management program promotes psychosocial recovery after stroke (Kendall et al., 2007)	Self-management Chronic disease management RCT Peer-reviewed journal	*Participants:* 100 people from Australia who were several mo poststroke (71 participants remained in the study at 12 mo) *Intervention:* Chronic disease self-management course (6 wk, 2 hr/wk) and a control group of standard follow-up from rehab *Outcomes:* Stroke Specific Quality of Life, Self-Efficacy Scale	• The control group reported decreased function in family roles, ADLs, self-care, and productivity compared with the intervention group. • Neither group showed significant improvement in self-efficacy.	Self-management programs may serve a protective function poststroke in preventing decline in specific quality-of-life domains.

(Continued)

Table 13.5. Evidence That Provides Direction for Occupational Therapy Practice *(cont.)*

Purpose and Reference	Type of Study and Publication	Method	Results	Conclusions and Recommendations
To determine whether training of caregivers reduces the burden of stroke (Kalra et al., 2004)	Caregiver and family Single-blind RCT Peer-reviewed journal *(British Medical Journal)*	*Participants:* 300 people with stroke and their caregivers. *Intervention:* Intervention group—instruction in stroke-related problems and prevention and hands-on training program in basic care and ADLs on stroke rehabilitation unit; conventional care—information and advice. *Outcomes:* Health and social services costs; functional status of participants and caregivers (Barthel Index, Frenchay Activities Index); psychological status (anxiety and depression); quality of life (EuroQol), institutionalization, mortality	• Training reduced burden of care and improved quality of life for people poststroke and their caregivers at 3 and 12 mo. • Costs of stroke care also decreased, with people achieving higher levels of independence earlier.	Developing structured training programs for caregivers may be an effective strategy to improve outcomes and decrease costs.
To determine whether interventions for family caregivers of people poststroke are effective (Brereton et al., 2007)	Caregiver and family Systematic review Peer-reviewed journal	An extensive review of databases, literature, and unpublished materials. A systematic review of 8 articles was completed	• Current interventions for family carers are heterogeneous and may include training, education, counseling, and a variety of social support strategies. • Stress-coping theories formed the basis for about half the interventions. • Most studies were low quality. • Training was associated with decreased depression, anxiety, and caregiving burden in caregivers along with improved well-being and quality of life; education and counseling improved knowledge and family function; support groups improved coping skills and self-efficacy.	Health professionals should work toward standard interventions and outcome measures to increase the consistency across studies and, thus, determine the degree to which interventions are effective.

(Continued)

Table 13.5. Evidence That Provides Direction for Occupational Therapy Practice *(cont.)*

Purpose and Reference	Type of Study and Publication	Method	Results	Conclusions and Recommendations
To determine whether interventions that address psychosocial functioning are effective in decreasing caregiver burden (Eldred & Sykes, 2008)	Caregiver and family Systematic review Peer-reviewed journal	Extensive review of health-related databases and specific journals Seven articles met all criteria and were included in the systematic review	• Four psychological models were used to develop interventions that addressed psychosocial needs: (1) family systems, (2) cognitive behavior, (3) social problem solving, and (4) stress coping. Interventions also included various formats: individual, group, telephone conferencing. Thus, direct comparisons of the studies were not appropriate. • Results provided tentative support for psychosocial interventions to improve family functioning, promote problem solving, provide a protective effect for psychosocial problems, improve function of people poststroke, and prevent personal adjustment decline.	Short-term interventions that promote problem solving and coping by caregivers may be beneficial. Consideration of outcome measures for people poststroke and caregivers is particularly important when providing interventions with limited evidence.
To determine what qualities should be considered in developing intervention programs for caregivers and how future research might lead to improved outcomes (Zarit & Femia, 2008)	Caregiver and family Continuing education article in peer-reviewed journal Family Caregiver Alliance	Review of literature	• Four characteristics were identified in many caregiver interventions: (1) psychological and educational approaches included, (2) multi-dimensional in nature, (3) flexible to respond to individual needs, and (4) sufficient dosage to adequately address needs.	Future research should address issues related to the 4 characteristics identified: (1) improve research design to match intervention goals and caregiver needs, (2) identify client-centered goals, (3) address needs of different types of caregivers, and (4) incorporate preventive and adaptive intervention approaches.

(Continued)

Table 13.5. Evidence That Provides Direction for Occupational Therapy Practice *(cont.)*

Purpose and Reference	Type of Study and Publication	Method	Results	Conclusions and Recommendations
To determine caregivers' self-identified interests in 12 technologies (National Alliance for Caregiving & AARP, 2009)	Caregiver and family Cross-sectional survey funded by United Healthcare National Alliance for Caregiving report	A quantitative online survey of 1,000 family caregivers who used technology examined the benefits of and receptivity to 12 technologies	• Approximately 75% of respondents identified benefits related to saving time, making caregiving easier and safer, increasing feelings of competence, and reducing stress. • Three technologies were rated as being helpful or very helpful by at least 70% of respondents: (1) personal health record tracking, (2) caregiving coordination system, and (3) medication support system. These technologies were identified as having barriers to trying them by fewer than 50% of respondents. • Three other technologies were identified as having potential for use: (1) symptom monitor and transmitter; (2) interactive system for physical, mental, and leisure activities; and (3) video phone system. • Caregivers most likely to use technologies were younger than age 50, early adopters of technology, racial/ethnic minorities, and caregivers with increased burden of care.	Understanding caregiver perspectives regarding technologies may help in designing technology-based interventions that may relieve caregiver burden. Findings of this study may assist in developing intervention studies to determine the effectiveness of technologies as part of an overall care plan.

(Continued)

Table 13.5. Evidence That Provides Direction for Occupational Therapy Practice *(cont.)*

Purpose and Reference	Type of Study and Publication	Method	Results	Conclusions and Recommendations
To determine whether a telephone-based intervention was effective in addressing caregiver needs and building caregiving skills (Bakas et al., 2009)	Caregiver and family RCT Peer-reviewed journal	*Participants:* 40 caregivers. *Intervention:* Intervention group— Telephone Assessment and Skill-Building Kit (TASK), an 8-wk program to increase knowledge, skill, and confidence in caregiving areas. Conventional care— 8-wk phone call from nurse. *Outcomes:* Caregiver optimism, task difficulty, threat appraisal, depression, life changes, general health perceptions	• Outcomes were measured at 4, 8, and 12 wk. • Optimism increased in the TASK group over the length of the study, and changes were significantly greater than the comparison group. The TASK group also had significant improvements in perceptions of task difficulty and threat appraisal (expectation of safety issues or losses).	A structured telephone-based intervention may effectively address caregiver needs in the 3 mo immediately poststroke. Studies of longer term outcomes are warranted.
To determine whether an occupation-based, client-centered, community-based occupational therapy program is effective in improving participation for people ≤6 mo poststroke (Egan et al., 2007)	Community Pilot RCT Peer-reviewed journal	*Participants:* 14 people at least 6 mo poststroke (6 in intervention group and 8 in control group). *Intervention:* Intervention group—8 visits by occupational therapist over 2–4 mo to develop a plan related to goals identified on the COPM and provide coaching, education, environmental modification, and resources; control—no services. *Outcomes:* Occupational performance (COPM), quality of life (SF–36), participation (Reintegration to Normal Living Index)	• After 6 mo, perception of performance in valued activities was similar for both intervention and control groups. However, the intervention group was significantly more satisfied with performance. No differences in well-being and participation were noted between the 2 groups.	Occupational therapy interventions may improve satisfaction, which may be related to self-efficacy. Additional research is needed to address measurement issues and the diversity of the sample.

Note. ADLs = activities of daily living; COPM = Canadian Occupational Performance Measure; CVA = cerebrovascular accident; FAME = Fitness and Mobility Exercise; hr = hour/hours; IADLs = instrumental activities of daily living; LE = lower extremity; MCI = myocardial infarction; min = minutes; mo = month/months; RCT = randomized controlled trial; UE = upper extremity; VO2 max = maximal oxygen consumption; wk = week/weeks; yr = year/years.

Table 13.6. Methods of Service Delivery and Interventions for Staying Active, Fitness, Self-Management, Caregivers and Families, and Community Services

Examples of Methods of Service Delivery and Interventions and Approaches	Examples of Settings, Positions, and Abbreviated Job Description
Types of Occupational Therapy Interventions and Service Delivery	
	Health care system: Community rehabilitation professional. Support stroke survivors in the community using a personalized team approach that includes health and social services.
Therapeutic use of occupations and activities: Address lifestyle issues that put people and communities at risk for stroke.	*Stroke association: Healthy initiatives director.* Promote healthier lifestyles through a plan that coordinates education, health care, and community resources.
Consultation process: Consult with employers who offer on-site health promotion programs and Americans With Disabilities Act (Pub. L. 101–336) services for employees with chronic disease and disabilities.	*Local hospital: Stroke center coordinator.* Conduct community outreach efforts for prevention of stroke. Serve as consultant to local employers for stroke-related initiatives.
Education and training: Provide educational programs to caregivers and families to address objective and subjective caregiver burden.	*Caregiver organization: Education coordinator.* Organize and coordinate workshops, classes, and conferences for caregivers in collaboration with local governments, health care organizations, and social services agencies.
Advocacy: Encourage community supports for people living with stroke and their families through public awareness campaigns.	*Health system: Stroke coordinator.* Participate in stroke outreach programs in the community. Develop public relations and educational programs for public officials and community members.
Occupational Therapy Intervention Approaches	
Create or promote (health promotion): Develop and implement evidence-based community education on healthy lifestyles and behavioral strategies.	*State department of health: Program coordinator.* Develop, implement, and evaluate heart disease and stroke prevention programs for diverse local communities.
Establish or restore (remediation, restoration): Identify community-based interventions that establish or restore skills for priority stroke outcomes.	*Academic institution: Clinical research associate.* Coordinate policies, procedures, and regulations related to stroke outcomes.
Maintain: Develop chronic disease or self-management programs for stroke that address long-term goals to maintain health and quality of life.	*Department of community health: Self-management program coordinator.* Develop and implement self-management programs. Conduct training and provide support for group facilitators.
Modify (compensation, adaptation): Identify environmental barriers to participation for people with physical and cognitive impairments.	*Small business: Universal design consultant.* Provide information on environmental planning and modification to improve accessibility and universal design.
Prevent (disability prevention): Study the role of occupational engagement in decreasing risk factors for stroke across the lifespan.	*Federal government: Behavioral scientist.* Work with public health officials on research initiatives and programs to address chronic diseases, such as stroke.

Note. Intervention types and approaches are based on the *Occupational Therapy Practice Framework: Domain and Process* (3rd ed.; American Occupational Therapy Association, 2014) and adaptations of job postings (from a variety of online and print sources) from August 2012.

age 56. The primary care provider referred Steve to a lifestyle coach who was also an occupational therapist. Although this service was not currently reimbursable under Steve's health insurance, he realized that he needs professional help if he is going to make a significant change in how he lives his daily life.

Steve met with the lifestyle coach for the first session. By the end of the session, Steve identified goals related to fitness and overall activity levels and explored occupations of interest that would support a healthy lifestyle. The lifestyle coach then referred Steve to a stroke recovery exercise and wellness program at a local fitness center. An interdisciplinary team of professionals, including an occupational therapist, designed the evidence-based program at this fitness center to include an individualized exercise program, educational sessions on healthy living, nutrition counseling, and an interactive website and mobile app that people can use to track their levels of physical activity and exercise, document measures of health, and monitor progress toward wellness goals. At the end of 6 months, Steve had significantly shifted his daily routines to increase participation in fitness center exercise programs, leisure occupations with his children and brothers, volunteering with local organizations, and regular breaks during his workday.

Mary: Self-Management and Community Resources

After discharge from rehabilitation services, Mary was referred to a new self-management program for people with stroke and diabetes. This multicenter evidence-based program was developed by an interdisciplinary research team that includes an occupational therapist who works as a health educator for the county public health department. The program offers people like Mary a small stipend, transportation, and assistive technology for self-care in exchange for their participation in a research study of the program. The occupational therapist who coordinates the new self-management program uses a train-the-trainer model; participants with stroke and diabetes are selected to become facilitators of small groups that address educational, support, motivational, and experiential needs.

After Mary completes the self-management program, she concludes that she wants to take control of the decision related to her living situation. Although she loves her home and neighborhood, she realizes that the stress and demands associated with keeping up a home are limiting her recovery. However, she does not know where to begin regarding next steps. She contacts the coordinator of the self-management program and asks for ideas on community resources. Mary is referred to a local realtor who is also an occupational therapist; the realtor has established a specialty practice that serves older adults who need emotional and physical support as they prepare to sell their home and envision a new lifestyle. Mary participates in individual planning sessions and small-group experiences offered by the realtor to help develop a plan, grieve over moving from her longtime home, and embrace her goals for change. At the end of 6 months, Mary has sold her home and is living in a nearby residential community that supports her engagement in meaningful occupations and provides services that improve her health and quality of life.

Walter and Adele: Caregiver and Community Resources

Walter and Adele remain committed to each other despite the life changes that have resulted from Walter's stroke. Adele has told Walter's general practitioner that she wants to continue as Walter's primary caregiver no matter where he lives. She has been faithfully at his side ever since the stroke happened. Adele has stated that she is confident that she can assist Walter in their condominium, despite his severe impairments. She asks for community resources to help her meet Walter's needs at home. The general practitioner refers Adele to a caregiver program offered by a stroke association.

The stroke association offers a variety of programs and services for caregivers and families. An occupational therapist serves as one of the outreach coordinators and develops evidence-based online programs that respond to caregiver needs. Adele eagerly participates in webinars, online support groups, and chats with professionals as she plans for Walter's discharge from the skilled nursing facility to home.

Through her online learning on the stroke association website, Adele realizes that having Walter at home will require significant support. If caregivers such as Adele encounter unique needs, the association provides links to health professionals in their geographic area. By entering her address and zip code on the website, Adele found a local nonprofit agency that will coordinate services in the home. The interdisciplinary team at the agency, including an occupational therapist, identified the supports and resources that Adele and Walter will need in the home environment. Adele works with the occupational therapist to modify the home environment, obtain additional training on providing assistance with self-care and mobility, plan meaningful occupations for respite from caregiving, and coordinate help given by other formal and informal caregivers. At the end of 6 months, Adele is implementing a caregiving plan for Walter, who was recently discharged to the home.

Conclusion

In this chapter, I have explored emerging areas of practice for occupational therapy. People living with stroke often have lifelong needs related to staying active, fitness, chronic disease and self-management, caregiver and family supports, and community supports and resources. An overview of each area provides an understanding of concepts, current research, community initiatives, and outcomes. Occupational therapists have many opportunities to provide leadership in improving the health and quality of life of this population.

References

American Heart Association & American Stroke Association. (2012). *Healthy living after stroke: Physical activity.* Retrieved July 2012 from http://www.strokeassociation.org/STROKE-ORG/LifeAfterStroke/HealthyLivingAfterStroke/PhysicalActivity/Physical-Activity_UCM_310896_Article.isp

American Medical Association. (2008). *Health care careers directory 2008–2009: Occupational therapy.* Retrieved July 2012 from http://www.ama-assn.org/amal/pub/upload/mm/40/occupther0809.pdf

American Occupational Therapy Association. (2014a). Occupational therapy practice framework: Domain and process (3rd ed.). *American Journal of Occupational Therapy, 68*(Suppl. 1), S1–S48. http://dx.doi.org/10.5014/ajot.2014.682006

American Occupational Therapy Association. (2014b). The role of occupational therapy in primary care. *American Journal of Occupational Therapy, 68*(Suppl. 3).

Bakas, T., & Champion, V. (1999). Development and psychometric testing of the Bakas Caregiving Outcomes Scale. *Nursing Research, 48,* 250–259. http://dx.doi.org/10.1097/00006199-199909000-00005

Bakas, T., Farran, C. J., Austin, J. K., Given, B. A., Johnson, E. A., & Williams, L. S. (2009). Stroke caregiver outcomes from the Telephone Assessment and Skill-Building Kit (TASK). *Topics in Stroke Rehabilitation, 16,* 105–121. http://dx.doi.org/10.1310/tsr1602-105

Barlow, J., Wright, C., Sheasby, J., Turner, A., & Hainsworth, J. (2002). Self-management approaches for people with chronic conditions: A review. *Patient Education and Counseling, 48,* 177–187. http://dx.doi.org/10.1016/S0738-3991(02)00032-0

Baum, C., & Edwards, D. (2008). *Activity Card Sort* (2nd ed.). Bethesda, MD: AOTA Press.

Brazzelli, M., Saunders, D. H., Greig, C. A., & Mead, G. E. (2012). Physical fitness training for patients with stroke: Updated review. *Stroke, 43,* e39–e40. http://dx.doi.org/10.1161/STROKEAHA.111.647008

Brereton, L., Carroll, C., & Barnston, S. (2007). Interventions for adult family carers of people who have had a stroke: A systematic review. *Clinical Rehabilitation, 21,* 867–884. http://dx.doi.org/10.1177/0269215507078313

Buchman, A. S., Boyle, P. A., Yu, L., Shah, R. C., Wilson, R. S., & Bennett, D. A. (2012). Total daily physical activity and the risk of AD and cognitive decline in older adults. *Neurology, 78,* 1323–1329. http://dx.doi.org/10.1212/WNL.0b013e3182535d35

Bugge, C., Alexander, H., & Hagen, S. (1999). Stroke patients' informal caregivers: Patient, caregiver, and service factors that affect caregiver strain. *Stroke, 30,* 1517–1523. http://dx.doi.org/10.1161/01.STR.30.8.1517

Carretero, S., Garcés, J., Ródenas, F., & Sanjosé, V. (2009). The informal caregiver's burden of dependent people: Theory and empirical review. *Archives of Gerontology and Geriatrics, 49,* 74–79. http://dx.doi.org/10.1016/j.archger.2008.05.004

Chu, K. S., Eng, J. J., Dawson, A. S., Harris, J. E., Ozkaplan, A., & Gylfadóttir, S. (2004). Water-based exercise for cardiovascular fitness in people with chronic stroke: A randomized controlled trial. *Archives of Physical Medicine and Rehabilitation, 85,* 870–874. http://dx.doi.org/10.1016/j.apmr.2003.11.001

Corbin, C. B., & Frank, B. D. (2012). *PCPFS Research Digests. Definitions: Health, fitness, and physical activity.* Retrieved July 2012 from https://www.presidentschallenge.org/informed/digest/docs/200003digest.pdf

Cott, C. A., Wiles, R., & Devitt, R. (2007). Continuity, transition and participation: Preparing clients for life in the community post-stroke. *Disability and Rehabilitation, 29,* 1566–1574. http://dx.doi.org/10.1080/09638280701618588

Danielsson, A., Willén, C., & Sunnerhagen, K. S. (2012). Physical activity, ambulation, and motor impairment late after stroke. *Stroke Research and Treatment, 2012,* Article ID 818513. http://dx.doi.org/10.1155/2012/818513

Deeken, J. F., Taylor, K. L., Mangan, P., Yabroff, K. R., & Ingham, J. M. (2003). Care for the caregivers: A review of self-report instruments developed to measure the burden, needs, and quality of life of informal caregivers. *Journal of Pain and Symptom Management, 26,* 922–953. http://dx.doi.org/10.1016/S0885-3924(03)00327-0

Department of Health. (2001). *The expert patient: A new approach to chronic disease management for the 21st century.* London: Crown Copyright.

Dewey, H. M., Thrift, A. G., Mihalopoulos, C., Carter, R., Macdonell, R. A., McNeil, J. J., & Donnan, G. A. (2002). Informal care for stroke survivors: Results from the North East Melbourne Stroke Incidence Study (NEMESIS). *Stroke, 33,* 1028–1033. http://dx.doi.org/10.1161/01.STR.0000013067.24300.B0

Dunn, A. L., Marcus, B. H., Kampert, J. B., Garcia, M. E., Kohl, H. W., 3rd, & Blair, S. N. (1999). Comparison of lifestyle and structured interventions to increase physical activity and cardiorespiratory fitness: A randomized trial. *JAMA, 281,* 327–334. http://dx.doi.org/10.1001/jama.281.4.327

Egan, M., Kessler, D., Laporte, L., Metcalfe, V., & Carter, M. (2007). A pilot randomized controlled trial of community-based occupational therapy in late stroke rehabilitation. *Topics in Stroke Rehabilitation, 14,* 37–45. http://dx.doi.org/10.1310/tsr1405-37

Eldred, C., & Sykes, C. (2008). Psychosocial interventions for carers of survivors of stroke: A systematic review of interventions based on psychological principles and theoretical frameworks. *British Journal of Health Psychology, 13,* 563–581. http://dx.doi.org/10.1348/135910707X236899

Feinberg, L. F. (2003). The state of the art of caregiver assessment. *Generations, 27,* 24–32.

Fredman, L., & Daly, M. P. (1997). Patient–Caregiver Functional Unit Scale: A new scale to assess the patient–caregiver dyad. *Family Medicine, 29,* 658–665.

Gordon, N. F., Gulanick, M., Costa, F., Fletcher, G., Franklin, B. A., Roth, E. J., & Shephard, T.; American Heart Association Council on Clinical Cardiology, Subcommittee on Exercise, Cardiac Rehabilitation, and Prevention; the Council on Cardiovascular Nursing; the Council on Nutrition, Physical Activity, and Metabolism; and the Stroke Council. (2004). Physical activity and exercise recommendations for stroke survivors: An American Heart Association scientific statement from the Council on Clinical Cardiology, Subcommittee on Exercise, Cardiac Rehabilitation, and Prevention; the Council on Cardiovascular Nursing; the Council on Nutrition, Physical Activity, and Metabolism; and the Stroke Council. *Stroke, 35,* 1230–1240. http://dx.doi.org/10.1161/01.STR.0000127303.19261.19

Greenwood, N., Mackenzie, A., Cloud, G. C., & Wilson, N. (2008). Informal carers of stroke survivors—Factors influencing carers: A systematic review of quantitative studies. *Disability and Rehabilitation, 30,* 1329–1349. http://dx.doi.org/10.1080/09638280701602178

Hammel, J., Jones, R., Gossett, A., & Morgan, E. (2006). Examining barriers and supports to community living and participation after a stroke from a participatory action research approach. *Topics in Stroke Rehabilitation, 13,* 43–58. http://dx.doi.org/10.1310/5X2G-V1Y1-TBK7-Q27E

Han, B., & Haley, W. E. (1999). Family caregiving for patients with stroke: Review and analysis. *Stroke, 30,* 1478–1485. http://dx.doi.org/10.1161/01.STR.30.7.1478

Hartman-Maeir, A., Soroker, N., Ring, H., Avni, N., & Katz, N. (2007). Activities, participation and satisfaction one-year post stroke. *Disability and Rehabilitation, 29,* 559–566. http://dx.doi.org/10.1080/09638280600924996

Haskell, W. L. (2003). Cardiovascular disease prevention and lifestyle interventions: Effectiveness and efficacy. *Journal of Cardiovascular Nursing, 18,* 245–255. http://dx.doi.org/10.1097/00005082-200309000-00003

Hildebrand, M., Brewer, M., & Wolf, T. (2012). The impact of mild stroke on participation in physical fitness activities. *Stroke Research and Treatment, 2012,* 548682. http://dx.doi.org/10.1155/2012/548682

Hu, G., Sarti, C., Jousilahti, P., Silventoinen, K., Barengo, N. C., & Tuomilehto, J. (2005). Leisure time, occupational, and commuting physical activity and the risk of stroke. *Stroke, 36,* 1994–1999. http://dx.doi.org/10.1161/01.STR.0000177868.89946.0c

James, B. D., Wilson, R. S., Barnes, L. L., & Bennett, D. A. (2011). Late-life social activity and cognitive decline in old age. *Journal of the International Neuropsychological Society, 17,* 998–1005. http://dx.doi.org/10.1017/S1355617711000531

Joice, S. (2012). Self-management following stroke. *Nursing Standard, 26,* 39–46. http://dx.doi.org/10.7748/ns2012.02.26.22.39.c8919

Jones, F., Mandy, A., & Partridge, C. (2009). Changing self-efficacy in individuals following a first time stroke: Preliminary study of a novel self-management intervention. *Clinical Rehabilitation, 23,* 522–533. http://dx.doi.org/10.1177/0269215508101749

Jones, F., & Riazi, A. (2011). Self-efficacy and self-management after stroke: A systematic review. *Disability and Rehabilitation, 33,* 797–810. http://dx.doi.org/10.3109/09638288.2010.511415

Kalra, L., Evans, A., Perez, I., Melbourn, A., Patel, A., Knapp, M., & Donaldson, N. (2004). Training carers of stroke patients: Randomised controlled trial. *British Medical Journal, 328,* 1099. http://dx.doi.org/10.1136/bmj.328.7448.1099

Kendall, E., Catalano, T., Kuipers, P., Posner, N., Buys, N., & Charker, J. (2007). Recovery following stroke: The role of self-management education. *Social Science and Medicine, 64,* 735–746. http://dx.doi.org/10.1016/j.socscimed.2006.09.012

Law, M., Baptiste, S., Carswell, A., McColl, M. A., Polatajko, H., & Pollock, N. (2005). *The Canadian Occupational Performance Measure* (4th ed.). Ottawa, Ontario: CAOT Publications.

Lindsay, P., Bayley, M., McDonald, A., Graham, I. D., Warner, G., & Phillips, S. (2008). Toward a more effective approach to stroke: Canadian best practice recommendations for stroke care. *Canadian Medical Association Journal, 178,* 1418–1425. http://dx.doi.org/10.1503/cmaj.071253

Lutz, B. J., & Young, M. E. (2010). Rethinking intervention strategies in stroke family caregiving. *Rehabilitation Nursing, 35,* 152–160. http://dx.doi.org/10.1002/j.2048-7940.2010.tb00041.x

Matuska, K. (2012). Description and development of the Life Balance Inventory. *OTJR: Occupation, Participation and Health, 32,* 220–228. http://dx.doi.org/10.3928/15394492-20110610-01

McCullagh, E., Brigstocke, G., Donaldson, N., & Kalra, L. (2005). Determinants of caregiving burden and quality of life in caregivers of stroke patients. *Stroke, 36,* 2181–2186. http://dx.doi.org/10.1161/01.STR.0000181755.23914.53

McGraw-Hill Concise Dictionary of Modern Medicine. (2002). Physical activity. Retrieved July 2012 from http://medical-dictionary.thefreedictionary.com/physical+activity

McKevitt, C., Fudge, N., Redfern, J., Sheldenkar, A., Crichton, S., Rudd, A. R., . . . Wolfe, C. D. (2011). Self-reported long-term needs after stroke. *Stroke, 42,* 1398–1403. http://dx.doi.org/10.1161/STROKEAHA.110.598839

Mosby's Medical Dictionary. (2009). Caregiver. Retrieved July 2012 from http://medical-dictionary.thefreedictionary.com/caregiver

National Alliance for Caregiving & AARP. (2009). *Caregiving in the U.S. 2009.* Retrieved July 18, 2012, from http://immn.org/nac/research/general

National Organization on Disability. (2004). *NOD/Harris Survey of Americans With Disabilities.* Retrieved June 29, 2013, http://nod.org/research_publications/surveys/harris/

Oakley, F., Kielhofner, G., Barris, R., & Reichler, R. K. (1986). The Role Checklist: Development and empirical assessment of reliability. *OTJR: Occupation, Participation and Health, 6,* 157–170.

Olney, S. J., Nymark, J., Brouwer, B., Culham, E., Day, A., Heard, J., . . . Parvataneni, K. (2006). A randomized controlled trial of supervised versus unsupervised exercise programs for ambulatory stroke survivors. *Stroke, 37,* 476–481. http://dx.doi.org/10.1161/01.STR.0000199061.85897.b7

Packer, T. (Ed.). (2011). An occupation-focused approach to self-management [Special issue]. *Occupational Therapy Now, 11*(5).

Pang, M. Y. C., Eng, J. J., Dawson, A. S., McKay, H. A., & Harris, J. E. (2005). A community-based fitness and mobility exercise program for older adults with chronic stroke: A randomized, controlled trial. *Journal of the American Geriatrics Society, 53,* 1667–1674. http://dx.doi.org/10.1111/j.1532-5415.2005.53521.x

Pang, M. Y. C., Harris, J. E., & Eng, J. J. (2006). A community-based upper-extremity group exercise program improves motor function and performance of functional activities in chronic stroke: A randomized controlled trial. *Archives of Physical Medicine and Rehabilitation, 87,* 1–9. http://dx.doi.org/10.1016/j.apmr.2005.08.113

Patient Protection and Affordable Care Act, Pub. L. No. 111–148, 42 U.S.C. §§ 18001-18121 (2010).

Pearson, M. L., Mattke, S., Shaw, R., Ridgely, M. S., & Wiseman, S. H. (2007). *Patient self-management support programs: An evaluation* (No. 08-0011).Washington, DC: Agency for Healthcare Research and Quality.

Pierce, L. L., Gordon, M., & Steiner, V. (2004). Families dealing with stroke desire information about self-care needs. *Rehabilitation Nursing, 29,* 14–17. http://dx.doi.org/10.1002/j.2048-7940.2004.tb00294.x

Robison, J., Wiles, R., Ellis-Hill, C., McPherson, K., Hyndman, D., & Ashburn, A. (2009). Resuming previously valued activities post-stroke: Who or what helps? *Disability and Rehabilitation, 31,* 1555–1566. http://dx.doi.org/10.1080/09638280802639327

Rogers, J. C. (1984). Why study human occupation? *American Journal of Occupational Therapy, 38,* 47–49. http://dx.doi.org/10.5014/ajot.38.1.47

Rombough, R. E., Howse, E. L., & Bartfay, W. J. (2006). Caregiver strain and caregiver burden of primary caregivers of stroke survivors with and without aphasia. *Rehabilitation Nursing, 31,* 199–209. http://dx.doi.org/10.1002/j.2048-7940.2006.tb00136.x

Saunders, D. H., Greig, C. A., Young, A., & Mead, G. E. (2004). Physical fitness training for stroke patients. *Stroke, 35,* 2235. http://dx.doi.org/10.1161/01.STR.0000137413.94706.ba

Scholte op Reimer, W. J., de Haan, R. J., Pijnenborg, J. M., Limburg, M., & van den Bos, G. A. (1998). Assessment of burden in partners of stroke patients with the Sense of Competence Questionnaire. *Stroke, 29,* 373–379.

Scholte op Reimer, W. J., de Haan, R. J., Rijnders, P. T., Limburg, M., & van den Bos, G. A. (1998). The burden of caregiving in partners of long-term stroke survivors. *Stroke, 29,* 1605–1611.

Schwamm, L. H., Pancioli, A., Acker, J. E., 3rd, Goldstein, L. B., Zorowitz, R. D., Shephard, T. J., . . . Adams, R. J.; American Stroke Association's Task Force on the Development of Stroke Systems. (2005). Recommendations for the establishment of stroke systems of care: Recommendations from the American Stroke Association's Task Force on the Development of Stroke Systems. *Circulation, 111,* 1078–1091. http://dx.doi.org/10.1161/01.CIR.0000154252.62394.1E

Struchen, M. A., Atchison, T. B., Roebuck, T. M., Caroselli, J. S., & Sander, A. M. (2002). A multidimensional measure of caregiving appraisal: Validation of the Caregiver Appraisal Scale in traumatic brain injury. *Journal of Head Trauma Rehabilitation, 17,* 132–154. http://dx.doi.org/10.1097/00001199-200204000-00005

Ulmer, C., Ball, J., McGlynn, E., & Bel Hamdounia, S. (Eds.). (2012). *Essential health benefits: Balancing coverage and costs.* Washington, DC: National Academies Press.

U.S. Department of Health and Human Services. (2011). *National strategy for quality improvement in health care: Report to Congress.* Retrieved July 2012 from http://www.healthcare.gov/law/resources/reports/quality03212011a.html

U.S. Department of Health and Human Services. (2012). *Chronic disease management.* Retrieved July 2012 from https://www.healthcare.gov/glossary/chronic-disease-management/

U.S. Department of Health and Human Services, Office of Disease Prevention and Health Promotion. (2008). *2008 physical activity guidelines for Americans.* Retrieved July 2012 from http://www.health.gov/PAGuidelines/guidelines/default.aspx

van Exel, N. J. A., Brouwer, W. B. F., van den Berg, B., Koopmanschap, M. A., & van den Bos, G. A. M. (2004). What really matters: An inquiry into the relative importance of dimensions of informal caregiver burden. *Clinical Rehabilitation, 18,* 683–693. http://dx.doi.org/10.1191/0269215504cr743oa

Verghese, J., Lipton, R. B., Katz, M. J., Hall, C. B., Derby, C. A., Kuslansky, G., . . . Buschke, H. (2003). Leisure activities and the risk of dementia in the elderly. *New England Journal of Medicine, 348,* 2508–2516. http://dx.doi.org/10.1056/NEJMoa022252

Visser-Meily, A., van Heugten, C., Post, M., Schepers, V., & Lindeman, E. (2005). Intervention studies for caregivers of stroke survivors: A critical review. *Patient Education and Counseling, 56,* 257–267. http://dx.doi.org/10.1016/j.pec.2004.02.013

White, J. H., Mackenzie, L., Magin, P., & Pollack, M. R. P. (2008). The occupational experience of stroke survivors in a community setting. *OTJR: Occupation, Participation and Health, 28,* 160–167. http://dx.doi.org/10.3928/15394492-20080901-05

Wolf, T. J., Baum, C., & Connor, L. T. (2009). Changing face of stroke: Implications for occupational therapy practice. *American Journal of Occupational Therapy, 63,* 621–625. http://dx.doi.org/10.5014/ajot.63.5.621

World Health Organization. (2012). *Health topics: Physical activity.* Retrieved July 2012 from http://www.who.int./topics/physical_activity/en/

Zarit, S., & Femia, E. (2008). Behavioral and psychosocial interventions for family caregivers. *American Journal of Nursing, 108*(Suppl.), 47–53, quiz 53. http://dx.doi.org/10.1097/01.NAJ.0000336415.60495.34

Zarit, S. H., Orr, N. K., & Zarit, J. M. (1985). *The hidden victims of Alzheimer's disease.* New York: New York University Press.

Points to Ponder
Answer Key

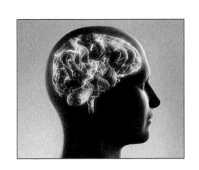

Chapter 2

Environmental Modifications, page 26: Examples: (1) A ramp to enter and exit the home and (2) an external aid, for example, a cell phone alarm, to remind the patient of appointments.

Therapy Adaptations, page 27: Example: Ask the patient whether he or she would typically cook at home and what type of food he or she would like to prepare during a therapy session instead of proceeding with a meal prep activity you already have planned.

Chapter 4

What Are the Physiological Concerns for Emma? page 82: The physiological concerns for occupational therapy at this time are preexisting diagnoses (diabetes, hypertension), obesity, high resting heart rate, and shortness of breath. These physiological concerns might affect Emma's occupational performance in limited energy to perform meaningful activities, inability to climb the steps, fatigue during ADL and IADL performance, safety when performing physically taxing activities, and an inability to hold objects close when lifting as a result of her large abdomen.

What Should the Therapist Do With Emma? page 87:
- Ensure that Emma has been taking her hypertension medication consistently.
- Ask Emma what she had been doing and thinking about just before the practitioner's visit.
- Retake Emma's blood pressure.

• If Emma had been resting comfortably without any emotional strain, have her call her physician to tell him or her of the blood pressure readings.

What Assessments Are Necessary for Emma? page 91: As stated in the text, if improving isotonic strength is a goal of treatment, isotonic strength should be measured instead of isometric strength. Many functional activities require movement, so an isotonic strength assessment will be more valid and predictive of function than an isometric assessment. Moreover, it may not be safe to perform an isometric manual muscle test because it may increase blood pressure; the client may use the Valsalva maneuver.

It is doubtful that Emma could safely step up and down from a 12-inch step or keep up with the fast metronome pace required to use the norms for the YMCA step test because of the moderate weakness in her left lower extremity and cardiovascular deconditioning.

Chapter 6

Measuring Weakness in a Clinically Relevant Manner, page 122: Comparable weakness across joints means that the occupational therapist should get similar manual muscle testing scores at each joint. Knowing this information, the therapist could choose to perform manual muscle testing of 3–4 joint movements vs. each joint movement. For instance, the therapist could test shoulder abduction, elbow flexion, wrist flexion, and finger flexion. Additionally, the Motricity Index is an example of a standardized assessment that measures the strength of 3 joint movements (shoulder abduction, elbow flexion, and pinch). This quick assessment could be performed instead of traditional manual muscle testing to save the therapist time and provide him or her with assessment results to measure progress over the course of therapy.

Applying Different Types of Practice During Treatment Sessions, page 135: When considering which types of practice to use during a treatment session, it is important to remember that massed, variable, whole-task, and random practice are generally considered the most effective for the improvement of movement. In Sally's case, the occupational therapist might change the order of the morning grooming, bathing, and dressing routine each day to create a random practice schedule.

A massed practice session would include very few rest breaks, with most of the time spent performing functional activities. For instance, the therapist might have Sally perform all grooming activities followed by standing at the sink to brush her hair, brush her teeth, and apply deodorant. By doing all of these activities at one time without a rest break, she would be performing massed practice. An example of distributed practice would be having Sally stand to brush teeth and then sit to take a rest break, stand to brush hair and then take a rest break, gather items for dressing then rest, and so forth. The idea is to make sure that treatment sessions have more practice time than rest time.

Chapter 8

Approaching Clients Recovering From a Stroke, page 192: For Mr. Jones, one can infer that the disruptions in the emotion domain are impairing his cognition domain (attention and focus on therapy), which is slowing his progress and ultimately limiting his participation in the therapy environment. If this perturbation in the emotion domain continues over time, his environmental domain will also be negatively affected (e.g., a decreased number of available opportunities for social support). The resulting interactions among emotion, cognition, and environment will then feed back to his participation domain, subsequently restricting it, and thereby continuing the disability process. Conversely, Mr. Anderson was able to work through his emotional and cognitive challenges to maintain equilibrium in all of the domains; by attending therapy and making timely progress, he was able to return to everyday participation in his occupations, for instance, returning to work and resuming his family roles.

An occupational therapist could inquire about the emotional disruption in an interview and with a general screen of emotions. After determining that Mr. Jones was experiencing emotional consequences of his stroke, the therapist could refer him for psychiatric evaluation and treatment. Moreover, the occupational therapy professional could engage Mr. Jones in a conversation about his meaningful occupations, and therapy could be refocused on participating in crucial occupations for him that may, in turn, have a positive impact on his emotional domain.

Collaborating With Other Disciplines to Manage Poststroke Emotional Consequences, page 195: Using a screen to assess for depression is the most appropriate and least intrusive method. Many clients may not want to discuss their emotions or may feel more vulnerable poststroke. Consulting with other health care professionals would require evidence. Results from the screen would be sufficient to provide and allow appropriate documentation of depression if present. Of course, a positive screening for depression should result in reporting the information gathered to an attending physician.

Chapter 10

Discharge Determination, page 225: Inpatient rehabilitation.

Environmental Influences on Performance, page 237: Examples may include increasing lighting, decreasing clutter, or reducing noise.

Chapter 11

Case Study—Steve, page 251: Tying a tie, opening mail, typing on a computer, texting on the phone, using tools with both hands as he would need to in restoring cars, cutting up food, opening containers, opening a briefcase, carrying a briefcase in one hand and opening a door with the other, buttoning shirts, tying shoes, and zipping up a jacket.

Case Study—Mary, page 257:
- *Personal or body neglect:* Does not comb left side of head; does not adjust left sleeve.
- *Near extrapersonal neglect (within arm's reach):* Cannot find objects on left side of sink or left side of plate.
- *Far extrapersonal neglect:* Cannot navigate doorways; cannot locate source of voice.

Some paper-and-pencil assessments of unilateral left neglect are the Star Cancellation Test, Albert's Test, Line Bisection Test, Single Letter Cancellation Test, Clock

Drawing Test, Draw-a-Man test, and so forth. These types of tests measure near extrapersonal neglect because the paper is on the table in front of the patient at midline within arm's reach. The paper is not a part of the patient's body, so the tests do not measure body neglect. Because the paper is within arm's reach, it does not measure far extrapersonal neglect.

Chapter 12

Home Exercise Compliance, page 278:
- Identify what type of delivery of plan works best for the patient: written, illustrated, or video.
- Have the patient demonstrate the exercise activity after the plan has been issued to evaluate the patient's understanding of the plan.
- Assign and check homework.
- Provide exercise tools or information on how to access tools.
- Use an activity journal.
- Educate others involved in the patient's care.

Lack of Awareness and Cognitive Intervention, page 279: Using the Model of Awareness (Barco, Crosson, Bolesta, Werts, & Stout, 1991; Crosson et al., 1989), the occupational therapist would not expect more of the patient than what he or she is neurologically capable of. The therapist would proceed to work with the patient and significant others in using external compensations. Because the patient is not aware of the existence of cognitive deficits, he or she will likely not see a need to compensate for problems that he or she believes do not exist. In such cases, the therapist will begin working with significant others on how best to assist the patient as well as on various environmental modifications so that the patient is best able to achieve a level of satisfactory productivity and participation.

Cognitive Intervention Within an Interdisciplinary Team, page 281: Although each team member has his or her unique focus, it is also likely that overlap exists between professions. For example, organization and memory may be addressed by all therapists with a unique focus by discipline. The occupational therapist may address how the client plans and organizes daily activities; the speech–language pathologist may address how organized the client's speech is and whether the client is able to maintain or remember the main focus of conversation; and the physical therapist may address the ability to remember a home exercise program from day to day. This overlap is viewed as positive because the client will benefit from the treatment continuity and subsequent use of strategies that occurs between professions.

Attendance, page 287: Potential barriers to attendance in the outpatient therapy setting may include the following:
- Weather
- Transportation
- Medical status
- Availability of caregiver
- Intensity of schedule and need for recovery time
- Motivation and depression
- Psychosocial stressors in the home environment.

Chapter 13

Occupations That Support Staying Active, page 314: Some nonexercise occupations that support staying active and could be incorporated into a weekly routine include the following:

- Stocking shelves at the local emergency food pantry
- Weeding in a community garden
- Delivering neighborhood flyers or newspapers
- Coaching youth sports
- Walking a dog
- Playing a musical instrument or singing in a choir.

Self-Management Program Activities, page 319: Some individual or group activities for each of the 5 core skills in a self-management program for people with stroke are as follows:

1. *Problem solving:* Develop a medication management routine that eliminates errors.
2. *Decision making:* Select the transportation options that are safest for given situations.
3. *Resource utilization:* Learn about the health promotion services provided by your health care system.
4. *Formation of a patient–professional partnership:* Practice communicating your goals with a rehabilitation professional.
5. *Taking action:* Engage in making healthy meals.

Objective (O) and Subjective (S) Caregiver Burden, page 321:

- Absences from work or school: O
- Loss of friendships: S
- Depletion of savings to purchase needed equipment: O
- Frustration with health care system: S
- Back injury associated with providing physical assistance: O
- Grief related to unrealized dreams and goals: S.

Information related to subjective caregiving burden could be obtained through interviews, focus groups in small-group sessions, and qualitative research methods.

References

Barco, P. P., Crosson, B., Bolesta, M. M., Werts, D., & Stout, R. (1991). Training awareness and compensation in postacute head injury rehabilitation. In J. S. Kreutzer & P. H. Wheman (Eds.), *Cognitive rehabilitation for persons with traumatic brain injury* (pp. 129–146). Baltimore: Brookes.

Crosson, B., Barco, P. P., Velozo, C. A., Bolesta, M. M., Cooper, P. V., Werts, D., & Brobeck, T. C. (1989). Awareness and compensation in postacute head injury rehabilitation. *Journal of Head Trauma Rehabilitation, 4,* 46–54. http://dx.doi.org/10.1097/00001199-198909000-00008

Glossary

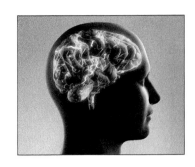

acetylcholine—A neurotransmitter involved in both the peripheral and the central nervous systems (Stahl, 2008).

acquired brain injury—Injury to the brain that is not congenital or degenerative and that incorporates traumatic brain injuries and nontraumatic brain injuries (such as stroke, hypoxia, and tumor; Fleming & Nalder, 2011).

active range of motion—The maximum amount of motion at a given joint achieved by the muscles that act on that joint (Killingsworth, Pedretti, & Pendleton, 2013).

activities of daily living—Activities related to taking care of one's own body, such as self-feeding, bathing, grooming, dressing, sexual activity, toilet use, and hygiene (American Occupational Therapy Association [AOTA], 2014).

agnosia—Failure to recognize a visual or other sensory stimulus (e.g., sound) or specific stimulus types (e.g., faces; see *prosopagnosia*). Agnosia affects one sensory system, but the person may retain the ability to recognize the stimulus using other sensory systems (Lezak, Howieson, Bigler, & Tranel, 2012; Milner & Teuber, 1968).

alexia—An acquired inability to read as a result of brain dysfunction (from the Greek, "no reading"; Lezak et al., 2012).

allocortex—Areas of cerebral cortex with fewer than six distinct layers of neurons ("other cortex"). Examples include the three-layered *archicortex* ("original cortex") of the hippocampal formation, the *paleocortex* ("old cortex") of the olfactory area, and the transitional or *mesocortex* ("middle cortex") of the limbic cortex (Blumenfeld, 2010; Nolte, 2009; Purves et al., 2012).

Alzheimer's disease—Disease causing progressive mental deterioration manifested by memory loss, aphasia, confusion, and disorientation; the most common neurodegenerative brain disorder. Brains of patients with Alzheimer's disease evidence atrophic changes in the temporoparietal area (and, to a lesser degree, in frontal areas) and the characteristic neuropathological signs confirmed on autopsy of neurofibrillary tangles, neuritic plaques, and granulovacuolar degeneration (American Psychiatric Association [APA], 2013).

amygdala—Collection of nuclei in the anteromedial part of the temporal lobe that form part of the limbic system; the major functions of the amygdala include autonomic, emotional, and sexual behavior (Blumenfeld, 2010; Nolte, 2009; Purves et al., 2012).

anger—An emotional reaction that may include outbursts, decreased impulse control, increased irritability, hostility, and insult (Scarpa & Raine, 1997).

anosodiaphoria—Lack of concern regarding the presence of impairment or disease (Ergh, Rapport, Coleman, & Hanks, 2002).

anosognosia—Explicit verbal denial of the presence of impairment or disease (Ergh et al., 2002); also called *denial of deficit* (Lezak et al., 2012).

antecedent—A precursor or cue; an event that precedes and increases or decreases the likelihood that a behavior will occur (Giles, 2011).

anterior cerebral artery—Major paired artery that sweeps across the medial surface of each hemisphere in the longitudinal fissure, supplying the medial surface of the frontal and anterior parietal lobes (Purves et al., 2012).

anterior cingulate gyrus—Area of cerebral cortex in the prefrontal lobe that is hypothesized to have executive control over information processing, especially target detection, and is linked to frontal lobe regions involved in working memory and to posterior regions for visual orienting and feature identification (Blumenfeld, 2010; Nolte, 2009; Purves et al., 2012).

anterior nucleus of the thalamus—Relay nucleus of the thalamus that primarily functions in the limbic system; receives inputs from the mammillary bodies and other limbic structures and sends outputs to the cingulate gyrus (Blumenfeld, 2010; Nolte, 2009; Purves et al., 2012).

anxiety—An overwhelming sense of worry or fear that may involve physical changes such as decreased energy and concentration, tachycardia, nausea, tense muscles, shortness of breath, and headache (National Stroke Association, 2006).

apathy—A reduction in motivation or a lack of initiative (Starkstein, Fedoroff, Price, Leiguarda, & Robinson, 1993).

aphasia—Impaired production or comprehension of speech or ability to communicate because of brain pathology (Lezak et al., 2012).

apraxia—Inability to organize and skillfully execute purposeful movements (Lezak et al., 2012).

arrhythmia—A problem with the rate or rhythm of the heartbeat (National Heart, Lung, and Blood Institute, 2011).

aspiration—Entry of food, fluid, or a foreign body below the vocal cords and into the lungs (Avery, 2010).

aspiration pneumonia—Pneumonia caused by entry of food, fluid, or a foreign body below the vocal cords and into the lungs (Avery, 2010).

association cortex—Portions of the cerebral cortex that receive and integrate sensory or motor information. This higher order information processing can involve single *(unimodal)* or multiple *(heteromodal)* sensory or motor modalities (Blumenfeld, 2010; Martini, 2009; Nolte, 2009; Purves et al., 2012).

astrocytes—One of the major types of glial cell found in the central nervous system. Among the major roles of astrocytes are regulation of the ionic milieu of neurons, metabolic and mechanical support of neurons, response to injury, and maintenance of the blood–brain barrier (Blumenfeld, 2010; Martini, 2009; Nolte, 2009; Purves et al., 2012).

ataxia—A movement disorder related to uncoordinated movements and postural instability (Armutlu, 2013).

atrial fibrillation—A relatively common form of heart arrhythmia characterized by rapid and uncoordinated heart rate that may lead to a range of associated medical conditions including fatigue and increased risk for stroke (Huntley, 2014).

attention—Focused awareness—a necessary precondition for most activities; ability to detect and orient to stimuli (Lezak et al., 2012).

attitude—Pervasive affective stance or preference for an event or object (Fox, 2008).

automaticity—Characteristic of a behavior whereby it is initiated and executed with minimal conscious decision making (Giles, 2011).

axon—Neuronal process that conducts the action potential away from the cell body (soma) and toward the target (most frequently, the axon terminals that make synaptic connections with other neurons; Hall, 2011; Martini, 2009; Purves et al., 2012; Rhoades & Bell, 2009; Widmaier, Raff, & Strang, 2006).

basal nuclei—Group of subcortical nuclei (historically referred to as *basal ganglia*), most prominently including the striatum, globus pallidus, substantia nigra, and subthalamic nucleus. The basal nuclei collectively organize motor behavior. Damage to these nuclei has traditionally been considered to cause disorders characterized by involuntary movements, difficulty initiating movement, and alterations in muscle tone. Damage to certain parts of the basal ganglia can also cause disturbances of cognition and motivation (Blumenfeld, 2010; Nolte, 2009; Purves et al., 2012).

basilar artery—Large vessel formed by the union of the two vertebral arteries. It runs upward along the anterior median surface of the pons, giving rise to many penetrating branches that supply the pons and caudal midbrain (Blumenfeld, 2010; Moore, Dalley, & Agur, 2010; Nolte, 2009; Purves et al., 2012).

blob cells—The color-processing cells of the primary visual cortex (Purves et al., 2012).

blood–brain barrier—The anatomical and transport barriers that collectively isolate the extracellular fluids of the central nervous system from those of the general circulation. The blood–brain barrier controls the entry and rates of transport of substances into the brain's extracellular space from the capillary blood, primarily as the result of astrocytes and capillary permeability (Martini, 2009; Purves et al., 2012).

body mass index—A common method for estimating adult body composition on the basis of height and weight (Keys, Fidanza, Karvonen, Kimura, & Taylor, 1972).

brainstem—Region of the brain that lies between the diencephalon and the spinal cord consisting of the midbrain, pons, and medulla (Blumenfeld, 2010; Nolte, 2009; Purves et al., 2012).

Brodmann's areas—Fifty-two regions of the cortex, described and numbered by Korbinian Brodmann (a German neurologist) in 1909 on the basis of observed structural differences. Many of the numbers continue to be used in reference to cortical areas because they correlate with functional divisions of the cortex (Purves et al., 2012).

calcarine sulcus (or fissure)—A major groove or furrow within the cerebral cortex on the medial aspect of the occipital lobe and the location of the primary visual cortex. The calcarine sulcus originates anteriorly in the temporal lobe near the splenium of the corpus callosum and continues posteriorly into the occipital lobe (Moore et al., 2010; Nolte, 2009).

carotid canals—The two foramina in the petrous part of the temporal bone of the skull through which the internal carotid arteries travel to enter the middle cranial fossa (Moore et al., 2010).

caudate nucleus—One of the nuclei that compose the basal nuclei (together with the putamen, globus pallidus, subthalamic nucleus, and substantia nigra); forms the most medial part of the striatum. It receives input from widespread association areas of the cerebral cortex and is therefore thought to be more involved in cognitive functions and less directly in movement (Blumenfeld, 2010; Nolte, 2009; Purves et al., 2012).

central nervous system—Brain and spinal cord (Posner, Saper, Schiff, & Plum, 2007).

central sulcus (of Rolando)—A major groove or furrow on the lateral aspect of the cerebral hemispheres that forms the boundary between the frontal and parietal lobes. The central sulcus is also the transition zone between primary motor and primary somatosensory cortex. The anterior bank (precentral gyrus) contains the primary motor cortex, and the posterior bank (postcentral gyrus) contains the primary sensory cortex (Moore et al., 2010; Nolte, 2009).

cerebellum—Large, highly convoluted subdivision of the brain ("little brain") that lies behind the forebrain and above the brainstem. It receives inputs from sensory systems, the cerebral cortex, and other sites and participates in the planning and coordination of movement and cognitive functions (Moore et al., 2010; Nolte, 2009).

cerebral cortex—Extensive, superficial gray matter layer covering the surfaces of the cerebral hemispheres. The majority of the cerebral cortex is composed of neocortex, which has six cell layers (I–VI) designated from the surface inward (Nolte, 2009).

cerebral hemisphere—Right or left half of the cerebral cortex as divided by the longitudinal fissure (Moore et al., 2010; Nolte, 2009).

cerebrospinal fluid—The fluid that permeates the ventricles and cavities of the brain and spinal cord (Posner et al., 2007).

cerebrovascular accident—Brain cell death resulting from lack of oxygen when the blood flow to the brain is impaired by blockage or rupture of an artery to the brain (MedicineNet.com, 2013).

cerebrum—Largest and most rostral (i.e., near the front or nose) part of the brain composed of two cerebral hemispheres. Together with the diencephalon, it forms the forebrain (Moore et al., 2010; Nolte, 2009).

cingulate gyrus—Prominent gyrus on the medial aspect of the cerebral hemisphere, partially surrounding the corpus callosum and considered part of the limbic system; involved in emotional processing, learning and memory, reward anticipation, decision making, and impulse control (i.e., executive functions; Blumenfeld, 2010; Nolte, 2009).

Circle of Willis—The arterial anastomosis at the base of the brain, connecting the anterior and posterior cerebral circulations and supplying arterial blood to the brain. Components include the internal carotid arteries and the anterior and posterior cerebral arteries, interconnected by the anterior and posterior communicating arteries. The anatomy of the Circle of Willis allows for redundancies such that should one part of the circle become blocked or narrowed, perfusion may continue (Moore et al., 2010; Nolte, 2009).

cognition—Information-processing functions of the brain, including attention, memory, and executive functions (e.g., problem solving, planning, self-awareness, self-monitoring; AOTA, 2013).

coma—State of unconsciousness and unarousability (even with vigorous stimuli) in which the patient lies with eyes closed (Posner et al., 2007).

commissural fibers—Bundles of axons (white matter) that interconnect and permit communication between the two cerebral hemispheres by crossing over from one hemisphere and into the other. Commissural fibers are predominantly located in the corpus callosum (Martini, 2009; Purves et al., 2012).

concentration—Direction of thoughts and actions toward a given stimulus and suppression of awareness of competing distractions (Lezak et al., 2012).

consciousness—State of full awareness of the self and the environment (Posner et al., 2007).

constraint-induced movement therapy—The forced use of the affected limb in functional activities via restraint of the unaffected limb; used to encourage return of motor function and control of the affected limb (Hayner, Gibson, & Giles, 2010; Taub, Uswatte, & Pidikiti, 1999).

continuous positive airway pressure machine—A machine that provides continuous positive airway pressure that prevents the airway from collapsing and facilitates breathing by providing continuous mild pressure; the patient must initiate the breaths (Chestnutt, Prendergast, & Tavan, 2013).

contracture—Loss of muscle-group tissue length (shortening) limiting range of motion (Gillen, 2013a).

contralateral—On the opposite side (e.g., each hemisphere controls the contralateral extremities; Purves et al., 2012).

coping—Sum of attempts, regardless of success, by which a person tries to manage a stressful situation (Lazarus & Folkman, 1984).

corona radiata—Bundles of fibers entering or leaving the internal capsule (Blumenfeld, 2010; Nolte, 2009; Purves et al., 2012).

corpus callosum—A massive curvilinear bundle of commissural fibers that bridges most cortical areas of the two cerebral hemispheres and serves to join them functionally, allowing for a unitary consciousness (Blumenfeld, 2010; Nolte, 2009; Purves et al., 2012).

cortical column—Functional unit of the cerebral cortex at the microscopic level that receives inputs from and sends signals within and outside the cortex; layers of neurons within a column all share a specific aspect of a neurological task (e.g., a column in the visual cortex may be responsible for detecting an edge at a certain angle at a small spot of the retina; Purves et al., 2012).

corticothalamic fibers—Axons of neurons located in the cerebral cortex (usually Layer VI) that project to the thalamus (Purves et al., 2012).

covert visual orienting network—One of the brain's attentional systems that is active in shifting attention from one focus to another in the external environment without shifting visual orientation (Purves et al., 2012).

deep vein thrombosis—Occlusion of a major vein caused by the formation of a clot *(thrombus)* most often occurring in the lower extremity, abdomen, or pelvic area (Atkins, 2014).

delirium—Temporary condition characterized by acute change in cognition with a disturbance in consciousness; characterized by sudden onset and clouded alertness (APA, 2013).

dementia—State of deteriorated mental function involving the presence of multiple cognitive deficits (including memory impairment) with significant impairment in occupational performance. The term *dementia* was replaced in the fifth edition of the *Diagnostic and Statistical Manual of Mental Disorders* by the term *major neurocognitive disorder* (APA, 2013).

dendrite—Neuronal process (fiber) that receives sensory information through synaptic input and transmits these electrical signals toward the cell body (Martini, 2009; Purves et al., 2012; Rhoades & Bell, 2009; Widmaier et al., 2006).

detection—Conscious recognition that an object is present, along with recognition of the object's identity and its significance; detection plays a special role in selecting a target from many alternatives, a process known as *target detection* (Posner & Petersen, 1990).

diaschisis—Transient suppression of brain activity outside the brain region that is the immediate site of damage (Lezak et al., 2012).

diencephalon ("in-between brain")—The caudal subdivision of the embryonic forebrain, lying just rostral to the midbrain. The diencephalon includes the epithalamus, thalamus, and hypothalamus (Blumenfeld, 2010; Nolte, 2009; Purves et al., 2012).

discrepancy score—The standard method of rating lack of awareness as a difference between the client and either the caregiver or the clinician (Visser-Keizer, Meyboom-de Jong, Deelman, Berg, & Gerritsen, 2002).

diurnal rhythms—Cyclic repetition (intensification and weakening) of biological phenomena or processes that occurs at daily intervals (Purves et al., 2012).

divided attentional deficit—An attentional system breakdown in which a person fails to process information necessary for optimal task performance (Schneider, Dumais, & Shiffrin, 1984).

dynamometry—Use of a dynamometer to measure hand grip strength (Kasch & Walsh, 2013).

dysarthria—Impaired articulation attributable to paralysis, incoordination, or spasticity of the muscles used for speaking (Lezak et al., 2012).

dysmetria—A condition in which a movement either overshoots the target *(hypermetria)* or fails to reach the target *(hypometria;* Preston, 2013).

dysphagia—Disorder of swallowing (Avery, 2010).

embolism—The obstruction of a blood vessel by a mass, which may be a blood clot, a colony of bacteria, a foreign body, or air (Gillen, 2013a).

emotion—A short-term affective state triggered by an event or object that causes global change in the brain, body, and behavior (Dalgleish, 2000; Dalgleish & Power, 1999).

emotional lability—A neurological syndrome that is characterized by uncontrollable emotional expressions of excessive or spontaneous crying or laughing; common after stroke or traumatic brain injury (House, Dennis, Molyneux, Warlow, & Hawton, 1989; Work, Colamonico, Bradley, & Kaye, 2011).

enteral feeding—Tube feeding directed into the stomach or duodenum (Avery, 2010).

episodic memory—Memory of discrete events with perceptual and temporal correlates still attached to them (Tulving, 1983, 2002).

errorless learning—Method of learning in which client errors are prevented by providing sufficient cueing to enable the client to achieve correct performance (Kessels & de Haan, 2003).

executive attention network—Detection network that provides conscious recognition that an object is present, along with its identity and significance, playing a special role in selecting a target from alternatives (Purves et al., 2012).

executive function—Higher-level mental processing that includes initiation, organization, sequencing, and problem solving (Stuss, 1991).

expanding-retrieval technique—Strategy for increasing a client's ability to learn information by recalling material at spaced intervals; often used with clients exhibiting memory disorders (Clare et al., 2000).

explicit memory—Memory that is available to awareness and involves a conscious and intentional recollection process (Tulving, 2002).

extracellular fluid—Liquid containing proteins and electrolytes found between the cells of the body that provides much of the liquid environment of the body (Hall, 2011; Martini, 2009; Rhoades & Bell, 2009; Widmaier et al., 2006).

extrastriate visual cortex—Areas of the occipital, temporal, and parietal lobes involved in processing visual information after initial reception in the striate (or primary visual) cortex (Purves et al., 2012).

feeling—The internal, subjective mental representation of the emotion (Dalgleish, 2000; Dalgleish & Power, 1999).

FIM™—Assessment measure (Hamilton, Granger, Sherwin, Zielezny, & Tashman, 1987) consisting of 18 items that grades the level of cognitive and physical assistance necessary for function. Item scores range from 1 *(completely dependent)* to 7 *(completely independent),* and total scores range from 18 to 126 (Uniform Data System for Medical Rehabilitation, 1997).

foramen magnum—The inferior aperture of the skull through which the spinal cord passes (Moore et al., 2010).

fovea (of the macula lutea)—The portion (of the macula lutea) of the retina that provides the sharpest vision because it has a high density of cones (Martini, 2009; Purves et al., 2012).

frontal lobe—Most anterior region of the brain; controls motor, cognitive, and executive functions (Blumenfeld, 2010; Moore et al., 2010; Nolte, 2009).

functional impairment—Interference with independence in everyday activity (Ganguli et al., 2011).

ganglia—Collection of neuronal cell bodies located in the peripheral nervous system that are anatomically discrete and typically serve a specific function (Blumenfeld, 2010; Purves et al., 2012).

gastric tube—Tube placed through the abdominal wall and into the stomach that may be used for enteral feeding; also called *gastrostomy tube* or *percutaneous endoscopic gastrostomy* (Avery, 2010).

genome—The complete DNA sequence of an organism containing its entire genetic information (Nussbaum, McInnes, & Willard, 2007).

glia—Diverse collection of non-neuronal cell types in the peripheral and central nervous systems that perform a wide variety of metabolic, electrical, and mechanical functions to support and protect the neurons; also called *neuroglia* or *glial cells* (Hall, 2011; Martini, 2009; Purves et al., 2012).

globus pallidus—One of the nuclei that compose the basal nuclei (together with the caudate, putamen, subthalamic nucleus, and substantia nigra), lying medial to the putamen. It is named "pale globe" because of the many myelinated fibers passing through it. Together with the putamen, it composes the lenticular nucleus. The globus pallidus has two segments, the internal (GPi) and external (GPe) segments (Blumenfeld, 2010; Nolte, 2009; Purves et al., 2012).

goniometric measurement—The measurement of angles and range of motion of a joint (Killingsworth et al., 2013).

gray matter—Regions of the central nervous system composed of neuronal cell bodies, neuroglia, and unmyelinated axons, including the cerebral and cerebellar cortices, as well as the various nuclei of the brain (Purves et al., 2012).

gyrus—Ridge or complex convolution; gyri are of varying widths and form the surface of the cerebral hemisphere, separated by grooves called *sulci*. Some gyri are consistently located from person to person and others are not, but nonetheless the gyri often form the basis for the division of the hemispheres into lobes (Blumenfeld, 2010; Nolte, 2009; Purves et al., 2012).

habit—Consistent response to stimuli that develops through repetition (AOTA, 2014).

hemianesthesia—Loss of sensation on one side of the body (Lezak et al., 2012).

hemiplegia—Paralysis of one side of the body (Lezak et al., 2012).

hemorrhage—Bleed; loss of blood from the vascular compartment into extravascular space (Kumar, Abbas, Fausto, & Aster, 2010).

heteromodal association areas—Sensory processing areas of the brain that receive input from several unimodal sensory areas (Purves et al., 2012).

heterotypic isocortex—Areas of cortex that do not display the prototypical six layers of cells present in isocortex (Nolte, 2009; Purves et al., 2012).

homonymous hemianopsia—A visual deficit in which the same (right or left) half of the visual field of both eyes is lost as a result of destruction of the right or left primary visual cortex or destruction or interruption of the fibers leading to it (Lezak et al., 2012; Moore et al., 2010; Purves et al., 2012).

homotypic isocortex—Cortical areas that display the prototypical six layers of varying thickness and differing proportions of neurons (Nolte, 2009).

hydrocephalus—The accumulation of cerebrospinal fluid in the brain, contributing to increased intracranial pressure and resulting from impaired reabsorption or obstruction of the flow of cerebrospinal fluid (Lezak et al., 2012).

hypertension—Blood pressure in the arterial system that is persistently at or above 140 mm Hg systolic or 90 mm Hg diastolic. The heart must work harder than normal to circulate blood through the constricted artery system (American Heart Association, 2014).

hypertonicity—A state of increased muscle tension (Preston, 2013).

hypotonicity—A reduction in the stiffness of a muscle to lengthening (Schumway-Cook & Woollacott, 2012).

hypoxic brain damage—Damage to the brain attributable to lack of oxygen caused either by decreased oxygenation of the blood (e.g., carbon monoxide poisoning) or by decreased blood flow to the brain (Posner et al., 2007).

immediate memory—Automatic learning and retrieval system of sensory information (also called *sensory memory*) that serves to mentally maintain how a stimulus looked (*iconic* or *visual sensory memory*) or sounded (*echoic* or *auditory sensory information*) for only a very short period of time (i.e., seconds) and dependent on the visual and auditory cortices, respectively (Cohen & Conway, 2008).

implicit memory—Knowledge that is expressed in performance without one's awareness that one possesses it (Giles, 2011).

instrumental activities of daily living—Activities that relate to independent living in the home and community, such as care of others, community mobility, meal preparation, and shopping (AOTA, 2014).

insular lobe—Central lobelike portion of the cerebral cortex that lies deep to the lateral fissure; its functions are not well understood but are known to include gustatory and autonomic areas (also called *insula;* Nolte, 2009).

international normalized ratio—A method for standardizing *prothrombin time* (the ratio of the time it takes a patient's plasma to clot to that of a normal control) across different tissue factor reagents used to perform the test (Kirkwood, 1983; van den Besselaar, 1996).

ischemia—A lack of blood supply that may result from a clot or a narrowing of blood vessels either globally, as after a cardiac arrest, or locally, as after vascular occlusion (Posner et al., 2007).

isocortex—Area of the brain consisting of a huge number of columnar functional modules organized into primary sensory and motor areas, unimodal association areas, multimodal association areas, and limbic areas (Blumenfeld, 2010; Nolte, 2009; Purves et al., 2012).

kyphosis—Increased posterior convexity of the spine that may be generalized over the extent of the spine or localized to one area (Hertling & Kessler, 2006).

lateral geniculate nucleus—One of the major thalamic relay nuclei, the role of which is to relay visual information from the retina via the optic tract to the primary visual cortex. The lateral geniculate nucleus is located within, above, and below the calcarine sulcus (Blumenfeld, 2010; Nolte, 2009; Purves et al., 2012).

lateral sulcus (Sylvian fissure)—A long, deep groove or furrow on the lateral aspect of each cerebral hemisphere arising during fetal development; it separates the frontal lobes from the temporal lobes inferiorly and laterally. The insula lies hidden within the depths of this sulcus (Blumenfeld, 2010; Moore et al., 2010; Nolte, 2009; Purves et al., 2012).

lateral ventricles—The first and second ventricles (right and left lateral ventricles); the largest cavities of each cerebral hemisphere, following a *C*-shaped course and containing cerebrospinal fluid (Moore et al., 2010; Nolte, 2009).

learned nonuse—The inability to use reemerging motor activation as a result of the extinction of use when the central nervous system was in shock or other processes made movement impossible (Taub et al., 1999).

leisure—Nonobligatory activity that is intrinsically motivating and takes place during time not committed to other occupations (AOTA, 2014).

limbic lobe—Region of the cortex that lies superior to the corpus callosum on the medial aspect of the cerebral hemispheres and forms the cortical component of the limbic system (Nolte, 2009; Purves et al., 2012).

locus coeruleus—A column of pigmented, blue-black neurons near the floor of the fourth ventricle, extending through the rostral pons. Neurons in this region provide most of the noradrenergic innervation of the cerebrum (Purves et al., 2012).

long and short association fibers—Axons that interconnect various sites within the same cerebral hemisphere (Martini, 2009).

longitudinal fissure—Extensive, sagittally oriented vertical cleft separating the two cerebral hemispheres (Blumenfeld, 2010; Moore et al., 2010; Nolte, 2009).

major neurocognitive disorder—Significant decline in cognitive functioning in two or more higher order cognitive domains (i.e., complex attention, executive ability, learning and memory, language, visuoconstructional–perceptual ability, social cognition; Ganguli et al., 2011).

mammillary bodies—Small, paired prominences that form the posterior portion of the hypothalamus and the ventral aspect of the diencephalon. The mammillary bodies are functionally part of the caudal hypothalamus and play a role in memory (Blumenfeld, 2010; Nolte, 2009).

mediodorsal nucleus—A thalamic relay nucleus that receives its main inputs from the amygdala, olfactory cortex, and basal nuclei. The mediodorsal nucleus sends its main outputs to the frontal cortex, and its main roles are in the limbic pathways and as a major relay to the frontal cortex (Blumenfeld, 2010; Nolte, 2009; Purves et al., 2012).

medulla oblongata—The most caudal portion of the brainstem, extending from the pons to the spinal cord. The medulla is crucial to many vital functions (respiratory, cardiovascular, visceral activity) and integrative activities and also transmits signals from most sensory and motor tracts of the central nervous system (Blumenfeld, 2010; Nolte, 2009; Purves et al., 2012).

memory—Acquisition, storage, and retrieval of knowledge (Cohen & Conway, 2008).

mesocortex—Transitional region of the cerebral cortex ("middle cortex") that is three to six cell layers deep and is found in the limbic cortex of the parahippocampal gyrus and the anterior inferior insula (Blumenfeld, 2010).

metabolic equivalent—The activity metabolic rate divided by the resting metabolic rate; indicates the intensity of physical activities. One metabolic equivalent is equal to the consumption of 3.5 milliliters of oxygen per kilogram of body mass per minute or expending approximately 1 kilocalorie per kilogram of body weight per hour, which correlates with lying or sitting quietly. Metabolic equivalent values range from 1 to 18 (About.com, 2014).

metabolic syndrome—A cluster of major cardiovascular risk factors related to obesity, insulin resistance, and dyslipidemia (Centers for Disease Control and Prevention, 2009).

middle cerebral artery—Major paired artery that arises from the carotid artery and turns laterally and enters the lateral sulcus (Sylvian fissure), where it bifurcates into a *superior division,* which provides blood to the lateral surface of the frontal and anterior parietal lobes, and an *inferior division,* which supplies the superior part of the temporal lobe. Branches of the middle cerebral artery known as *lenticulostriate arteries* supply the basal nuclei and internal capsule and are the most common sites for a stroke (Purves et al., 2012).

middle cranial fossa—Large depressions formed by the sphenoid and temporal bones of the skull that lie along the internal surface of the cranial base and house the temporal lobes of the brain. The middle cranial fossa also transmits the internal carotid artery as well as numerous cranial nerves (Moore et al., 2010; Nolte, 2009).

mild cognitive impairment—Cognitive changes in excess of the normal cognitive changes of aging but not reaching the level of major neurocognitive disorder. *Mild cognitive impairment* has been replaced in the fifth edition of the *Diagnostic and Statistical Manual of Mental Disorders* by the term *mild neurocognitive disorder* (APA, 2013).

mild neurocognitive disorder—Mild cognitive deficits in one or more higher cognitive domains (i.e., complex attention, executive ability, learning and memory, language, visuoconstructional–perceptual ability, social cognition); the person can function independently, often through increased effort or compensatory strategies (Ganguli et al., 2011). The generally accepted criteria for mild neurocognitive disorder are presence of a memory or other cognitive limitation, objective deficits on standardized objective cognitive tests, intact general intellectual function, and lack of significant deficits in social or occupational function (Brooks & Loewenstein, 2010).

Mini-Mental State Examination—Widely used assessment of global cognition (Folstein, Folstein, & McHugh, 1975).

mood—A general state of lesser intensity and of longer duration that can be caused by an emotion (Dalgleish, 2000; Dalgleish & Power, 1999).

motor association cortex (primary motor cortex)—The area of the frontal lobe that is involved in motor planning of intended movements (Blumenfeld, 2010; Nolte, 2009; Purves et al., 2012).

muscle paresis—The partial or incomplete paralysis of the muscle (Lezak et al., 2012).

myelin—Fatty, membranous, multilayered axonal sheath produced by either Schwann cells (in the peripheral nervous system) or oligodendrocytes (in the central nervous system) interrupted periodically by nodes of Ranvier. Myelination increases the conduction velocity of the axon it surrounds by insulating it and enabling saltatory conduction (Hall, 2011; Martini, 2009; Purves et al., 2012).

nasogastric tube—Tube introduced through the nose and guided into the stomach; may be used for enteral feeding (Avery, 2010).

National Institutes of Health Stroke Scale—A method to assess stroke-related neurological impairment. Scores range from 0 *(no deficit)* to 42 *(severe deficit).*

Interrater reliability for the total score is high (intraclass correlation = .80) with good predictive validity (r = .70; Brott et al., 1989).

neural network—Group of neurons that share a similar function and therefore are organized into specific groups (Nolte, 2009).

neurocognitive disorder—Acquired condition characterized by progressively deteriorating cognitive functioning (APA, 2013).

neuromodulation—Physiological adjustment of some chemical neurotransmitters to the sensitivities of multiple neurons, thereby either facilitating or inhibiting signaling, synaptic transmission, or growth of the neuron. Neuromodulators are secreted by a small group of neurons but diffuse through large areas of the nervous system and are therefore more systemic and slower acting than classical synaptic transmission, in which a presynaptic neuron directly influences a postsynaptic neuron (Hall, 2011; Martini, 2009; Rhoades & Bell, 2009).

neuron—Excitable cell of the nervous system that is electrically active and specialized for intercellular communication. Most typically, motor neurons are *multipolar,* with numerous dendrites and a single axon emerging from an axon hillock, whereas sensory neurons are *unipolar* (i.e., only one protoplasmic process extends from the cell body), and special sensory neurons are *bipolar* (i.e., only two protoplasmic processes extend from the cell body; Blumenfeld, 2010; Nolte, 2009; Purves et al., 2012).

neuroplasticity—The brain's ability to structurally and functionally adapt in response to damage as a result of its history of activation; includes the processes of neurogenesis and rerouting of connections (Lezak et al., 2012; Nolte, 2009; Purves et al., 2012).

neuroscience—A general term encompassing a wide range of scientific disciplines and approaches focusing on the functioning of the nervous system (Krebs, Weinberg, & Akesson, 2012).

neurotransmitter—Chemical compound synthesized and released by neurons into the synaptic cleft that affects the transmembrane potential of another nearby neuron. The purpose is to transmit information from one neuron to another, and the result may lead to neuronal excitation or inhibition depending on the type of neurotransmitter and the magnitude of its activity. Most neurotransmitters are small amine molecules, amino acids, or neuropeptides, but some are gases that simply diffuse across neuronal membranes (Hall, 2011; Martini, 2009; Rhoades & Bell, 2009; Widmaier et al., 2006).

nonsynaptic diffusion neurotransmission—Diffusion through the extracellular fluid of neurotransmitters and other neuroactive substances released at sites that may be remote from the target cells, with the resulting activation of extrasynaptic receptors (Purves et al., 2012).

nuclei—Collection of neuronal cell bodies located in the central nervous system that are anatomically discrete and typically serve a specific function (Blumenfeld, 2010; Purves et al., 2012).

occipital lobe—Most posterior lobe of the cerebral hemisphere; includes the primary visual cortex. The occipital lobe is specifically located within the borders of the calcarine sulcus and adjoining areas of visual association cortex (Blumenfeld, 2010; Moore et al., 2010; Nolte, 2009).

occlusion (cerebral)—Blockage of a blood vessel resulting in diminished perfusion of brain tissue (Posner et al., 2007).

olfaction—Sense of smell (Hall, 2011; Purves et al., 2012).

optic radiation—A heavily myelinated bundle of visual fibers originating in the lateral geniculate nucleus, departing the thalamus through the retrolenticular and sublenticular parts of the internal capsule and terminating in the primary visual cortex on the upper and lower banks of the calcarine sulcus (Purves et al., 2012).

orientation—Ability to identify person, place, and time (see also *spatial orientation;* Lezak et al., 2012).

overlearning—Practice of a skill beyond the point at which mastery has been achieved to make the skill less susceptible to forgetting (Rohrer, Taylor, Pashler, Wixted, & Cepeda, 2005).

parietal lobe—A central lobe of the brain that is bounded by the frontal lobe anteriorly, the temporal lobe laterally, and the occipital lobe posteriorly (Blumenfeld, 2010; Moore et al., 2010; Nolte, 2009).

passive range of motion—Maximum amount of motion at a given joint achieved when the joint is moved by an outside force (e.g., the therapist; Killingsworth et al., 2013).

percutaneous endoscopic gastrostomy—Tube introduced though the abdominal wall into the stomach for enteral feeding (Avery, 2010).

perfusion (cerebral perfusion)—The dispersion of blood to brain tissue; the degree to which blood suffuses brain tissue. Cerebral perfusion pressure is the blood pressure minus intracranial pressure (Posner et al., 2007).

peripheral nervous system—Anatomically, the collection of neurons and nervous tissue that lies outside of the brain and spinal cord; physiologically, the neurons that carry information toward and away from the central nervous system (Nolte, 2009; Purves et al., 2012).

perseveration—Continuation or repetition of a response once it is no longer appropriate (Lezak et al., 2012).

posterior cerebral artery—Major paired artery and terminal branch arising from the bifurcation of the basilar artery at the level of the midbrain and forming the posterior part of the Circle of Willis. The posterior cerebral artery supplies the inferior surface of the brain and the occipital pole (Moore et al., 2010; Nolte, 2009).

posterior inferior cerebellar artery—A long, circumferential branch of the vertebral artery, supplying much of the inferior surface of the cerebellum (Moore et al., 2010; Nolte, 2009).

poststroke depression—A poststroke sequela that includes having five or more symptoms (e.g., fatigue or loss of energy, insomnia or hypersomnia, thoughts of death or suicide, significant weight loss or gain, reduced ability to think) in a 2-week interval, a change in function, and one required symptom being either depressed mood or loss of interest (APA, 2013).

postsynaptic—A term of reference designating a neuron downstream to a synapse (Hall, 2011; Martini, 2009; Rhoades & Bell, 2009; Widmaier et al., 2006).

prefrontal cortex—Most anterior region of the cerebrum and the part of the frontal lobe immediately anterior to the primary and supplementary (association) motor cortices; important for working memory, planning, expression of personality, and choice of appropriate social behavior (Blumenfeld, 2010; Purves et al., 2012).

premotor cortex—Cortical areas on the lateral surface of the frontal lobe immediately anterior to the primary motor cortex. Premotor cortex is important for the planning of voluntary movements (Blumenfeld, 2010; Purves et al., 2012).

presynaptic—A term of reference designating a neuron upstream to a synapse (Hall, 2011; Martini, 2009; Rhoades & Bell, 2009; Widmaier et al., 2006).

primary visual cortex (striate cortex)—Cortical region in the occipital lobe (Brodmann's area 17) that lies on the banks of the calcarine fissure. The role of primary visual cortex is to sort visual information and distribute it to other cortical areas (Purves et al., 2012).

priming (cognitive or perceptual)—Process in which memory recall is facilitated by means of prior exposure to the stimulus that elicits it (Squire & Schacter, 2002).

projection fibers—Axons (white matter) that carry information from the thalamus to the cerebral cortex (Martini, 2009; Purves et al., 2012).

proprioception—Awareness of joint position in space, independent of vision (Cooper & Canyock, 2013).

prosody—The expressive intonations of speech including variation in pitch, stress, and duration of speech sounds. Loss of appreciation and production of speech prosody is particularly associated with right hemisphere damage (Lezak et al., 2012).

prosopagnosia—Difficulty in identifying familiar faces and impairment in learning new faces (Lezak et al., 2012).

prospective memory—The ability to remember to do things in the future, to carry out future intentions (Gillen, 2013b).

putamen—One of the major nuclei that compose the basal nuclei; the part of the striatum that is involved most prominently in the motor functions of the basal nuclei and that receives its inputs from the cerebral cortex (Blumenfeld, 2010; Nolte, 2009; Purves et al., 2012).

range of motion—Maximum amount (arc) of motion at a given joint (Killingsworth et al., 2013).

rating of perceived exertion—Method of measuring the intensity of physical activity based on a total feeling of exertion and fatigue. It is a behavior-anchored scale used to describe exertion levels, ranging from 6 *(no exertion at all)* to 20 *(maximal exertion;* Borg, 1998).

rehabilitation—Services provided to people with physical or cognitive deficits that limit their participation in daily life activities and important social roles. Interventions are designed to assist people to resume these life activities and roles (AOTA, 2014).

self-efficacy—A person's belief in his or her functional capability to perform as required to influence how events affect his or her life (Bandura, 1977).

self-esteem—A person's appraisal of his or her self-worth typically containing beliefs about himself or herself (Fox, 2008; Heatherton & Polivy, 1991).

self-management of chronic conditions—Active participation in efforts to protect and promote one's own health through various activities and to organize daily life (Wiersma et al., 2011).

semantic memory—Memory of general knowledge without acquisition context (Tulving, 2002).

short-term memory—Processing and temporary storage of information needed to carry out activities as diverse as understanding, learning, and reasoning for a limited amount of material to be readily accessible for a brief period of time (i.e., several seconds); also called *active* or *primary memory* (Cohen & Conway, 2008).

social participation—Activities associated with organized patterns of behavior in interaction with others (AOTA, 2014).

somatic sensation—Sensations and perceptions arising from skin, muscle, and bones (sense of the body; Hall, 2011; Purves et al., 2012).

somatosensory cortex—The region of the cerebral cortex in the parietal lobe in which nerve fibers transmitting somatic sensory information synapse (Purves et al., 2012).

somatotopic map—A representation of the systematic arrangement of different regions of the body and the neurons of the cerebral cortex that serve them (e.g., precentral and postcentral gyri; Purves et al., 2012).

spaced-retrieval techniques—Strategy for maximizing recall of relatively limited amounts of information (e.g., face–name associations) in people with severe memory disorder by recalling material at spaced intervals of increasing duration (Cermak, Verfaellie, Lanzoni, Mather, & Chase, 1996; Davis, Massman, & Doody, 2001; Schacter, Rich, & Stampp, 1985).

spasticity—A state of hypertonicity with velocity-dependent increase in tonic stretch reflexes (Preston, 2013).

spatial orientation—Ability to sense the location or direction of movement of objects or of points in space in relation to one another or to oneself (Lezak et al., 2012).

Specific Adaptation to Imposed Demand principle—The principle that the body will adapt specifically to the form of biomechanical or neurological stress or training that is performed, resulting in increased ability to withstand that specific form of stress or activity in the future (Knight & Draper, 2012).

stereognosis—The identification of an object through touch (Lezak et al., 2012).

stereopsis (asteriopsis)—Stereoscopic vision (or its absence); important in depth perception (Lezak et al., 2012).

stress—Negative emotional states (e.g., fear, sadness, anxiety, frustration, anger, depression) evoked by a situation (Taylor, 2006).

striate cortex—Primary visual cortex in the occipital lobe (Brodmann's area 17), named for its striped appearance when observed with the naked eye that results from the prominence of Layer IV in myelinated sections (Purves et al., 2012).

striatum—An inclusive term referring to the caudate nucleus and putamen of the basal nuclei. The striatum is the major point of entry into the basal nuclei circuitry, receiving inputs from large cortical areas and projecting inhibitory outputs to the globus pallidus and substantia nigra (Blumenfeld, 2010; Nolte, 2009).

stroke—Cerebrovascular accident in which blood flow to a region of the brain is impaired by hemorrhage, embolism, or ischemia (Gillen, 2013a).

subarachnoid hemorrhage—A bleed adjacent to the brain; an acute medical emergency often the result of an aneurysm and often preceded by severe headache and leading to alteration in consciousness, coma, or death (Posner et al., 2007).

subcortical—Pertaining to the portion of the brain that lies below the cerebral cortex; this region is responsible for the fast, unconscious activities involving structures of the diencephalon and brainstem (Nolte, 2009; Purves et al., 2012).

subluxation—Incomplete dislocation in which contact remains between joint surfaces, often of the glenohumeral joint after cerebrovascular accident (Gillen, 2013a).

substantia nigra—Large nucleus at the base of the midbrain positioned between the red nucleus and cerebral peduncle that receives input from several cortical and subcortical structures. The *substantia nigra pars compacta* contains closely packed, pigmented dopaminergic neurons that send their output to the striatum, and the *substantia nigra pars reticulata* contains more loosely arranged GABAergic neurons that receive inputs from the striatum and send their output to the thalamus (Blumenfeld, 2010; Purves et al., 2012).

subthalamic nucleus—Large nucleus at the base of the midbrain, medial and superior to the junction of the internal capsule and cerebral peduncle; the basis of the indirect route through the basal nuclei, receiving input from the striatum and participating in the modulation of motor control (Blumenfeld, 2010; Purves et al., 2012).

sulcus—A groove or furrow of varying depth along the surface of the cerebral hemisphere. Some sulci are consistently located and others are not, but they often form the basis for the division of the hemispheres into lobes (Moore et al., 2010; Nolte, 2009).

superior colliculus—A large, rounded mass of gray matter that forms the roof of the midbrain. It receives input from the retina and visual cortex, sends outputs to the pulvinar and other structures, and plays an important role in orienting movements of the head and eyes (Nolte, 2009; Purves et al., 2012).

suprachiasmatic nucleus—A rice grain–sized hypothalamic nucleus that lies above the optic chiasm and receives direct input from the retina. Suprachiasmatic nucleus neurons are sensitive to light via the retina and serve as the "master clock" of circadian rhythms (Blumenfeld, 2010; Purves et al., 2012).

synapse—Point of contact between neurons at which one neuron is able to influence the other (electrically or, most often, chemically; Hall, 2011; Martini, 2009; Rhoades & Bell, 2009; Widmaier et al., 2006).

temporal lobe—Most inferior lobe of each cerebral hemisphere, lying inferior to the lateral sulcus (Sylvian fissure) and anterior to the occipital lobe. The temporal lobe contains auditory sensory and association cortex, part of the posterior language cortex, visual and higher order association cortex, primary and association olfactory cortex, the amygdala, and the hippocampus (Blumenfeld, 2010; Moore et al., 2010; Nolte, 2009).

thalamus—Collection of nuclei that form the majority of the diencephalon. The thalamus has numerous functions, but its primary role is to relay sensory information from lower centers of the central nervous system to the various regions of the cerebral cortex (Blumenfeld, 2010; Nolte, 2009; Purves et al., 2012).

third ventricle—One of four spaces in the brain that are formed as the lumen from the embryonic neural tube. The third ventricle is a vertically oriented cavity within the diencephalon separating the thalamus and hypothalamus and is confluent anteriorly with both lateral ventricles via the interventricular foramina and posteriorly with the fourth ventricle through the aqueduct (Moore et al., 2010; Nolte, 2009).

thrombosis—Formation or presence of a blood clot *(thrombus)* in the cardiovascular system, often leading to stroke or transient ischemic attack (Gillen, 2011).

tissue plasminogen activator (t-PA)—An antithrombotic drug that can reduce some of the functional deficits associated with a stroke (Saver et al., 2013).

tone—The resting state of muscle (mild contraction), ready for movement (Preston, 2013).

unilateral neglect—A condition in which a person fails to report, respond to, or orient to novel stimuli or maintain attention to stimuli presented unilaterally (Lezak et al., 2012).

unimodal association cortices—Areas of sensory cortex specialized for processing information from one specialized primary sensory receptive area (Purves et al., 2012).

vascular neurocognitive disorder—Cognitive and functional impairment resulting from one or more large cerebrovascular accidents (hemorrhagic, embolic, or ischemic) or small vessel disease; previously known as *vascular dementia* (APA, 2013).

vertebral artery—One of the two major arteries that supply the brainstem, cerebellum, and occipital lobe of the cerebrum. The vertebral artery originates as the first branch of the subclavian artery, courses cranially via the transverse foramina of cervical vertebrae, enters the base of the skull through the foramen magnum, and finally ascends along the medulla and pons where the two vertebral arteries join to form the basilar artery (Moore et al., 2010; Nolte, 2009).

vertebral–basilar system—The system of arteries that supplies the brainstem, cerebellum, and occipital lobe (Nolte, 2009).

vigilance network—Network of the brain involving the right frontal and parietal regions that enables the maintenance of a sustained state of alertness (Purves et al., 2012).

visual field—The area visible to one eye. Because the optics of the eye reverse and invert the image on the retina, the temporal field is seen by the nasal retina, the superior part of the field is seen by the inferior retina, and the blind spot (corresponding to the optic disk) is temporal to the fovea in the visual field (Moore et al., 2010; Nolte, 2009; Purves et al., 2012).

white matter—Regions of the central nervous system that contain mostly myelinated axons and therefore appear white (Purves et al., 2012).

working memory—Knowledge briefly held in awareness while a mental operation (e.g., planning, organizing, problem solving, paying attention) is performed (Cohen & Conway, 2008).

References

About.com. (2014). *MET—The standard metabolic equivalent.* Retrieved from http://sportsmedicine.about.com/od/glossary/g/MET.htm

American Heart Association. (2014). *What is high blood pressure?* Retrieved May 29, 2013, from http://www.heart.org/HEARTORG/Conditions/HighBloodPressure/AboutHighBloodPressure/What-is-High-Blood-Pressure_UCM_301759_Article.jsp

American Occupational Therapy Association. (2013). Cognition, cognitive rehabilitation, and occupational performance. *American Journal of Occupational Therapy, 67*(Suppl.), S9–S31. http://dx.doi.org/10.5014/ajot.2013.67S9

American Occupational Therapy Association. (2014). Occupational therapy practice framework: Domain and process (3rd ed.). *American Journal of Occupational Therapy, 68*(Suppl. 1), S1–S48. http://dx.doi.org/10.5014/ajot.2014.682006

American Psychiatric Association. (2013). *Diagnostic and statistical manual of mental disorders* (5th ed.). Arlington, VA: Author.

Armutlu, K. (2013). Ataxia: Physical therapy and rehabilitation applications for ataxic patients. In J. H. Stone & M. Blouin (Eds.), *International encyclopedia of rehabilitation.* Buffalo, NY: Center for International Rehabilitation Research Information and Exchange. Retrieved from http://cirrie.buffalo.edu/encyclopedia/en/article/112

Atkins, M. S. (2014). Spinal cord injury. In M. V. Radomski & C. A. Trombly Latham (Eds.), *Occupational therapy for physical dysfunction* (7th ed., pp. 1168–1214). Philadelphia: Wolters Kluwer.

Avery, W. (2010). *Dysphagia care and related feeding concerns for adults* (2nd ed.). Bethesda, MD: American Occupational Therapy Association.

Bandura, A. (1977). Self-efficacy: Toward a unifying theory of behavioral change. *Psychological Review, 84,* 191–215. http://dx.doi.org/10.1037/0033-295X.84.2.191

Blumenfeld, H. (2010). *Neuroanatomy through clinical cases* (2nd ed.). Sunderland, MA: Sinauer Associates.

Borg, G. (1998). *Borg's Perceived Exertion and Pain Scales.* Champaign, IL: Human Kinetics.

Brooks, L. G., & Loewenstein, D. A. (2010). Assessing the progression of mild cognitive impairment to Alzheimer's disease: Current trends and future directions. *Alzheimer's Research and Therapy, 2,* 28.

Brott, T., Adams, H. P., Olinger, C. P., Marker, J. R., Barsan, W. G., & Biller, J. (1989). Measurements of acute cerebral infarction: A clinical examination scale. *Stroke, 20,* 864–870. http://dx.doi.org/10.1161/01.STR.20.7.864

Centers for Disease Control and Prevention. (2009). *Prevalence of metabolic syndrome among adults 20 years of age and over, by sex, age, race and ethnicity, and body mass index: United States, 2003–2006* (National Health Statistics Reports No. 13). Retrieved September 10, 2013, from http://www.cdc.gov/nchs/data/nhsr/nhsr013.pdf

Cermak, L. S., Verfaellie, M., Lanzoni, S., Mather, M., & Chase, K. A. (1996). Effects of spaced repetitions on amnesia patients' recall and recognition performance. *Neuropsychology, 10,* 219–227. http://dx.doi.org/10.1037/0894-4105.10.2.219

Chestnutt, M. S., Prendergast, T. J., & Tavan, E. T. (2013). Pulmonary disorders. In M. A. Papadakis, S. J. McPhee, & M. W. Rabow (Eds.), *Current medical diagnosis and treatment* (52nd ed., pp. 242–323). New York: McGraw-Hill Medical.

Clare, L., Wilson, B. A., Carter, G., Breen, K., Gosses, A., & Hodges, J. R. (2000). Intervening with everyday memory problems in dementia of Alzheimer's type: An errorless learning approach. *Journal of Clinical and Experimental Neuropsychology, 22,* 132–146. http://dx.doi.org/10.1076/1380-3395(200002)22:1;1-8;FT132

Cohen, G., & Conway, M. A. (2008). *Memory in the real world* (3rd ed.). Hove, England: Psychology Press.

Cooper, C., & Canyock, J. D. (2013). Evaluation of sensation and intervention for sensory dysfunction. In H. M. Pendleton & W. Schultz-Krohn (Eds.), *Pedretti's occupational therapy: Practice skills for physical dysfunction* (7th ed., pp. 575–589). St. Louis: Mosby.

Dalgleish, T. (2000). Roads not taken: The case for multiple functional-level routes to emotion. *Behavioral and Brain Sciences, 23,* 196–197. http://dx.doi.org/10.1017/S0140525X00272427

Dalgleish, T., & Power, M. J. (1999). *Handbook of cognition and emotion.* Chichester, England: Wiley.

Davis, N. R., Massman, P. J., & Doody, R. S. (2001). Cognitive intervention in Alzheimer disease: A randomized placebo-controlled study. *Alzheimer Disease and Associated Disorders, 15,* 1–9.

Ergh, T. C., Rapport, L. J., Coleman, R. D., & Hanks, R. A. (2002). Predictors of caregiver and family functioning following traumatic brain injury: Social support moderated caregiver distress. *Journal of Head Trauma Rehabilitation, 17,* 155–174. http://dx.doi.org/10.1097/00001199-200204000-00006

Fleming, J., & Nalder, E. (2011). Transition to community integration for persons with acquired brain injury. In N. Katz (Ed.), *Cognition, occupation, and participation across the life span* (3rd ed., pp. 51–70). Bethesda, MD: AOTA Press.

Folstein, M. F., Folstein, S. E., & McHugh, P. R. (1975). "Mini-Mental State": A practical method for grading the cognitive state of patients for the clinician. *Journal of Psychiatric Research, 12,* 189–198. http://dx.doi.org/10.1016/0022-3956(75)90026-6

Fox, E. (2008). *Emotion science: Cognitive and neuroscientific approaches to understanding human emotions.* Basingstoke, England: Palgrave Macmillan.

Ganguli, M., Blacker, D., Blazer, D. G., Grant, I., Jeste, D. V., Paulsen, J. S., . . . Sachdev, P. S.; Neurocognitive Disorders Work Group of the American Psychiatric Association *DSM–5* Task Force. (2011). Classification of neurocognitive disorders in *DSM–5:* A work in progress. *American Journal of Geriatric Psychiatry, 19,* 205–210. http://dx.doi.org/10.1097/JGP.0b013e3182051ab4

Giles, G. M. (2011). A neurofunctional approach to rehabilitation following brain injury. In N. Katz (Ed.), *Cognition, occupation, and participation across the life span* (3rd ed., pp. 351–381). Bethesda, MD: AOTA Press.

Gillen, G. (2011). *Stroke rehabilitation: A function-based approach* (3rd ed.). St Louis: Mosby.

Gillen, G. (2013a). Cerebrovascular accident/stroke. In H. M. Pendleton & W. Schultz-Krohn (Eds.), *Occupational therapy: Practice skills for physical dysfunction* (7th ed., pp. 844–880). St. Louis: Mosby.

Gillen, G. (2013b). Evaluation and treatment of limited occupational performance secondary to cognitive dysfunction. In H. M. Pendleton & W. Schultz-Krohn (Eds.), *Occupational therapy: Practice skills for physical dysfunction* (7th ed., pp. 648–677). St. Louis: Mosby.

Hall, J. E. (2011). *Guyton and Hall textbook of medical physiology* (12th ed.). Philadelphia: Saunders/Elsevier.

Hamilton, B. B., Granger, C. V., Sherwin, F. S., Zielezny, M., & Tashman, J. S. (1987). A uniform national data system for medical rehabilitation. In M. J. Fuhrer (Ed.), *Rehabilitation outcomes: Analysis and measurement* (pp. 137–147). Baltimore: Paul H. Brookes.

Hayner, K., Gibson, G., & Giles, G. M. (2010). Comparison of constraint-induced movement therapy and bilateral treatment of equal intensity in people with chronic upper-extremity dysfunction after cerebrovascular accident. *American Journal of Occupational Therapy, 64,* 528–539. http://dx.doi.org/10.5014/ajot.2010.08027

Heatherton, T., & Polivy, J. (1991). Development and validation of a scale for measuring state self-esteem. *Journal of Personality and Social Psychology, 60,* 895–910. http://dx.doi.org/10.1037/0022-3514.60.6.895

Hertling, D., & Kessler, R. M. (2006). *Management of common musculoskeletal disorders* (4th ed.). Philadelphia: Lippincott Williams & Wilkins.

House, A., Dennis, M., Molyneux, A., Warlow, C., & Hawton, K. (1989). Emotionalism after stroke. *British Medical Journal, 298,* 991–994. http://dx.doi.org/10.1136/bmj.298.6679.991

Huntley, N. (2014). Cardiac and pulmonary diseases. In M. V. Radomski & C. A. Trombly Latham (Eds.), *Occupational therapy for physical dysfunction* (7th ed., pp. 1300–1326). Philadelphia: Wolters Kluwer.

Kasch, M. C., & Walsh, J. M. (2013). Hand and upper extremity injuries. In H. M. Pendleton & W. Schultz-Krohn (Eds.), *Occupational therapy: Practice skills for physical dysfunction* (7th ed., pp. 1037–1073). St. Louis: Mosby.

Kessels, R. P. C., & de Haan, E. H. F. (2003). Mnemonic strategies in older people: A comparison of errorless and errorful learning. *Age and Ageing, 32,* 529–533. http://dx.doi.org/10.1093/ageing/afg068

Keys, A., Fidanza, F., Karvonen, M. J., Kimura, N., & Taylor, H. L. (1972). Indices of relative weight and obesity. *Journal of Chronic Diseases, 25,* 329–343. http://dx.doi.org/10.1016/0021-9681(72)90027-6

Killingsworth, A. P., Pedretti, L. W., & Pendleton, H. M. (2013). Joint range of motion. In H. M. Pendleton & W. Schultz-Krohn (Eds.), *Pedretti's occupational therapy: Practice skills for physical dysfunction* (7th ed., pp. 529–574). St. Louis: Mosby.

Kirkwood, T. B. (1983). Calibration of reference thromboplastins and standardisation of the prothrombin time ratio. *Thrombosis and Haemostasis, 49,* 238–244.

Knight, K. L., & Draper, D. O. (2012). *Therapeutic modalities: The art and science.* Philadelphia: Lippincott Williams & Wilkins.

Krebs, C., Weinberg, J., & Akesson, E. (2012). *Neuroscience*. Baltimore: Lippincott Williams & Wilkins.

Kumar, V., Abbas, A. K., Fausto, N., & Aster, J. (2010). *Robbins and Cotran pathologic basis of disease* (8th ed.). Philadelphia: Saunders/Elsevier.

Lazarus, R. S., & Folkman, S. (1984). *Stress, appraisal, and coping.* New York: Springer.

Lezak, M. D., Howieson, D. B., Bigler, E. D., & Tranel, D. (2012). *Neuropsychological assessment* (5th ed.). New York: Oxford University Press.

Martini, N. (2009). *Fundamentals of anatomy and physiology* (8th ed.). San Francisco: Pearson Benjamin Cummings.

MedicineNet.com. (2013). *Definition of cerebrovascular accident.* Retrieved from http://www.medterms.com/script/main/art.asp?articlekey=2676

Milner, B., & Teuber, H.-L. (1968). Alteration of perception and memory in man. In L. Weiskrantz (Ed.), *Analysis of behavioral change* (pp. 268–375). New York: Harper & Row.

Moore, K. L., Dalley, A. F., & Agur, A. M. R. (2010). *Clinically oriented anatomy* (6th ed.). Baltimore: Lippincott Williams & Wilkins.

National Heart, Lung, and Blood Institute. (2011). *What is an arrhythmia?* Retrieved from http://www.nhlbi.nih.gov/health/health-topics/topics/arr/

National Stroke Association. (2006). *Recovery after stroke: Coping with emotions.* Retrieved June 19, 2012, from http://www.stroke.org/site/DocServer/NSAFactSheet_Emotions.pdf?docID=990

Nolte, J. (2009). *The human brain: An introduction to its functional anatomy* (6th ed.). Philadelphia: Elsevier.

Nussbaum, R., McInnes, R. R., & Willard, H. F. (2007). *Thompson and Thompson genetics in medicine* (7th ed.). Philadelphia: Saunders/Elsevier.

Posner, J. B., Saper, C. B., Schiff, N. D., & Plum, F. (2007). *Plum and Posner's diagnosis of stupor and coma* (4th ed.). Oxford, England: Oxford University Press.

Posner, M. I., & Petersen, S. E. (1990). The attention system of the human brain. *Annual Review of Neuroscience, 13,* 25–42. http://dx.doi.org/10.1146/annurev.ne.13.030190.000325

Preston, L. A. (2013). Evaluation of motor control. In H. M. Pendelton & W. Schultz-Krohn (Eds.), *Occupational therapy: Practice skills for physical dysfunction* (7th ed., pp. 461–488). St. Louis: Mosby.

Purves, D., Augustine, G. J., Fitzpatrick, D., Hall, W. C., LaMantia, A. S., & White, L. E. (2012). *Neuroscience* (5th ed.). Sunderland, MA: Sinauer Associates.

Rhoades, R. A., & Bell, D. R. (2009). *Medical physiology: Principles for clinical medicine* (3rd ed.). Baltimore: Lippincott Williams & Wilkins.

Rohrer, D., Taylor, K., Pashler, H., Wixted, J. T., & Cepeda, N. J. (2005). The effect of overlearning on long-term retention. *Applied Cognitive Psychology, 19,* 361–374. http://dx.doi.org/10.1002/acp.1083

Saver, J. L., Fonarow, G. C., Smith, E. E., Reeves, M. J., Grau-Sepulveda, M. V., Pan, W., . . . Schwamm, L. H. (2013). Time to treatment with intravenous tissue plasminogen activator and outcome from acute ischemic stroke. *JAMA, 309,* 2480–2488. http://dx.doi.org/10.1001/jama.2013.6959

Scarpa, A., & Raine, A. (1997). Psychophysiology of anger and violent behavior. *Psychiatric Clinics of North America, 20,* 375–394. http://dx.doi.org/10.1016/S0193-953X(05)70318-X

Schacter, D. L., Rich, S. A., & Stampp, M. S. (1985). Remediation of memory disorders: Experimental evaluation of the spaced-retrieval technique. *Journal of Clinical and Experimental Neuropsychology, 7,* 79–96. http://dx.doi.org/10.1080/01688638508401243

Schneider, W., Dumais, S. T., & Shiffrin, R. M. (1984). Automatic and control processing and attention. In R. Parasuraman & D. R. Davis (Eds.), *Varieties of attention* (pp. 1–27). London: Academic Press.

Schumway-Cook, A., & Woollacott, M. H. (2012). *Motor control: Translating research into clinical practice* (4th ed.). Philadelphia: Lippincott Williams & Wilkins.

Squire, L. R., & Schacter, D. L. (Eds.). (2002). *Neuropsychology of memory* (3rd ed.). New York: Guilford Press.

Stahl, S. M. (2008). *Stahl's essential psychopharmacology* (3rd ed.). Cambridge, England: Cambridge University Press.

Starkstein, S. E., Fedoroff, J. P., Price, T. R., Leiguarda, R., & Robinson, R. G. (1993). Apathy following cerebrovascular lesions. *Stroke, 24,* 1625–1630. http://dx.doi.org/10.1161/01.STR.24.11.1625

Stuss, D. T. (1991). Self-awareness and the frontal lobes: A neuropsychological perspective. In J. Strauss & G. R. Goethals (Eds.), *The self: Interdisciplinary approaches* (pp. 255–278). New York: Springer-Verlag.

Taub, E., Uswatte, G., & Pidikiti, R. (1999). Constraint-induced movement therapy: A new family of techniques with broad application to physical rehabilitation—A clinical review. *Journal of Rehabilitation Research and Development, 36,* 237–251.

Taylor, S. E. (2006). *Health psychology* (6th ed.). Boston: McGraw-Hill.

Tulving, E. (1983). *Elements of episodic memory.* Oxford, England: Clarendon Press.

Tulving, E. (2002). Episodic memory: From mind to brain. *Annual Review of Psychology, 53,* 1–25. http://dx.doi.org/10.1146/annurev.psych.53.100901.135114

Uniform Data System for Medical Rehabilitation. (1997). *Guide for the Uniform Data Set for Medical Rehabilitation (including the FIM™ instrument), version 5.1.* Buffalo, NY: Author.

van den Besselaar, A. M. (1996). Precision and accuracy of the international normalized ratio in oral anticoagulant control. *Haemostasis, 26*(Suppl.), 248–265.

Visser-Keizer, A. C., Meyboom-de Jong, B., Deelman, B. G., Berg, I. J., & Gerritsen, M. J. (2002). Subjective changes in emotion, cognition, and behaviour after stroke: Factors affecting the perception of patients and partners. *Journal of Clinical and Experimental Neuropsychology, 24,* 1032–1045. Retrieved from http://dx.doi.org/10.1076/jcen.24.8.1032.8383

Widmaier, E. P., Raff, H., & Strang, K. T. (2006). *Vander's human physiology: The mechanisms of body function* (11th ed.). New York: McGraw-Hill.

Wiersma, E., Kelly, M. L., Wilford, R., Dupuis, S., LeClair, K., & Puxty, J. (2011). *Self-management of dementia.* Retrieved from http://www.akeresourcecentre.org/files/HealthyLiving/CDRAKE.AKE_SelfManageDementia_ElaineWiersma_Jan2012.pdf

Work, S. S., Colamonico, J. A., Bradley, W. G., & Kaye, R. E. (2011). Pseudobulbar affect: An under-recognized and under-treated neurological disorder. *Advances in Therapy, 28,* 586–601. http://dx.doi.org/10.1007/s12325-011-0031-3

Subject Index

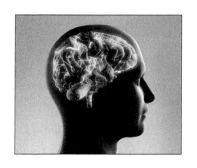

Boxes, case studies, exhibit, figures, and tables are indicated by "b," "cs," "e," "f," and "t," respectively, following page numbers.

Citation Index

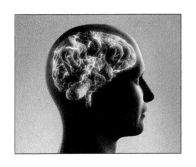

Boxes, figures, Points to Ponder, and tables are indicated by "b," "f," "ptp," and "t," respectively, following page numbers.